Textbook of Human Embryology

with Clinical Cases and 3D Illustrations

Yogesh Sontakke MBBS, MD

Associate Professor
Department of Anatomy
Jawaharlal Institute of Postgraduate Medical Education and Research (JIPMER)
(An institute of national importance under the Ministry of Health and Family Welfare, Government of India)
Pondicherry, India

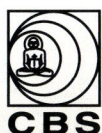

CBS Publishers & Distributors Pvt Ltd

New Delhi • Bengaluru • Chennai • Kochi • Kolkata • Mumbai
Bhopal • Bhubaneswar • Hyderabad • Jharkhand • Nagpur • Patna • Pune • Uttarakhand • Dhaka (Bangladesh)

> *Disclaimer*
> Science and technology are constantly changing fields. New research and experience broaden the scope of information and knowledge. The author has tried his best in giving information available to him while preparing the material for this book. Although all efforts have been made to ensure optimum accuracy of the material, yet it is quite possible some errors might have been left uncorrected. The publisher, the printer and the author will not be held responsible for any inadvertent errors, or inaccuracies.

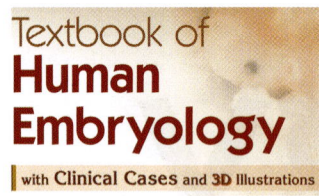

ISBN: 978-93-88108-37-9

Copyright © Yogesh Sontakke and Publisher

Illustrations: © Yogesh Sontakke

First Edition: 2019
Reprint: 2020

All rights reserved. No part of this book may be reproduced or transmitted in any form or by any means, electronic or mechanical, including photocopying, recording, or any information storage and retrieval system without permission, in writing, from the author and the publisher.

Published by Satish Kumar Jain and produced by Varun Jain for

CBS Publishers & Distributors Pvt Ltd
4819/XI Prahlad Street, 24 Ansari Road, Daryaganj, New Delhi 110 002, India.
Ph: 23289259, 23266861, 23266867   Fax: 011-23243014   Website: www.cbspd.com
e-mail: delhi@cbspd.com; cbspubs@airtelmail.in.
Corporate Office: 204 FIE, Industrial Area, Patparganj, Delhi 110 092
Ph: 4934 4934   Fax: 4934 4935   e-mail: publishing@cbspd.com; publicity@cbspd.com

Branches

- **Bengaluru:** Seema House 2975, 17th Cross, K.R. Road,
  Banasankari 2nd Stage, Bengaluru 560 070, Karnataka
  Ph: +91-80-26771678/79   Fax: +91-80-26771680   e-mail: bangalore@cbspd.com

- **Chennai:** 7, Subbaraya Street, Shenoy Nagar, Chennai 600 030, Tamil Nadu
  Ph: +91-44-26680620, 26681266   Fax: +91-44-42032115   e-mail: chennai@cbspd.com

- **Kochi:** 42/1325, 1326, Power House Road, Opposite KSEB Power House,
  Ernakulam 682 018, Kochi, Kerala
  Ph: +91-484-4059061-65   Fax: +91-484-4059065   e-mail: kochi@cbspd.com

- **Kolkata:** 6/B, Ground Floor, Rameswar Shaw Road, Kolkata-700 014, West Bengal
  Ph: +91-33-22891126, 22891127, 22891128   e-mail: kolkata@cbspd.com

- **Mumbai:** 83-C, Dr E Moses Road, Worli, Mumbai-400018, Maharashtra
  Ph: +91-22-24902340/41   Fax: +91-22-24902342   e-mail: mumbai@cbspd.com

Representatives

• **Bhopal**	0-8319310552	• **Bhubaneswar**	0-9911037372	• **Hyderabad**	0-9885175004
• **Jharkhand**	0-9811541605	• **Nagpur**	0-9421945513	• **Patna**	0-9334159340
• **Pune**	0-9623451994	• **Uttarakhand**	0-9716462459	• **Dhaka (Bangladesh)**	01912-003485

Printed at Magic International Pvt. Ltd. Greater Noida, UP, India

Preface

This *Textbook of Human Embryology* has been written keeping in mind the requirements of students and teachers. Due to the complexity of the subject, readers face difficulty in understanding and imagining the developing human structures. Hence, in the present book, the attempt has been made to provide all necessary information for easy understanding.

User-friendly features of this book with their purposes are as follows:

- **Concise text** is given in easy language; unnecessary details are avoided.
- **3D illustrations** to provide easy imagining of developing structures.
- **Flowcharts** to revise and memorise the developmental sequence.
- **Tables** to summarise essential facts.
- **Summary (examination guide)** to overcome the difficulty of summarising the facts in theory examinations.
- **Neet, MCQ, Viva Voce and Clinical facts** markings for preparation of various upcoming academic entrance examinations.
- **Boxes** to focus on important topics.
- **Interesting facts** to isolate them from the main text, so that these facts should not be missed by readers.
- **40 Scanning electron micrographs** to give real insight in developing structures.
- **70 Clinical cases** for early clinical exposure of various clinical anomalies encountered by eminent clinicians.
- **Special topics** such as assisted reproductive techniques (including *in vitro* fertilisation) and ultrasonography in embryology are also included to give orientation towards clinical aspects.

I am hopeful that this book will help to fulfil all the requirements of students and teachers.

Students are suggested to read in the following sequence:

> Illustrations → Stages of development → Flowchart → Table → Summary (examination guide) → Practice Figure

Any suggestions from the readers for rectification and improvement are welcome at dryogeshas@rediffmail.com

Yogesh Sontakke

Acknowledgements

I am thankful to Professors Dr SC Parija (Former Director), Dr B Vishnu Bhat (Former Director), Dr S Vivekanandan (Director), Dr RP Swaminathan (Dean Academics), Dr Ashok Badhe (Medical Superintendent), Jawaharlal Institute of Postgraduate Medical Education and Research (JIPMER), Pondicherry, and Professor Dr GK Pal, Dean, JIPMER, Karaikal, for encouraging and inspiring me for writing this book. I am greatly indebted to Professor Dr Parkash Chand (Retd.) and Dr K Aravindhan (Additional Professor and Head), Department of Anatomy, JIPMER, for their encouragement, invaluable support and suggestions.

I am grateful to Dr SD Joshi (Indore), Dr SS Joshi (Indore), Dr GP Pal (Indore), Dr Shipra Paul (Delhi), Dr Sunetra Naidu (Nagpur), Dr Manik Chaterjee (Raipur), Dr RR Marathe (Akola), Dr Manisha Rajanand Gaikwad (AIIMS, Bhubaneswar), Dr BS Lala (Indore) for suggestions and support.

I am obliged to Prof Kathleen Sulik (Chapel Hill, North Carolina, USA), Dr Kumaravel S (Paediatric Surgery, JIPMER), Dr Bibekanand Jindal (Paediatric Surgery, JIPMER), Dr Adhisivam B (Neonatology, JIPMER), Dr Subashini Kaliaperumal (Ophthalmology, JIPMER), Dr Haritha Sagili (OBGY, JIPMER), Dr Mamatha Gowda (OBGY, JIPMER), Dr Keshav Malhotra (Rainbow IVF, Agra), Dr Saikat Chakraborty (Oral Pathology, Pondicherry), Dr Rohit Rao (Ophthalmology, Raipur), Dr Prakhar Mohniya (Paediatrics, Jhansi) for contribution of scanning electron micrographs, clinical images and suggestions.

I acknowledge the supports from Dr M Sivakumar, Dr Suma HY, Dr Sarasu J, Dr Raveendranath V, Dr Suman Verma, Dr Sulochana Sakthivel, Dr Rajasekhar SSSN, Dr Dinesh Kumar V (JIPMER), Dr Nagaraj S, Dr Vishwajit Deshmukh (JIPMER, Karaikal) for their continuous unconditional support. Especially thankful to Dr V Gladwin and Dr Dharmaraj Tamgire for their suggestions.

A special thank of mine goes to my colleagues and friends who helped me by exchanging their views, interesting ideas, thoughts and made it possible to complete this book. I acknowledge the supports from Dr Mukesh Mittal (Indore), Dr PS Mittal (Greater Noida), Dr Jagruti Agarwal (Raipur), Dr Natwar Agrawal (Jabalpur), Dr Prashant Chaware (AIIMS, Bhopal), Dr V Dharani (Villupuram), Dr Praveen Kurrey (Raipur), Dr Rupa Chhaparwal (Indore), Dr Amit Kumar (Bilaspur), Dr R Sarah (Pondicherry), Dr Shrikant Verma (Raipur), Dr Garima Pardhi (Bhopal), Dr Harsh Kumar Chawre (Reva), Dr Aparna Muraleedharan (Pondicherry), Dr Vishal Bhadkaria (Sagar), Dr M Siva Kumar (Tiruvannamalai), Dr Kashish Singh Chakraborty (Pondicherry).

I also acknowledge Dr Thuslima M, Dr Vijaykishan Bheemavarapu, Dr Sujithaa N, Dr Praveena R, Dr Vani PC, Dr Chandan Lal Gupta, Dr Surraj S (senior residents) for their support. I also acknowledge Dr Anitha B, Dr Sujithaa N, Dr Ariyanachi K, Dr Vidhya Meena S, Dr Kiran K, Dr Shanthini S, Dr Phoebe Johnson, Dr Challa Ravi, Dr Rajeev Panwar, Dr G Dhivya Lakshmi, Dr Saleena N Ali, Dr Tom J Nallikuzhy, Dr Arun Prasad, Dr Sabin Malik, Dr Kavitha T, Dr Sankaranarayanan G, Dr Jahira Banu T, Dr Lavanya R, Dr CH Chaitanya Kumar, Dr Raju Kumaran T, Dr Srinivasan S (junior residents) for their help. I am thankful to Mr U Sakthivelu, graphic designer (Pondicherry) for teaching me the graphic designing and helping in the initial stages of this book.

I am thankful for the acceptability of views and support of Mr SK Jain (CMD) and Mr Varun Jain (Director), CBS Publishers & Distributors Pvt Ltd.

I am obliged for continuous support from Mr YN Arjuna (Senior Vice-President—Publishing, Editorial and Publicity) and his entire team, specially Ms Ritu Chawla (AGM—Production), Ms Ritu Tiwari (DTP operator), Mr Neeraj Prasad (graphic artist) and Mr Paul (copyeditor). I appreciate the entire team of CBS Publishers & Distributors in shaping this book to its present from.

I thank my wife Dr Anindita for editing, proofreading and support. I appreciate my little daughter, Aripra, for her unconditional love. My sincere regards to my family for moral support. I thank the Almighty for giving me the strength and patience to work.

Acknowledgements for Image Courtesy

I am greatful to the following academicians for their suggestions and contributions of clinical images (indicated in front of their names) in the present book.

- **Professor Kathleen Sulik**, PhD, Emeritus Professor, University of North Carolina School of Medicine, Department of Cell Biology and Physiology, Chapel Hill, North Carolina, USA.
  Scannning electron micrographs: 7.1 to 7.5, 8.1 to 8.5, 11.1 to 11.3, 12.1 to 12.4, 13.1, 14.1, 14.2, 15.1, 18.1 to 18.4, 19.1, 20.1, 21.1 to 21.3, 22.1 to 22.4, 23.1, 23.2, 24.1, 24.2, 26.1, 26.2.
- **Dr Kumaravel S**, MBBS, MS, MCh (Paediatric Surgery), Additional Professor and Head, Department of Paediatric Surgery, JIPMER, Pondicherry, 605 006, India.

Clinical images: 7.2, 9.5, 10.1 to 10.3, 11.1, 14.2 to 14.7, 17.1, 18.3, 20.1, 20.2, 21.1 to 21.5, 22.1 to 22.3, 26.1 to 26.4, 30.1.

- **Dr Adhisivam B**, Additional Professor, Department of Neonatology, JIPMER, Pondicherry, 605 006, India.
  Clinical images: 12.2, 14.1, 22.4A, 22.5 to 22.7.
- **Dr Subashini Kaliaperumal**, MBBS, MS (Ophthalmology), FRCS, DNB (Ophthalmology), Additional Professor, Department of Ophthalmology, JIPMER, Pondicherry. 605 006, India.
  Clinical images: 23.5, 23.6 to 23.9.
- **Dr Haritha Sagili**, MBBS, MD, MRCOG, MFSRH, European University Diploma in Operative Gynaecological Endoscopy, FICS, CIMP, FIMSA, Additional Professor, Department of Obstetrics and Gynaecology, JIPMER, Pondicherry, 605 006. India.
  Clinical images: 9.1 to 9.4, 18.1, 28.1, 30.2.
- **Dr Mamatha Gowda**, Assistant Professor, Department of Obstetrics and Gynaecology, JIPMER, Pondicherry, 605 006, India.
  Clinical images: 7.1, 18.1, 18.2, 22.8 to 22.11, 29.1 to 29.4, 30.3.
- **Dr Keshav Malhotra**, MBBS MCE, Director, Rainbow IVF, Rainbow Hospitals, Agra, Uttar Pradesh, 282007.
  Clinical images: 2.1, 4.1, 4.2, 4.3, 5.1.
- **Dr Rohit Rao**, MBBS, MS (Ophthalmology), IOL and Anterior Segment Fellowship (Aravind Eye Hospital), Anterior Segment Surgeon, Shri Ganesh Vinayak Eye Hospital, Raipur, Chhattisgarh, India.
  Clinical images: 23.1 to 23.4.
- **Dr Prakhar Mohniya**, MBBS, MD (Paediatrics), Fellowship in Neonatology. Senior Resident, Maharani Laxmi Bai Medical College, Jhansi, UP, 284128. India.
  Clinical images: 12.1, 22.4B.
- **Dr Saikat Chakraborty**, Resident, MDS (Oral Pathology), Mahatma Gandhi Postgraduate Institute of Dental Sciences, Pondicherry, 605 006, India.
  Clinical images: 13.1.

Neet markings are given only to indicate important facts that may be useful for the preparation for National Eligibility cum Entrance Test (NEET).

Reader should not get confused for the spellings of terminologies due to the difference between British and American English. For the reference purpose, a few of the differences are shown in the following table.

Table: Difference in terminologies in British and American English.

British English	American English
amenorrhoea	amenorrhea
caecum	cecum
caesarean	cesarean
canalise	canalize
centre	center
characterise	characterize
colour	color
dysmenorrhoea	dysmenorrhea
favourable	favorable
fertilisation	fertilization
fibre	fiber
foetus	fetus
grey	gray
hypomenorrhoea	hypomenorrhea
keratinisation	keratinization
luteinising	luteinizing
masculinise	masculinize
oedema	edema
oesophagus	esophagus
oestrogen	estrogen
oligomenorrhoea	oligomenorrhea
polymenorrhoea	polymenorrhea
towards	toward

Grey and white are **matter** in brain, whereas pia, arachnoid and dura are **mater** covering the brain.

Yogesh Sontakke

Contents

Preface   *iii*

1. **Introduction**   1
2. **Gametogenesis**   6
3. **Menstrual Cycle**   16
4. **First Week of Development**   24
5. **Assisted Reproduction Technology**
   In vitro Fertilisation and Intracytoplasmic Sperm Injection   34
6. **Second Week of Development**   40
7. **Third Week of Development**   49
8. **Embryonic Period**
   Four to Eight Weeks of Development   61
9. **Placenta and Umbilical Cord**   73
10. **Integumentary System**
    Skin, its Appendages and Mammary Gland   86
11. **Pharyngeal Apparatus**   96
12. **Alimentary Tract I**
    Development of Face, Nose, Palate   109
13. **Alimentary Tract II**
    Development of Teeth, Pharynx, Tongue and Salivary Glands   117
14. **Alimentary Tract III**
    Development of Intestine   126
15. **Alimentary Tract IV**
    Development of Liver, Gallbladder, Pancreas and Spleen   141
16. **Respiratory System**   149
17. **Development of Body Cavities and Diaphragm**   158
18. **Cardiovascular System I**
    Development of Heart   168
19. **Cardiovascular System II**
    Blood Vessels and Foetal Circulation   184
20. **Urinary System**
    Kidney, Ureter, Urinary Bladder, Urethra   203
21. **Reproductive System**
    Male and Female Reproductive Organs   215
22. **Nervous System**   231
23. **Development of Eye**   257
24. **Development of Ear**   266
25. **Endocrine System**   273
26. **Skeletal System and Limbs**   279
27. **Muscular System**   293
28. **Foetal Period**
    Nine Weeks to Birth   297
29. **Clinical Applications and Ultrasonography in Embryology**   300
30. **Multiple Pregnancy (Twinning)**   305

Annexures   310
  I. Embryonic Remnants   310
  II. Placenta Previa   311
  III. Hermaphrodite   312
  IV. Derivatives of Neural Crest Cells   313

Index   *315*

1

Introduction

Chapter Outline

- Basic terminology
- Periods of human embryology
- Periods of postnatal development
- Need of embryology
- Chromosomes
- Cell division
  - Mitosis
  - Meiosis
- Non-disjunction
- Organiser and induction

BASIC TERMINOLOGY

Embryology
- Embryology is a branch of science that deals with the study of formation and development of an organism.

Reproduction
- Sexual reproduction involves fusion of male and female gametes to produce an offspring.
- It helps in maintenance of species.

Ontogeny
- Ontogeny is a branch of science that deals with complete life cycle (prenatal and postnatal growth and development) of an organism.

Phylogeny
- Phylogeny deals with an evolutionary history and relationship among organisms.
- Phylogenetically, organisms are classified as fishes, amphibians, reptiles, birds and mammals.
- Mammals are classified as Protheria (lay eggs), Metatheria (produce extremely young offspring that mature in pouch of mother, marsupials) and Eutheria (deliver mature young ones, receive nutrition through placenta till birth).
- Humans are eutherian or placental mammals.
- During human development, it is found that ontogeny recapitulates phylogeny (Ernst Haeckel, 1866).
- It can be explained by the developing human kidney: Pronephric kidney → mesonephric kidney → metanephric kidney.

Development
- Development of a human from a single cell stage of life involves growth and differentiation.
- **Development** is a broad term that involves transformation of a simple single cell into a complex multicellular organism.
- **Growth** is a mere increase in the number and size of cells.
- Growth is of three types:
  1. *Multiplicative growth*: It is an increase in cell number by cell division.
  2. *Auxetic growth*: It is an increase in cell size.
  3. *Accretionary growth*: It is an increase in intracellular substances.
- **Differentiation** is a process of cell transformation to acquire specific character and function.
- Zygote divides to form many undifferentiated cells as follows:
  1. *Totipotent cells*: Cells of zygote or morula can form all differentiated cell types of an organism. These are called totipotent cells.
  2. *Pluripotent*: For example, inner cell mass of blastocyst can form all types of differentiated cells of an organism except placenta.
- **Gametogenesis** is a process of formation of gametes (ovum and sperms) from germ cells.

PERIODS OF HUMAN EMBRYOLOGY

- Most of the clinicians divide human prenatal development as first, second and third trimesters (each of three-month period) (Fig. 1.1).
- Embryologically, prenatal growth is divided into:
  1. *Germinal/ovular period*: First three weeks of development after fertilisation.
  2. *Embryonic period*: From fourth to eighth week of development.[Neet]
  3. *Foetal period (organ growth)*: From third month till termination of the pregnancy.
- *Period of egg*: It extends for one week from fertilisation to implantation into uterine wall.
- *Conceptus* (product of conception) is also called preimplantation conceptus. In *in vitro* fertilisation, *pre-implantation conceptus* needs to be transferred to uterus for further growth.
- Further, on implantation, conceptus is called *postimplantation conceptus*.

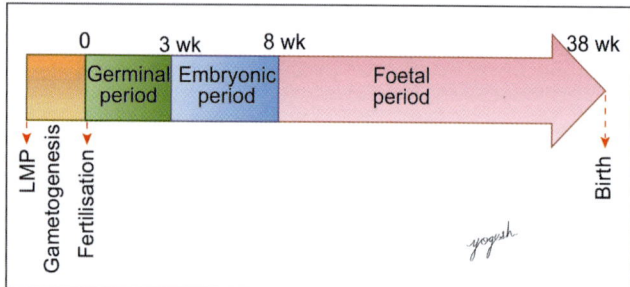

Fig. 1.1: Periods of human embryology. *Abbreviations:* wk: Week; LMP: Last menstrual period

PERIODS OF POSTNATAL DEVELOPMENT

- Postnatal period is divided into the following phases of life:
  1. *Infancy*: From birth till 1 year of age
  2. *Childhood*: From 1 to 12 years of age
  3. *Puberty*: After childhood till 16 years of age
  4. *Adolescence*: After puberty till 18 years of age
  5. *Adulthood*: From 18 years to 25 years of age

NEED OF EMBRYOLOGY

1. Usually 3–4% of live births children suffer from birth defects. Understanding of this malformation is essential before treatment.
2. All structures in the human body develop from a single cell. Studying embryology will help to understand the gross anatomy and histological structures of body.
3. Deviated growth and development may lead to many diseases. Genes controlling the development may have mutation that results into a disease.

Some Interesting Facts
- Aristotle (384–322BC) is the founder of embryology, whereas Karl Ernst von Baer is the father of modern embryology.
- Louise Brown (1978) is the first born test-tube baby.
- Dolly, a female sheep (1996), is the first cloned mammal.
- Y chromosome is acrocentric and smaller in size, whereas X chromosome is large submetacentric.[Neet]

---

4. In the field of reproductive medicine, embryology helps for better practice for well-being of mother and newborn.
5. Knowledge of embryology can be applied in infertility cases (*in vitro* fertilisation, intrauterine insemination).

Box 1.1: Chromosomes
- Each human cell has 46 chromosomes except ovum (22 + X chromosomes) and sperms (22 + X or 22 + Y chromosomes).
- Out of 46 human chromosomes, 22 pairs are *autosomes* and one pair is *sex chromosomes* (X and Y chromosome).
- Sex chromosomes determine sex characteristics of an individual.
- *Structure* (Fig. 1.2)
  - Each chromosome consists of deoxyribonucleic acid (DNA) tightly coiled around histone proteins.
  - Each chromosome has sister chromatids connected at centromere.
  - Chromosome shows two arms: Short arm (p arm, p for *petit* means small) and long arm (q arm).
  - This typical structure of chromosome appears only during cell division.
  - In interphase, chromosomes form a thin thread-like structure called *chromatin*.

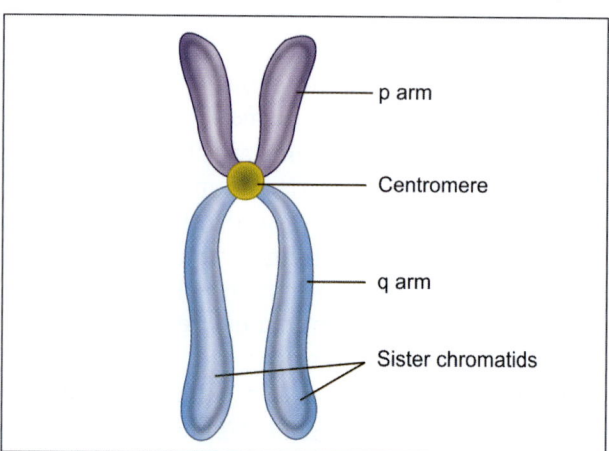

Fig. 1.2: Structure of chromosome

6. Knowledge of embryology is essential for prenatal diagnosis and fetal therapy (amniocentesis, chorionic villus sampling).

CELL DIVISION

- Cell division is a process of cell multiplication.
- It is of two types: Mitosis and meiosis.

Mitosis

- Mitosis is a cell division that maintains constant number of chromosomes in parent and offspring cells.
- Mitosis is always preceded by S phase where DNA duplicates.

Phases of Mitosis (Fig. 1.3)

1. *Prophase:* Events—chromosomes condense and become visible; spindle fibres emerge from centrosomes, nuclear envelope breaks down, and centrosome moves toward the opposite pole.
2. *Prometaphase:* Events—continued condensation of chromosomes, centromeres become visible, attachment of microtubules to the centromere.
3. *Metaphase:* Events—chromosomes arranged at metaphase plate, attachment of each sister chromatids to spindle fibres from the opposite pole.
4. *Anaphase:* Events—centromeres split in two, sister chromatids are pulled towards the opposite poles.
5. *Telophase:* Events—chromosomes arrive at the opposite poles; mitotic spindle breaks, nuclear membrane starts forming.

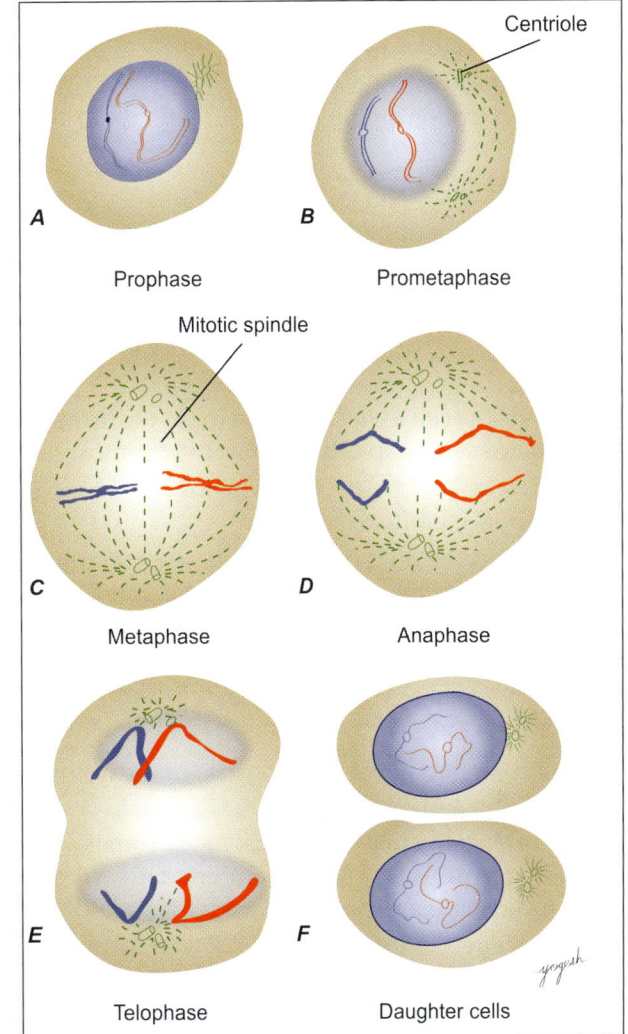

Fig. 1.3: Stages of mitosis

Differences between Mitosis and Meiosis

Q. Write the differences between mitosis and meiosis.

Table 1.1	Differences between mitosis and meiosis	
Event	Mitosis	Meiosis
Occurrence	All cells of body	Only in germ cells
Process	It is equational division	It is a reductional division
Prophase	No crossover of genetic material No synapsis	Crossover of genetic material takes place Synapsis occurs in zygotene phase
Metaphase	No chiasmata formation Chromosomes arrange at the equator	Chiasmata formation Homologous chromosome arranges on either side of equator
Anaphase	Centromere divides Chromatids move to the opposite pole	No division of centromere Whole chromosome moves to the opposite pole
Telophase	Daughter cells with the same number of chromosomes (46)	Daughter cells with a haploid number of chromosomes (23)
Number of daughter cells	Two	Four

6. *Cytokinesis:* Event—cleavage furrow appears to separate daughter cells.
   - At the end of one mitotic cycle, two cells are formed from a single cell.

Significance of Mitosis

- It helps in development and growth of an organism.
- It helps in replacing the damaged body cells.
- It contributes to replace old body cells.

Meiosis

- Meiosis is the cell division that helps in the formation of gametes with haploid number of chromosomes.
- Meiosis consists of two cell divisions as first meiotic and second meiotic divisions.
- The first meiotic division has prophase I, metaphase I, anaphase I and telophase I, whereas second meiotic division has prophase II, metaphase II, anaphase II and telophase II.

Prophase I

- It is a prolonged phase and consists of the following phases (Fig. 1.4):^{Neet}
  1. **Leptotene:** Events—chromosome becomes visible and condensed, sister chromatids of each chromosome are closely placed.
  2. **Zygotene:** Events—synapsis or conjugation (pairing of homologous chromosomes), paired chromosomes are called **bivalent** or **tetrad chromosomes**.^{MCQ}
  3. **Pachytene:** Events—crossing over (there is an exchange of chromatin material in between approximated chromatids of homologous bivalent chromosomes). The point of contact of chromatids during crossing over is called **chiasmata**.^{MCQ}
  4. **Diplotene:** Events—homologous chromosomes separate apart from each other.

- Diplotene phase is followed by metaphase I, anaphase I and telophase I. In anaphase I, there is no division of centromere.
- Homologous chromosome moves towards opposite poles. Hence, resultant daughter cells receive only haploid number of chromosomes.
- The second meiotic division is equivalent of mitosis and just form two cells.
- Thus, at the end of meiosis, four daughter cells with haploid number of chromosomes are produced.

Significance of Meiosis

1. Formation of gametes is the prime aim of meiosis.
2. Meiosis helps to maintain constant chromosome number during sexual reproduction.
3. Exchange of maternal and paternal genes that are carried by homologous chromosomes takes place.
4. Meiosis (crossing over) helps to maintain genetic diversity and mixing of characters.

> **Box 1.2:** Non-disjunction
>
> *Non-disjunction*
> - Usual separation of chromosomes in first meiotic division or sister chromatids in second meiotic division is called disjunction.^{MCQ}
> - If segregation is not normal, it is called *nondisjunction*.
> - On nondisjunction, resultant cells may receive less number of chromosomes or extra chromosomes.
> - Cells of non-disjunction on fertilisation may form foetus with an abnormal number of chromosomes (trisomy or monosomy).
> - *Examples:*
>   – Down syndrome: Trisomy of chromosome 21.
>   – Klinefelter syndrome: Extra X chromosome in males (phenotypically male case).
>   – Turner syndrome: Lack of Y chromosome (phenotypically female case).

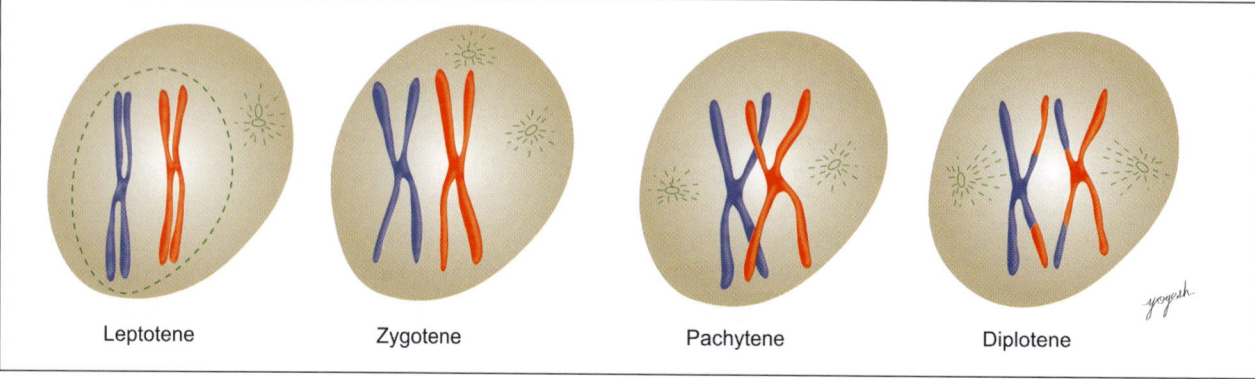

Fig. 1.4: Stages of prophase of first meiotic division

Box 1.3: Organiser and induction

- Organiser is a cluster of cells in developing embryo that can determine differentiation of other regions.
- Primary organiser is a dorsal lip of blastopore that is self-differentiating and its removal results in total failure of embryonic development. *MCQ*
- Influence of an organiser on another area of development is called **induction**.
- Inductors are substances that exert the same effects as that of organiser.
- Hans Spemann was awarded the Nobel Prize in 1935 for his discovery of embryonic induction.

For example:
1. Optic vesicle acts as an organiser and it induces formation of lens on overlaying skin.
2. Primary organiser—dorsal lip of primitive streak
   Secondary organiser—notochord
   Tertiary organiser—neutral tube

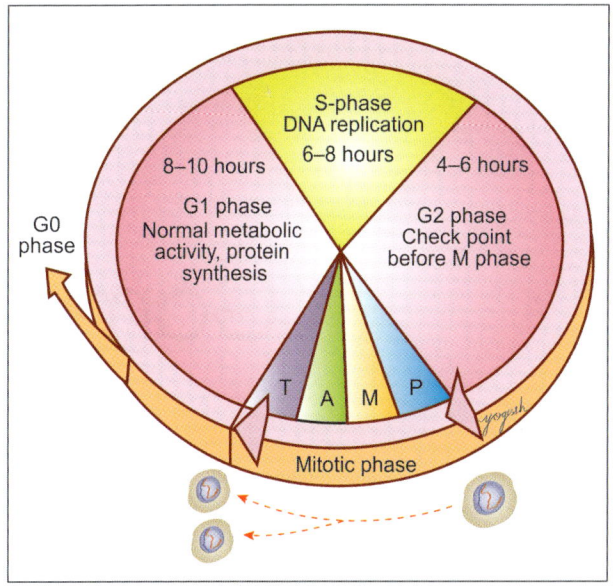

Fig. 1.5: Phases of cell division. *Abbreviations:* P: Prophase; M: Metaphase; A: Anaphase; T: Telophase

Some Interesting Facts

Phases of Cell Life (Fig. 1.5)
- *G1 phase:* It follows M phase. Events: Cytoplasm increases in volume; damaged DNA gets repaired.
- *S phase:* It follows G1 phase. Events: DNA gets replicated to form two sister chromatids of each arm of the chromosome. Each cell contains 4n (double 2n) number of chromosomes.
- *G2 phase:* It follows S-phase. Event: It is a check point before mitosis or meiosis for the confirmation of duplicated chromatin.
- *G0 phase:* It is a nondividing phase of cell cycle.
- *M phase:* It is the cell division phase.

2
Gametogenesis

Chapter Outline

- Primordial germ cells
- Teratoma
- Gametogenesis
- Spermatogenesis
- Capacitation of spermatozoa
- Structure of spermatozoa
- Abnormal spermatozoa and its counts
- Oogenesis
- Ovulation
- Tests for ovulation
- Disorders of ovulation
- Structure of ovum

INTRODUCTION

Primordial Germ Cells

- Primordial germ cells (PGC) give rise to sperm in males and ovum in females.
- PGC resides in yolk sac (extraembryonic membrane) and can be identified by fourth week of gestation (Fig. 2.1).^{MCQ}
- PGC are derived from epiblast (old concept: PGC are derived from endoderm of yolk sac).^{Neet}
- PGC migrates with amoeboid movement from yolk sac to wall of gut from fourth to sixth weeks.
- Later, these cells migrate through mesentery of gut to dorsal body wall and colonise to form gonadal ridge (primitive gonads).
- Cells of the gonadal ridge are invaded by somatic supporting cells from coelomic epithelium.
- Migration of PGC and invasion of coelomic epithelium are essential in the formation of gonads.

GAMETOGENESIS

- Gametogenesis is a process of formation of gametes (sperms in male and ovum in female) from germ cells by cell division.
- In men, PGCs remain dormant from sixth week of intrauterine life till puberty.

Box 2.1: Teratoma

- Teratoma is a tumour that consists of tissues derived from all germ layers
- Sacrococcygeal teratoma is the most common tumour in newborns (1 in 20,000–70,000 births). It arises from primordial germ cells.^{Neet}
- It occurs more frequently in females than in males.
- It constitutes 3% of childhood malignancies.
- Gonadal teratomas occur due to the capability of germ cells to form many cell types (pluripotency).
- Teratoma shows the presence of hairs, teeth, bone and so on.

- At puberty, seminiferous tubules undergo maturation to form *spermatogonia* that on meiosis form *spermatozoa* until death.
- In females, PGCs differentiate to form *oogonia*. By *fifth month* of intrauterine life, all oogonia enter in meiosis and get arrested in prophase of the first meiotic division to form primary oocytes.^{MCQ}
- Primary oocytes undergo dormancy until puberty.^{MCQ}
- After puberty, each month few primary oocytes form ovarian follicles out of which the only one completes first meiotic division to form *secondary oocyte* and gets ovulated.

Gametogenesis

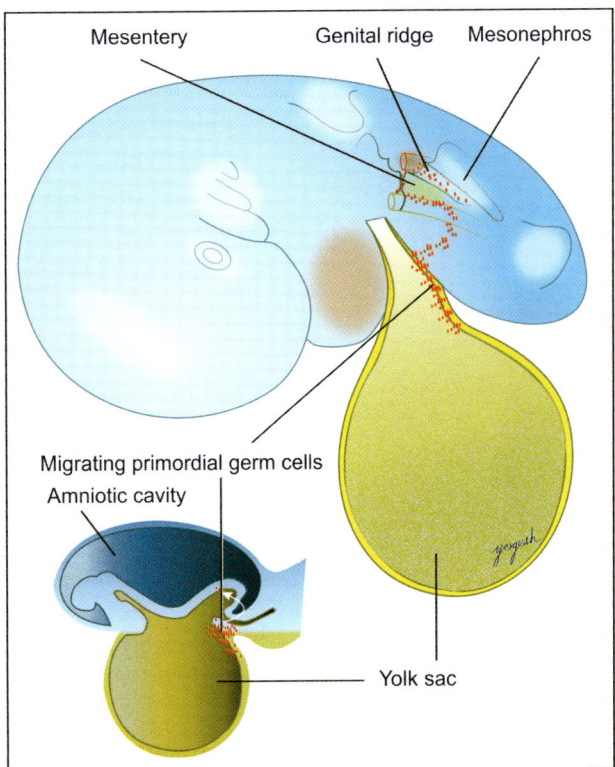

Fig. 2.1: Primordial germ cells (PGC) and formation of gonads. PGC resides in the yolk sac and migrates to the wall of the gut during fourth to sixth weeks. Later these cells migrate through mesentery of the gut to the dorsal body wall and colonise to form gonadal ridge and subsequently gonads (testis or ovaries)

- Only after fertilisation, the second meiotic division can be completed.^MCQ These cycles continue until menopause (45–50 years of age).
- Meiosis of PGCs is essential to half the number of chromosomes in gametes.

SPERMATOGENESIS

Q. Write short note on spermatogenesis.

- *Definition*: Spermatogenesis is a process of formation of sperms (male gametes) from spermatogonia in seminiferous tubules of testis.
- Site: Seminiferous tubules of testis
- Time: Occurs after puberty and continue even in old age.
- Duration: 64–74 days.^Viva
- Responsible hormone: Testosterone

Process

- It occurs in three steps as follows (Flowchart 2.1, Fig. 2.2):
- **Spermatocytosis**
    - It is a conversion of *spermatogonia → primary spermatocyte*.
    - Primary spermatocyte is the largest germ cell in seminiferous tubules.

Flowchart 2.1: Stages in spermatogenesis

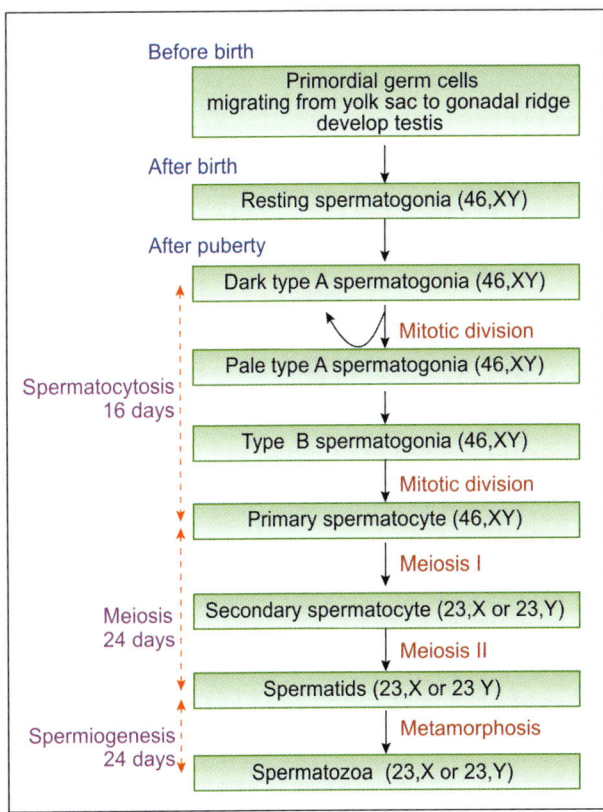

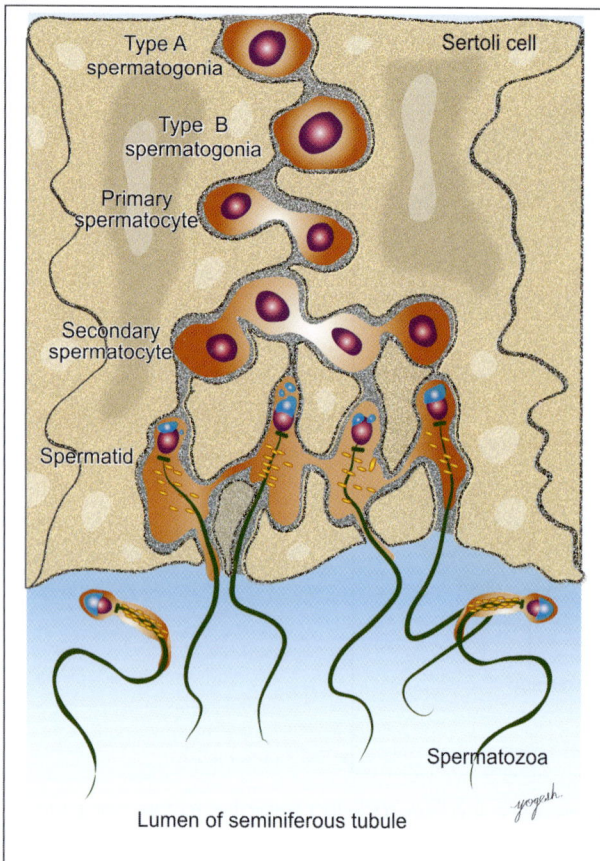

Fig. 2.2: Process of spermatogenesis. Sertoli cells support developing spermatogonia and other cells and finally phagocytose residual bodies

- At puberty, testosterone stimulates primordial germ cells to develop and differentiate into *spermatogonia* (*type A dark*).
- Spermatogonia are located immediately under the basement membrane.
- Spermatogonia are supported by Sertoli cells.
- Dark type A spermatogonia undergo **mitosis** to form *pale type A spermatogonia*.[Neet]
- Further pale type A spermatogonia on **mitosis** form *type B spermatogonia* (46,XY).[Neet]
- Type B spermatogonia undergo mitosis to form *primary spermatocyte* (46,XY).

- **Meiotic division**
    - It is the conversion of *primary spermatocyte* (46, XY) → *spermatids* (23,X and 23,Y).
    - Each primary spermatocyte (46,XY) undergoes first **meiotic** division to form **secondary** spermatocyte (23,X and 23,Y) that later undergoes to form four **spermatids** (23,X; 23,X; 23,Y; 23,Y).[Neet]

Spermiogenesis

Q. Write a short note on spermiogenesis.

- Definition: Spermiogenesis is the process of **metamorphosis** of spermatids by which they get converted into a *spermatozoon*.[MCQ, Viva]
- Metamorphosis is the change in the form of the cell.

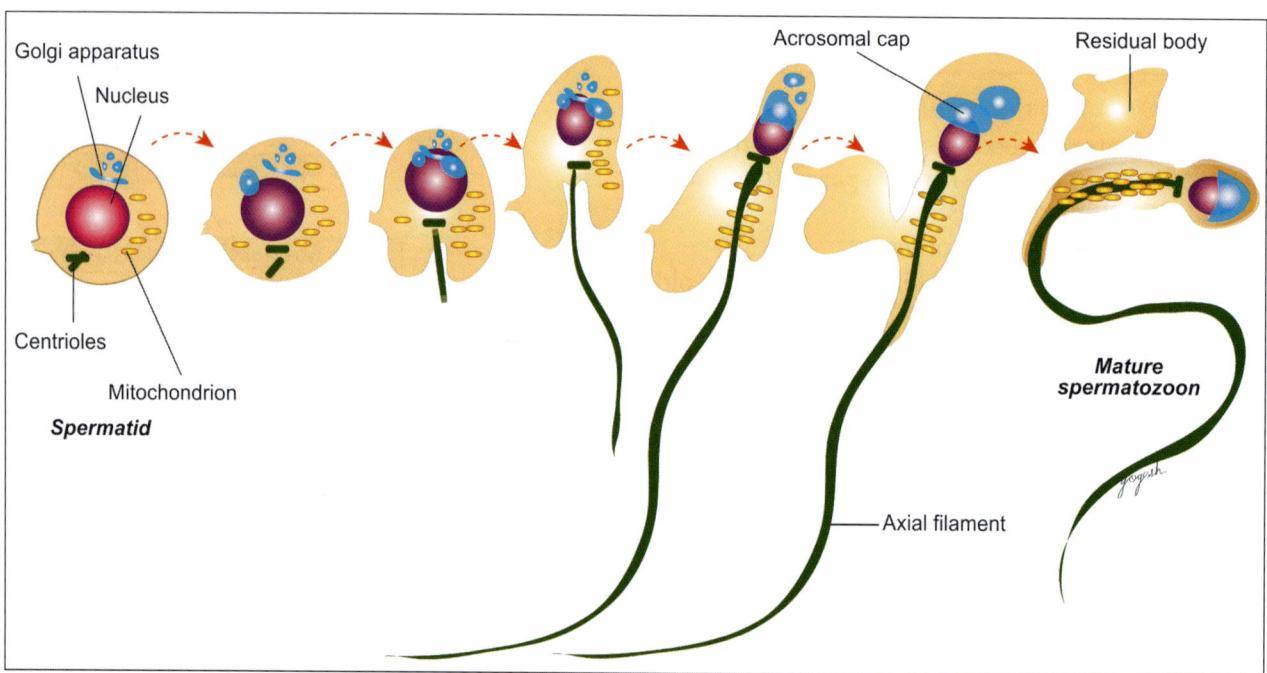

Fig. 2.3: Process of spermiogenesis

Gametogenesis

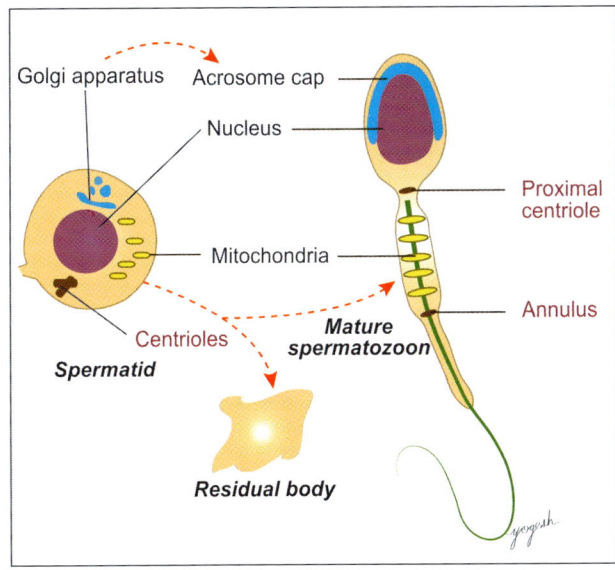

Practice Fig. 2.1: Process of spermiogenesis

- **Process of spermiogenesis** (Fig. 2.3, Practice Fig. 2.1)
  – Nucleus condenses and move towards one pole.
  – Golgi apparatus forms an acrosomal cap and covers two-thirds of the nucleus.
  – Centromere divides into proximal centriole and distal centriole comes to lie near nucleus (in the neck of sperm) and gives rise to axial filament.
  – Distal centriole lies at the junction of the middle piece with tail.
  – Mitochondria develop spiral sheath around axial filament to form a middle piece of sperm.
  – Most of the cytoplasm of spermatid is shaded as *Renaud's residual body*. [Sertoli cells phagocytose residual bodies].[MCQ]
  – Release of spermatozoa: Finally, spermatozoa are released into lumen of seminiferous tubules. This is **spermiation**.[MCQ]

Timings of Spermatogenesis

- Spermatogenesis of one sperm: 64 days (70–75 days also given by some authors).[MCQ]
- It includes mitoses—16 days, meiosis I—8 days, meiosis II—16 days and spermiogenesis—24 days.[MCQ]

Some Interesting Facts

- Spermatogenesis occurs in a continual wave throughout seminiferous tubules.
- During spermatogenesis, because of incomplete cytokinesis, daughter cells produced by mitosis or meiosis are connected with each other by slender cytoplasmic bridges.
- Secretion of fluid in seminiferous tubules pushes immature spermatozoa towards epididymis.

- Sperms start motility in epididymis.[Neet] Sperm acquires full motility only on ejaculation with the help of prostatic and seminal secretions.
- Reduction division (meiosis I) or independent assortment of chromosomes occurs in spermatogenesis during conversion of primary to secondary spermatocyte; hence, secondary spermatocyte onwards haploid number of chromosomes are seen.[Neet]
- Spermatogonia and primary spermatocytes have diploid number of chromosomes (46,XY). Secondary spermatocytes, spermatids and sperms have haploid number of chromosomes.[Neet]
- Spermatogenesis requires temperature that is ~2°C below body temperature.[Neet]
- Differences between spermatid and spermatozoon are listed in Table 2.1.

Box 2.2: Capacitation of spermatozoa

Q. Write short note on capacitation.
- Capacitation is a process of conversion of immature spermatozoa to mature spermatozoa.
- Capacitation is discovered by Chang and Austin (1951).
- Site: Female reproductive tract (uterus and uterine tubes).[Neet,Viva]
- Capacitation involves the following events:
  – Removal of acrosomal membrane
  – Alteration of glycoprotein coat over head of sperm.
  – Removal of seminal proteins from head of sperm.
- Effect of capacitation:
  – Increases sperm motility
  – Destabilises acrosomal membrane and allows it to penetrate outer layer of egg.

Q. List the differences between spermatid and spermatozoon.

Table 2.1	Differences between spermatid and spermatozoon
Spermatid	Spermatozoon
It is immature male gamete.	It is mature male gamete.
Nucleus: Big, central.	Nucleus: Condensed, lies in head portion.
Golgi apparatus is not fused to form acrosomal cap.	Golgi apparatus fuse to form acrosomal cap.
It has dispersed mitochondria in the cytoplasm.	Mitochondria are arranged spirally in the middle piece.
It does not have tail or axial filament.	It has tail and axial filament.
It has abundant cytoplasm.	It has scanty cytoplasm.

Some Interesting Facts

- Spermatozoa are artificially capacitated and used for *in vitro* fertilisation (IVF).
- In assisted reproduction technology (ART) for a patient with defective acrosome, sperm is injected directly into oocyte.
- Sperm with Y chromosome swims faster due to smaller size of Y chromosome.[Neet]
- Sperms are stored in seminiferous tubules after formation.[Neet]

STRUCTURE OF SPERMATOZOA

Q. Write short note on the structure of spermatozoa or sperm.
Q. Draw a well-labelled diagram of sperm.

- Matured spermatozoa have head, neck, middle piece and tail.
- Length: 50–60 µm.
- Count: In a single ejaculation, 200–300 million sperms are emitted in a volume of 2–5 ml semen.

Parts of Spermatozoa (Fig. 2.4, Practice Fig. 2.2)

- It has the following parts:

Head

- Shape: Pyriform
- Length: 4 µm
- Contains haploid condensed nucleus (23,X or 23,Y chromosomes).
- *Acrosomal cap* (galea capitis) cover two-thirds of nucleus (derived from Golgi apparatus).
- Acrosome contains digestive enzymes (hyaluronidase and acrosine) that help to break the outer wall of the ovum.[MCQ]

Neck

- Length: 0.3 µm
- Contains proximal centriole with transverse and longitudinal cylinders.
- The longitudinal cylinder has nine thick filaments that are continuous with axial filaments of body and tail of spermatozoon.

Middle Piece/Body

- Length: 4 µm.
- Axial filament passes from neck into middle piece and tail.
- At the junction of a middle piece with tail, distal centriole is present in the form of an *annulus* (ring-like structure).

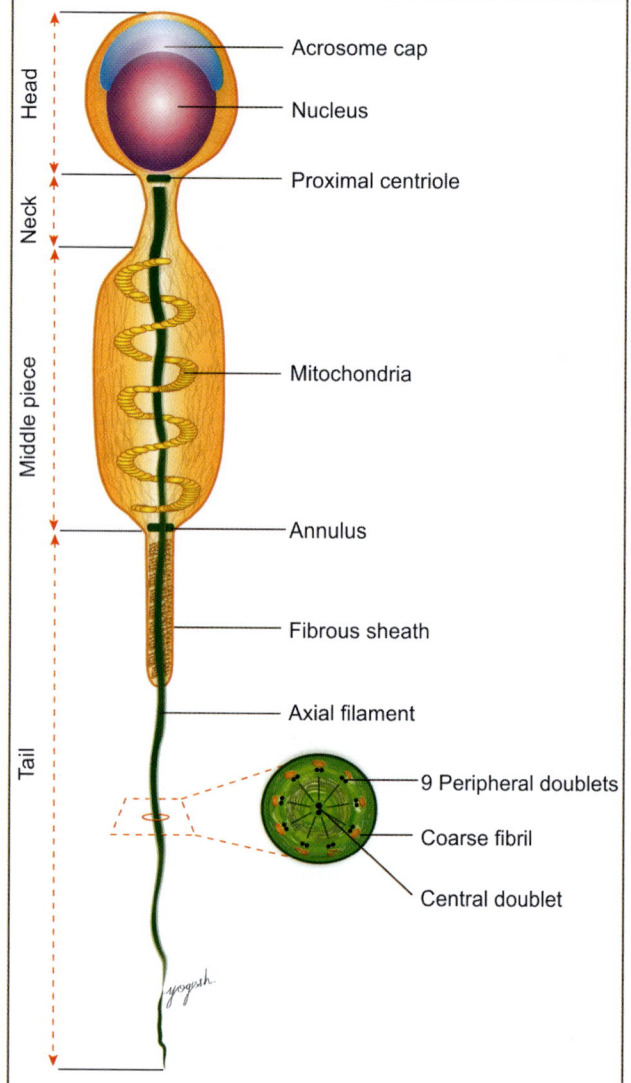

Fig. 2.4: Structure of sperm

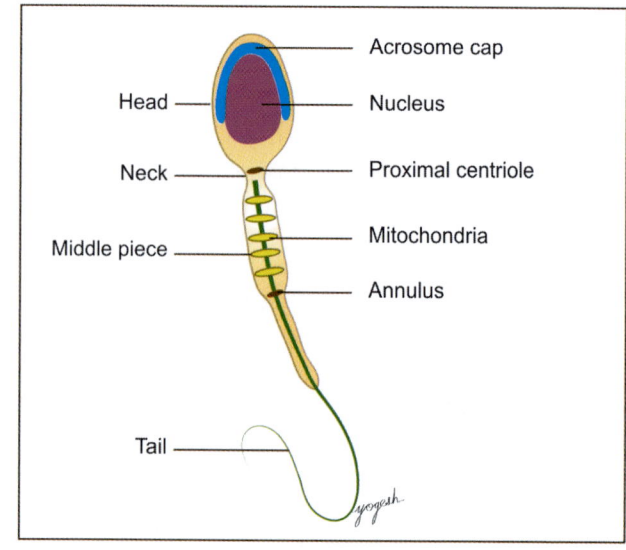

Practice Fig. 2.2: Structure of sperm

- The axial filament is surrounded spirally by mitochondrion.
- Axial filament is made up of central doublet of fibril surrounded by nine doublets of fibrils. Each peripheral doublet is associated with coarser, petal-shaped fibril.

Tail

- Length: 40 μm.
- Parts:
  - In *principal piece*, axial filament is surrounded by plasma membrane and the fibrous sheath.
  - In *end piece*, the fibrous sheath is absent.

Life

- Usual period of viability after ejaculation is 48 hours, but may survive up to 4 days in female genital tract.

Box 2.3: Abnormal spermatozoa and its counts (Fig. 2.5)[MCQ,Viva]

- *Oligozoospermia*: Sperm count <15 millions/ml of semen is called oligozoospermia (WHO).
- *Azoospermia*: It is the absence of sperms in semen. It affects about 1% of male population and 20% of male infertility cases.
- *Aspermia*: It is the complete lack of semen. It may be due to retrograde ejaculation, prostatectomy, ejaculatory duct obstruction.
- *Asthenozoospermia*: It is reduced sperm motility.
- *Hyperspermia* is large semen volume and *hypospermia* is small semen volume.
- *Teratozoospermia*: It is the abnormal morphology of sperms that affects fertility in males. It includes giant or dwarf sperms, double head or body of sperm. Even during semen analysis of healthy individuals, 10% of abnormal spermatozoa have been observed.

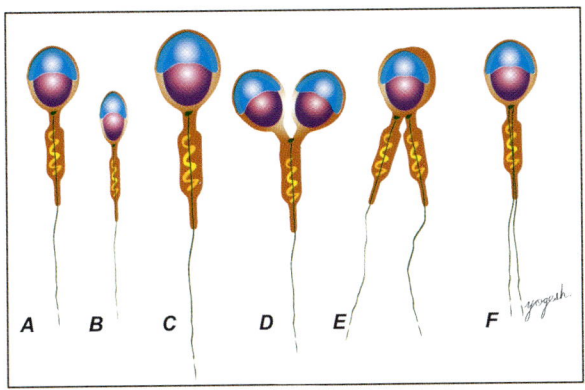

Fig. 2.5: Morphology of sperms: (A) Normal sperm; (B) Microsperm; (C) Giant sperm; (D) Double-headed sperm; (E) Sperm with double body; (F) Sperm with double tail

OOGENESIS

Q. Write short note on oogenesis.

- Definition: Oogenesis is a process of formation of a mature ovum from primordial germ cells.
- Location: Ovarian cortex.

Process of Oogenesis (Flowchart 2.2)

- It takes in three phases—before birth, after puberty, after fertilisation.

Before birth

- Before third month of IUL, the PGCs undergo mitosis to form *oogonia*.
- Before 7th month of IUL, oogonia multiply *mitotically* and enlarge to form *primary oocytes* that get surrounded by epithelial cells.[Neet]
- 7th month to birth, *primary oocytes* complete prophase I of meiotic division and get arrested at **dictyotene (diplotene) stage** at birth by *oocyte maturation inhibitor* (OMI) factor till puberty.[Neet]
- Out of 2 million primary oocytes (primordial follicles), 400,000 persist up to puberty and only 500 ovulate.[Neet]
- From birth to puberty follicles remain in dormant phase.

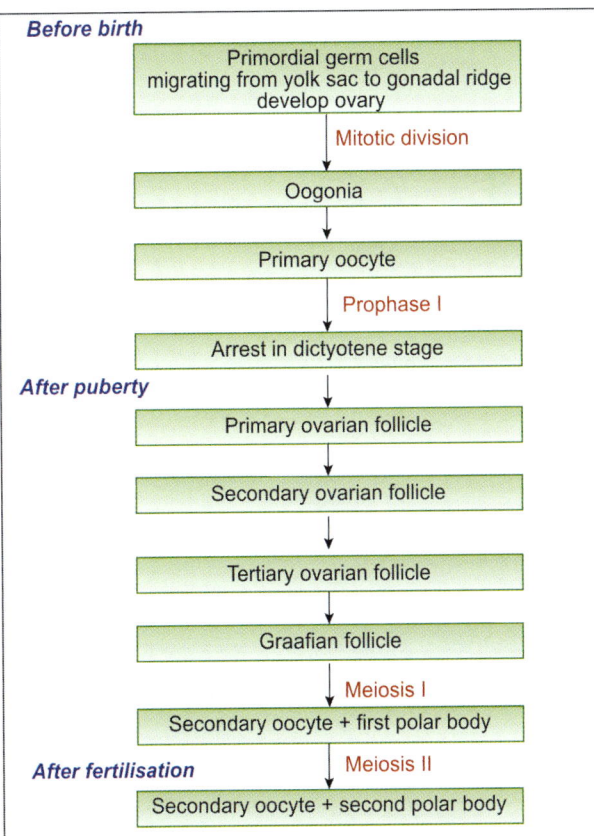

Flowchart 2.2: Stages in oogenesis

After puberty (Fig. 2.6)
- Due to hormonal changes, ovary shows cyclic changes called *ovarian cycle*.
- Primary oocyte (46,XX) undergoes maturation and increase in size.
- Surrounding flattened follicular cells mature and form cuboid cells. Then this follicle is called **primary follicle**.
- Follicular cells multiply to form multilayered *granulosa layer*. Then, this follicle is called **secondary follicle**.

- Fluid-filled cavity (follicular antrum) appears in the follicular cells and forms **tertiary follicle** and fluid is called *liquor folliculi*.
- Antrum folliculi separates granulosa cells as outer *stratum granulosum* and inner *cumulus ovaricus* layers that surround primary oocyte.[Neet]
- Finally, stromal cells surround the follicle and condenses to form vascular inner layer *theca interna* (theca = membrane) and outer fibrous layer, *theca externa*. Then this follicle is called **matured graafian follicle** (named after the Dutch anatomist R. de Graaf, 1641–73) (Fig. 2.7).
- Theca interna secretes estrogen hormone.
- **Zona pellucida:** Accumulated amorphous **glycoprotein** forms a layer between the primary oocyte and follicular cells called zona pellucida.[MCQ]
- Primary oocyte completes first meiotic division without cytoplasmic division. Primary oocyte retains one nucleus (23,X) and expels another nucleus (23,X) as a *first polar body* in perivitelline space.
- Thus, the primary oocyte is converted into **secondary oocyte**. Secondary oocyte enters in second meiotic division and gets arrested at metaphase (Fig. 2.8).
- Graafian follicle ovulates secondary oocyte.[MCQ]

After fertilisation
- If ovum gets fertilised, secondary oocyte completes second meiotic division.
- During second meiosis, secondary oocyte retains cytoplasm and one nucleus (23,X) and expels another nucleus as a *second polar body* in perivitelline space.
- If fertilisation does not occur, secondary oocyte does not complete second meiotic division and undergo degeneration within **24 hours** after ovulation.[MCQ]
- After ovulation graafian follicle collapses and forms *corpus luteum*.

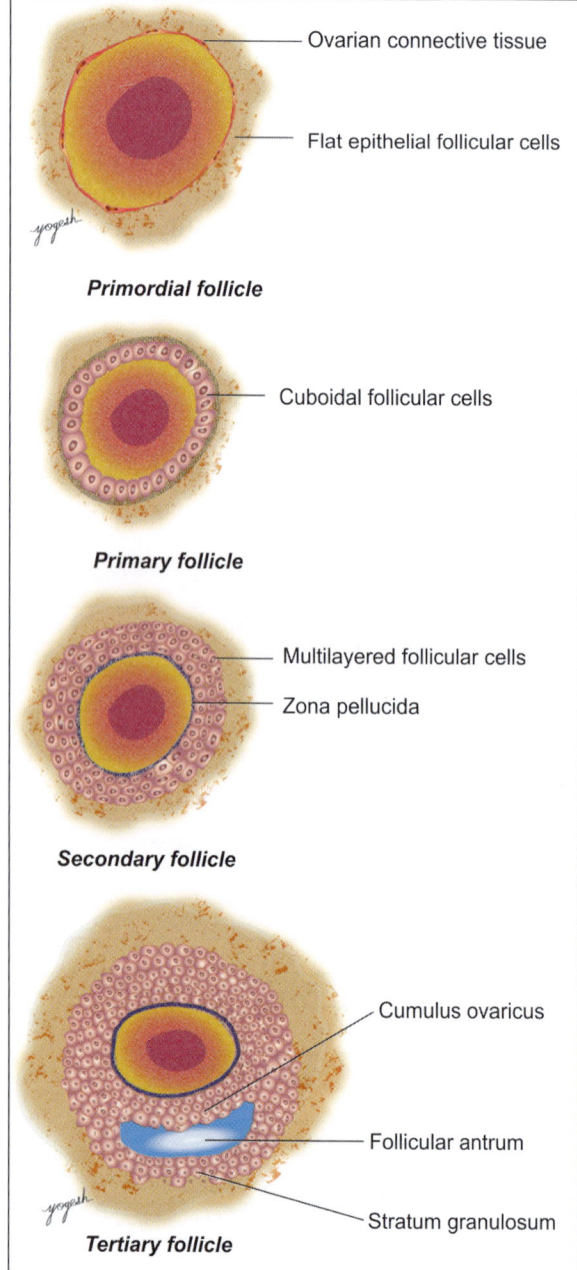

Fig. 2.6: Follicular development

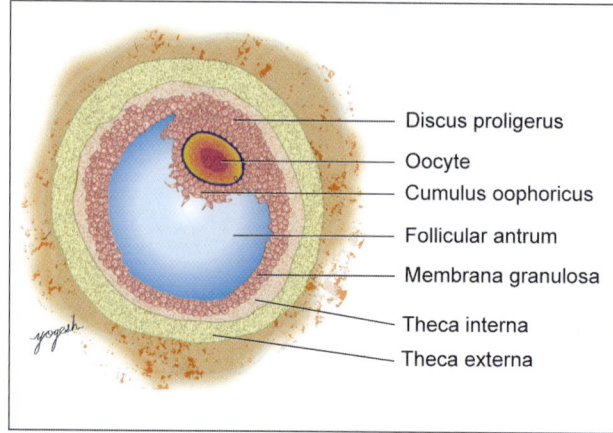

Fig. 2.7: Graafian follicle

Gametogenesis

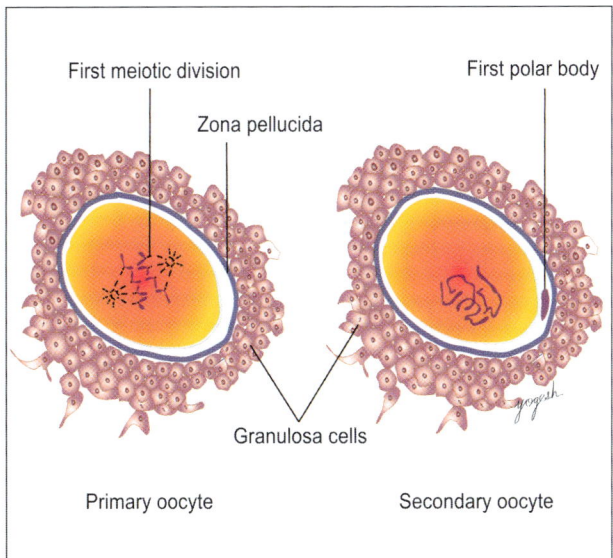

Fig. 2.8: Maturation of oocyte. Primary oocyte completes first meiotic division to form secondary oocyte and first polar body

Some Interesting Facts
- In females, formation of gametes occurs at puberty (10–14 years of age) to 45–50 years of age (menopause).
- In males, formation of gametes continues up to old age.
- In each menstrual cycle, 5–30 primary oocytes mature but only one ovulates and other denaturates.
- Polar bodies are formed during oogenesis (not in spermatogenesis).[Neet]

OVULATION

Q. Write short note on ovulation.

- Definition: Ovulation is a process of *release of ovum* from graafian follicle.
- Time: 14 days prior to onset of next menstrual bleeding.[MCQ]

Responsible Factors

1. LH surge: High concentration of luteinising hormone (LH) prior to ovulation → increase collagenase activity → digestion of collagen fibres surrounding graafian follicle.
2. Prostaglandins: Increased concentration of prostaglandins → causes contraction of smooth muscles of wall of ovary.
3. Follicular fluid: Increased amount of follicular fluid → increased follicular pressure.

Events (Flowchart 2.3)

Flowchart 2.3

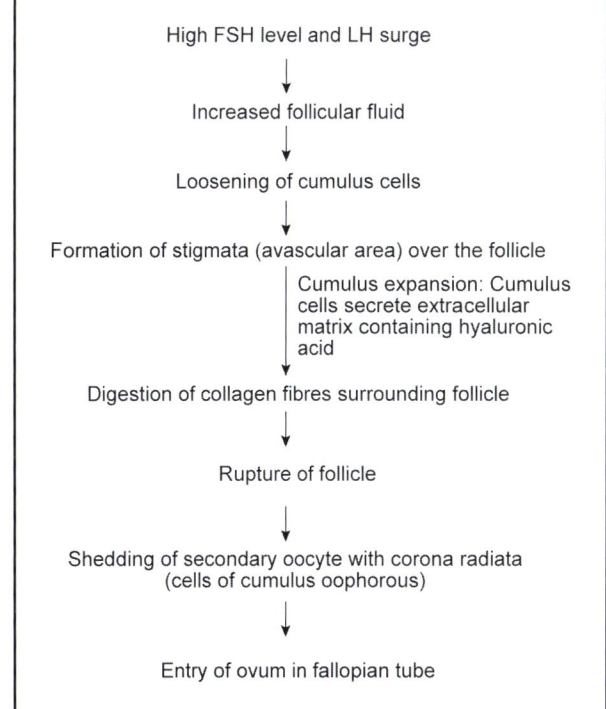

Some Interesting Facts
- After fertilisation, first polar body also undergoes a second meiotic division.
- Why do only a few follicles develop during menstrual cycle?
  Explanation: Some follicles become progressively sensitive to the effect of FSH and develop earlier than other follicles.
- Ovulation occurs about 38 hours after beginning of LH and FSH surge.
- First polar body is extruded 24 hours prior to the ovulation.[Neet]
- Differences between spermatogenesis and oogenesis are listed in Table 2.2.

Box 2.4: Tests for ovulation[MCQ,Viva]

1. Calendar method: Ovulation occurs 14 days prior to onset of next menstrual cycle.
2. *Raise in basal body temperature*: Record the temperature every day in morning. Temperature increases 0.3°–0.5°C during ovulation due to thermogenic effect of the progesterone.
3. Spinnbarkeit [cervical mucus method (Billings method)]: Cervical mucous is watery and sticky at the

Contd.

Human Embryology

Q. List the differences between spermatogenesis and oogenesis.

Table 2.2 Differences between spermatogenesis and oogenesis

Spermatogenesis	Oogenesis
It is a process of formation of male gametes (sperms).	It is a process of formation of female gamete (ovum).
Site: Seminiferous tubules in testis.	Site: Cortex of ovary.
It continues from puberty till death.	It continues from puberty till menopause.
It starts only after puberty.	It starts during intrauterine life.
In spermatogenesis, one spermatocyte forms four gametes (sperms).[Neet]	In oogenesis, one primary oocyte forms only one gamete (ovum).[Neet]
Fertilisation is not required for second meiotic division.	Fertilisation is required for completion of second meiotic division.
Most of the cytoplasm is shed from spermatozoon as residual body.	Cytoplasm is conserved in ovum for nutritional need after fertilisation.

Contd.

time of ovulation and it shows a fern pattern. A drop of the cervical muscous can be streatched about 10 cm or more like a thread at the time of ovulation. This elastic nature of cervical mucous is called *spinnbarkeit*. Elasticity is less before and after this period.
4. Hormonal estimation: Increased LH and estrogen with a decrease in FSH at the time of ovulation. Ovulation kits (ELISA strips, similar to pregnancy test kits) help in the detection of LH surge.
5. Ultrasonography monitoring contributes to keep follow-up of ovulation.
6. Endometrial biopsy (nowadays it is not done routinely.)
7. **Mittelschmerz** (short-lived lower abdominal pain): It occurs due to peritoneal irritation by small amount of blood that escapes from follicles during ovulation.
8. Vaginal discharge or spotting: There is transient increase in vaginal discharge during ovulation.

Box 2.5: Disorders of ovulation[MCQ]
- **Anovulation**: It is absence of ovulation. It may be due to menopausal or due to hormonal imbalances.
- **Oligo-ovulation:** It is infrequent or irregular ovulation.
- **Induced ovulation:** In assisted reproductive technology, **clomiphene citrate** and a low dose of **human chorionic gonadotropin** are used for induced ovulation.
- **Suppressed ovulation**: Contraceptive hormonal pills suppress folliculogenesis and ovulation.

STRUCTURE OF OVUM

Q. Write short note on the structure of ovum.
- Ovum is also called the **secondary oocyte**.
- Size: 140 μm.

Structure (Fig. 2.9, Practice Fig. 2.3)
- It consists of a nucleus, ooplasm, vitelline membrane, zona pellucida and corona radiata.

Nucleus
- Nucleus of ovum is called germinal vesicle that has proximal nucleolus (germinal spot).
- It contains 23,X chromosomes.[MCQ]

Ooplasm/cytoplasm/yolk
- Ooplasm contains droplets of **lecithin-like** substances that forms **deutoplasm**.[MCQ]
- Two centrioles are present near the nucleus but they disappear during fertilisation.

Vitelline membrane
- It is a cell membrane that is surrounded by perivitelline space.
- First polar body lies within the perivitelline space.

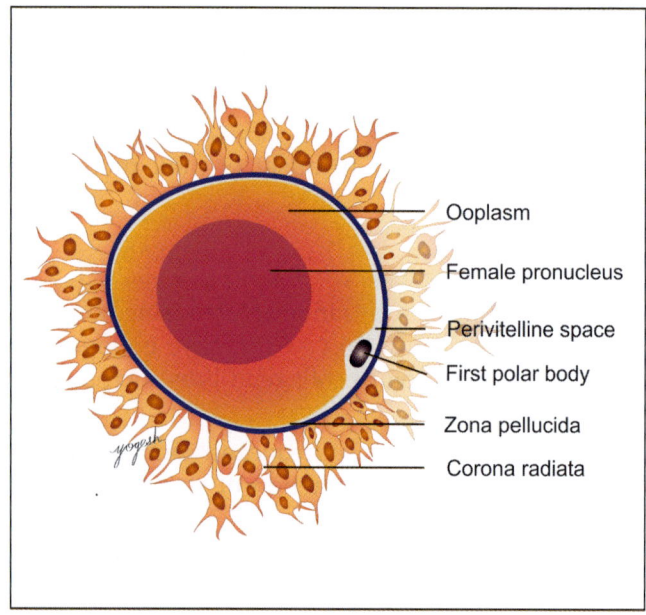

Fig. 2.9: Ovum

Gametogenesis

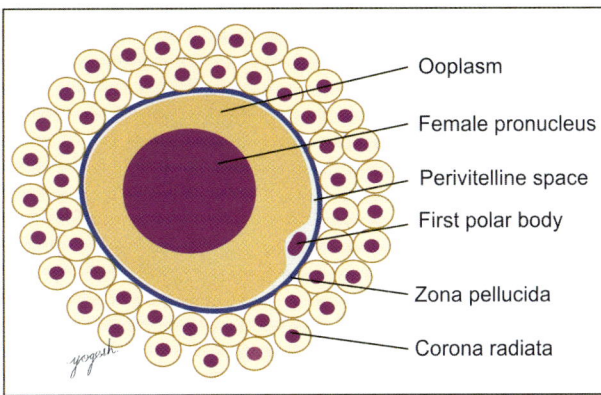

Practice Fig. 2.3: Structure of ovum

Zona pellucida

- It is a glycoprotein coat that surrounds vitelline membrane. Barrier in zona pellucida is provided by fertilin.^{Neet}
- Zona pellucida glycoprotein (ZP3) facilitates binding of sperms and induces an acrosomal reaction.^{MCQ}
- Zona pellucida prevents implantation. Zona pellucida disappears on the fifth or sixth day after fertilisation to permit implantation.^{MCQ,Viva}

Corona radiata

- A few cells of cumulus oophorous remain attached to outer surface of ovum and that forms corona radiata.
- Acrosomal enzyme (hyaluronidase) disintegrates corona radiata cells during fertilisation.

Some Interesting Facts

- Zona pellucida prevents implantation.
- Deutoplasm provides nutrition to developing embryo in early stages.
- Human ovum is **microlecithal** as it has scanty amount of deutoplasm.^{MCQ}
- Eggs of birds are **macrolecithal** as they contains large amount of deutoplasm.
- Differences between sperm and ovum are listed in Table 2.3.

Q. List the differences between sperm and ovum.

Table 2.3 Differences between sperm and ovum

Sperm	Ovum
It is male gamete.	It is female gamete.
It has less width (2 μm) than ovum.	It has more width (120 μm) than sperm.
It is motile.	It is immotile.
It has very less cytoplasm.	It has abundant cytoplasm.
It has X or Y chromosome.	It has only X chromosome.
It undergoes capacitation.	It does not undergo capacitation.
It does not undergo second meiotic division after fertilization.	It undergoes second meiotic division after fertilization.
It is not surrounded by any cell layer.	It is surrounded by corona radiata cells.
It has acrosome cap, spirally arranged mitochondrion, axial filament and tail.	It has zona pellucida.

CLINICAL EMBRYOLOGY

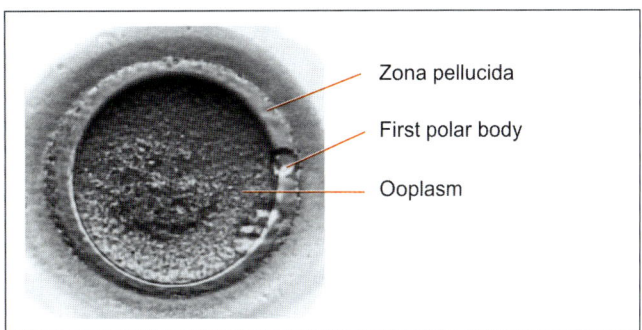

Clinical image 2.1: Human ovum (secondary oocyte) is collected for *in vitro* fertilisation. It consists of a nucleus, ooplasm, thin vitelline membrane, thick zona pellucida and first polar body (Image courtesy: *Dr Keshav Malhotra*)

3

Menstrual Cycle

Chapter Outline

- Duration of menstrual cycle
- Phases of menstrual cycle
  - Follicular phase
  - Luteal phase
- Changes in reproductive organs
  - Changes in follicular phase
  - Changes in luteal phase
- Strata of endometrium
- Mechanism of menstrual bleeding
- Hormonal changes in menstrual cycle
  - Oestrogen
  - Progesterone
  - Luteinising hormone
- Disorders of menstrual cycle
- Amenorrhoea

INTRODUCTION

- Reproductive system in females consists of pair of ovaries, uterine tubes, uterus, vagina and external genitalia.
- *Fertile period* of the female extends from the age of puberty to menopause.
- *Puberty* is a period of adolescence in which a female reaches sexual maturity and becomes capable of reproduction. It occurs by the age of 11–14 years.
- *Menopause* is the absence of menstrual cycle for a period of 12 months or more in the later life of a female and by then she is no longer able for reproduction. It occurs between 49 and 52 years of age.
- A fertile female shows monthly periodic changes in the ovary and uterus from puberty till menopause.
- The periodic structural and functional changes of female reproductive organs are under the control of hormones of the pituitary gland (hypothalamo–pituitary–ovarian axis).
- These periodic changes are grouped as follows:
  a. *Ovarian cycle*: Rhythmic changes in the ovary involves formation and maturation of ovarian follicles, release of gamete (ovum) and secretion of ovarian hormones.
  b. *Uterine cycle* or *menstrual cycle*: It consists of the periodic changes in the endometrium of uterus. It is mainly targeted towards the preparation of uterus for implantation, to nourish fertilised gametes after implantation and shedding of endometrium in absence of fertilisation.
- Ovarian cycle and ovulation are covered in Chapter 2. This chapter deals with the uterine or menstrual cycle.
- *Menstrual cycle* is a rhythmic change in uterus starting from puberty until menopause.
- Menstruation is a cyclic bleeding that occurs due to the shedding of endometrium in the absence of fertilisation.
- Menstrual cycle is studied as follows:
  1. Duration of cycle
  2. Phases of menstrual cycle
  3. Changes in reproductive organs
  4. Mechanism of menstrual bleeding
  5. Hormonal changes
  6. Disorders of menstrual cycle

DURATION OF MENSTRUAL CYCLE

- Length of menstrual cycle varies from female to female. Even in one female, it is not always the same.
- Usually, average menstrual cycle consists of 28 days. Menstrual means lunar month of 28 days in Latin (Flowchart 3.1, Fig. 3.1).
- Factors affecting the duration of menstrual cycle:
  - Emotional status
  - Nutritional status

Menstrual Cycle

Flowchart 3.1: Phases of menstrual cycle

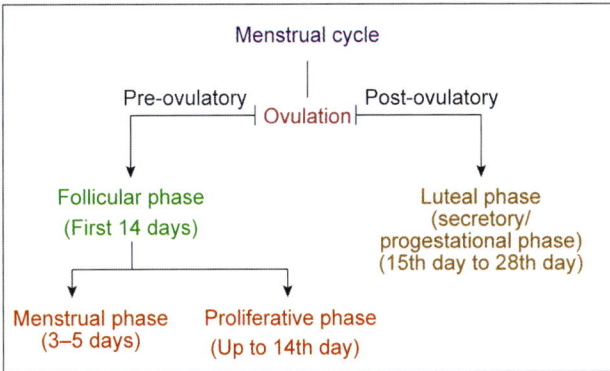

- Psychological and social aspects
- Environmental factors
- Hormonal status
- Near menopause

- The normal range of menstrual cycle: 21–35 days.
- Each menstrual cycle extends from the first day of beginning of the menstrual bleeding up to the first day of beginning of the next menstrual bleeding.
- Because of hormonal influence, menstrual cycles are absent during pregnancy and lactation.

PHASES OF MENSTRUAL CYCLE

Q. Write short note on the phases of menstrual cycle.

- Menstrual cycle shows follicular (post-menstrual) phase, proliferative phase, secretory phase and menstrual phase (Flowchart 3.1).
- In this chapter, menstrual cycle is divided into two phases: Follicular phase (it includes menstrual phase) and luteal phase. These two phases are separated by ovulation.

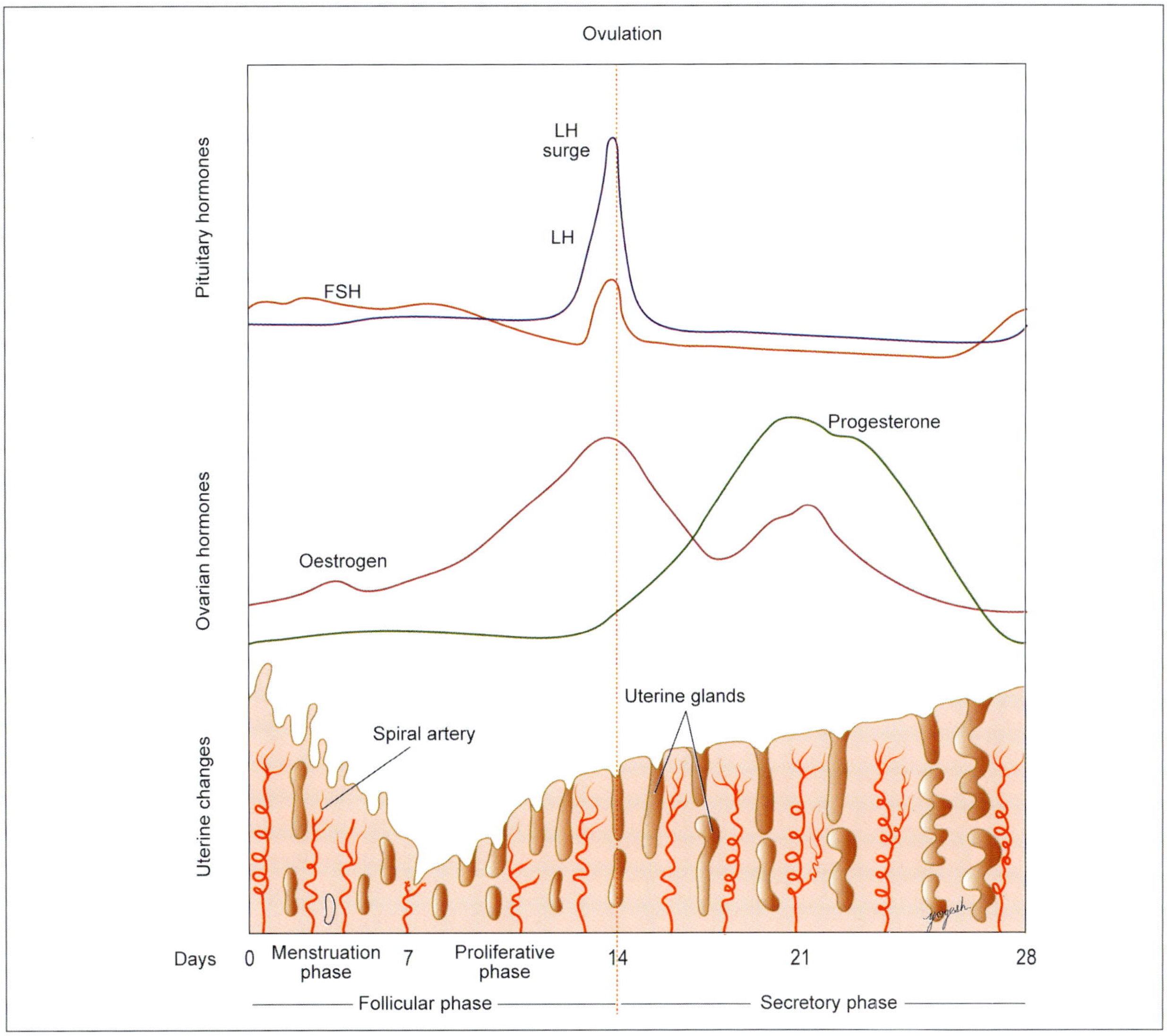

Fig. 3.1: Hormonal and uterine changes in the menstrual cycle
Abbreviations: FSH: Follicle stimulating hormone; LH: Luteinising hormone

Follicular Phase (Pre-ovulatory)

- Developing ovarian follicle secrete oestrogen that controls the changes in uterus. Hence, this phase of menstrual cycle is called *follicular phase*.
- Follicular phase lasts up to ovulation.
- In initial few days of follicular phase, superficial parts of the thickened endometrium (stratum compactum and stratum spongiosum) are shed off. It constitutes menstrual bleeding that lasts for 3–5 days. This part of follicular phase is also known as *menstrual phase*.
- In remaining part of the follicular phase, uterine endometrium proliferates, hence called *proliferative phase*.

Luteal Phase (Post-ovulatory)

- Following the ovulation, corpus luteum secretes progesterone that influences uterine changes. Hence, this phase is *luteal phase* or *progestational phase*.
- Uterine endometrium becomes secretory in the luteal phase; hence, this phase is also called *secretory phase*.

Box 3.1: Endometrium

Q. Write short note on endometrium.

- Uterine endometrium shows cyclic changes during menstrual cycle.
- Uterus has three layers: Endometrium, myometrium and perimetrium (inside outwards) (Fig. 3.2).
- *Myometrium* is very thick and consists of smooth muscles. *Perimetrium* is the outer connective tissue layer covered by visceral peritoneum.
- *Endometrium* is the inner mucous membrane. It is a functional layer of the uterus.
- It consists of columnar epithelium, connective tissue stroma and simple tubular uterine glands.
- The stroma of endometrium contains spiral arteries.
- Endometrium shows three strata as follows:
  a. *Stratum compactum*: Superficial layer containing necks of uterine glands.
  b. *Stratum spongiosum*: Middle layer, consists of loose areolar tissue.
  c. *Stratum basale*: Deep layer, lies adjacent to myometrium.
- During the phase of menstrual bleeding, stratum basale do not shed off, only stratum functionale (stratum compactum and stratum spongiosum) shed off.
- Stratum basale contains fundi of uterine glands
- Stratum basale is supplied by straight arteries that are the branches of arcuate artery, whereas stratum spongiosum and compactum are supplied by spiral arteries.

Some Interesting Facts

- Stratum functionale = stratum compactum + stratum spongiosum.
- Length of luteal phase remains constant (14 days). Thus, irrespective of length of the menstrual cycle, ovulation takes place 14 days prior to next menstrual bleeding. *Clinical fact*

CHANGES IN REPRODUCTIVE ORGANS

Q. Write short note on uterine changes in menstrual cycle.

- During menstrual cycle, ovary and uterus show cyclic changes specific to phases of the cycle (Figs 3.1 and 3.3).

Changes in Follicular Phase

Ovarian Changes

- In each ovarian cycle, one of the follicles reaches up to the stage of Graafian follicle.
- Some of the important changes occurring in the ovary are as follows (Fig. 3.3):
  1. Primary oocyte undergoes maturation and gets surrounded by follicular cells and subsequently forms primary, secondary and tertiary follicles.
  2. Liquor folliculi separates follicular (granulosa) cells into inner cumulus oophoricus and outer stratum granulosum.
  3. Stromal cells condense to form theca interna and theca externa.
  4. Granulosa cells secrete oestrogen that influences uterine changes.
  5. Primary oocyte completes first meiotic division and forms secondary oocyte and first polar body.
  6. At the end of follicular phase, secondary oocyte undergoes ovulation.

Uterine Changes

- The uterine changes in follicular phase can be grouped into *menstrual phase* and *proliferative phase* (Fig. 3.4).

Menstrual phase

- Degeneration of corpus luteum at the end of the previous menstrual cycle results in stoppage of secretion of progesterone and oestrogen.
- Absence of these hormones causes temporary spasm (contraction) of spiral arteries. It results in ischemia and necrosis of stratum compactum and spongiosum (superficial 2/3rd of endometrium) (Fig. 3.2 and Flowchart 3.2).
- Stratum basale has not been supplied by spiral arteries (but by straight arteries); hence, it does not shed off (Fig. 3.2).

Menstrual Cycle

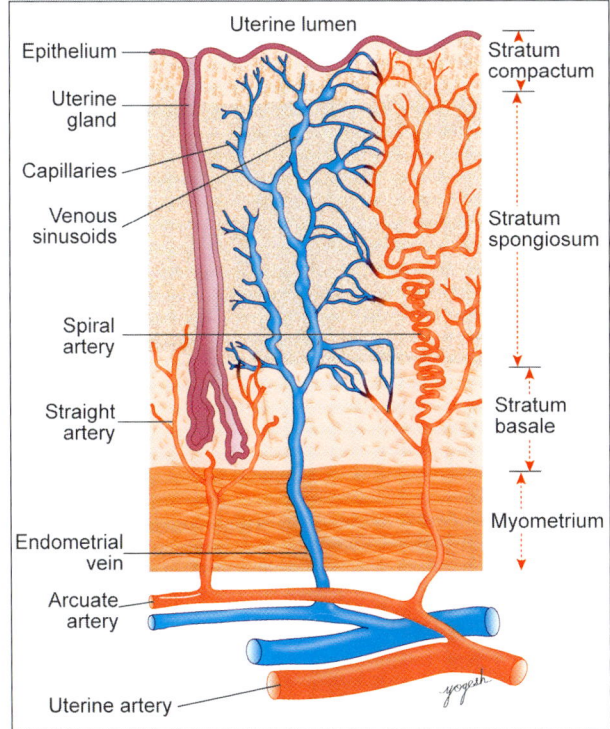

Fig. 3.2: Layers of uterine endometrium during proliferative phase of the menstrual cycle, and blood supply of endometrium

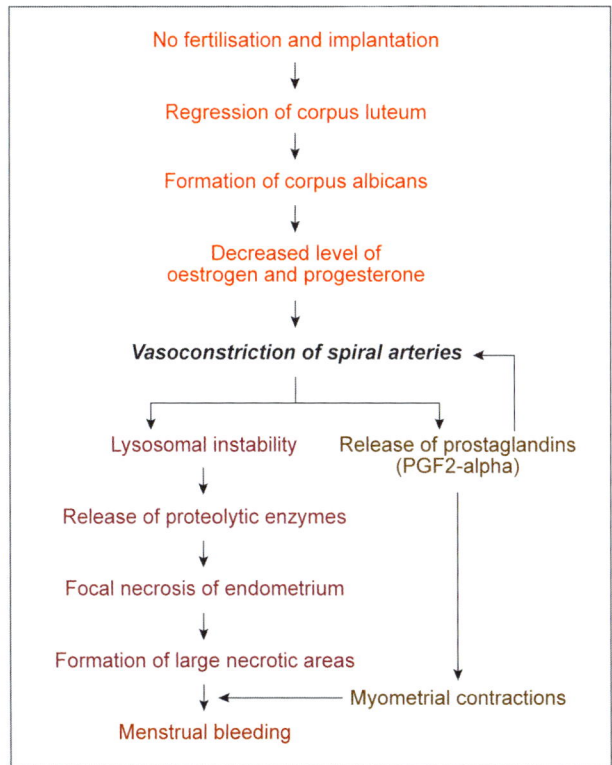

Note: Overproduction of prostaglandins causes excessive uterine contractions and produce dysmenorrhoea (painful menstruation).

- Average duration: 3–5 days.
- Menstrual blood does not clot due to the presence of proteolytic enzymes.^Clinical fact, MCQ

Proliferative phase (oestrogenic phase)
- On 5th day onwards, under the influence of oestrogen, the thickness of endometrium starts increasing due to regeneration.
- Uterine endometrium undergoes hypertrophy and hyperplasia.
- The length of uterine gland increases (Fig. 3.4).
- Uterine glands become straight, long, widely separated and they have scanty secretions.
- Number of spiral arteries increases and it enhances blood supply to the endometrium (Fig. 3.4).

- Under the influence of oestrogen, the volume, alkalinity and elasticity of cervical mucous increases. It makes cervical mucous favourable for the passage of sperms through cervix of the uterus.

Changes in Luteal (Progestational) Phase
Ovarian Changes
- Luteal phase starts after ovulation.
- Soon after the ovulation, ovarian follicle is filled with blood, hence called *corpus haemorrhagicus*.

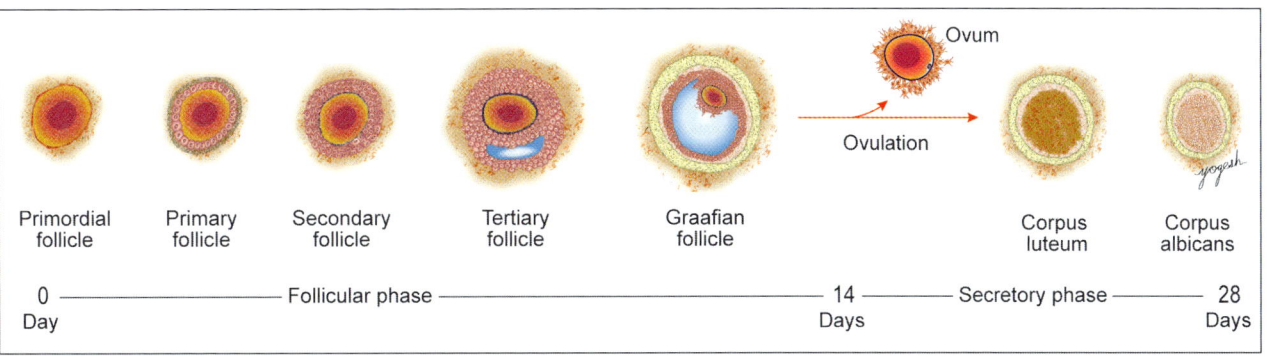

Fig. 3.3: Ovarian changes during the menstrual cycle

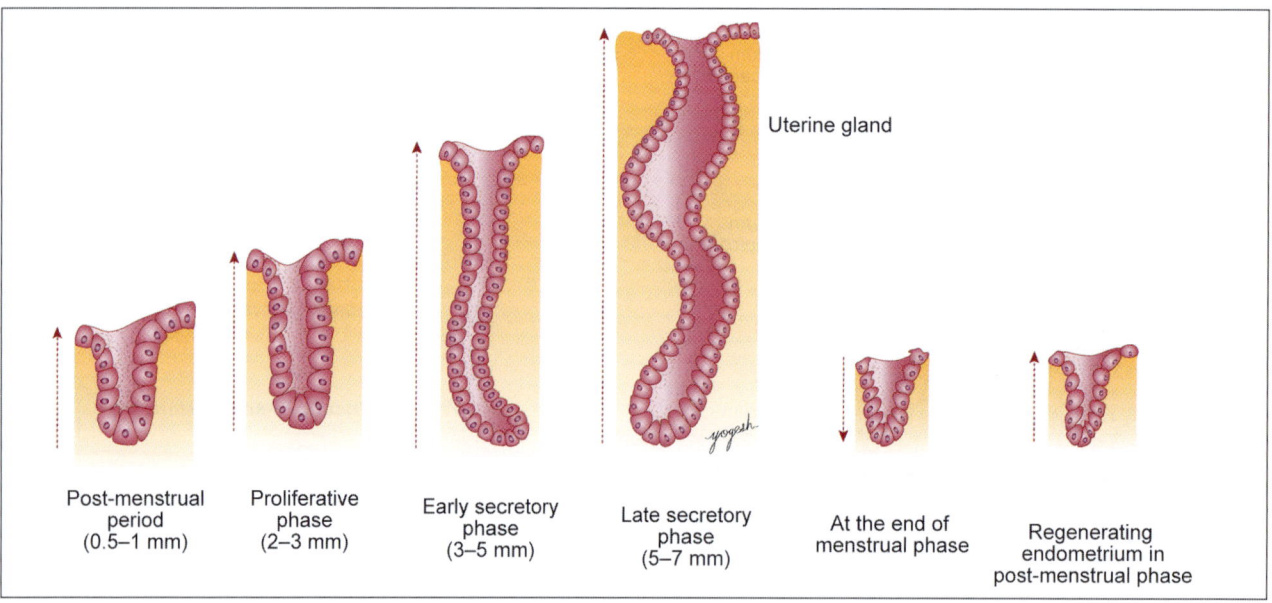

Fig. 3.4: Changes in the uterine endometrium during the menstrual cycle

- Granulosa cells start accumulating a yellow pigment (lutein), hence *luteal phase*. This process is *luteinisation* of granulosa and theca cells.
- Luteal cells secrete progesterone and oestrogen.
- If fertilisation does not occur, then corpus luteum degenerate by the 26th or 28th day.
- Corpus luteum undergoes luteolysis to form a scar tissue called *corpus albicans*.

Uterine Changes

During luteal phase, high level of progesterone enhances the growth of endometrium and induces the following changes:

1. Changes in glands
- Uterine glands become more coiled and tortuous (produces sawtooth appearance).
- Glandular epithelium starts accumulating glycogen. Glands secrete carbohydrate-rich fluid.

2. Changes in stroma
- Spiral arteries become more tortuous.
- Vascularity of endometrium enhances.
- Uterine fluid starts accumulating in stroma and makes it oedematous and thick.
- Stromal cells accumulate glycogen and lipid droplets in their cytoplasm. This is called *decidual reaction* (For details, read Chapter 9, Box 9.2).
- In the later part of the luteal phase, due to the absence of progesterone, vasospasm of spiral arteries begins to produce focal necrotic changes in endometrium. At the end of the luteal phase, menstruation begins in the absence of implantation.

3. Cervical mucus changes
- Under influence of progesterone, cervical mucus becomes thick and less elastic. These changes prevent entry of sperms through cervix.

MECHANISM OF MENSTRUAL BLEEDING

Q. Write short note on mechanism of menstrual bleeding.

- In absence of a pregnancy, steroid hormone levels begin to fall due to the degeneration of corpus luteum.
- Decreased steroid hormone levels cause increased coiling of spiral arteries and constriction. It results in decreased blood supply (ischemia) to endometrium.
- Ischemia of endometrium causes
  1. Destabilisation of lysosomal membranes and release of proteolytic enzymes from lysosomes.
  2. Release of prostaglandins, mainly PGF2α.^{MCQ}
- Loss of blood supply and action of proteolytic enzymes initially produce focal areas of necrosis that later fuse to form large necrotic areas in the endometrium.
- Prostaglandins induce smooth muscle (myometrium) contractions and it results into the beginning of menstrual bleeding.
- Because of the presence of proteolytic enzymes, menstrual blood does not form clots.
- Normal amount of menstrual bleed: 30–130 ml.

Menstrual Cycle

HORMONAL CHANGES IN MENSTRUAL CYCLE

Q. Write short note on hormonal control of menstrual cycle.

- Menstruation in female is under the influence of *hypothalamo-pituitary-ovarian axis* (HPO axis) (Flowchart 3.3).
- Pituitary gland secretes follicle stimulating hormone (FSH) and luteinising hormone (LH) (Fig. 3.1).
- Ovaries produce two steroid hormones, oestrogen and progesterone under influence of the LH and FSH.
- Secretion of LH and FSH by anterior pituitary is under the control of gonadotropin-releasing hormone (GnRH) of hypothalamus (Table 3.1).

Oestrogen

- Oestrogen hormone is involved in the uterine cycle as well as maintenance of secondary sexual characters.
- Oestrogen has two peaks in the menstrual cycle (Fig. 3.1).
  1. First peak: It occurs about 48 hours before ovulation.
  2. Second peak: It occurs in the middle of the luteal phase.
- Oestrogen level continuously rises during development of ovarian follicles. It decreases suddenly after ovulation.
- About two days after ovulation, oestrogen concentration starts increasing in the luteal phase and reaches again at high in middle luteal phase.

Progesterone

- Progesterone is the hormone of luteal phase and is secreted by corpus luteum. Hence, concentration of progesterone is less in proliferative phase and increases in luteal phase (Fig. 3.1).

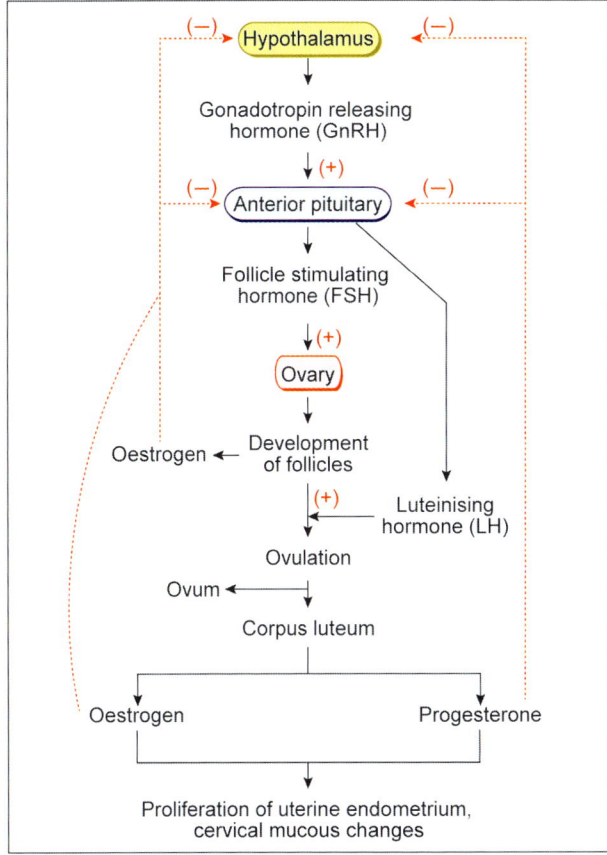

Flowchart 3.3: Hormonal changes in menstrual cycle

- Progesterone rises after ovulation and reaches to peak within 4–5 days after ovulation.
- At the end of luteal phase, progesterone level decreases due to lysis of corpus luteum.

Luteinising Hormone (LH)

- Luteinising hormone concentration increases a day prior to ovulation.
- This LH peak is *LH surge* that occurs typically 34–36 hours before ovulation.

Table 3.1	Hormones in menstrual cycle	
Endocrine gland	Hormone	Major functions
Anterior pituitary	FSH	• Stimulates follicular growth in ovaries. • Stimulates follicles for oestrogen secretion.
	LH	• LH surge causes ovulation. • LH surge, on ovulation, forms corpus luteum.
Ovaries	Oestrogen	• Stimulates endometrial proliferation. • Inhibits secretion of GnRH, FSH and LH.
	Progesterone	• Increases thickness of uterine endometrium and make it suitable for implantation. • Inhibits GnRH, FSH and LH secretion.
	Inhibin	• Inhibits secretion of FSH by anterior pituitary.

- LH levels reach its usual level within 24–48 hours after ovulation.
- High levels of oestrogen concentration in the later part of follicular phase induce *LH surge*.
- LH surge induces ovulation with help of the following changes:
  1. Increases prostaglandins and bradykinin secretion that increase blood flow to the developing follicle.
  2. Increased blood flow enhances accumulation of intercellular fluid and increases volume of antral fluid.
  3. Increased antral fluid enhances intra-follicular pressure.
  4. LH induces proteolytic activity by enhancing production of plasminogen activation (secreted by theca cells).
- All the above-mentioned changes (1–4) cause rupture of follicular wall and release of an ovum (ovulation).
- For tests/indicators of ovulation, refer to Chapter 2.

DISORDERS OF MENSTRUAL CYCLE

Q. List the disorders of menstrual cycle.
Q. Define amenorrhoea, oligomenorrhoea, dysmenorrhoea, menorrhagia and anovulation.

Disorders of menstrual cycle are grouped as
1. Disorders of flow: Amenorrhoea, hypomenorrhoea, oligomenorrhoea
2. Painful menstruation: Dysmenorrhoea, premenstrual syndrome
3. Disorders of timing: Menometrorrhagia, menorrhagia, metrorrhagia
4. Disorders of ovulation: Oligoovulation, anovulation

Definitions

- *Amenorrhoea* is the absence of menstrual cycle.
- *Hypomenorrhoea* is short or scanty periods (extremely light menstrual flow).
- *Oligomenorrhoea* is infrequent menstruation that occurs at intervals of greater than 35 days (only 4–9 menstruations/year).
- *Dysmenorrhoea* is painful menstruation. It involves sharp, intermittent pain or dull aching abdominal pain associated with the beginning of menstruation.
- *Premenstrual syndrome* (PMS) are non-specific symptoms that develop a week before onset of menstrual bleeding. It includes painful or swollen breast, depression, irritability, headache and so on. These symptoms disappear 1–3 days after the menstruation starts.
- *Menorrhagia* is excessive menstrual bleeding.
- *Metrorrhagia* is uterine bleeding that occurs at irregular intervals.
- *Menometrorrhagia* is excessive uterine bleeding at frequent and irregular intervals.
- *Anovulation* is the absence of ovulation.
- *Oligoovulation* is an irregular ovulation, usually if menstrual cycle is more than 36 days.
- *Polymenorrhoea* is frequent menstruation (cycle of less than 21 days).

Box 3.2: Amenorrhoea

Q. Write short note on amenorrhoea.
Q. Write short note on primary amenorrhoea.

Definition: Amenorrhoea is the absence of menstruation in a menstrual cycle in a woman of reproductive age.

Classification
- Amenorrhoea is classified as primary and secondary. It may be physiological or pathological.

Primary amenorrhoea
- Primary amenorrhoea is an absence of menstruation since birth of a woman. It can be physiological or pathological.

Physiological primary amenorrhoea
– It is normally occurring primary amenorrhoea due to physiological reasons.
– Causes
  1. Before puberty: Normally menstruations begin by the age of 12–14 years.
  2. Constitutional amenorrhoea is delayed onset of menstruation even up to the age of 18 years without any reason.

Pathological primary amenorrhoea
– In pathological primary amenorrhoea, menstruation does not start until the age of 18 years.
– Causes
  1. Congenital genetic disorders such as Turner syndrome (45,X).
  2. Congenital anomalies of reproductive tract such as imperforate hymen, absence of uterus, vaginal atresia.

Secondary amenorrhoea
- It occurs when menstrual cycle stops in a woman who had menstruation before. It can be physiological or pathological.

Physiological secondary amenorrhoea
– Causes
  1. Pregnancy
  2. Lactational amenorrhoea: Prolactin secreted during lactation inhibits release of gonadotropin-releasing hormone (GnRH) and prevents ovulation and menstruation.

Contd.

Contd.

3. Menopause (ceasing of menstruation by the age of 45–50 years).
4. Emotional and environmental factors, such as stress, exposure to extreme climates and so on.

Pathological secondary amenorrhoea
- **Causes**
    1. Hypothalamic disorders causing failure of GnRH release.
    2. Pituitary disorders causing failure of LH and FSH production.
    3. Ovarian diseases causing failure of production of oestrogen and progesterone.
    4. Uterine diseases.
    5. Systemic diseases.
    6. Drugs and medication (contraceptive pills).

4

First Week of Development

Chapter Outline

- Fertilisation
  - Stages of fertilisation
    - Approximation of gametes
    - Contact and fusion of gametes
    - Effects of fertilisation
- Parthenogenesis
- Cleavage
- Hydatidiform mole
- Functions of zona pellucida
- Implantation
  - Site of implantation
  - Process of implantation
  - Abnormal implantation
- Changes in trophoblast during implantation

INTRODUCTION

- A period of first week of development starts with fertilisation (fusion of an ovum and a spermatozoon) and ends with implantation (process of penetration of product of conceptus into an uterine endometrium).
- Major events of the first week of human development are listed in Table 4.1 and Fig. 4.1.

Table 4.1	Events in the first week of development
Day	Event
Day 0	Approximation of ovum and sperms Fertilisation of ovum
Day 1	Two-celled stage
Day 2	Four-celled stage
Day 3	Eight-celled stage
Day 4	Formation of morula
Day 5	Formation of blastocyst
Day 6	Beginning of implantation

FERTILISATION

Q. Write short note on fertilisation.

- **Definition**
  Fertilisation is the process of fusion of two mature germ cells, an ovum and a spermatozoon (haploid cells) to form a single cell, *zygote* (diploid cell).

- Fertilisation is a process of fusion or anti-thesis of cell division.^{MCQ} Haploid gametes fuse to form a diploid undifferentiated zygote.
- Usual site of fertilisation: Ampulla of uterine (fallopian) tube.^{Neet,Viva}

Stages of Fertilisation (Practice Fig. 4.1)

- Fertilisation involves three basic steps:
  1. Approximation of gametes

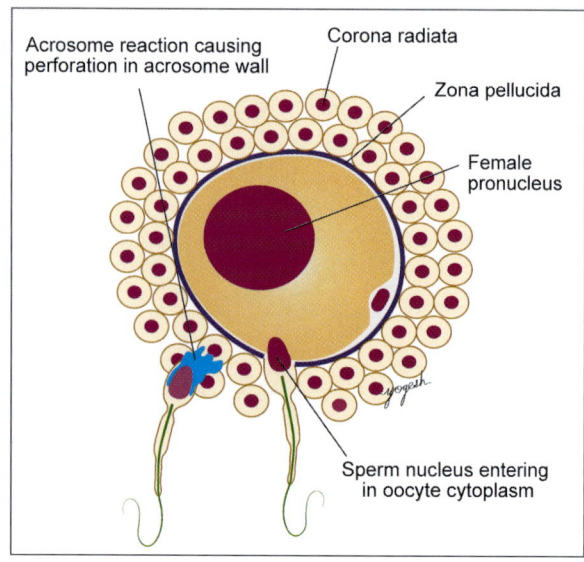

Practice Fig. 4.1: Fertilisation

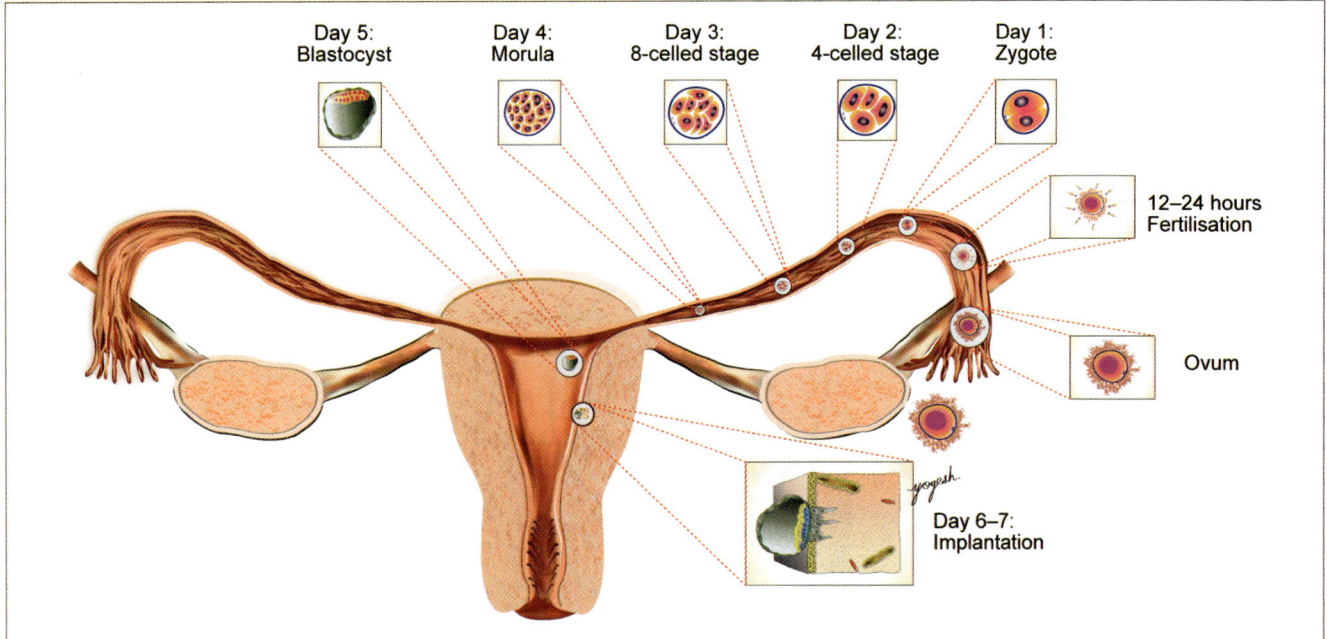

Fig. 4.1: Events in the first week of development

2. Contact and fusion of gametes
3. Effects of fertilisation.

1. Approximation of Gametes (Fig. 4.2)

- It involves transport of spermatozoa and ovum in female genital tract towards the ampulla of uterine tube (usual site of fertilisation).
- Spermatozoa transport is affected by the following factors:
  - Liquefaction of semen: Semen contains fibrinolysin that liquefies semen within 30 minutes after ejaculation.
  - Contractions of uterine muscles: Prostaglandins of semen stimulate peristaltic contractions in the female genital tract.
  - Effect of oxytocin: Sexual intercourse stimulates secretion of oxytocin from neurohypophysis that also produces uterine contractions.
  - Aspiration of sperms: Repeated uterine contractions generates vacuum (syringe-like action) that aspirates sperm into uterine cavity and later into uterine tube.
  - Only 1% of deposited sperms in vagina enter the uterine cervix and only 300–500 sperms reach the fallopian tube (at the site of fertilisation).[MCQ,]
  - Sperms require 2–7 hours for transport from cervix to fallopian tube.
  - Chemotaxis: Sperm is attracted towards ovum by chemicals secreted by corona radiata cells that surround the ovum.
- Lifespan of sperm: After ejaculation, sperms are viable for 24–48 hours in female reproductive tract (maximum up to 4 days).[Neet,Viva]
- Transport of ovum
  - Ovum enters the fimbriated part of fallopian tube due to ciliary beats and rhythmic contractions of uterine tube musculature.
  - Transcoelomic migration: Sometimes ovum released by an ovary aspirated into fallopian tube on opposite side by transcoelomic migration.
  - Duration: Ovum takes 25 minutes to reach ampulla of uterine tube.
  - Lifespan of ovum: Ovum is viable for 24–48 hours after ovulation.[Neet,Viva]

Some Interesting Facts
Clinical Facts
- Non-steroidal anti-inflammatory drugs (like aspirin) have anti-prostaglandin effects. Their regular intake by female reduces sperm transport in female reproductive tract and may impart reduced fertility.

2. Contact and Fusion of Gametes (Fig. 4.3)

- Three barriers: Sperm must break three barriers (corona radiata, zona pellucida and vitelline membrane) of secondary oocyte for fertilisation.[MCQ,Viva]
- Capacitation: During transport of sperm in female reproductive tract, they undergo capacitation. It is a

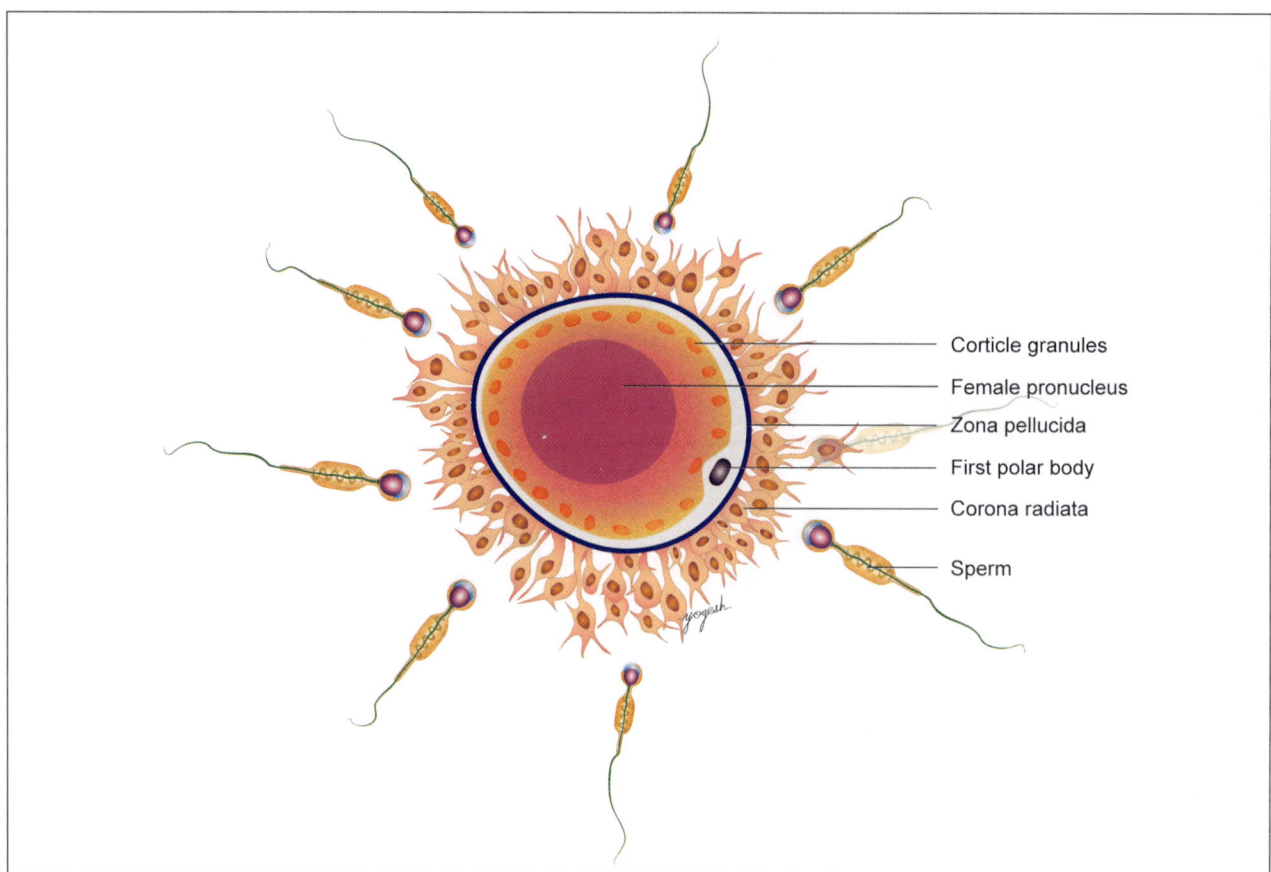

Fig. 4.2: Fertilisation. Phase of approximation of gametes

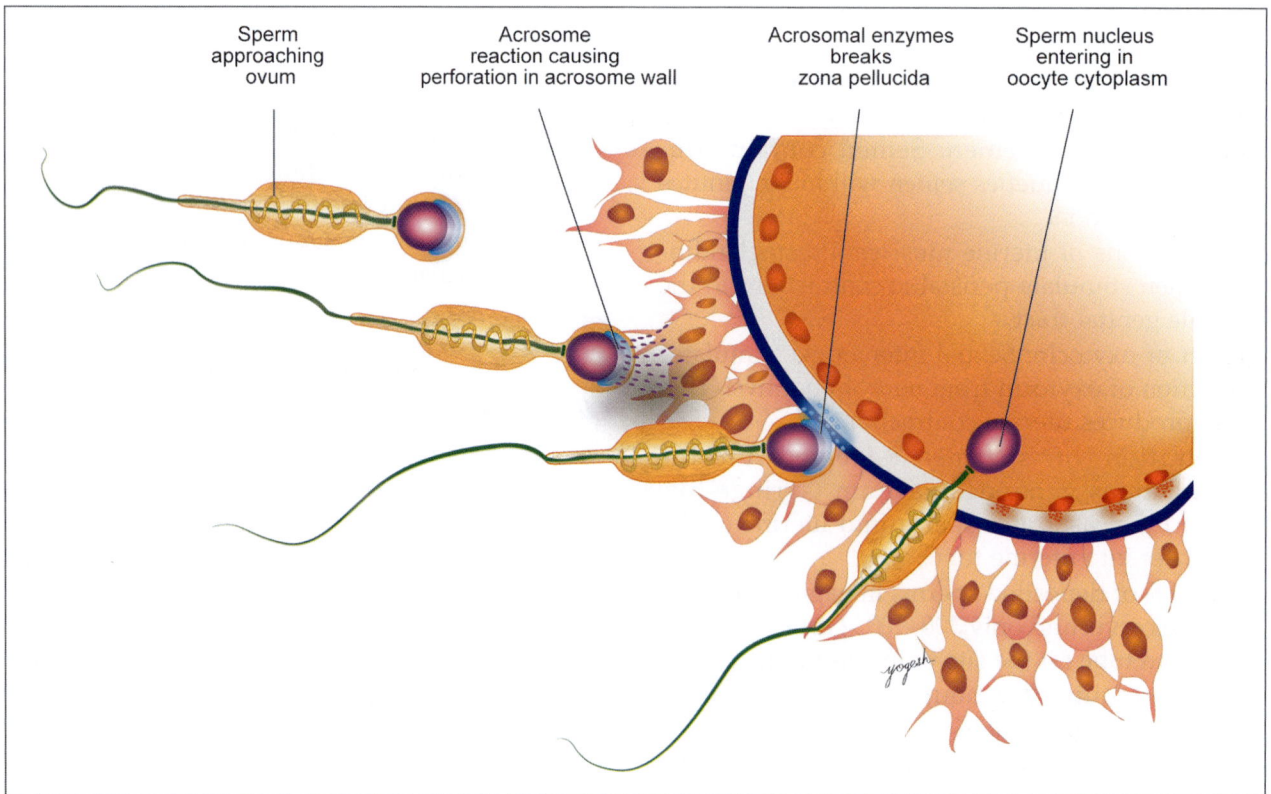

Fig. 4.3: Fertilisation. Phase of sperm penetration through coverings of the ovum

process of maturation of spermatozoa. During capacitation, coat of glycoproteins from head of spermatozoa is removed to enhance sperm motility.^MCQ,,Viva
- Four phases are involved in the penetration of sperm into ovum as follows:^Neet

Phase I: Acrosome reaction
- Acrosome cap establishes multiple contacts with plasma membrane sperm head and releases acrosomal enzymes.
- Acrosome enzymes include hyaluronidase, acrosine (protease enzyme and acid phosphatase).^MCQ,,Viva

Phase II: Disintegration of barriers (Fig. 4.4)
- Hyaluronidase (acrosomal enzyme) disintegrates corona radiata.
- Sperm head binds with Zp2 and Zp3 receptor proteins of zona pellucida (Zp = zona pellucida).
- Acrosine (protease enzyme from acrosome) disintegrates zona pellucida.
- Disintegrin peptides of sperms and integrin of vitelline membrane of ovum help in fusion of sperm plasma membrane with vitelline membrane.
- Phase II takes about 30 minutes to complete.

Phase III: Calcium wave for the depolarisation of oocyte
- Sperm fusion with vitelline membrane of oocyte induces calcium wave and depolarises vitelline membrane.
- Calcium wave is responsible for the following changes:
  i. Secondary oocyte completes second meiotic division and one set of chromosomes as a female pronucleus, whereas expel another set as a *second polar body* in perivitelline space.
  ii. *Calcium* wave triggers release of cortical granules to form oocyte that hydrolyses Zp3 receptors on zona pellucida and prevents further binding of sperms.^Neet
  iii. Release of cortical granules alter the vitelline membrane and induce *vitelline block* that prevents *polyspermy* (entry of multiple sperms in ovum).^Neet

Phase IV: Nuclear fusion (Fig. 4.5)
- Only nucleus and tail of sperm enter cytoplasm of oocyte (ooplasm) leaving behind body and cytoplasm.
- Male pronucleus (sperm nucleus) approaches towards the female pronucleus. Tail of the sperm degenerates.

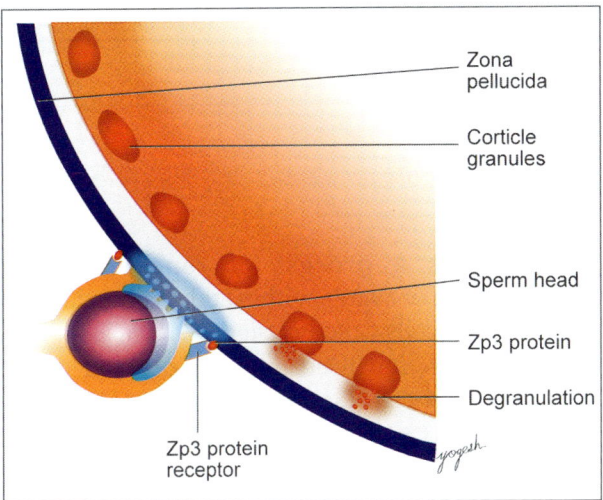

Fig. 4.4: Role of Zp3 proteins. Zp3 proteins of zona pellucida bind with Zp3 receptors of sperm

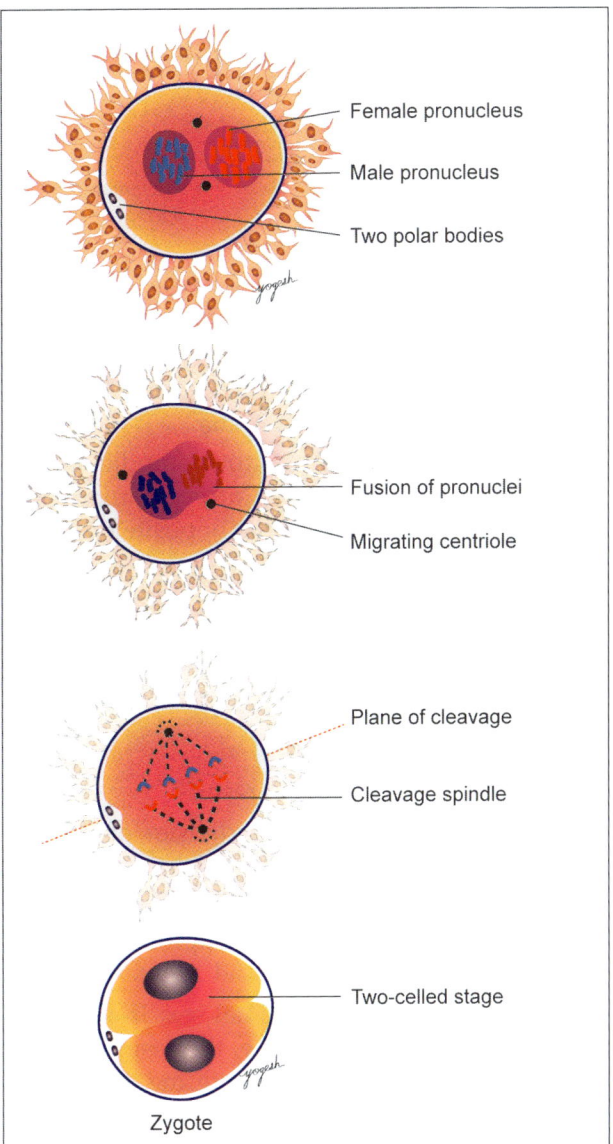

Fig. 4.5: Formation of zygote

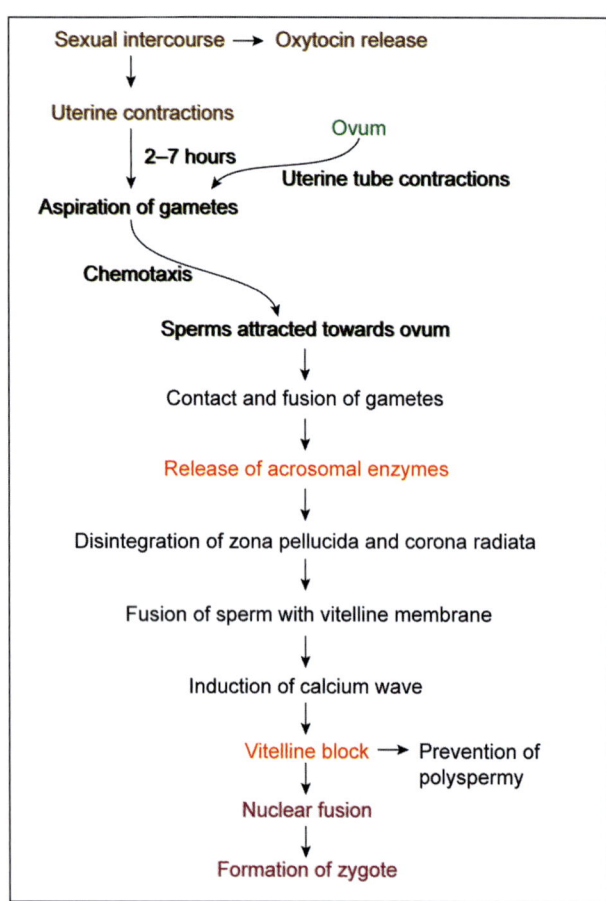

Flowchart 4.1: Fertilisation

- Both male and female pronuclei replicate their DNA and lose their nuclear membrane.
- DNA condenses to form mitotic spindle and later with longitudinal splitting at centromere, sister chromatids move towards the opposite poles.

Formation of zygote: Finally, cytoplasm divides to form two cells with a diploid number of chromosomes. It is called *zygote*.

3. Effects of Fertilisation

Q. List the effects of fertilisation.

Fertilisation has the following results: *(Viva)*

1. Completion of second meiotic division of secondary oocyte (female gamete).
2. Restoration of a diploid number of chromosomes (46). Haploid male (23) and haploid female (23) pronuclei fuse to form a diploid zygote (46).
3. Determination of chromosomal sex: If a fertilising sperm carries X chromosome, the resultant zygote forms a female foetus and if a fertilising sperm carry Y chromosome, the resultant zygote forms a male foetus.
4. Initiation of cleavage: Fertilisation provides energy for repetitive cell divisions of zygote.

Some Interesting Facts

1. Embryo receives mitochondria from ooplasm (mother) only. Sperm does not contribute any mitochondria. Hence, abnormal mitochondrial DNA shows *maternal inheritance*. ^{MCQ}
2. Sex determination entirely depends on sex chromosome of sperm (male partner) only.
3. Fallopian tubes are lined by ciliated columnar epithelium. ^{Neet}
4. Secondary oocyte has haploid number of chromosomes (2N). ^{Neet}
5. Fertilisation takes place within 1–2 days after ovulation. ^{Neet}
6. In *in vitro* fertilization, fertilisation is considered as complete on the appearance of second polar body. ^{Neet}
7. Mosaics and chimera are the individuals that have more than one genetically distinct population of cells. All cell lines arise from single zygote in mosaic, whereas from more than one zygote in chimeras. ^{Neet}

Box 4.1: Parthenogenesis

Definition
- Parthenogenesis is a method of asexual reproduction that involves development of embryo by cleavage division of female gamete without fertilisation.
- *Parthenas* means *virgin* and *genesis* means *creation* in Greek.
- Parthenogenesis occurs in many plants, some invertebrate animals and a few vertebrates (some fish and reptiles).
- In human, parthenogenesis may occur as an ovarian teratoma, but a complete viable foetus cannot be formed.

CLEAVAGE

Q. Write short note on cleavage.
Q. Write short note on morula.

- **Definition**
  Cleavage is a process of repeated mitotic segmentation of zygote within zona pellucida to give rise to small cells called *blastomeres*. ^{Viva}
- In a cleavage, fertilised ovum is divided to form 2-cell, 3-cell, 4-cell stage and so on.
- *Duration*: Up to 6–7 days after fertilisation till implantation.
- *Site*: It continues from the ampulla of fallopian tube till conceptus reaches the site of implantation in uterus.

Events or Stages (Fig. 4.6, Practice Fig. 4.2)

- In each division of cleavage, zygote divides the cytoplasm unequally to form one large and another small cell. Larger cell divides first followed by a smaller one.
- Cleavage aims at formation of morula and later blastocyst.

A. Formation of morula
- Zygote continues divisions one after another to form various stages as follows:

  1st cleavage: 2-cell stage (30 hours after fertilisation)

  2nd cleavage: 4-cell stage (40–50 hours after fertilisation)

  3rd cleavage: 12-cell stage (72 hours after fertilisation)

  4th cleavage: 16-cell stage (96 hours after fertilisation)

- *Morula*
  - 16-cell stage looks similar to mulberry; hence, called *morula*.[Neet]
  - Morula consists of
    - *Inner cell mass* or *embryoblast* that forms future embryo
    - Outer *trophoblast* that forms covering of embryo.[Neet] Trophoblast is also called **trophectoderm** (Gray's Anatomy, 41st Ed).[Neet]
    - Morula is covered by zona pellucida.[Neet]

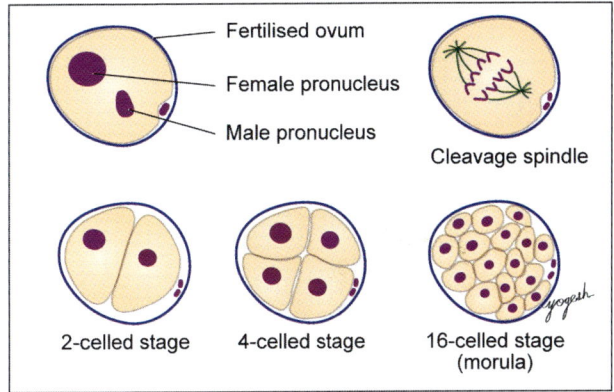

Practice Fig. 4.2: Cleavage and formation of morula

B. Formation of blastocyst (Figs 4.6, 4.7, Practice Fig. 4.3)
- Cells of morula continue to divide and form 32–64-cell stage.
- Uterine fluid slowly diffuses through zona pellucida and gets accumulated in intercellular spaces of morula.
- Accumulated fluid increases intercellular spaces, forms cavities that fuse to form a single cavity called *blastocoel*.
- Outer flattened lining cells of blastocoel form a *trophoblast* and the inner cell mass forms *embryoblast*.
- Thus, embryoblast with blastocoel and trophoblast form **blastocyst**.

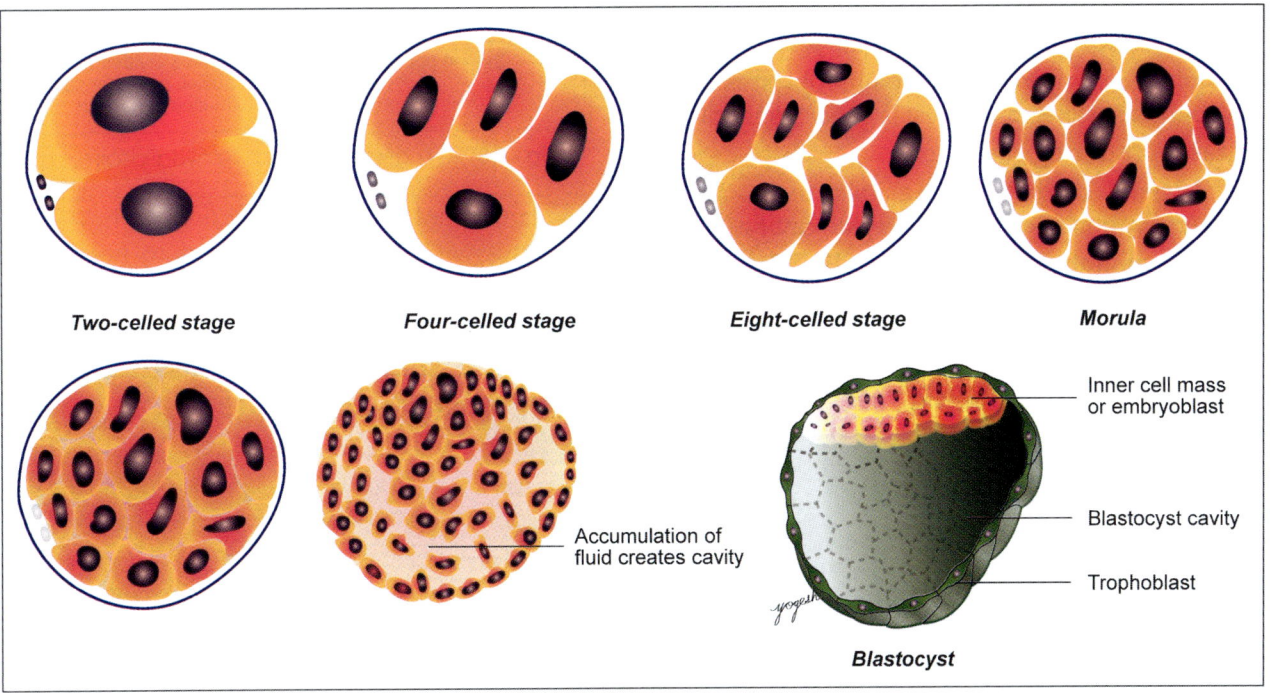

Fig. 4.6: Formation of morula and blastocyst

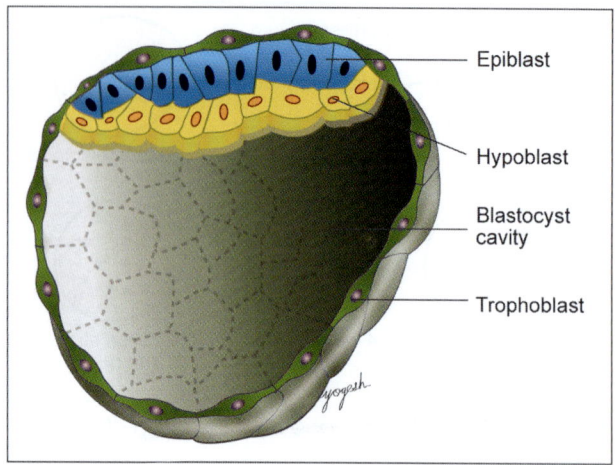

Fig. 4.7: Blastocyst. Differentiation of inner cell mass into epiblast and hypoblast

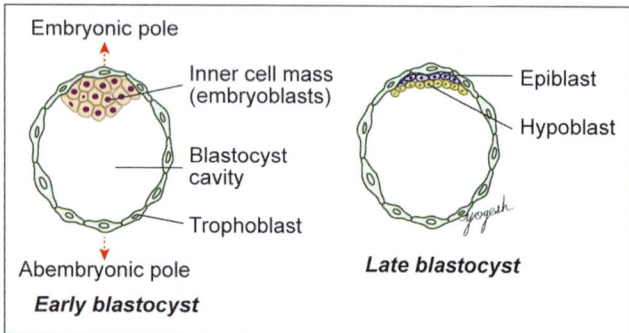

Practice Fig. 4.3: Blastocyst

- Side of the embryoblast attachment with the trophoblast is *embryonic* or *animal pole*, whereas the opposite side is an *abembryonic pole*.
- Trophoblast in contact with embryoblast is *polar* trophoblast, whereas the rest is *mural* trophoblast.
- Transport during cleavage:
  - Zygote gradually migrates away from fertilisation site towards uterine cavity.
  - This migration is assisted by **ciliary beats** and contraction of musculature of fallopian tube.[Neet]

Box 4.2: Hydatidiform mole

- Hydatidiform mole is also called *molar pregnancy* in which a non-viable fertilised ovum implants in the uterus.[MCQ]
- Pathology:
  - Complete mole: During fertilisation, female pronucleus disintegrate, and male chromosomes duplicate. Later, such fertilised egg having only paternal chromosomes can form only trophoblasts and fail to form an embryo (Fig. 4.8).

Flowchart 4.2: Formation of blastocyst

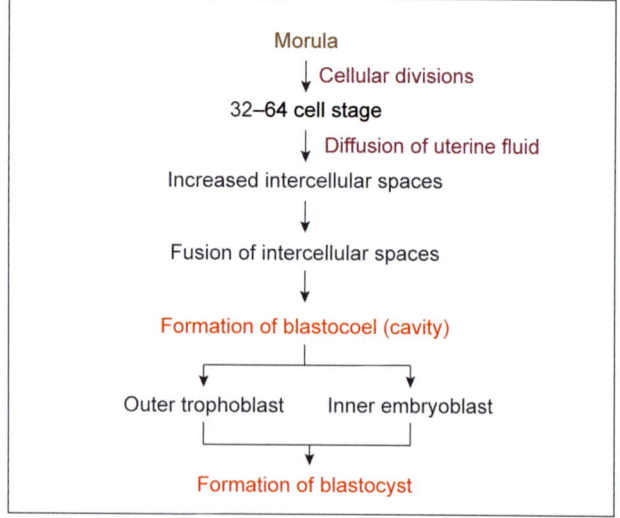

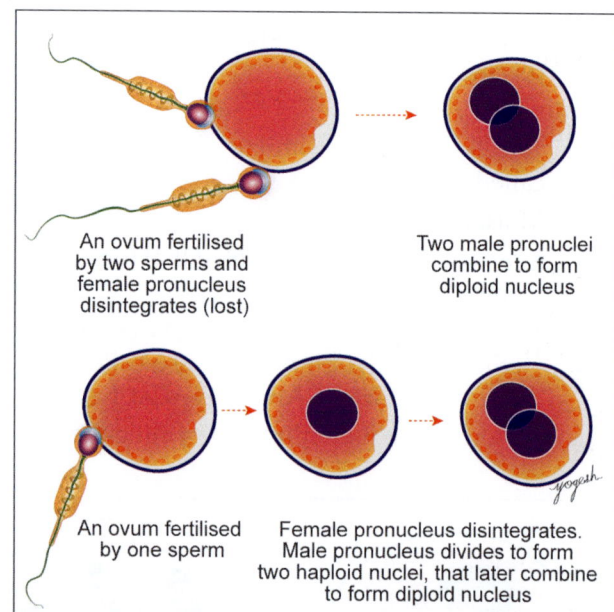

Fig. 4.8: Formation of complete hydatidiform mole

- Partial mole: Duplicated paternal chromosomes fuses with female pronucleus to form 69,XXY chromosomes (Fig. 4.9).[MCQ]
- The differences between complete and partial hydatidiform mole are listed in Table 4.2.

Table 4.2	Difference between complete and partial hydatidiform mole	
Difference	Complete mole	Partial mole
Karyotype	46,XX or 46,XY	69,XXY
Human chorionic gonadotropin	Very high levels	Elevated levels
Choriocarcinoma conversion	2% chance	rare
Pathology	2 sperms + empty egg	2 sperms + egg

Note: Choriocarcinoma is an invasive trophoblastic tumour.

First Week of Development

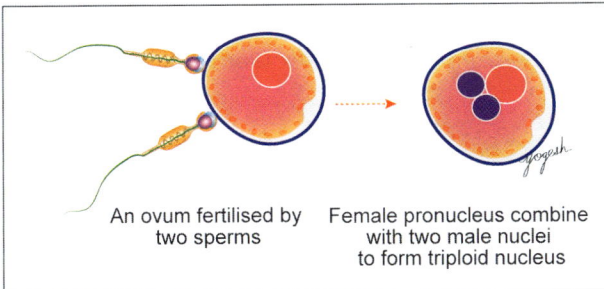

Fig. 4.9: Formation of partial hydatidiform mole

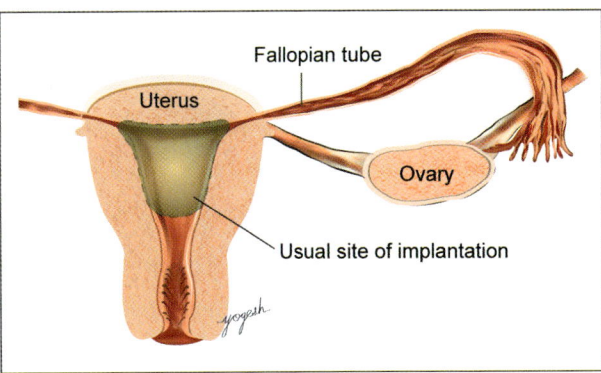

Fig. 4.10: Normal site of implantation. On seventh day after fertilisation, blastocyst usually implants in endometrium of uterus at the site shown by the shaded region (posterior wall of superior part of uterus)

IMPLANTATION

Q. Write short note on implantation.

- **Definition**
  Implantation is a process of penetration of product of conceptus (blastocyst) into the uterine endometrium (Fig. 4.9).
- *Time*: Implantation begins on 6th or 7th day after fertilisation and completes by the 12th day (20th–22nd day of the menstrual cycle).^{Neet}

Site of Implantation (Fig. 4.10)

- Usually, implantation occurs in the upper part of body of the uterus in mid-sagittal plane.^{MCQ, Viva}
- Mostly, it happens on the posterior uterine wall (55%) or anterior uterine wall (45%).
- In human, as blastocyst implants in endometrium, it is called *interstitial implantation*.^{MCQ, Viva}

Box 4.3: Functions of Zona Pellucida

Q. Write short note on functions of zona pellucida.

Zona pellucida is the acellular layer that surrounds ovum, zygote, morula and disappears on hatching of blastocyst in 4–7 days after fertilisation.^{Neet}

1. Prevents implantation: Zona pellucida prevents trophoblast from sticking with uterine epithelium.
2. Zp3 proteins of zona pellucida help in sperm binding.
3. Zona pellucida glycoproteins induce acrosomal reaction.
4. On penetration of sperm, it undergoes zona reaction to prevent polyspermy (entry of multiple sperms.)
5. Allows diffusion of uterine secretion for nourishment of blastomeres and formation of blastocyst cavity.
6. Disappearance of zona pellucida only on 6–7 days of fertilisation facilitates implantation in uterus and prevents ectopic pregnancy.

Process of Implantation (Fig. 4.11, Practice Fig. 4.4 and Flowchart 4.3)

- Hatching of blastocyst: Zona pellucida prevents implantation. By the sixth day of fertilisation, zona pellucida disappears.
- Polar trophoblast adheres with the uterine epithelium.
- Trophoblast secretes proteolytic enzymes that erode endometrium to make passage for blastocyst.
- Blastocyst burrows deep till it completely come to lie within the endometrium.
- *Note*: Binding of trophoblast is assisted by an interaction between the pentasaccharide-lato-N-fucopentose-1 of epithelial surface and its receptor on trophoblast.
- Closure of penetration defect by surface epithelium takes place by 9th day after fertilisation with the formation of fibrin plug.

Abnormal Implantation (Fig. 4.11)

Q. Enlist the abnormal sites of implantation.

- If conceptus does not implant at the usual site, that is, upper part of body of uterus in endometrium, it is called abnormal or ectopic implantation and it results in *ectopic pregnancy*.
- Ectopic pregnancy or implantation are classified according to their site of implantation as follows:
  A. Uterine abnormal implantation.
   - Placenta previa: It is an implantation in lower uterine segment.^{MCQ,}
  B. Tubal implantation: It is an implantation in uterine tube. It is the most common extrauterine implantation.^{MCQ,}
  C. Abdominal implantation: It is a rare ectopic implantation. It usually occurs in the ovary or mesentery (Fig. 4.12).

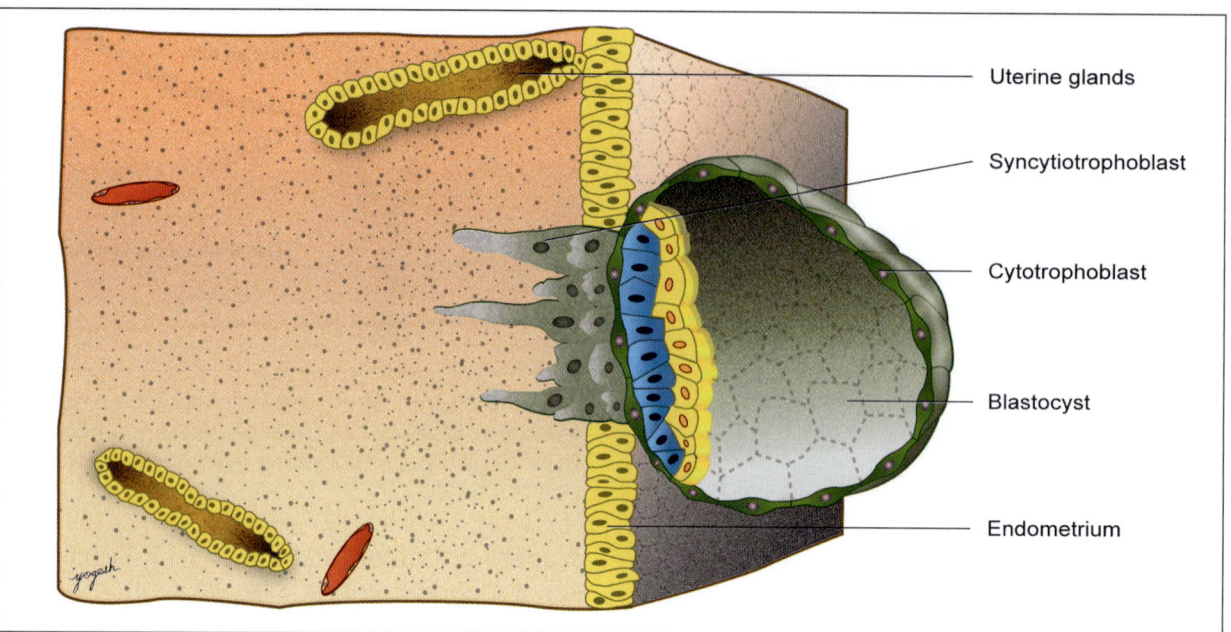

Fig. 4.11: Implantation—trophoblastic invasion. Trophoblastic cells start invading endometrium

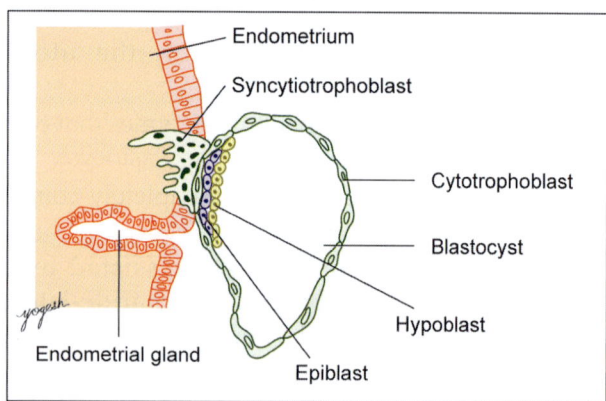

Practice Fig. 4.4: Implantation

Flowchart 4.3: Process of implantation

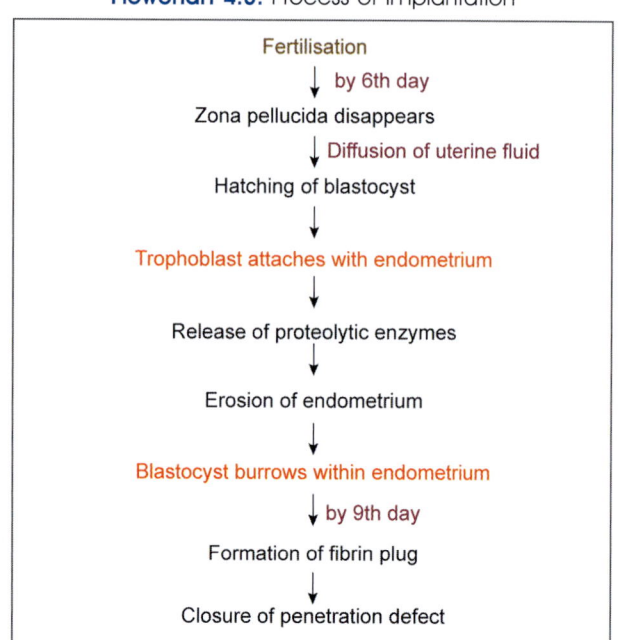

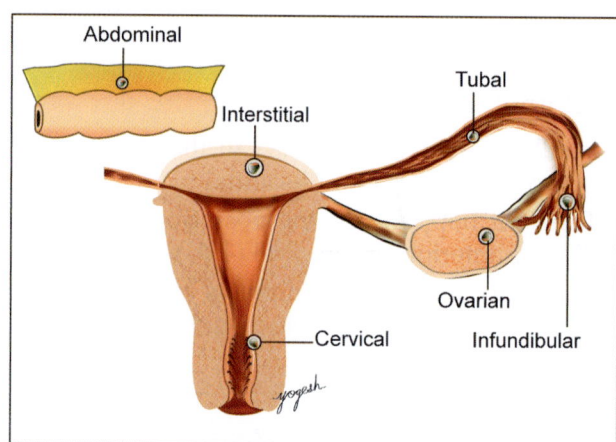

Fig. 4.12: Abnormal sites of implantation. Ovarian, tubal, infundibular, cervical, interstitial, abdominal

CHANGES IN TROPHOBLAST DURING IMPLANTATION

- As soon as polar trophoblast attaches to uterine endometrium, trophoblasts start differentiating into two layers on 6–8 days after fertilisation (Fig. 4.9).[Neet]
  - Cytotrophoblast forms inner cell layer.[Neet]
  - Syncytiotrophoblast forms outer layer. Cells of syncytiotrophoblast form multinucleated protoplasmic mass without distinct cell boundaries.
  - Fingerlike processes of syncytiotrophoblast help to invade endometrium.

Some Interesting Facts

- Humans are *viviparous animals*. Embryos of viviparous animals receive nutrition from mothers and retain scanty egg yolk.

Contd.

First Week of Development

Contd.

- Continuous expression of *Oct4* and *Nanog* transcription factor converts blastomeres into inner cell mass and repression (decreased expression) of these factors by eomesodermin convert blastomere trophoblasts.
- Fertilised ovum reaches the uterus in 3–4 days (at 32-celled stage).^{Neet}
- *Decidual reaction* is a change in uterine endometrium that occurs in secretory phase of menstrual cycle. These changes make endometrium favourable for implantation of blastocyst.
- Blastocyst makes contact with endometrium on 5–7 days (1–2 days prior to the implantation).^{Neet}

CLINICAL EMBRYOLOGY

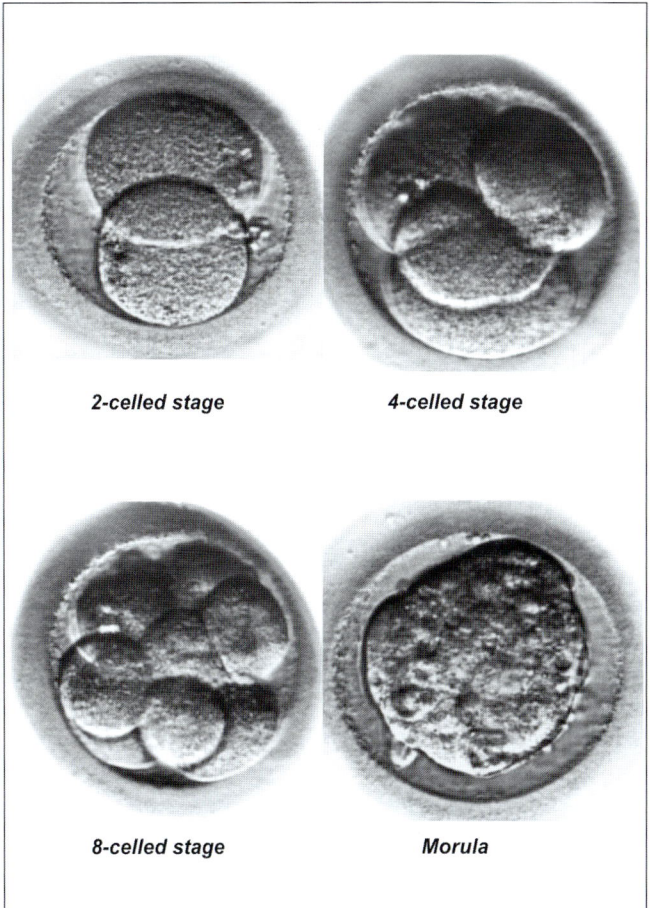

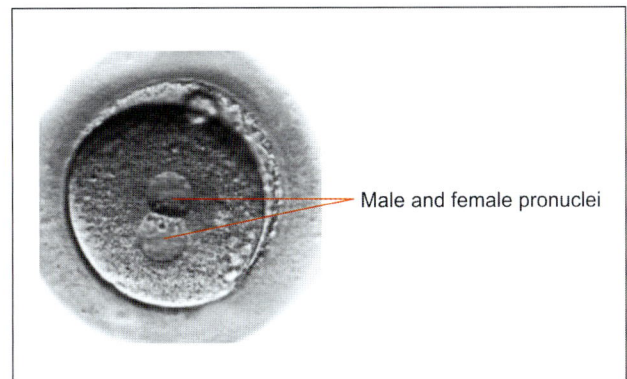

Clinical image 4.1: Human zygote. In fertilisation, fusion of two mature germ cells, an ovum and a spermatozoon (haploid cells) form a single cell, zygote (diploid cell) (Image courtesy: *Dr Keshav Malhotra*)

Clinical image 4.2: Human zygote continues division one after another. 1st cleavage: 2-cell stage (24–30 hours after fertilisation), 2nd cleavage: 4-cell stage (40–50 hours after fertilisation), 3rd cleavage: 8-cell stage (66 hours after fertilisation) and 4th cleavage: 16-cell stage (90–96 hours after fertilisation). Sixteen cell stage looks similar to mulberry; hence, called morula (Image courtesy: *Dr Keshav Malhotra*)

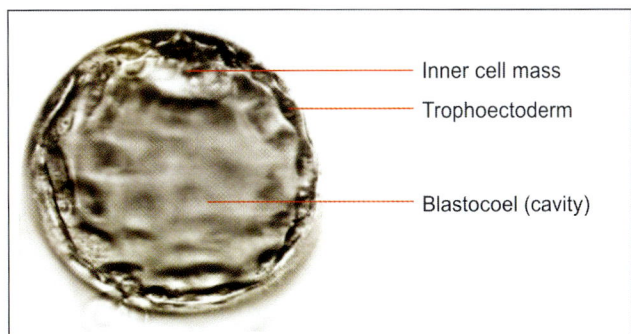

Clinical image 4.3: Cells of morula continue to divide and form 32–64 cell stage. Accumulated fluid increases intercellular spaces, forms a cavity called blastocoel. Outer flattened lining cells of blastocoel form trophoblast and inner cell mass forms embryoblast. Embryoblast with blastocoel and trophoblast form blastocyst (115–120 hours after fertilisation). (Image courtesy: *Dr Keshav Malhotra*)

5

Assisted Reproduction Technology
In vitro Fertilisation and Intracytoplasmic Sperm Injection

Chapter Outline

- *In vitro* fertilisation
  - Uses of *in vitro* fertilisation
  - Stages of IVF
- Ovarian hyperstimulation syndrome
- Surgical sperm extraction
- Success rate in ART
- Intracytoplasmic sperm injection (ICSI)
  - Indications
  - Protocol
- Artificial insemination
- Gamete intrafallopian transfer
- Zygote intrafallopian transfer
- Egg freezing (oocyte cryopreservation)

INTRODUCTION

- Having a child is always a great gift of nature to human beings.
- About 1 in 6 couples have difficulty in conceiving naturally on their own.
- About 90% of infertile couples can conceive with medical intervention.
- Assisted reproductive technology is used to support the infertile patients.
- Table 5.1 lists various assisted reproductive techniques.

Table 5.1	Methods of assisted reproductive technology
1. Counselling for reproduction
2. Fertility medications that help to form ovarian follicles. For example, gonadotropins and gonadotropin releasing hormone.
3. *In vitro* fertilization (IVF): It involves fertilisation of ovum outside the female body.
4. Gamete intrafallopian transfer (GIFT): It involves the direct transfer of sperms and ovum in the fallopian tube.
5. Zygote intrafallopian transfer (ZIFT): It involves the direct transfer of zygote in the fallopian tube.
6. Surgical approach: It involves surgical treatment of fallopian tube obstruction and vas deferens obstruction.

IN VITRO FERTILISATION

- *Definition:* In vitro fertilisation is a process of fertilising ovum outside the body.
- The first baby born by *in vitro* fertilisation was *Louise Brown* on 25th July 1978.
- Founders of IVF are Robert Edward (The Noble Prize, 2010) and Patrick Steptoe.
- IVF is also known as *test-tube baby*.

Uses (Indications) of IVF

- *In vitro* fertilisation is useful in the following conditions:
  1. Blockage of fallopian tube
  2. Problem with ovulation
  3. Endometriosis
  4. Polycystic ovarian syndrome
  5. Cervical problems

Stages of IVF

The basic steps involved in IVF are as follows (Flowchart 5.1 and Fig. 5.1):
Stage 1: Ovarian stimulation and monitoring
Stage 2: Oocyte retrieval
Stage 3: Fertilisation
Stage 4: Embryo development
Stage 5: Embryo transfer
Stage 6: Luteal phase support

Flowchart 5.1: Stages of *in vitro* fertilisation

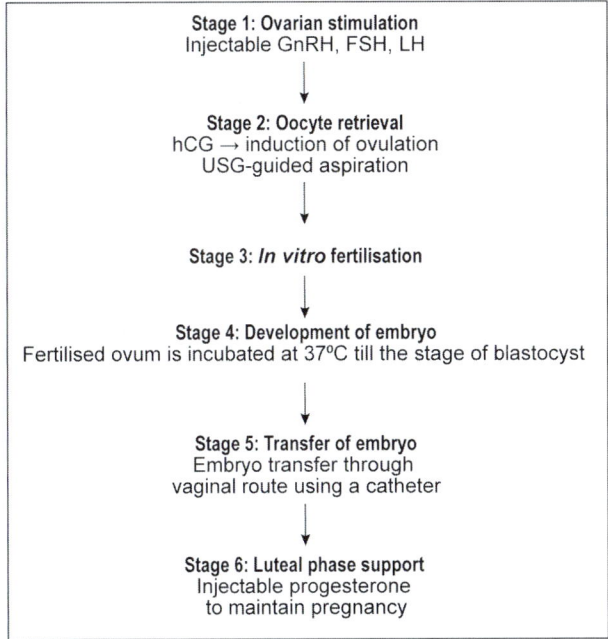

Abbreviation: GnRH: Gonadotropin releasing hormone; FSH: Follicle stimulating hormone; LH: Luteinizing hormone; hCG: Human chorionic gonadotropin; USG: Ultrasonography

Stage 1: Ovarian Stimulation and Monitoring

- During each menstrual cycle, the following hormones play important roles:
    i. Gonadotropin-releasing hormone (GnRH): It is secreted by hypothalamus (part of a brain) and stimulates pituitary gland to release follicle stimulating hormone (FSH).
    ii. Follicle stimulating hormone: It is secreted by pituitary on GnRH stimulus and promotes maturation of ovarian follicles and prepare endometrium for implantation.
    iii. Luteinising hormone (LH): It is secreted by pituitary gland and induces ovulation.
- *Medicine for follicle development:*
    - In assisted reproductive technology, injectable hormones are given to induce follicle development and ovulation. In each cycle, 5–10 secondary oocytes are collected.
    - For this purpose, the following treatments are usually given:
        a. FSH (gonadotropin): It is given in injectable form for the development of follicles.
        b. GnRH: It is given in injectable form on a daily basis for the first two weeks to prevent premature ovulation. It makes multiple eggs available for IVF.
        c. Nafarelin acetate: It has similar effects similar to GnRH. It is given on a daily basis (morning and night) as a nasal spray.
        d. Leuprorelin: It has similar effects similar to GnRH. It is given as subcutaneous injections.
        e. Cetrorelix and ganirelix: These are injectable GnRH antagonists and prevent premature ovulation.
        f. Luteinising hormone (LH): LH induces ovulation. In IVF, naturally occurring LH surge (that usually induces ovulation) needs to be avoided by suppressing pituitary gland's LH and FSH secretion. It is called *pituitary suppression* or *down regulation*.
           Protocol 1: It is achieved with the help of nafarelin or leuprorelin given for first 10 days of the cycle.
           Protocol 2: It can also be achieved with the help of GnRH antagonists (cetrorelix or ganirelix) given from fifth or sixth day after commencement of FSH injections and continued till ovulation induction.

Monitoring:

- Ultrasound examinations are used for monitoring follicle growth in ovaries.
- Oestrogen or oestradiol (E2) blood levels can be monitored. These hormones are produced by developing follicle in response to FSH treatment.
- Monitoring is required to determine the timing for induction of ovulation.

Stage 2: Oocyte Retrieval

- It is also called egg retrieval or egg pickup.
- Induction of ovulation: Injectable human chorionic gonadotropin or luteinising hormone is given 36–48 hours before preplanned egg pickup.
- Methods of egg pickup:
    1. Ultrasound-guided aspiration: Under mild sedation and local anaesthesia, eggs are aspirated with the ultrasound-guided fine needle. The needle is passed through the vaginal wall into mature follicle to collect egg.

Box 5.1: Ovarian hyperstimulation syndrome
- Stimulation of ovary by various fertility medicines may produce OHSS.
- Ovaries enlarge and produce a large quantity of fluids.
- Symptoms: Pain and blotting in abdomen.

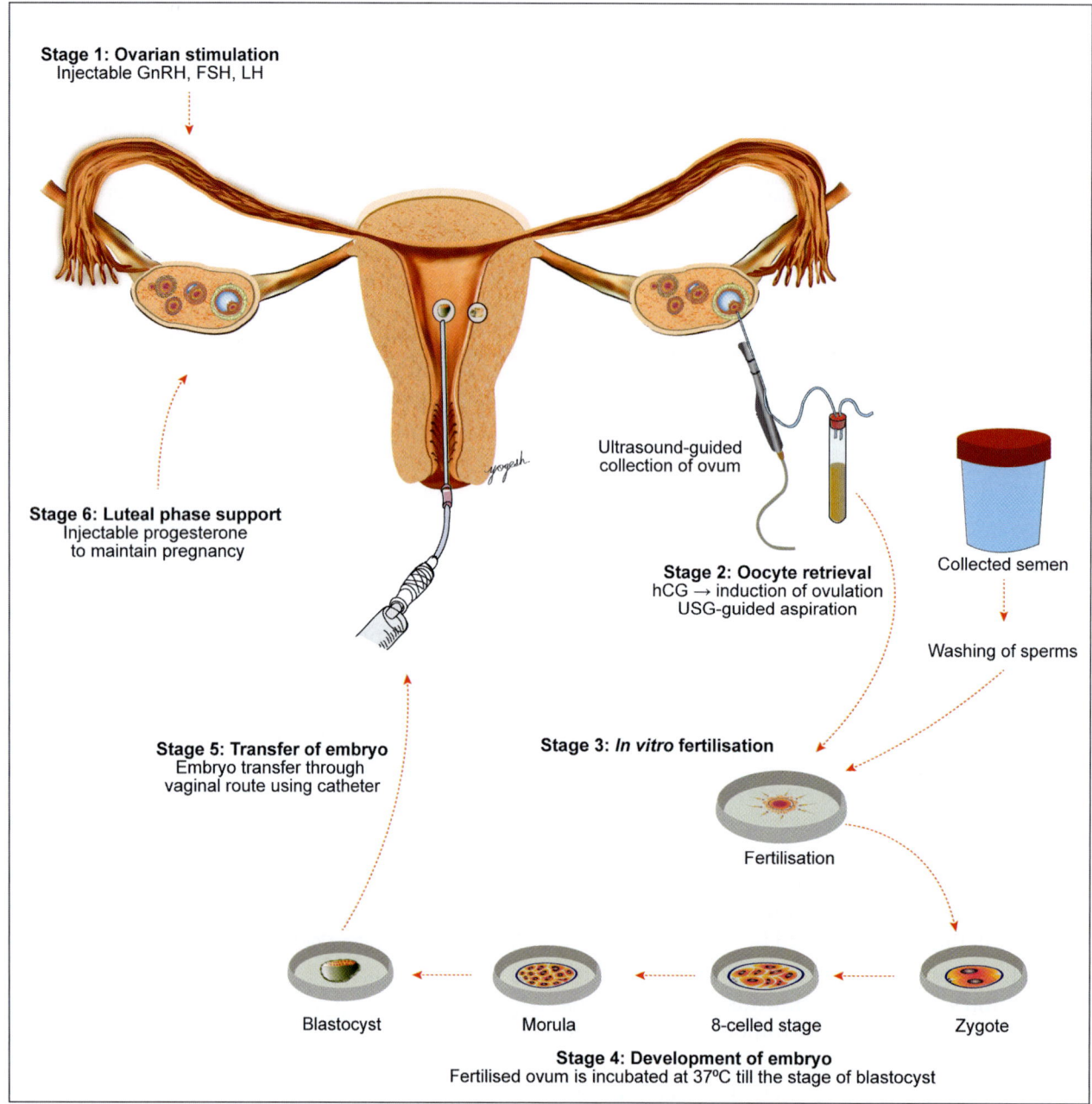

Fig. 5.1: *In vitro* fertilisation. It involves six stages as follows: Stage 1, ovarian stimulation and monitoring; Stage 2, oocyte retrieval; Stage 3, fertilisation; Stage 4, embryo development; Stage 5, embryo transfer; Stage 6, luteal phase support. Abbreviations: GnRH: Gonadotropin releasing hormone; FSH: Follicle stimulating hormone; LH: Luteinising hormone; hCG: Human chorionic gonadotropin; USG: Ultrasonography

2. Laparoscopy assisted aspiration: If ovaries are not readily available via transvaginal approach due to disorders, such as uterine fibroid, laparoscopy is used. Under general anaesthesia, eggs are aspirated with gentle suction from matured follicles.
   - Collected fluid is examined microscopically for eggs.
   - Collected eggs are placed in an incubator.

Stages 3: Fertilisation
- A collection of sperms: Sperms are collected at clinics 2–3 hours before egg collection.
- *Sperm washing*: It is a process to remove mucous and nonmotile sperms from semen to improve the chances of fertilisation.
- Procedure. Sperms are washed by density gradient centrifugation or direct swim-up technique. Washed

sperm are kept in Hams F10 media without L-glutamine at 37°C.
- IVF: Sperms and eggs are incubated at 37°C for overnight. Next day, eggs are examined microscopically to confirm fertilisation. One fertilised ovum is further processed as stage 4, whereas others are stored with cryopreservation for future use.

Box 5.2: Surgical sperm extraction

- In assisted reproductive technology, if male partner does not have sperms in semen, then it can be collected surgically from epididymis or testis.

Conditions requiring surgical sperm extractions:
1. Blockage in the ejaculatory duct or vas deferens
2. Vasectomy patients.

Stage 4: Embryo Development

- Fertilised ovum is nothing but a cell and it can be grown in a culture media at 37°C.
- *In vitro*, in culture media, zygote starts cleavage.
- A zygote is transferred on or before the day of development, at the stage of the blastocyst. Only one or two fertilised eggs are transferred to uterus for implantation and the remaining are stored with cryopreservation for future use.

Some Interesting Facts

1. Assisted hatching: Disappearance of zona pellucida (hatching) is essential for implantation. In case of repeated IVF failures, older females or cryopreserved egg, assisted hatching may be required. It is done with the help of treatment with a dilute acid to remove zona pellucida.
2. Preimplantation genetic diagnosis (PGD): In IVF, PGD can be performed to identify the genetic disorder. Before the transfer of blastocyst on day five to the uterus, one or more cells are collected from the blastocyst. DNA from these cells is analysed for genetic disorders such as Down syndrome, haemophilia A and so on.

Stage 5: Embryo Transfer

- Fertilised egg or blastocyst is transferred to the uterus using a catheter via vaginal route.
- In one cycle, one or two blastocysts are transferred, whereas remaining is stored with cryopreservation for future.

Stage 6: Luteal Phase Support

- In ART, a collection of ovum results in improper formation of corpus luteum. Hence, there will be lack of sufficient oestrogen and progesterone hormone.
- Hence, in IVF pregnancy should be supported at least for first two weeks after ovum collection with progesterone.
- Pregnancy can be confirmed by detection of hCG hormone in maternal blood or ultrasonography after two weeks of fertilisation date.

Success Rate in ART

- One study reported success rate of 17.9% of total treated cases with ART.
- The success rate is influenced by many factors, such as maternal age, cause of infertility, sperm quality and so on.

INTRACYTOPLASMIC SPERM INJECTION (ICSI)

- *Definition:* ICSI is a procedure that involves a direct transfer of a single sperm into a cytoplasm of oocyte.
- ICSI technique is developed by G Palermo (1991).

Indications for ICSI

1. Teratozoospermia: Abnormal sperm morphology
2. Poor sperm motility
3. Low sperm count
4. Vasectomy cases or obstruction in passage sperm.
5. Anti-sperm antibodies in male that inhibit sperm functions.

Protocol

- ICSI involves six steps as follows:
  Stage 1: Ovarian stimulation and monitoring
  Stage 2: Oocyte retrieval
  Stage 3: Fertilisation
  Stage 4: Embryo development
  Stage 5: Embryo transfer
  Stage 6: Luteal phase support
- All the above-mentioned steps are similar to the steps involved in IVF.
- In step 3: Fertilisation is carried out with the help of tiny glass tube (needle).
- A glass tool or pipette tip is used to hold the egg in place.
- A sperm is aspirated in a tiny glass tube and it is inserted in the cytoplasm of ovum under microscopic view.
- Fertilised egg is incubated overnight at 37°C and observed on next day for fertilisation. Later, fertilised egg is transferred to the uterus on sixth day.

ARTIFICIAL INSEMINATION

- Artificial insemination is a method of assisted reproductive technology.
- *Definition*: Artificial insemination is the deliberate introduction of sperm into uterus or cervix by means other than sexual intercourse.
- Artificial insemination is of two types:
  1. *Intrauterine insemination* (IUI), and
  2. *Intracervical insemination* (ICI).

Indications
Artificial insemination is preferred in the following conditions:
1. Sperm donation
2. Male infertility
3. Failure of reproduction on natural course

Technique
- Artificial insemination involves the following steps:
  1. Collection of sperms
  2. Transfer of sperms either into cervix (unwashed sperms) or into uterus (washed sperms) using a catheter.
- Female is asked to rest on the table for 15 minutes to increase the pregnancy rate.

Success rate
- The success rate for ICI is 10–15% per menstrual cycle and for IUI is 15–20% per cycle.
- In IUI about 60–70% females achieve pregnancy in 6 cycles.

Box 5.3: Gamete Intrafallopian Transfer (GIFT)
- In assisted reproductive technology, collected eggs and sperms are transferred into the fallopian tube using laparoscope.

Indications:
- Ovary and at least one of the fallopian tubes of the female should be normal.
- GIFT is preferred in cases of sperm dysfunction or couple with unknown cause of infertility.
- Success rate: Approximately 25–30%.

Box 5.4: Zygote Intrafallopian Transfer (ZIFT)
- In ART, *in vitro* fertilised egg is transferred to fallopian tube using a laparoscope.
- Success rate: 64.8%.

Table 5.2 lists the indications for commonly used methods of assisted reproductive techniques.

Table 5.2	Commonly used methods of assisted reproductive techniques and their indications
Method	Indications
In vitro fertilisation: It is a process of fertilising ovum outside the body.	• Blockage of fallopian tube • Problem with ovulation • Endometriosis • Polycystic ovarian syndrome • Cervical problems
Intracytoplasmic Sperm Injection (ICSI): It is a procedure that involves the direct transfer of a single sperm into a cytoplasm of oocyte.	• Teratozoospermia • Poor sperm motility • Low sperm count • Vasectomy cases or obstruction in passage sperm. • Anti-sperm antibodies in male
Artificial insemination: It is a method of assisted reproductive technology.	• Sperm donation • Male infertility • Failure of reproduction on natural course
Gamete intrafallopian transfer (GIFT): It is transfer of collected eggs and sperms into fallopian tube.	• Ovary and at least one of the fallopian tube should be normal. • Sperm dysfunction or couple with unknown cause of infertility.
Zygote intrafallopian transfer (ZIFT): It is zygote transfer to fallopian tube using a laparoscope.	

Box 5.5: Egg freezing (oocyte cryopreservation)
- Human oocyte cryopreservation or egg freezing is a procedure to preserve an ovum.
- Procedure:
  - Ovum are extracted from a female same as in IVF.
  - The extracted ova are frozen and stored in liquid nitrogen at –196°C.
- In the future, ova will be thawed, fertilised and transferred to the uterus as embryos to facilitate a pregnancy.
- Indications: As germ cell deteriorate but uterus remains active till middle age, egg freezing can be used to postpone maternity until suitable situations (to set carrier or medical conditions that require chemotherapy).
- Success rate:
  - Varies with the age of woman at the time of egg retrieval.
  - It ranges from 14.8 to 31.5%.

CLINICAL EMBRYOLOGY

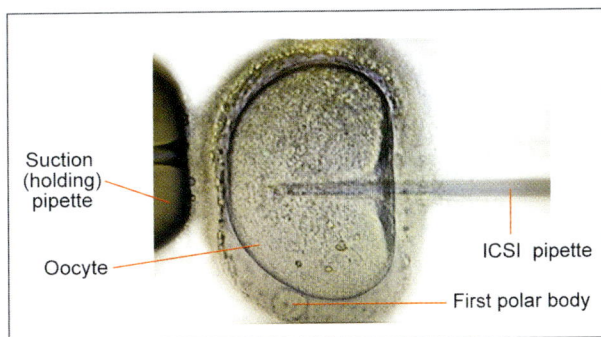

Clinical image 5.1: Intracytoplasmic sperm injection (ICSI) is a procedure that involves a direct transfer of a single sperm into a cytoplasm of oocyte. Oocyte is held with a suction pipette and ICSI pipette, containing a single sperm, is used to penetrate the zona pellucida and oocyte. After pressure injection of the sperm, the ICSI pipette is withdrawn (Image courtesy: *Dr Keshav Malhotra*)

6
Second Week of Development

Chapter Outline

- Day 8
  - Changes in trophoblasts
  - Changes in embryoblast
- Day 9–10
  - Changes in trophoblasts
  - Changes in embryoblast
- Day 11–12
  - Changes in trophoblasts
  - Changes in embryoblast
- Day 13–14
  - Changes in trophoblasts
  - Changes in embryoblast
- Yolk sac
- Foetus as graft
- Genomic imprinting
- X chromosome inactivation
- Endometrial changes

INTRODUCTION

- Process of implantation that begins in the first week gets completed in the second week.
- During implantation, blastocyst sinks in the endometrium due to the invading capacity of trophoblasts.
- Blastocyst completely embeds in the endometrial stroma by the 12th day of development.^{MCQ}
- Site of penetration is initially sealed by fibrin and coagulation plug and is later healed by the lining epithelial of endometrium.
- Developmental changes in the second week can be grouped as follows:
  1. Changes in the trophoblast
  2. Changes in the embryoblast
  3. Changes in the endometrium
- For study purpose, day by day changes in the second week are described in this chapter.

DAY 8 (Fig. 6.1)

Changes in Trophoblasts

- A blastocyst partially sinks in the endometrium.
- Trophoblast is differentiated into two layers.^{Viva}
  1. Inner cytotrophoblast
  2. Outer syncytiotrophoblast
- Cytotrophoblast on mitosis migrates outwards to form the syncytiotrophoblast.

Changes in Embryoblast

- Embryoblast (inner cell mass) differentiates into the following two layers:
  1. Hypoblast: It is a flat (low cuboidal) cell layer facing towards the blastocoel (cavity of blastocyst).
  2. Epiblast: Embryoblasts facing towards embryonic pole (attached to cytotrophoblast) forms a layer of columnar cells called *epiblast*.
- Epiblast cells get separated from some embryoblast by the formation of a cavity called *amniotic cavity*.
- Flat embryoblast lining a roof of amniotic cavity is called *amnioblasts* (amnion), whereas epiblasts line the floor of the amniotic cavity.^{MCQ}
- Upon formation of an amniotic cavity, hypoblasts, and epiblasts form a **bilaminar germ disc**.
- The junction of amnioblast with germ disc is called *amnio-ectodermal junction*.

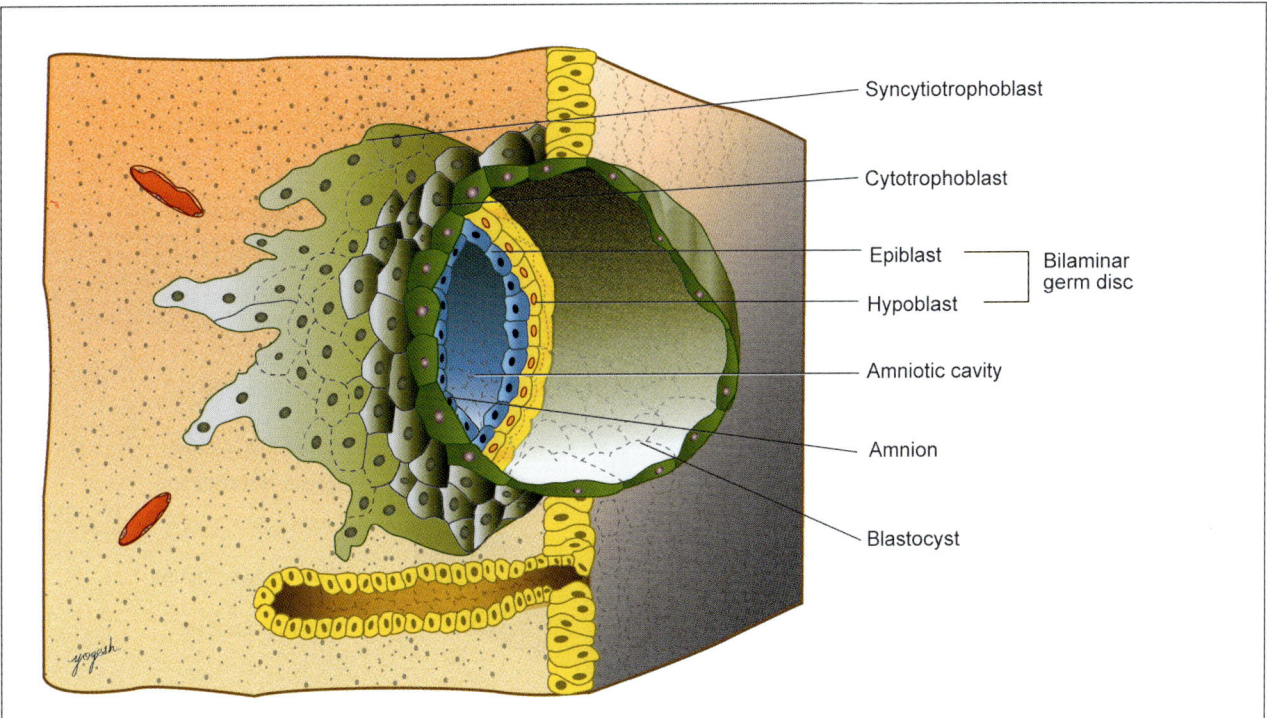

Fig. 6.1: Day 8: Implantation—formation of amniotic cavity. Epiblast cells multiply and amniotic cavity appears in between them as a small cleft. Trophoblast differentiates into the outer syncytiotrophoblast and inner cytotrophoblast. The embryoblast is formed by the epiblast and hypoblast layers

DAY 9–10 (Fig. 6.2, Practice Fig. 6.1)

Changes in Trophoblasts

- Blastocyst further penetrates endometrium.
- Penetration defect is closed by a fibrin coagulation plug.
- Syncytiotrophoblast develops more rapidly along embryonic pole.
- Cells of syncytiotrophoblast grow rapidly and lose their adjacent cell membrane to form multinucleated protoplasmic mass. *Viva*
- **Lacunar stage of trophoblast** *MCQ, Viva,*
- Several small lacunar spaces appear in syncytiotrophoblast. These lacunar spaces fuse with each other to form large lacunar spaces.

Changes in Embryoblast

- **Formation of exocoelomic or Heuser's membrane:** *MCQ*
  At the abembryonic pole, hypoblast cells proliferate to form flattened mesothelial cells. These mesothelial cells line the inner surface of the cytotrophoblast, (the surface facing the blastocyst cavity) and form *Heuser's membrane*.
- On lining of exocoelomic membrane, blastocoel cavity modifies to form *primary yolk sac or exocoelomic cavity*.

- Thus, bilaminar germ disc lies between the amniotic cavity and the primary yolk sac.

DAY 11–12 (Fig. 6.3, Practice Fig. 6.2)

Changes in Trophoblasts

- Endometrial epithelium completely heals the defect caused due to implantation.
- Lacunar spaces enlarge and form communication with each other. This change is more prominent along the embryonic pole.
- Cords of syncytiotrophoblasts form the trabeculae.
- Syncytiotrophoblast erodes maternal capillaries and other vessels; hence, lacunar spaces get filled with maternal blood.
- Erosion of maternal veins takes place earlier than the maternal arteries. *MCQ*
- Filling of lacunar spaces with maternal blood establish *uteroplacental circulation*.

Changes in Embryoblast

- Cells of yolk sac multiplies to form a layer of loosely arranged connective tissue called *extraembryonic mesoderm*. *Neet* Extraembryonic mesoderm forms structures that do not contribute to future body of embryo. *Neet*

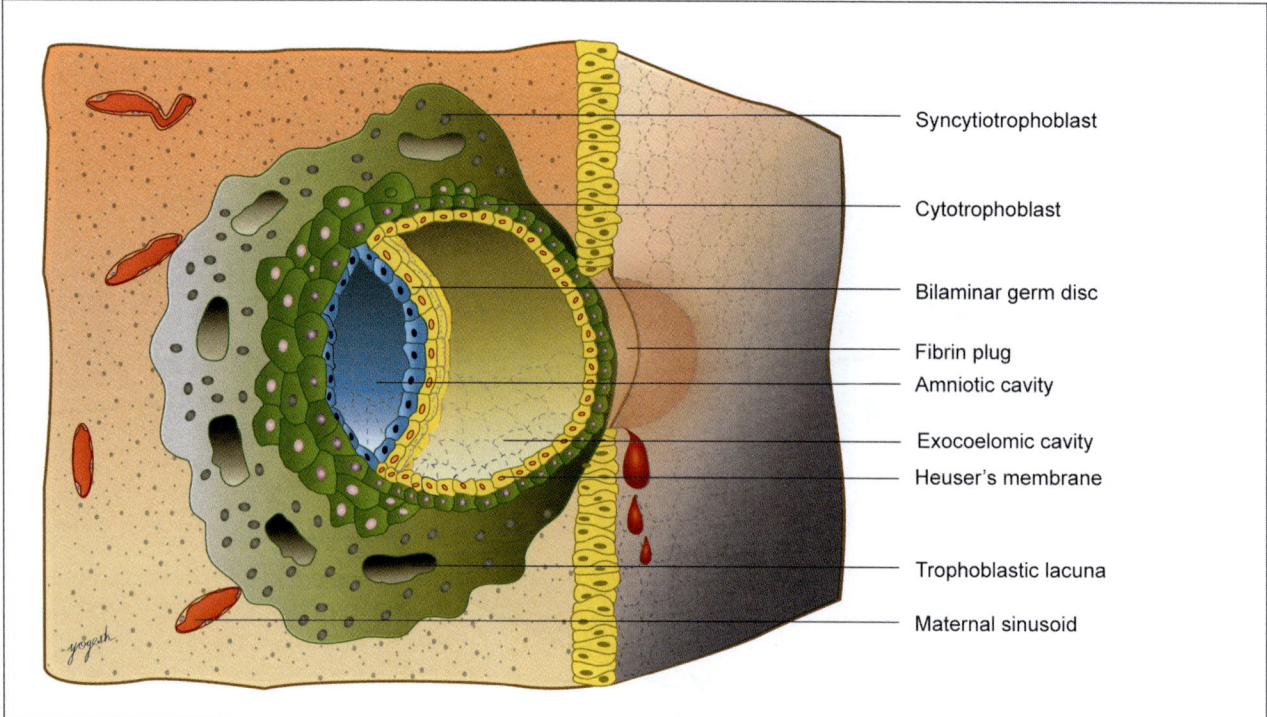

Fig. 6.2: Day 9 embryo. Formation of trophoblastic lacunae. Small lacunar cavities appear in syncytiotrophoblast. A layer of columnar epiblast cells and a layer of cuboidal hypoblast cells form bilaminar germ disc. The bilaminar disc lies between amniotic cavity and primary yolk sac. The endometrial surface defect is closed by a fibrin coagulum. Hypoblast cells multiply to form flat cell layer called Heuser's membrane that lines the yolk sac

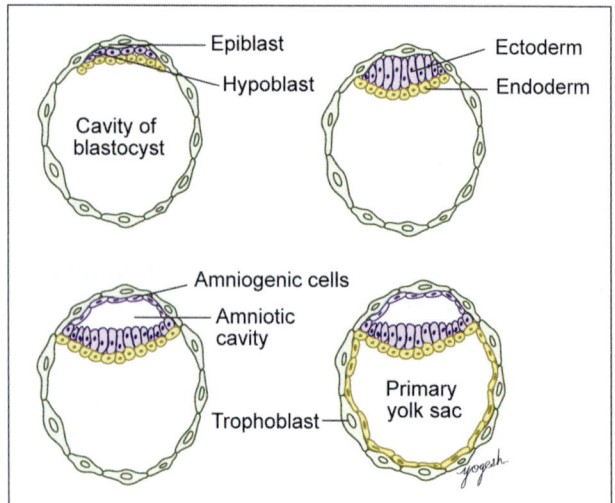

Practice Fig. 6.1: Formation of ectoderm, endoderm, amniotic cavity and primary yolk sac

- Extraembryonic mesoderm spreads underneath the cytotrophoblast.
- Spreading of the extraembryonic mesoderm separates the germ disc, amniotic cavity and yolk sac from the cytotrophoblast.
- Cavities start appearing in the growing extraembryonic mesoderm. These cavities soon fuse to form an *extraembryonic coelom*.
- Continuous increase in extraembryonic coelom isolates the yolk sac and amniotic cavity from the cytotrophoblast except at the caudal end of the germ disc where it forms a *connecting stalk* of extraembryonic mesoderm.
- Connecting stalk ultimately develops an *umbilical cord*.^MCQ
- Exocoelomic cavity divides extraembryonic mesoderm into *somatopleuric* and *splanchnopleuric mesoderm*.^MCQ
- Somatopleuric (somatic) extraembryonic mesoderm lines the amnion and cytotrophoblast, whereas splanchnopleuric extraembryonic mesoderm lines the yolk sac.

Chorion
Q. What is chorion?
- Trophoblast and somatopleuric layer of extraembryonic mesoderm together form a *chorion* and blastocystic cavity called the *chorionic cavity*.^MCQ, Viva

---

Some Interesting Facts
- Embryotroph is a fluid that appears in syncytiotrophoblastic lacunar spaces.
- Embryotroph nourishes bilaminar disc through diffusion before the development of uteroplacental circulation.

Second Week of Development

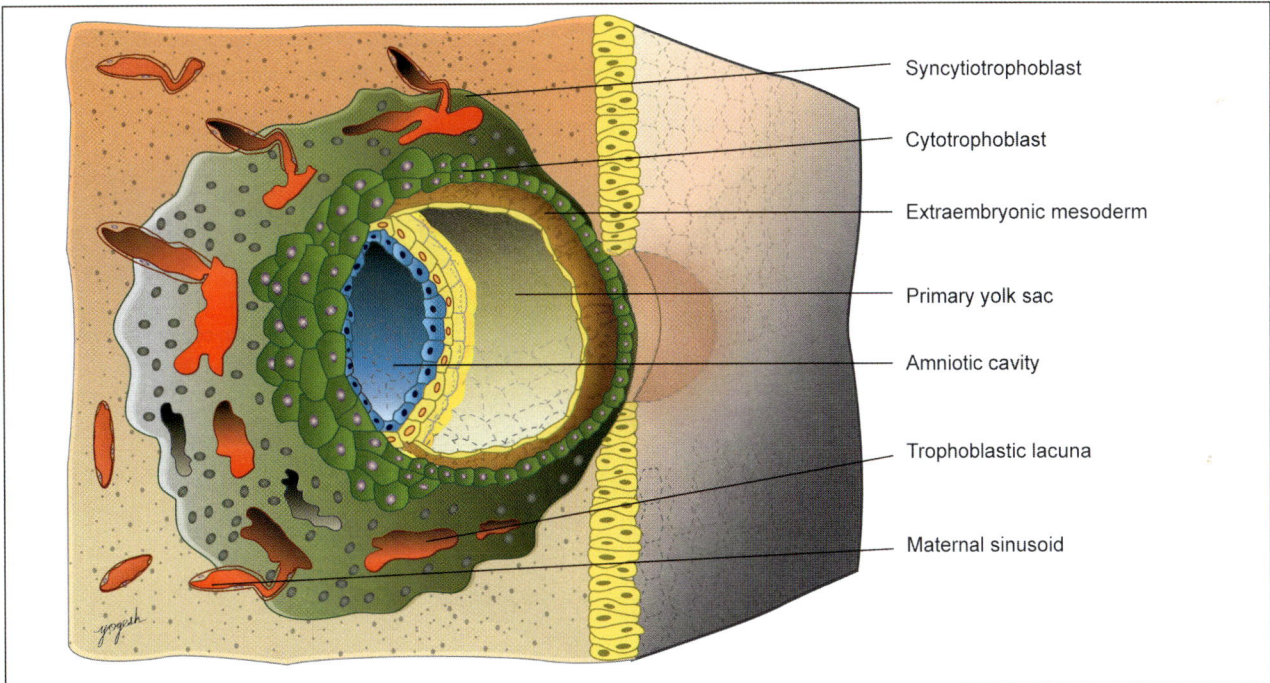

Fig. 6.3: Day 10–11: Formation of extraembryonic mesoderm. Establishment of communication between maternal blood vessels and trophoblastic lacunae. The trophoblastic lacunae get filled with maternal blood. The extraembryonic mesodermal cells separate Heuser's membrane from cytotrophoblast

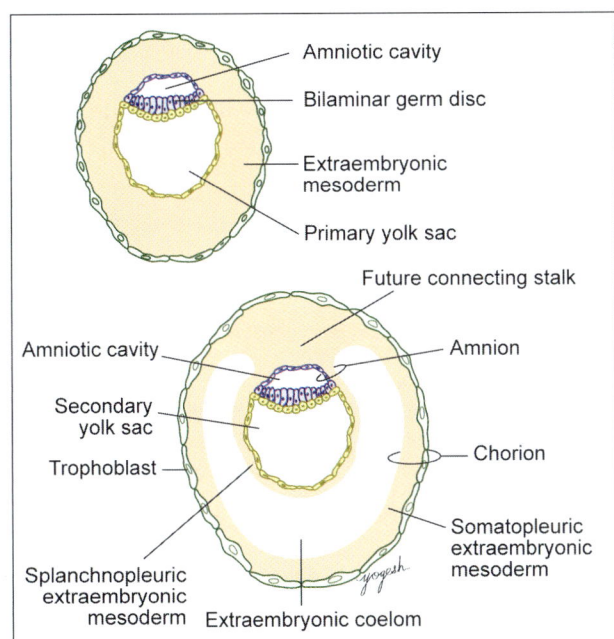

Practice Fig. 6.2: Formation of extraembryonic mesoderm, extraembryonic coelom, amnion and chorion

DAY 13–14 (Figs 6.4 to 6.8, Practice Fig. 6.2)

Changes in Trophoblasts

- Endometrial surface defect heals completely.
- Syncytiotrophoblast forms column-like structures called *villi*. The villi lie between adjacent lacunar spaces.
- Syncytiotrophoblastic villi are invaded by cytotrophoblastic cells to form *primary stem villi*. MCQ, Viva (Fig. 6.9).
- Primary stem villi have a central core of cytotrophoblast and peripheral syncytiotrophoblast.

Some Interesting Facts

- Occasional bleeding through endometrial surface defect may occur due to increased maternal blood to lacunar spaces.
- This bleeding may fall on the 28th day of menstrual cycle and may be confused with usual menstrual bleeding. MCQ

Changes in Embryoblast

- **Formation of secondary yolk sac**

  A portion of primary yolk sac is pinched off by developing extraembryonic coelom. Thus, the primary yolk sac results in the reduction in size to form smaller *secondary yolk sac*. MCQ

- A 14-day embryo is a flat, bilaminar germ disc. It is sandwiched between the floor of the amniotic cavity and roof of the yolk sac.

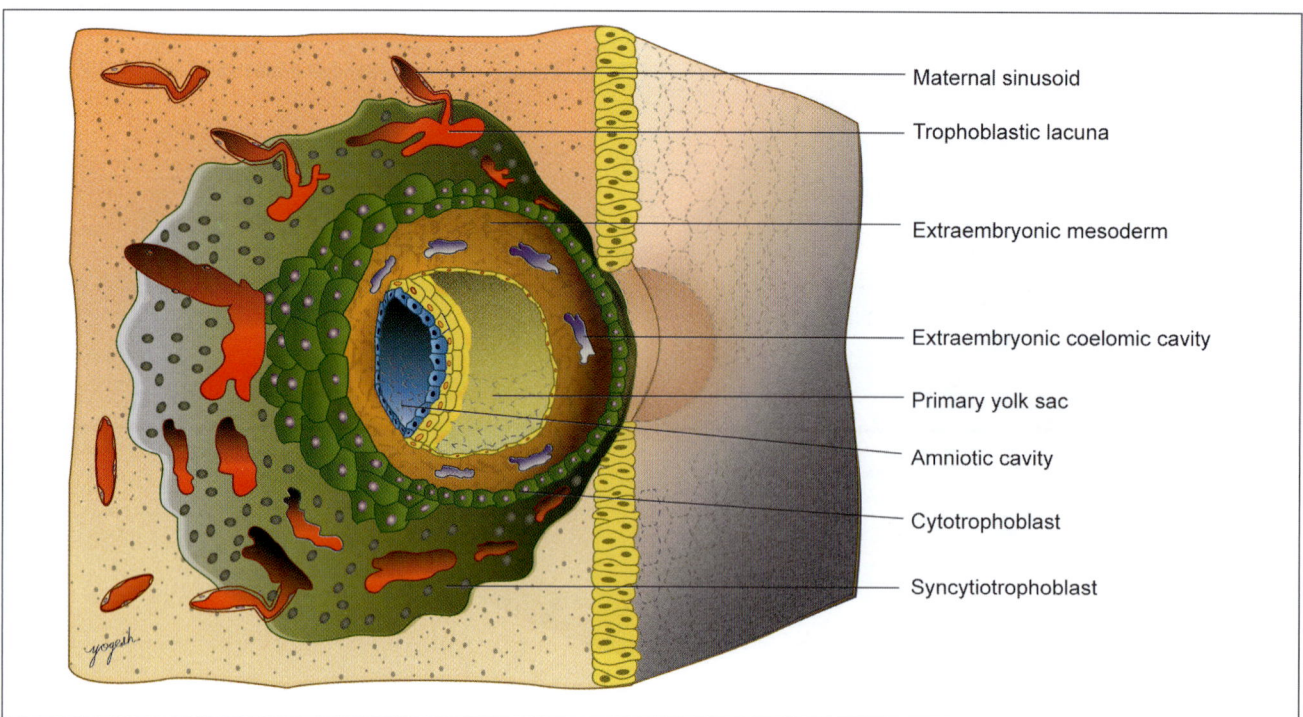

Fig. 6.4: Day 12: Formation of extraembryonic coelom. Extraembryonic coelomic cavities appear in extraembryonic mesoderm. The trophoblastic lacunae at the embryonic pole develop communication with maternal vessels. Extraembryonic mesoderm proliferates and separates bilaminar germ disc, amniotic cavity and yolk sac with exocoelomic membrane from trophoblastic shell

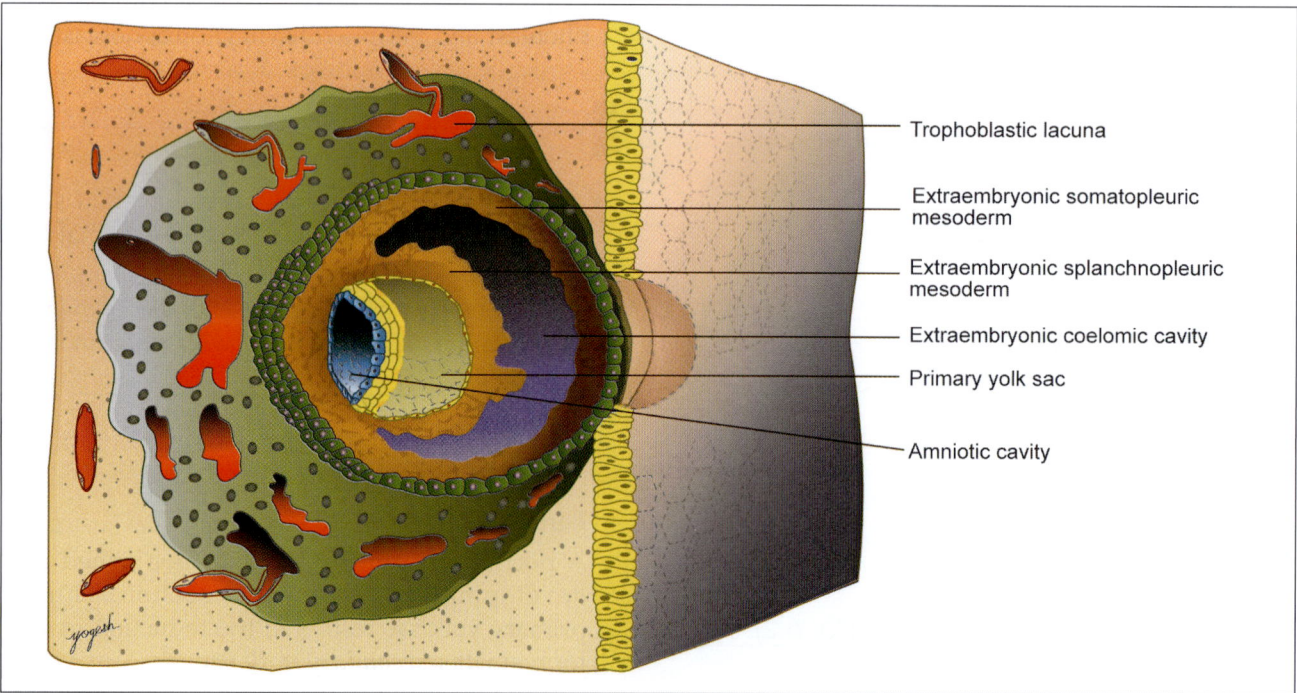

Fig. 6.5: Day 12–13: Formation of extraembryonic splanchnopleuric and somatopleuric mesoderm. Extraembryonic coelomic cavities fuse and divide extraembryonic mesoderm into two layers—somatopleuric and splanchnopleuric layers

Second Week of Development

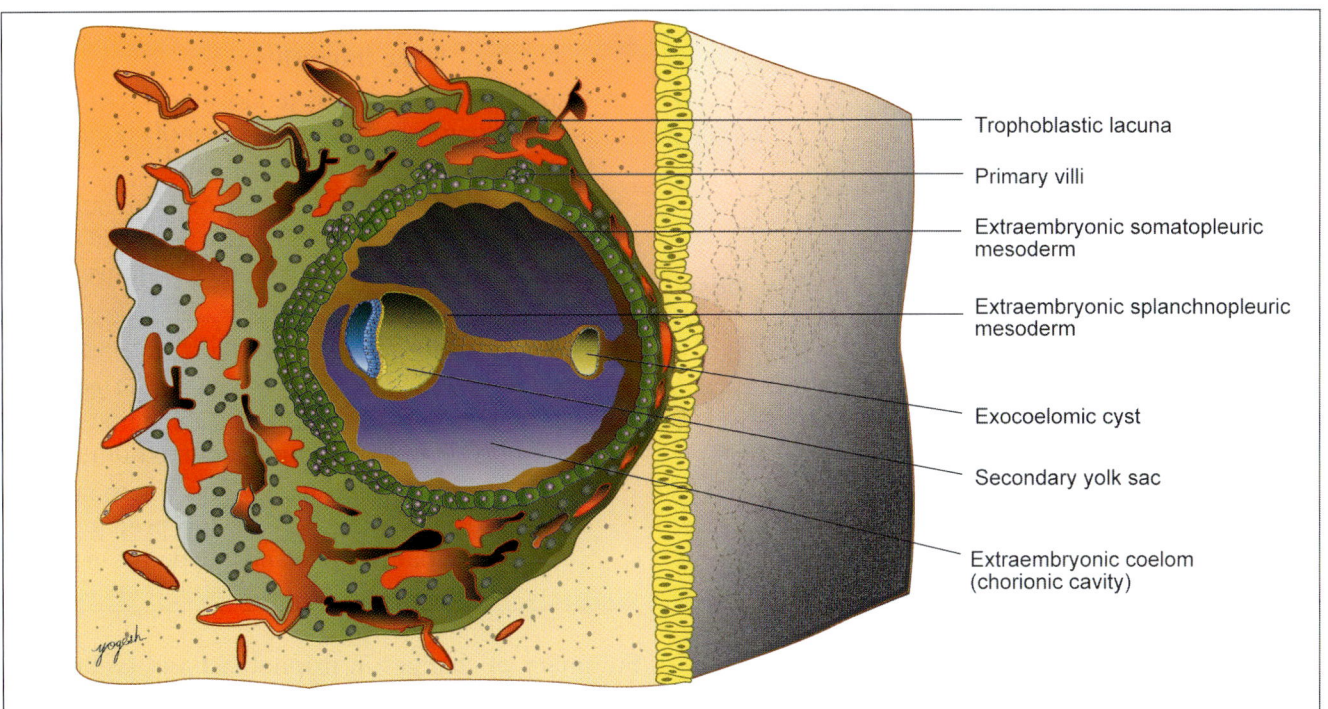

Fig. 6.6: Day 13: Development of extraembryonic coelom and formation of secondary yolk sac. Enlarged cavity of extraembryonic coelom pinch primary yolk sac and forms smaller secondary yolk sac and exocoelomic cyst. Developing embryo is connected with trophoblast by connecting stalk (future umbilical cord). Protruding cytotrophoblast forms primary villi. Cytotrophoblast proliferates in syncytiotrophoblast to form primary villi

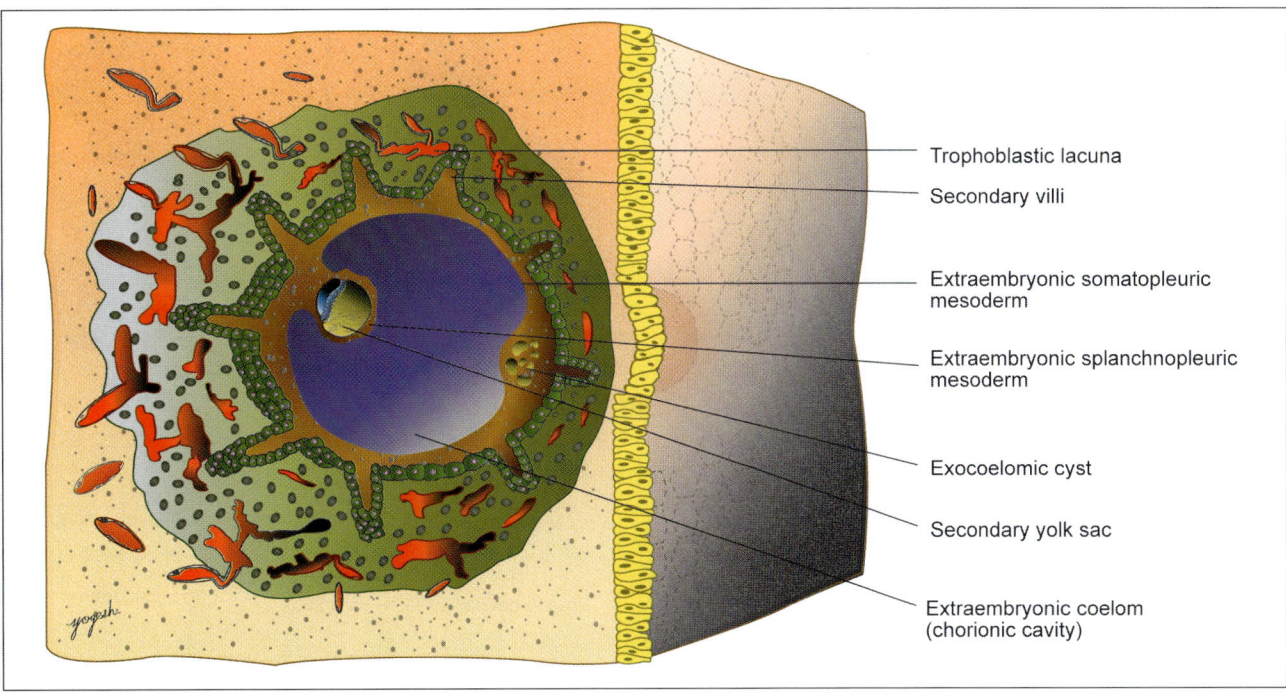

Fig. 6.7: Day 13–14: Exocoelomic cavity enlarges and push developing germ disc with yolk sac towards embryonic pole. Exocoelomic cysts break up to a collection of vesicles at the abembryonic end of the chorionic cavity and get absorbed slowly

- **Formation of prechordal plate** (Fig. 6.8, Practice Fig. 6.3)

Q. Write short note on prechordal plate.

Hypoblast cells become columnar in a small area near cranial end of germ disc (head end). This small circular area is called *prechordal plate*.

- **Significance of prechordal plate** [MCQ]
  - It shows the first sign of differentiation.
  - It establishes *cephalocaudal axis* (head and tail ends).
  - It is an important *organiser* of head region.

Some Interesting Facts

- Transvaginal sonography (endovaginal sonography) is useful for measuring the diameter of chorionic sac to evaluate embryonic development.
- Human chorionic gonadotrophin radio immunoassay or ultrasonography can be used for detection implantation (pregnancy) by the end of second week. [MCQ]
- **Prevention of implantation**
  - Implantation can be prevented in contraception by:
    - Using intrauterine devices (IUD): IUD (copper-T) inhibits implantation due to induction of local inflammation of uterine endometrium.
    - Using low dose estrogen pills (morning pills): These pills interfere with the preparation of endometrium for implantation during menstrual cycle.

Summary of changes in trophoblast and embryoblast is given in Flowcharts 6.1 and 6.2.

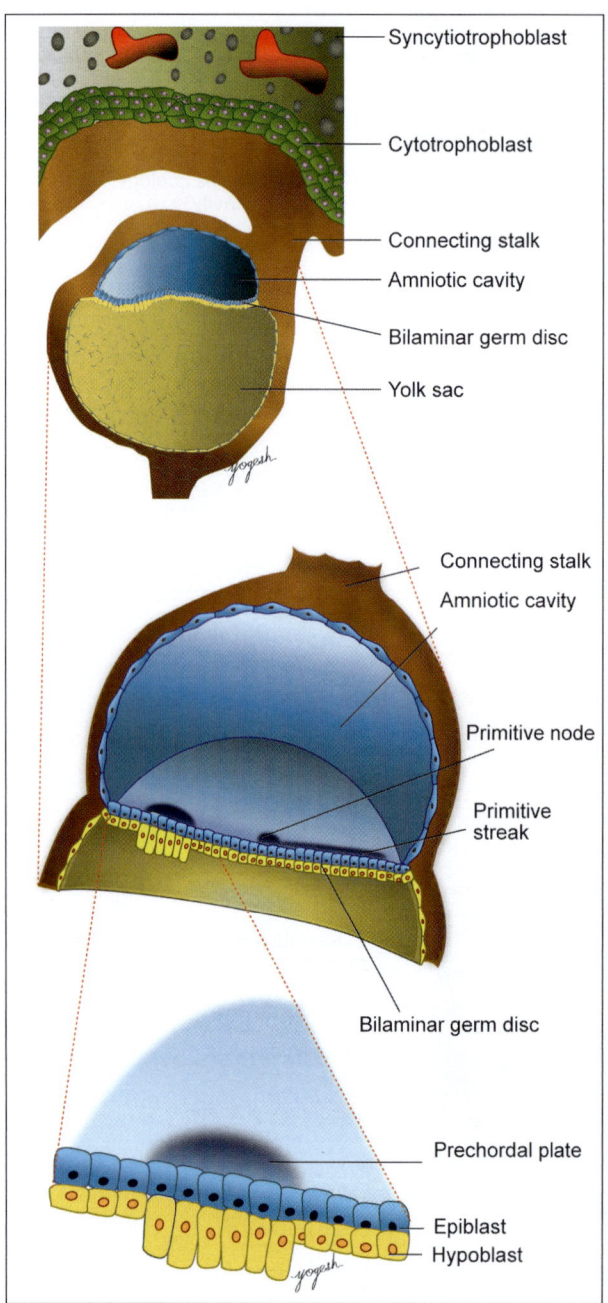

Fig. 6.8: Bilaminar germ disc seen on section through amnion and secondary yolk sac. Hypoblast cells become columnar in a small area near the cranial end of the germ disc (head end). This small circular area is called prechordal plate

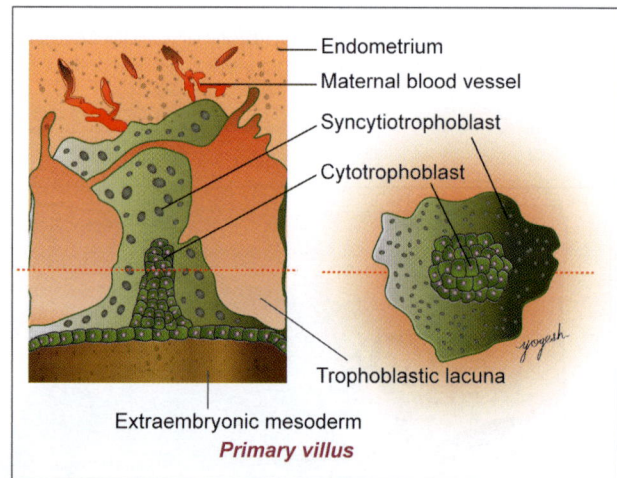

Fig. 6.9: Formation of primary villi. Cytotrophoblast invades syncytiotrophoblastic villi to form primary villi

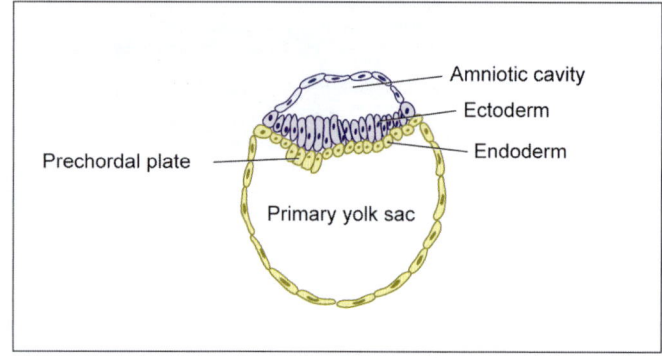

Practice Fig. 6.3: Formation of prechordal plate

Second Week of Development

Flowchart 6.1: Trophoblastic changes in the second week

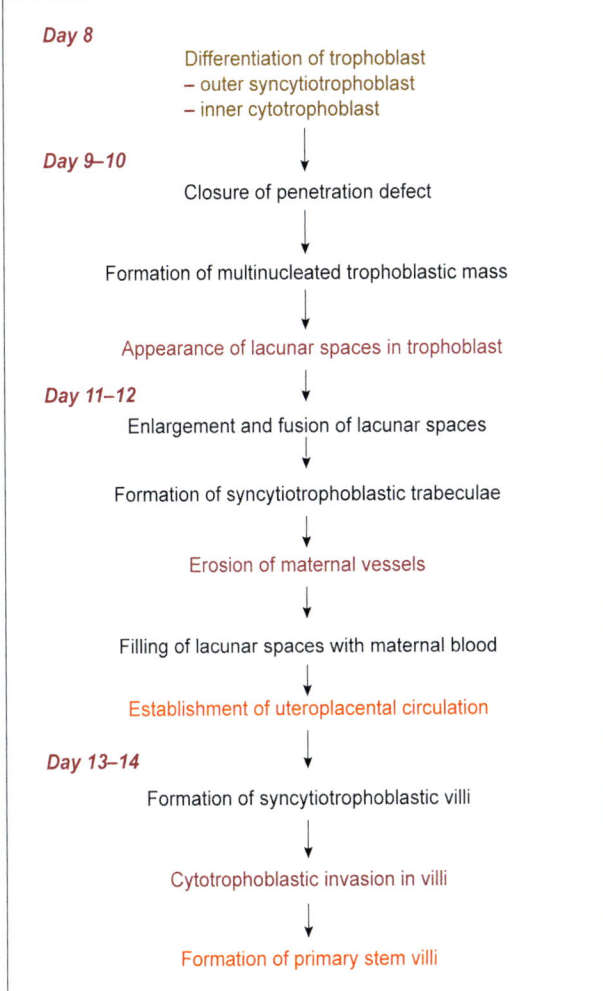

Flowchart 6.2: Changes in embryoblasts in the second week

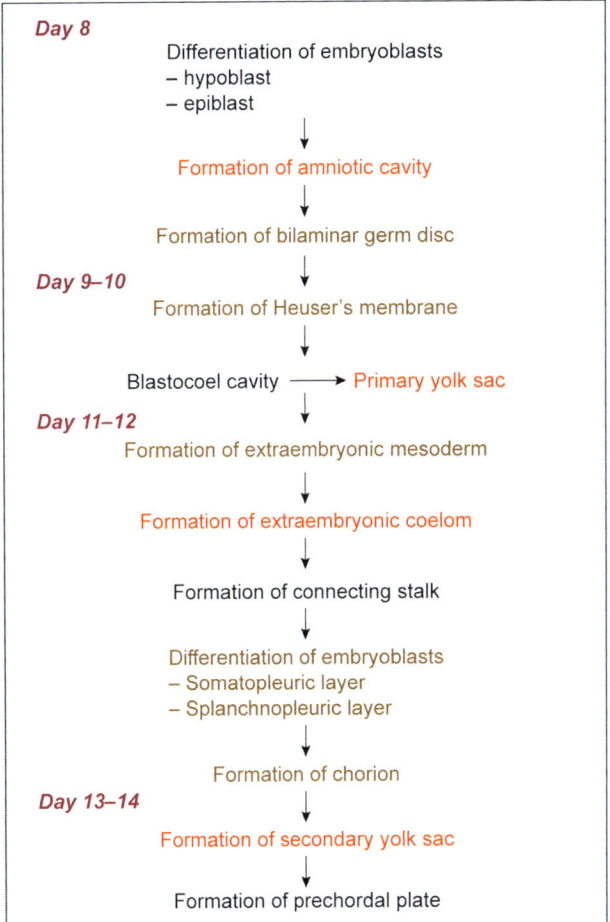

Box 6.1: Yolk sa

- Yolk sac (umbilical vesicle) attains full development and reaches its maximum size by 32nd day of IUL (4–5 weeks).[Neet]
- Yolk sac is visible from 5th to 20th week after which it becomes invisible on ultrasonography.
- Yolk sac in human is essential because
    1. It gives nutrition to embryo in 2nd and 3rd weeks.[Neet]
    2. It is a source for primordial germ cells.[Neet]
    3. It is the first organ for haematopoietic germ cells.[Neet]
    4. Incorporated part of the yolk sac forms gut tube endoderm and it gives rise to lung buds (trachea, bronchi, parenchyma of lungs) and gastrointestinal duct.[Neet]

Box 6.2: Foetus as graft

Q. Explain 'why conceptus is not rejected by its mother'.[Viva]

- Allograft is the transfer of tissue from one member of species to another member of species. Here, foetus is the allograft for mother (human to human).
- Mother accepts the foetus (conceptus) without inducing any immune reactions.
- Antigens (from conceptus) bound to the major histocompatibility complex (MHC) molecules that induce immune reaction on exposure to host's (mother) T cells, but there is no such response during pregnancy.
- Probable reasons (Medawar, 1953): (Fig. 6.10)
    1. Physical separation: Trophoblast separates foetus from mother. Trophoblast poorly expresses MHC molecules.
    2. Tolerant maternal immune system: Specific hormonal conditions make maternal immune

Contd.

Contd.

system nonresponsive to the foetal tissue, even for a few foetal circulating cells in maternal blood. Mother during pregnancy is not having suppressed immunity for infections.
3. **Antigenically immature conceptus:** Conceptus is not antigenically mature. Hence, conceptus cannot induce an antigenic reaction.
4. **Apoptosis of activated maternal T cells:** Trophoblast produces a tumour necrotic factor (TNF) that induces apoptosis in maternal activated T cells.

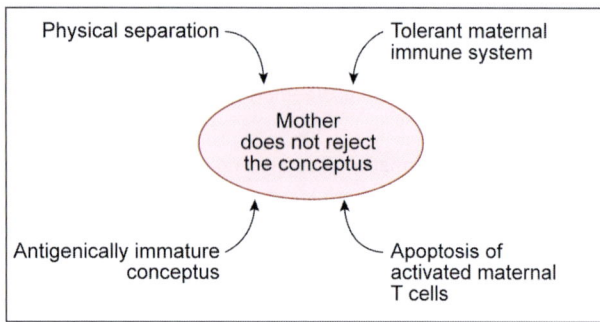

Fig. 6.10: Reasons for non-rejection of foetus by mother

GENOMIC IMPRINTING

Q. Write short note on genomic imprinting.

- In experimental studies, zygote containing two male pronuclei gives rise to only the trophoblastic mass (similar to hydatidiform mole), whereas zygote containing two female pronuclei gives rise to only nonsurviving embryoblast. This fact indicates that genomic contribution of both the parents is essential for healthy foetal development.
- **Cause**
  - Genomic imprinting is a phenomenon that involves expression of a gene depending on its maternal or paternal origin. (*Source*: Sontakke YA. *Clinical Genetics*, Chapter 4, Chromosomal aberration, 1st ed. 2017).
  - Basis of genomic imprinting is methylation of DNA that leads to gene silencing or activation.
  - DNA of female germline is more methylated than DNA of male germ lines.
  - In primordial germ cells, imprints (methylation) are erased and they again get established during gametogenesis. Hence, during spermatogenesis male specific patterns and oogenesis female-specific patterns (methylation) are formed.
- Genomic imprinting affects inheritance of congenital disease.
- For example, deletion of long arm of chromosome 15 (15q11.2–913) results in Prader-Willi syndrome if inherited from the father, whereas Angelman syndrome is inherited from the mother (*Source*: Sontakke YA. Clinical Genetics, Chapter 4, Chromosomal aberration, 1st ed. 2017).$^{MCQ, Viva}$

Box 6.3: X chromosome inactivation

Q. Write a short note on X chromosome inactivation.

- In female embryoblast, one of the two X chromosomes is inactivated irrespective of its parental source; however, in trophoblast of female blastocyst, paternal X chromosome is inactivated.
- **Process:** Inactivation of X chromosome involves expression of a particular X chromosome locus *Xist* (X inactive specific transcript gene) that produces methylation of X chromosome.^{MCQ}
- Inactivated X chromosome lacks histone H4 acetylation and it results in the condensation of X chromosome to form *Barr body*.
- Inactive X chromosome is reactivated only in the early foetal life and remains dormant throughout remaining life.

ENDOMETRIAL CHANGES

- During implantation, blastocyst sinks in the endometrium due to the invading capacity of trophoblasts.
- Blastocyst is completely embedded in the endometrial stroma by 12th day of development.^{MCQ}
- Site of penetration is initially sealed by fibrin and coagulation plug and later healed by lining epithelial of endometrium.
- Blastocyst lies in the stratum compactum of endometrium. Stratum compactum sheds off during child birth; hence, it is called *decidua*. Part of decidua that lies deep to blastocyst is *decidua basalis*, thus trophoblast invades only decicua basalis.^{Neet}
- **Decidual reaction:** ^{Viva}

  Q. Explain decidual reaction.

  It involves the following changes:
  - Increased hormonal levels during pregnancy increase glycogen and lipids deposited in decidual cells.^{MCQ}
  - Intracellular substances also increase.
  - Decidua becomes oedematous.
  - Tortuosity of endometrial gland increases.

7
Third Week of Development

Chapter Outline

- Gastrulation
- Notochord
- Allantois
- Development of chorionic villi
- Formation of neural tube
- Neural crest

INTRODUCTION

Q. Enlist the major events of third week of gestation.

- The third week of development begins after five weeks of onset of the last menstrual period.
- Characteristics of the third week of development are as follows:
  1. Formation of primitive streak[Neet]
  2. *Gastrulation*: Formation of three germ layers[Neet]
  3. Formation of notochord[Neet]
  4. Formation of allantois
  5. Formation of neural plate, neural tube and neural crest
  6. Development of chorionic villi
  7. Formation of somites
  8. Formation of intraembryonic coelom

GASTRULATION (FORMATION OF GERM LAYERS)

Q. Write short note on gastrulation.

Definition

- Gastrulation is a process of convention of **bilaminar** embryonic disc to **trilaminar** disc during the ***third week*** of development.[Neet,Viva]

Steps (Flowchart 7.1)

- Bilaminar embryonic disc of second week continue its development (Figs 7.1 to 7.4, Practice Figs 7.1 and 7.2).

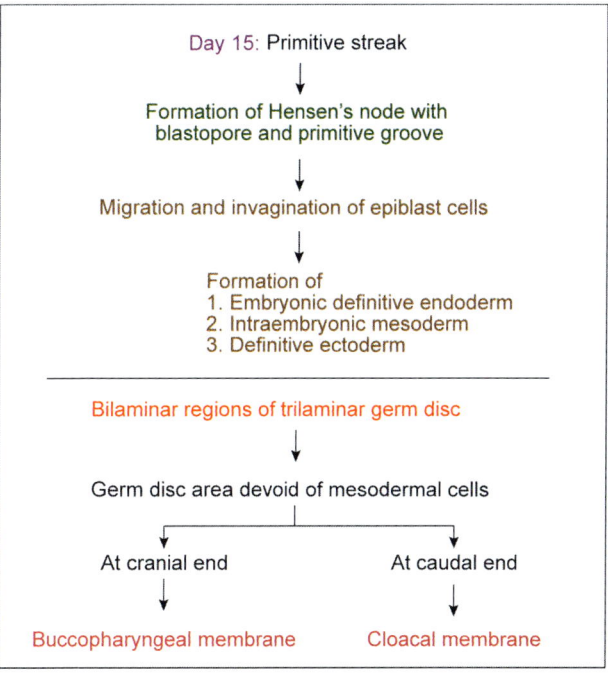

Flowchart 7.1: Process of gastrulation

- On 15th day, **primitive streak** appears that **induces** gastrulation. Primitive streak is a thickened linear band of **epiblast** in midline **at the caudal end** on the dorsal part of embryonic disc.[Neet] Formation of primitive streak is an indicator/first sign of the start of gastrulation.[Neet]
- Elevated cranial end of primitive streak form a primitive node (**Hensen's node** or primitive knot)

Human Embryology

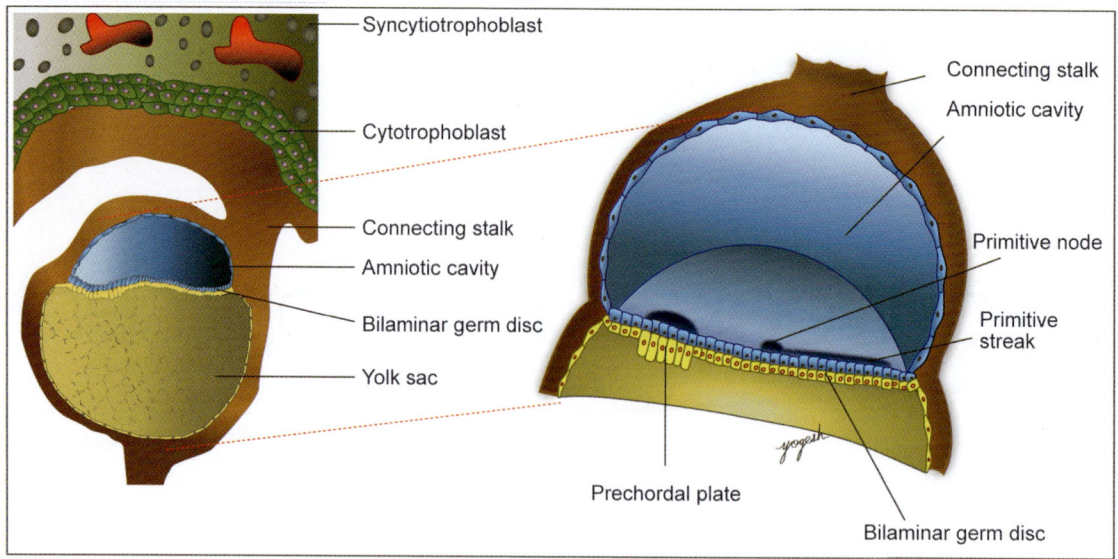

Fig. 7.1: Bilaminar germ disc at the end of second week. Hypoblast cells become columnar in a small area near the cranial end of the germ disc (head end). This small circular area is called prechordal plate

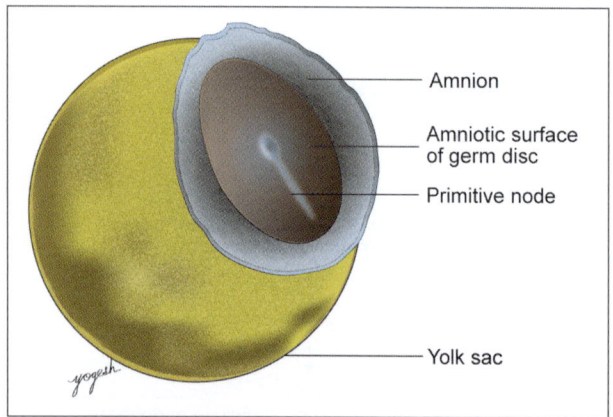

Fig. 7.2: Formation of the primitive streak (Day 16: Side view)

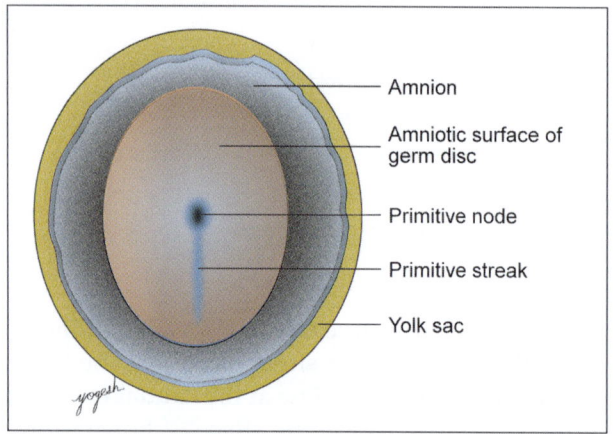

Fig. 7.3: Formation of primitive streak (Day 16: Top view)

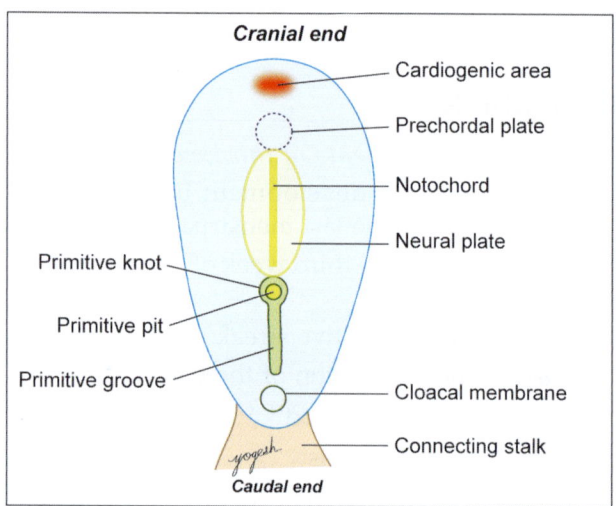

Practice Fig. 7.1: Germ disc showing notochord, primitive pit, primitive knot, primitive groove and cloacal membrane

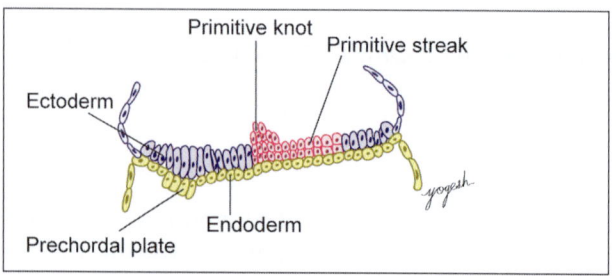

Practice Fig. 7.2: Bilaminar germ disc showing primitive knot and primitive streak

Third Week of Development

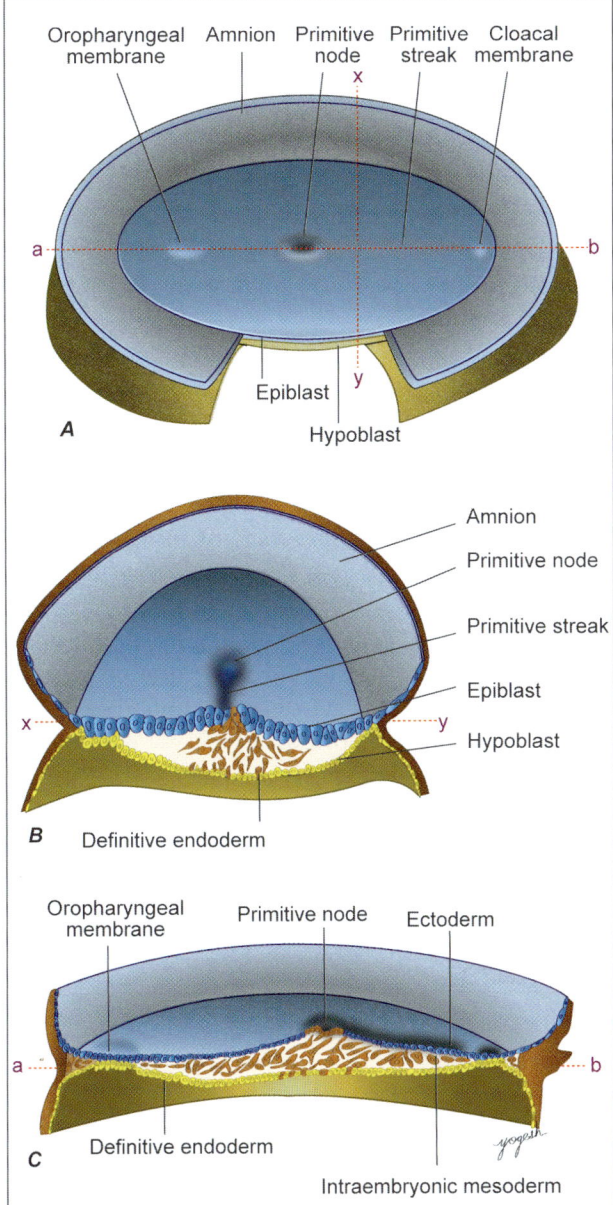

Fig. 7.4: 15–16-day embryo: (A) Gastrulation: Formation of intra-embryonic mesoderm and definitive endoderm. Cells migrate from primitive streak and node to invaginate between hypoblast and epiblast. Migrated cells replace cells of hypoblast to form definitive endoderm and remaining cells form intra-embryonic mesoderm; (B) Germ disc is cut along the transverse axis in between primitive node and cloacal membrane; (C) Germ disc is cut along the longitudinal axis

that surrounds a depressed pit called primitive pit or **blastopore.**
- Germ disc and primitive streak elongates craniocaudally.
- A narrow depressed central area of primitive streak called **primitive groove** develops.
- Epiblast cells **migrate** toward primitive streak. The migrating cells invaginate and detach from primitive streak.

- Invaginated cells (SEM 7.1 and 7.2)
  1. Displaces hypoblast cells to form embryonic definitive **endoderm.**
  2. Form a layer between endoderm and epiblast—known as **intraembryonic mesoderm** by the process of epithelial to mesenchymal transformation (EMT).
- Remaining cells (non-invaginating cells) of epiblast form definitive **ectoderm.**
- *Thus, epiblast forms all three germ layers by gastrulation.*[Neet, Viva]
- Migrating mesodermal cells establish contact with extra-embryonic mesoderm at lateral end of the germ disc.
- Migrating mesoderm separates ectoderm from endoderm except at two places: Cranially at buccopharyngeal membrane and caudally at cloacal membrane (Fig. 7.5, Practice Fig. 7.3[Neet]).
- **Buccopharyngeal membrane or oral membrane:**
  – It is a small oval depressed area at cranial end of the germ disc and it appears in prechordal plate.

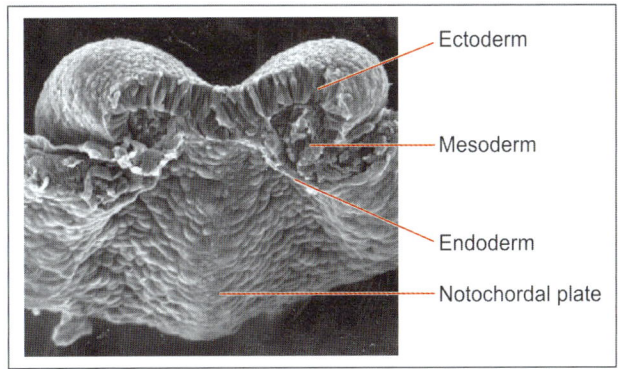

Scanning electron micrograph 7.1: SEM showing three germ layers. A cut through anterior end of embryo illustrates three germ layers: Ectoderm, mesoderm and intraembryonic endoderm. The mesoderm in ventral midline is notochordal plate [Species: Mouse, approximate human age: 17 days, ventral view]

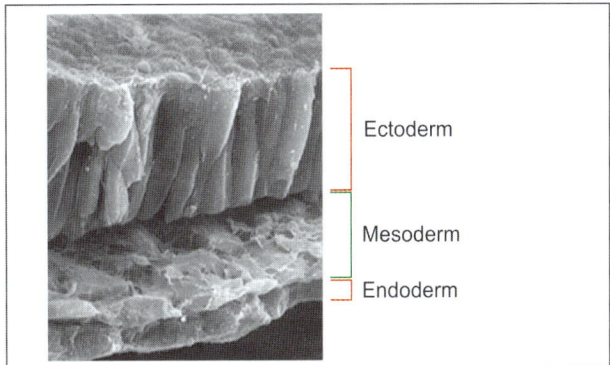

Scanning electron micrograph 7.2: SEM showing three germ layers in high magnification. A cut through the embryo illustrates the three germ layers: Ectoderm, mesoderm, and endoderm [Species: Mouse, approximate human age: 17 days, dorsal view]

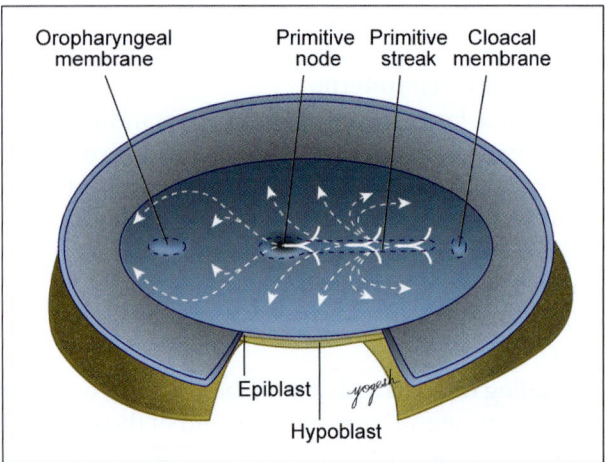

Fig. 7.5: Day 16: Germ disc showing a path for the movement of surface epiblast cells (white solid arrows) through the primitive streak and node and their subsequent migration between the hypoblast and epiblast (white dashed arrows) during gastrulation

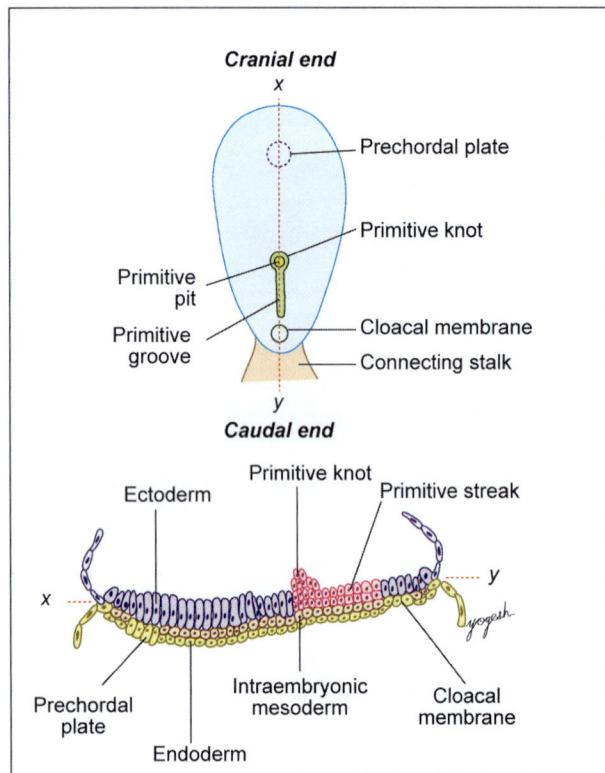

Practice Fig. 7.3: Formation of intraembryonic mesoderm

- In buccopharyngeal membrane, endodermal cells are firmly adherent with ectodermal cells.
- It is bilaminar as it is devoid of mesodermal cells.
- Oropharyngeal membrane breaks down in fourth week to form opening of oral cavity.^{MCQ}
- **Cloacal membrane**
  - At caudal end of primitive streak, germ disc remains bilaminar due to firm endodermal attachment with ectoderm. This small circular bilaminar area is called cloacal membrane.
  - Later, on further development, cloacal membrane divides into anal and urogenital membranes.
  - Cloacal membrane disintegrates in seventh week to form opening of anus, urethra and genital tracts.^{MCQ}
- **Pericardial bar**
  - It is midline horseshoe shaped mesodermal cell condensation that is cranial to the buccopharyngeal membrane.

Box 7.1: Cellular basis of primitive streak formation
- **Koller's sickle** or **Rauber's sickle** is a local thickening of extraembryonic tissue at the caudal edge of germ disc.^{MCQ}
- Koller's sickle induces adjacent epiblast to form primitive streak by cell–cell interactions at the caudal end of germ disc.
- Cellular basis of primitive streak formation involves four major processes, that is cell migration, oriented cell division, progressive delamination from epiblast and convergent extension.^{MCQ}
- Primitive streak formation is initiated and maintained by expression of nodal gene.^{Neet}
- Nodal gene is a member of transforming growth factor β (TGF-β) superfamily.^{Neet}

NOTOCHORD

Q. Write short note on notochord.

Definition

- Notochord is a midline embryonic structure that develops during **third week** of development from cells of primitive node, that is, **epiblast**.^{Neet}
- Axial mesoderm (chordamesoderm) is a mesoderm that lies along the central axis and it will give rise to notochord.^{Neet}

Extent

- From cranial end of primitive streak to prechordal plate.

Formation of Notochord (Fig. 7.6, Flowchart 7.2, Practice Fig. 7.4)

- Cells of primitive knot proliferate and from depression called *primitive pit*. In lower animals, primitive pit is also called *blastopore*.
- On 17th–18th day, proliferated cells invaginate between ectoderm up to prechordal plate to form **solid cord** called **notochordal process** or head process.

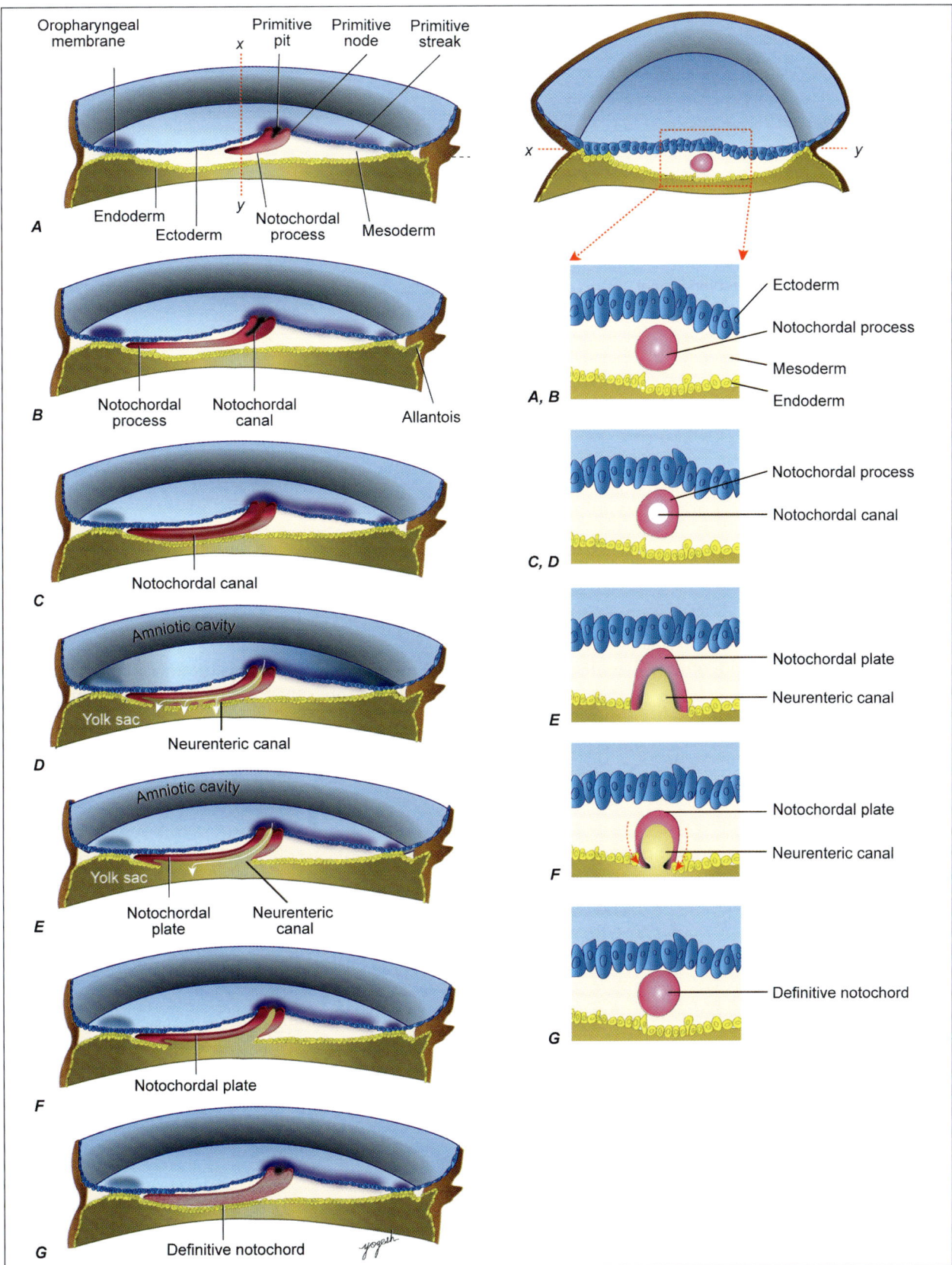

Fig. 7.6: Formation of notochord: (A) At 16th day, cells of primitive node proliferate and form notochordal process; (B) Notochordal process proliferates and extends up to oropharyngeal membrane; (C) Notochordal canal develops in the centre of notochordal process by extension of primitive pit; (D and E) Cells of the floor of notochordal plate and adjoining endodermal cells disappear to form neurenteric canal; (F) Cells of the roof of the neurenteric canal form notochordal plate; (G) Notochordal plate folds to form solid mass of cells *definitive notochord*

Flowchart 7.2: Formation of notochord

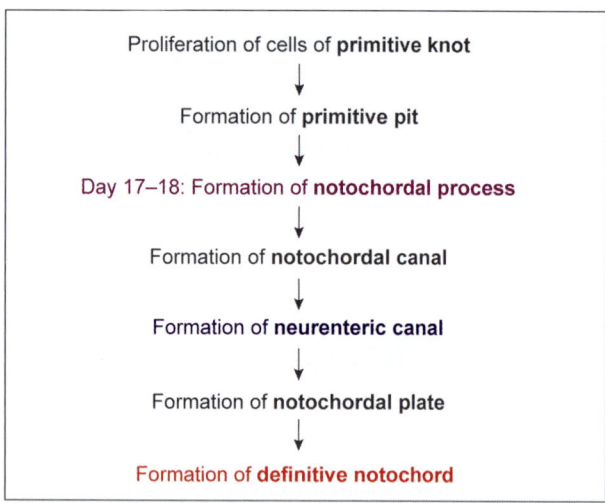

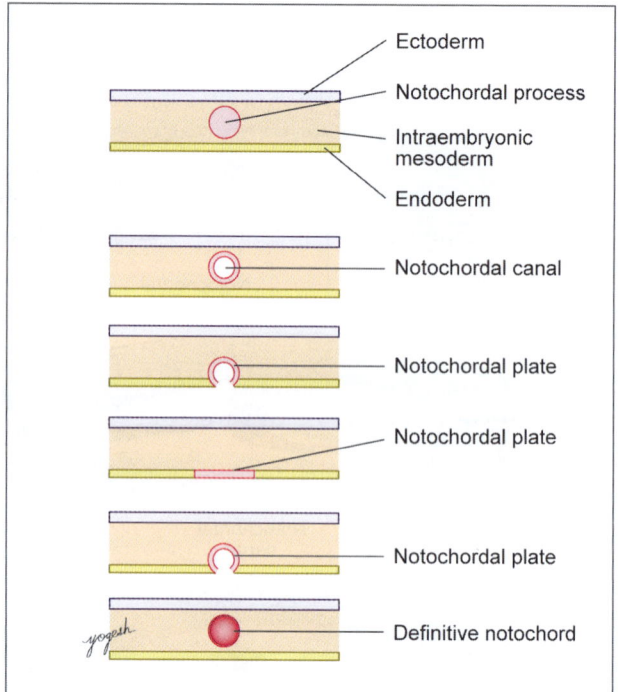

Practice Fig. 7.4: Formation of notochord

Box 7.2: Cellular basis of gastrulation

- During gastrulation, cells undergo morphogenetic movements as follows:
  1. **Epiboly**: Epiboly is spreading of an epithelial sheet.
  2. **Emboly**: Emboly or internalisation is movement of cells into interior of an embryo.
  3. **Convergence**: It is movement of cells toward midline.
  4. **Extension**: It is lengthening in cranial caudal plane.
- Morphogenetic changes include changes in cell shape, size, position, number, cell to cell and cell to extracellular matrix adhesion.
- Epithelial to mesenchymal transformation involves changes in cell to cell adhesion, cell shape and changes in cytoskeleton.
- **Snail gene *(zinc finger transcription factor)*** expression represses epithelial characteristics in mesenchymal cells.
- Snail gene ceases E-cadherin (cell to cell adhesion molecule) and induces expression of vimentin (cytoskeletal proteins) in mesodermal cells.

Establishing medial–lateral subdivisions of mesoderm

- Mesodermal patterning involves interaction between dorsalising factors (proteins of Noggin, Chordin, Nodal, Follistatin and Cerberus genes) and ventralising factors (Bmps and Wnts).
- Low Bmp and Wnt signalling dorsalises mesoderm and induces notochord formation, whereas high expression of Bmp and Wnt signalling ventralises mesoderm and converts it to lateral plate mesoderm.^{MCQ}

Some Interesting Facts

1. Embryonic disc remains bilaminar at two places, one at buccopharyngeal membrane (prechordal plate) and another at cloacal membrane.
2. Continuous migration of cells from primitive streak towards criminal region makes disc elongated craniocaudally.
3. Cilia of cells of the primitive node may be responsible for right–left visceral side determination. Its abnormality may cause **situs inversus** (major visceral organs are reversed from their normal positions).
4. Primitive streak regresses by 26th day of intrauterine life. ^{MCQ, Viva}
5. Anterior visceral endoderm (cells at cranial margin of germ disc) produces certain transcriptions factors (OTX2, cerebrus). Primitive streak also produces transforming growth factor β, bone morphogenic protein 4, fibroblast growth factor and so on. These factors determine body axes, anteroposterior, right–left, and dorsoventral sides.
6. During epithelial to mesenchymal transformation, epiblast cells often elongate, become flask or bottle shaped, and develop pseudopodia (foot-like processes), filopodia (thinner processes) or lamellipodia (flattened processes), which allow them to migrate through primitive streak into the space between epiblast and hypoblast.

Third Week of Development

- Cavity of primitive pit extend into notochordal process to form **notochordal canal**
- Cells of notochordal canal fuse with endoderm.
- The cells of the notochord canal disappear in a craniocaudal direction to form a **communication** between amniotic cavity (via primitive pit) and yolk sac. This communication is called **neurenteric canal.**
- Neurenteric canal flattens to form **notochordal plate** in the roof of yolk sac.
- Soon, flattening of notochordal plate reverses by folding of notochordal plate.
- Cells of notochordal plate get separated from endoderm to form solid cord of cells called **definitive notochord.**

Significance of Notochord

- Notochord is a characteristic feature of phylum Chordata animals.
- Notochord **defines axis of embryo**[Neet] and forms basis for developing axial skeleton, specifically vertebral body.
- It acts as primary inducer or inductor.[Neet]
- In humans, notochord disappears except its remnants in adult represent *nucleus pulposus* of intravertebral discs or *chordomas*.[Neet] (SEM 7.3)

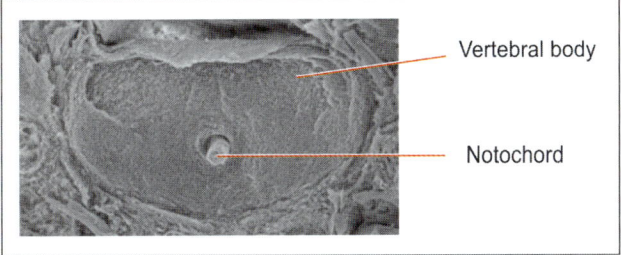

Scanning electron micrograph 7.3: SEM showing intervertebral disc and notochord that will form nucleus pulposus [Species: Mouse, approximate human age: 9 weeks, transverse view]

Box 7.3: Importance of neurenteric canal

- Neurenteric canal provides nutrition from yolk sac to rapidly differentiating ectoderm as intraembryonic blood circulation is not developed during the third week of development.[MCQ, Viva]

Box 7.4: Role of E-cadherin and FGF8

- E-cadherin is a transmembrane protein that play role in epiblast cell adhesion.
- Fibroblast growth factor 8 (FGF8) is expressed by epiblast cells. FGF8 acts as an **'organiser'** and controls cell migration.

- FGF8 inhibits E-cadherin production and thus, promotes cell migration at primitive streak and node.
- Hence, primitive node is known as **embryonic organizer** or *Spemann organizer* as it promotes formation of three germ layers (discovered by Hans Spemann and Hilda Mangold in 1924).[MCQ]

Box 7.5: Sacrococcygeal teratoma

- **Primitive streak regresses** at the end of third week of development and completely disappears by **26th day** of development.[Neet]

Cause

- Persistent **remnant** of primitive streak form tumour in coccygeal region of newborn known as *sacrococcygeal teratoma*.

Features

- It is the most common tumour in newborn (1 in 37,000 neonates).
- It is usually nonmalignant tumour.
- As derived from primitive streak (pluripotent cells), tumour contains incompletely differentiated derivatives of all the three germ layers; for example, hairs, bone, cartilage, muscles and so on.

Treatment

- Surgical removal of tumour.

Box 7.6: Teratogenic agents

- Teratogenesis is development of abnormality during germinal period (1–3 weeks of intrauterine life) or embryonic period (4–8 weeks) due to toxicity.
- Teratogenic agent exposure (radiation, infection or rays) between 15th and 18th day of development produces gross malformation.

ALLANTOIS

Q. Write short note on allantois.

Definition

- Allantois or **allantoenteric diverticulum** is an outpouching of yolk sac in connecting stalk (*allas* = sausage in Greek).

Development and Fate

- On day 16 of intrauterine life, outpouching of yolk sac in connecting stalk forms **allantois.**
- On formation of the embryonic tail fold, allantois is connected with cloaca (caudal part of hindgut).

- Part of allantois is absorbed in primitive urinary bladder, whereas the remaining part of allantois forms **urachus.**^{MCQ}
- After birth, urachus forms **median umbilical ligament.**^{MCQ}

Significance

- In birds, reptiles and some mammals, allantois acts as a reservoir of urine during embryonic life.
- In human, allantois remains small as placenta take over its function.
- Allantoic blood vessels of allantois later form umbilical vessels.

Clinical Aspects ^{MCQ,Viva}

- During second month of intrauterine life, extraembryonic part of allantois degenerates and intraembryonic portion forms urachus (median umbilical ligament after birth) and part of urinary bladder.
- **Urachal cyst**: It is a remnant of lining epithelium of urachus.
- **Urachal sinus**: It is a remnant of urachus that communicates with urinary bladder or outside the body.
- **Urachal fistula**: It is a persistent urachus that forms a passage from umbilicus to urinary bladder.

DEVELOPMENT OF CHORIONIC VILLI

Development of Fetoplacental Circulation
(Fig. 7.7)

- In second week of gestation, **primary chorionic villi** (inner cytotrophoblast and outer syncytiotrophoblast) appears.
- In the beginning of the third week, mesodermal cells penetrate in the core of primary villi to form **secondary villi.**
- By the end of the third week, mesodermal cells differentiate to form capillaries. Such villi with capillaries are called **tertiary** or **definitive chorionic villi.**
- **Anchoring villus** extends from chorionic plate to decidua basalis.
- Branches of anchoring villi forms **free villi** that floats in trophoblastic lacunar spaces. Free villi are main site for nutrient exchange.
- Development of communication between capillaries of villi, chorionic plate and connecting stalk and intraembryonic vessels form **fetoplacental circulation.**
- Cytotrophoblast cells penetrate syncytiotrophoblast and form **outer cytotrophoblast shell** that helps in the firm attachment with endometrial stroma.

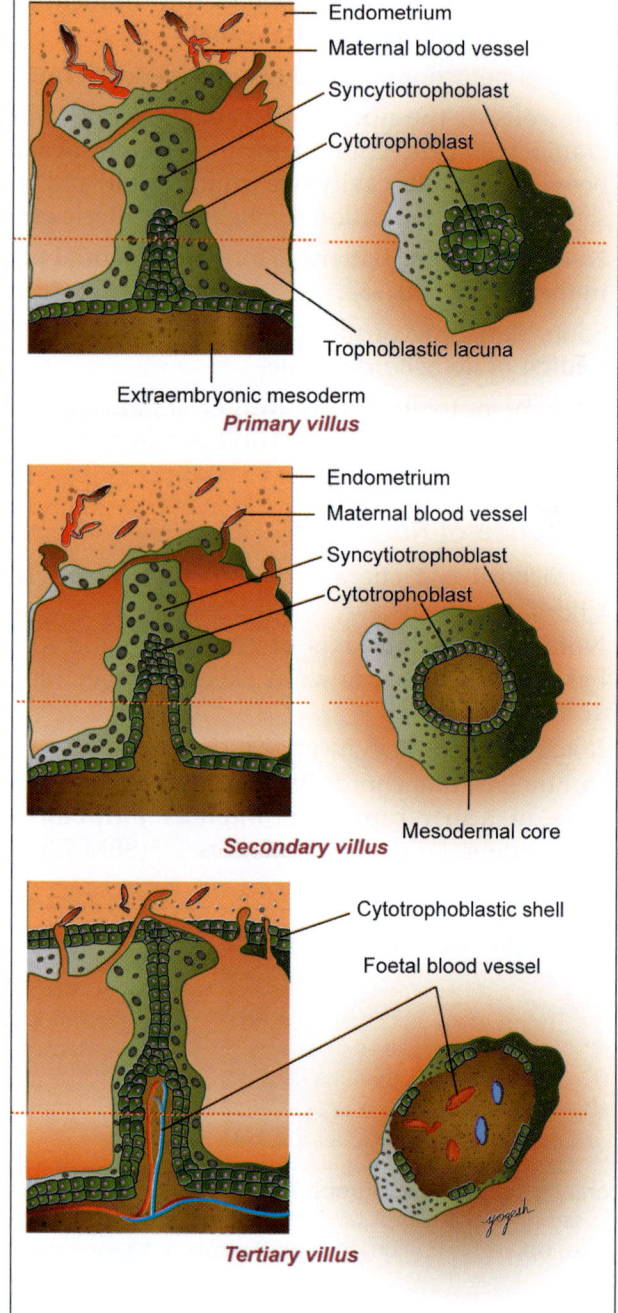

Fig. 7.7: Development of chorionic villi. Primary villi have core of cytotrophoblast under cover of syncytiotrophoblast. Secondary villi have core of mesoderm under cover of cytotrophoblast and syncytiotrophoblast. Foetal blood vessels develop in mesodermal core to form tertiary villi

Some Interesting Facts

Holoprosencephaly

- High alcohol consumption during period of gastrulation may result in holoprosencephaly.
- It includes small forebrain, fused lateral ventricles, hypotelorism (closely set eyes).

Contd.

Third Week of Development

Contd.

Sirenomelia/caudal dysgenesis
- It is also known as *mermaid syndrome*.
- Insufficient mesoderm in caudal portion of germ disc result in hypoplasia or fusion of lower limbs, anomalies of vertebrae, kidney and genital organs and imperforated anus.

Box 7.7: Fate of the germ layers
- Each of the three germ layers gives rise to specific structures as follows:
  - Ectoderm gives rise to epidermis, central and peripheral nervous system and retina.
  - Endoderm gives rise to epithelial lining of respiratory tract, gastrointestinal tract, glands opening in these tracts, pancreas, liver, gallbladder.
  - Mesoderm gives rise to musculature, bone, cartilage, cardiovascular, reproductive and excretory system.

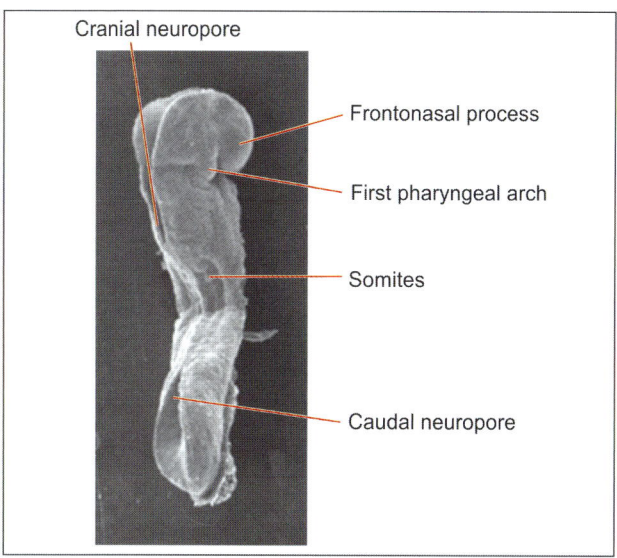

Scanning electron micrograph 7.4: SEM showing neural folding with cranial and caudal neuropores. The developing face is represented by the frontonasal region, and the first pharyngeal (branchial, visceral) arch. [Species: Mouse, approximate human age: 22 days, dorsolateral view]

FORMATION OF NEURAL TUBE/NEURULATION

Q. Define neurulation and list the steps involved in it.

Definition
- A process of formation of neural plate, neural folds and closure of these folds to form neural tube is called *neurulation*.

Process of Neurulation (Fig. 7.8, Flowchart 7.3)
- At the beginning of the third week, midline central part of **ectoderm** (in between primitive node and prechordal plate) lying above the developing notochord **thickens**. This thickened part forms **neural plate or medullary plate**.
- Elevation of edges of neural plate forms peripheral **neural folds** and central depressed part forms **neural groove**.
- Elevation of neural folds continue and starts fusion in a future cervical region and then extend in **craniocaudal direction (bidirectional)** to form neural tube. Conversion of neural plate into neural tube is called *neurulation.* Closure of neural tube begins in cervical region at the level of 5th somite.^{Neet} Recent concept: Closure of neural tube begins in multiple sites and proceeds simultaneously.
- **Cranial and caudal neuropores** are open ends of neural tube. (SEM 7.4).
- On 25th day, cranial neuropore closes, whereas on 27th day, caudal neuropore closes to form closed neural tube.^{MCQ,Viva} Closure of cranial neuropore occurs at the 20 somite stage and posterior neuropore at 25 somite stage. ^{MCQ, Viva}
- During detachment of neural tube from ectoderm, cells from lateral margins of neural plate/folds come to lie between neural tube and ectoderm and these detached cells are called **neural crest cells.** ^{MCQ, Viva}
- Neural crest cells undergo epithelial to mesenchymal transformation.^{Neet}
- Neural tube forms central nervous system and neural crest forms peripheral and autonomic nervous system.
- Prior to closer of neuropores, amniotic fluid circulates through developing neural tube to provide nutrition.

NEURAL CREST

Q. Write short note on neural crest.

Definition
- Neural crest is a portion of **lateral margins of the neural plate** at its junction with rest of ectoderm.

Process of Formation (Fig. 7.9, Practice Fig. 7.5, Flowchart 7.3)
- At the time of separation of neural tube from surface ectoderm, cells of neural crest also get separated and come to lie between ectoderm and neural tube.
- Thus, neural plate forms neural tube and neural crest cells.

Human Embryology

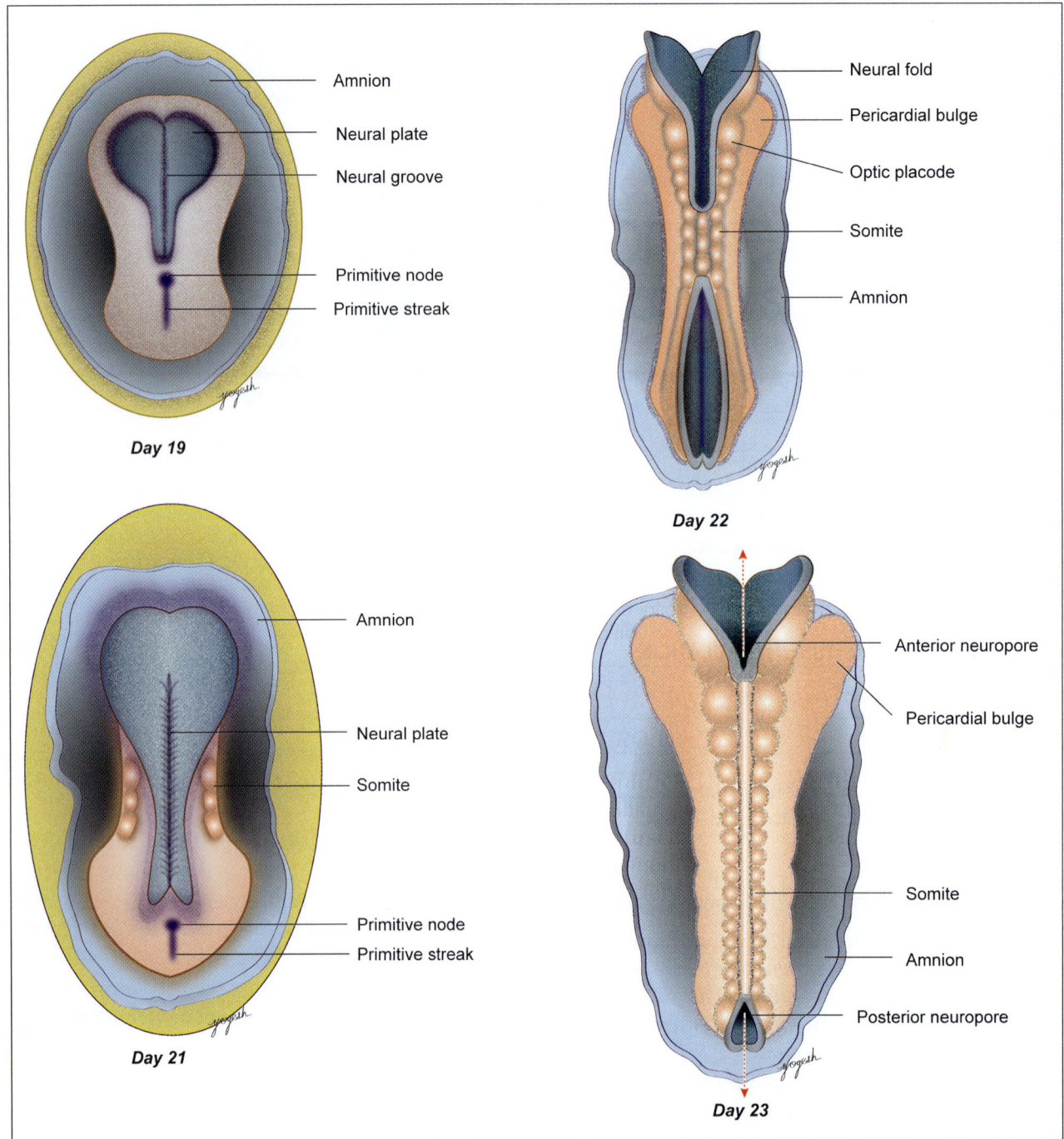

Fig. 7.8: Formation of the neural tube. Neural plate continues its folding to form neural tube

- Neural crest cells further divide to form dorsal mass and ventral mass.
- Further details about derivatives of neural crest cell are given in Chapter 22 (development of nervous system).

FURTHER DEVELOPMENT

- In the third week of IUL, neural tube formation begins and gets completed by 27th day.
- In the third week, mesodermal elements also differentiate to form paraxial mesoderm, intermediate mesoderm and lateral plate mesoderm (SEM 7.5).
- A cavity called intraembryonic coelom appears in mesoderm that divides lateral plate mesoderm into two layers (somatopleuric and splanchnopleuric).
- By the end of third week, folding of embryo begins.
- Further detailed development of mesodermal elements and folds of the embryo are included in Chapter 8.

Third Week of Development

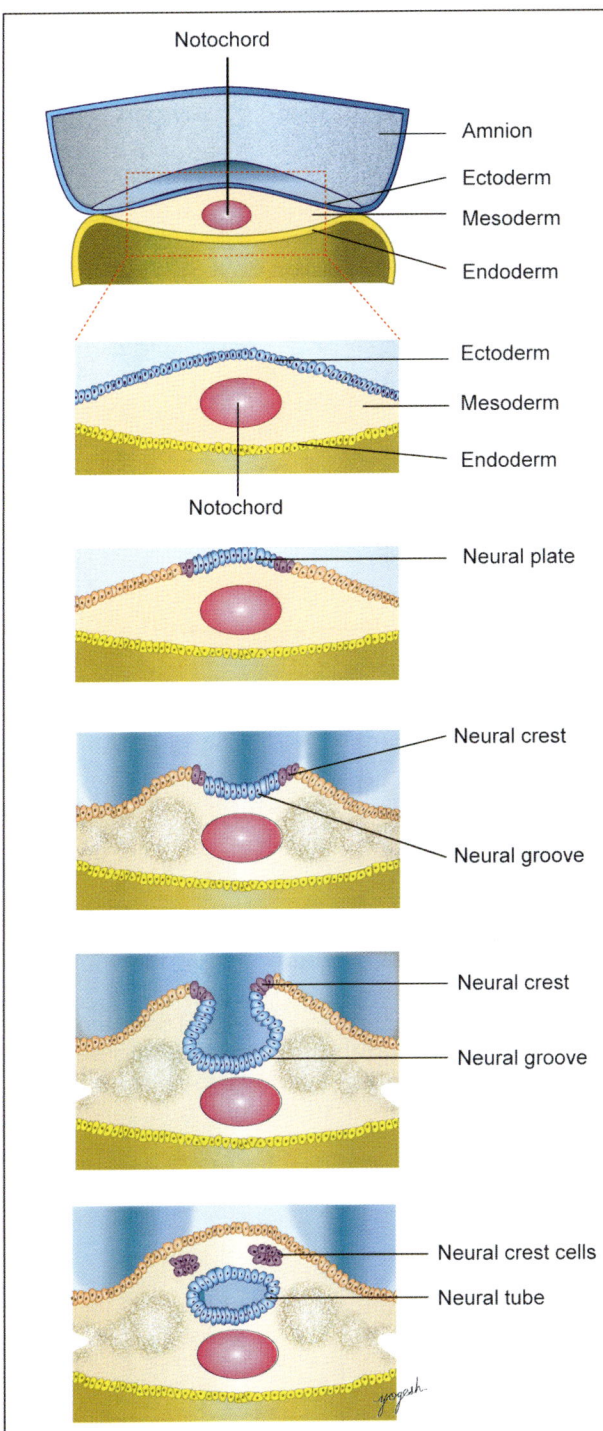

Fig. 7.9: Formation of neural tube and neural crest cells. The neural plate fold on itself to form neural tube. At the time of separation of the neural tube from the surface ectoderm, cells at the margin of the neural plate also separate to form neural crest cells. These cells lie between neural tube and the ectoderm

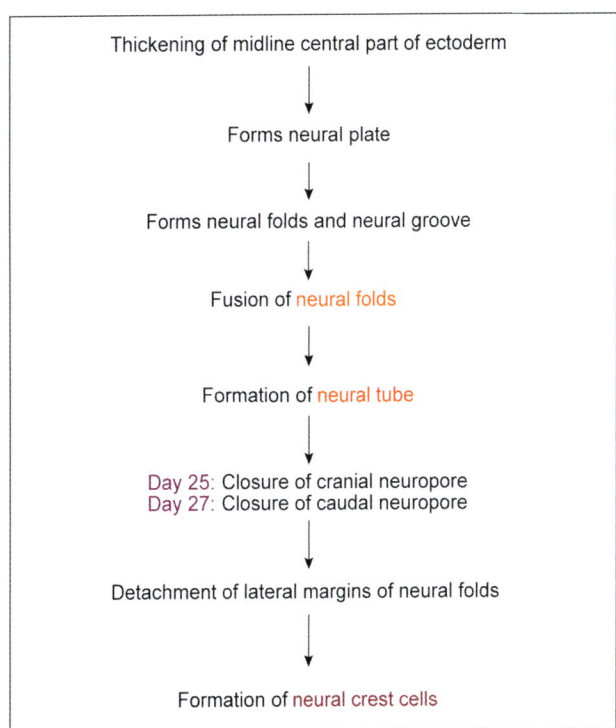

Flowchart 7.3: Process of neurulation

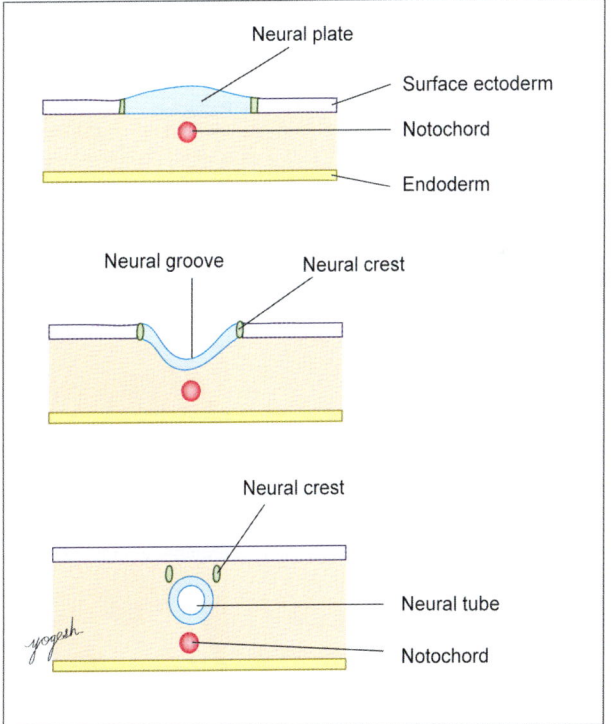

Practice Fig. 7.5: Formation of neural plate and neural crest

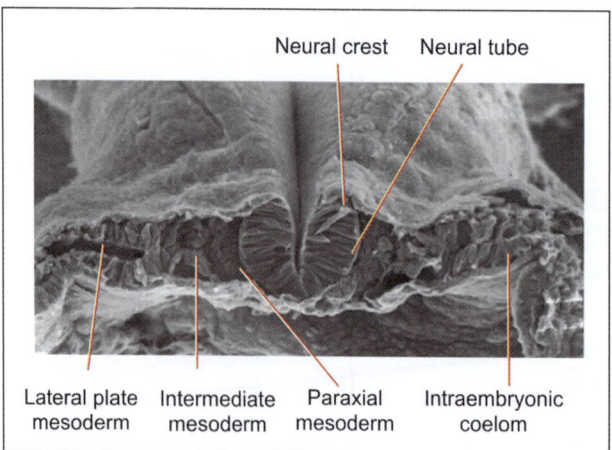

Scanning electron micrograph 7.5: SEM showing differentiation of intraembryonic mesoderm. The intraembryonic mesoderm differentiates into paraxial, intermediate and lateral plate mesoderm [Species: Mouse, approximately human age: 22 days, transverse section]

CLINICAL EMBRYOLOGY

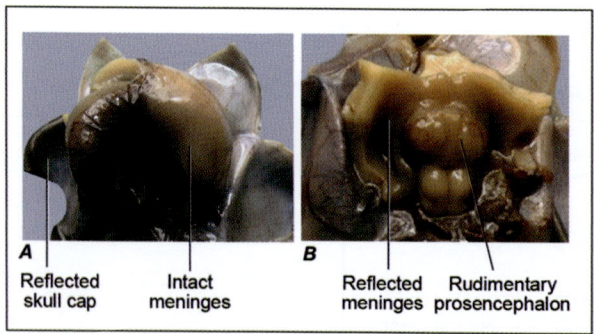

Clinical image 7.1: Holoprosencephaly (HPE) is a cephalic disorder with failure of prosencephalon (the forebrain of the embryo) development. Normally, the forebrain is formed and face begins to develop in 5th–6th weeks of intrauterine life: (A) Skull coverings are dissected to show the intact meninges. (B) Meninges are dissected to expose brain–holoprosencephaly (Image courtesy: *Dr Mamatha Gowda*)

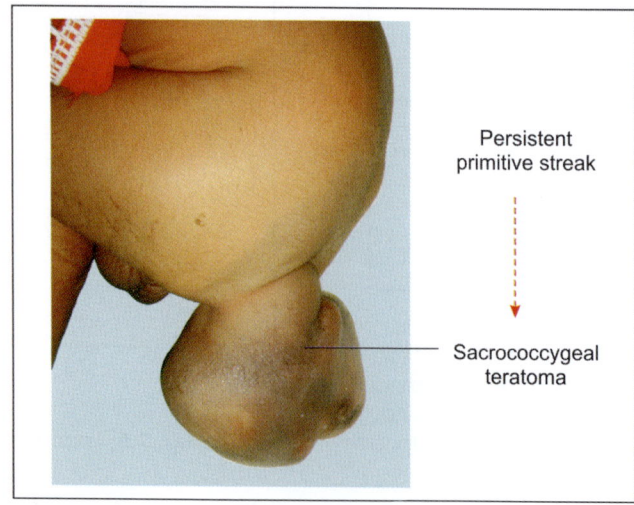

Clinical image 7.2: Sacrococcygeal teratoma. Sacrococcygeal teratoma is a tumour derived from primitive streak and it develops at the base of coccyx. Its incidence is 1 in 40,000 live births. Prenatally it can be diagnosed using sonography. Treatment of choice is the surgical removal. *Note*: Teratoma is a tumour made up of derivatives of all germ layers (ectoderm, endoderm and mesoderm) such as hairs, muscle, bone, tooth, cartilages and so on. Sometime sacrococcygeal teratoma may contain embryonic connective tissue (Image courtesy: *Dr Kumaravel S*)

8
Embryonic Period
Four to Eight Weeks of Development

Chapter Outline

- Ectodermal differentiation
  - Neuroectoderm
  - Surface ectoderm
- Mesodermal differentiation
  - Paraxial mesoderm
  - Intermediate mesoderm
  - Lateral plate mesoderm
- Embryonic folding
  - Headfold
  - Tail fold
  - Lateral fold
- Endodermal differentiation
- Changes in embryonic period

INTRODUCTION

- Period of 4th week to 8th week of development is *embryonic period*.
- During the embryonic period (4th–8th week), all derms are changing and assigning fate for further development and organ formation. Hence, the embryonic period is also called *organogenic period*.^{Neet}
- During the embryonic period, germ disc gets folded to form identifiable shape of human embryo.
- For understanding, the events of embryonic period are grouped under the following headings:
  - Ectodermal differentiation
  - Mesodermal differentiation
  - Embryonic folding
  - Endodermal differentiation
- Teratogens (factor causing embryonic malformation) affect the developing embryo to produce congenital anomalies.

Differentiation of Ectoderm

- At the beginning of the third week, the central part of ectoderm overlying the developing notochord thickens to form a neural plate or *neuroectoderm*.
- Remaining part of the ectoderm is called *surface ectoderm*.
- Ectoderm = neuroectoderm + surface ectoderm

Neuroectoderm

- Neural plate grows to form peripheral *neural folds* and a central depressed area called *neural groove* (Fig. 8.1).
- Neural folds start fusion in the central (cervical) region. Fusion extends craniocaudally to form *neural tube*.
- Cranial open end of neural tube called *anterior neuropore* closes by the 25th day of IUL (Figs 8.2 and 8.3).
- Caudal open end of neural tube called *posterior neuropore* closes by the 27th day.
- Cells at the margin of neural plate form the *neural crest*.
- Neural tube gets separated from surface ectoderm, whereas neural crest cells come to lie between ectoderm and neural tube.
- Cephalic part of neural tube shows dilations as forebrain vesicle, midbrain vesicle, and hindbrain vesicle, whereas distal part of neural tube forms spinal cord (for details, read Chapter Development of Nervous System).
- Neuroectoderm forms entire central and peripheral nervous system and autonomic ganglia.

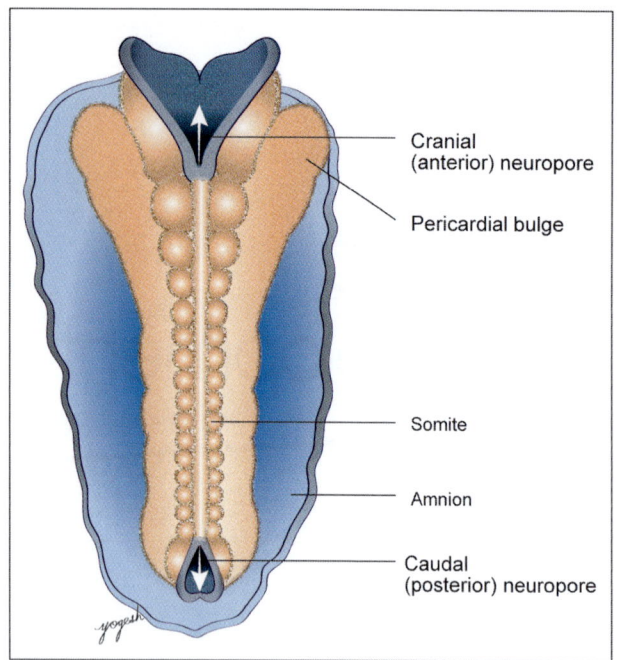

Fig. 8.1: Day 23: Top view of the developing embryo. Anterior and posterior neuropores are open

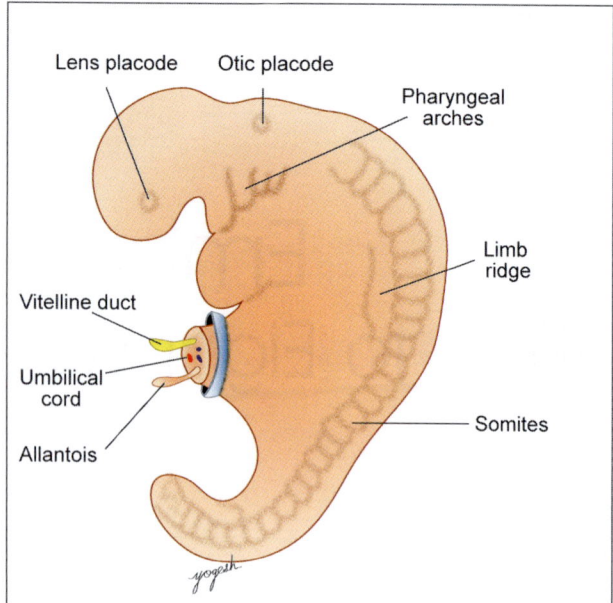

Fig. 8.3: Embryo by day 28: Side view of developing embryo. At the end of the fourth week, first four pharyngeal arches, limb ridge, otic placode and lens placode are seen

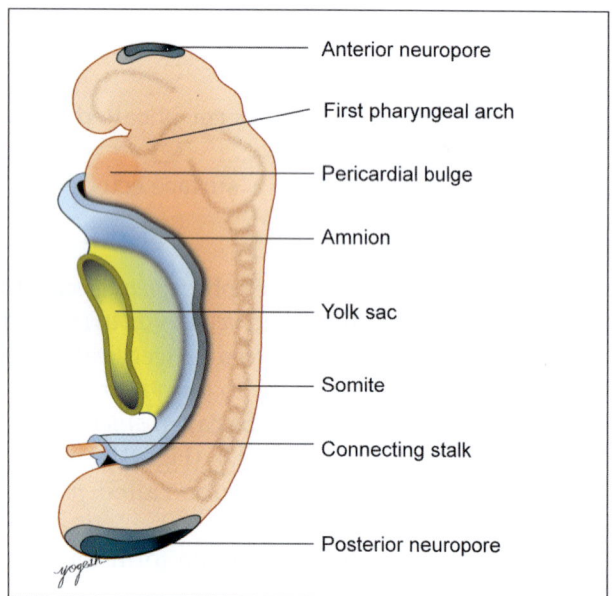

Fig. 8.2: Embryo by day 24: Side view

Surface Ectoderm

- Surface ectoderm shows depression at *buccopharyngeal membrane* and *cloacal membrane*. At these two depressions, ectoderm is firmly adherent to endoderm.

Buccopharyngeal membrane (oropharyngeal membrane)

- In the third week, it lies cranial to the prechordal plate. On development of head fold, prechordal plate comes to lie between forebrain vesicle and pericardial bulging.

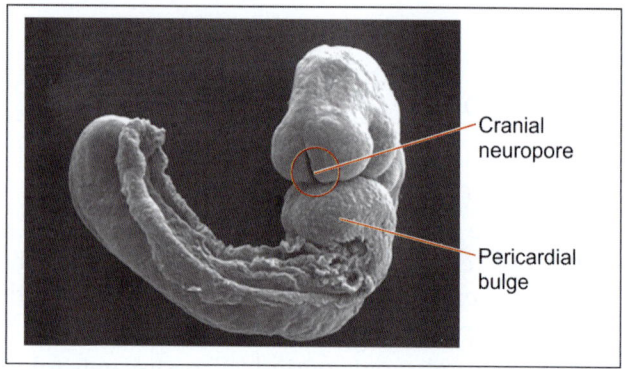

Scanning electron micrograph 8.1: SEM showing embryo at 25th day with closing anterior neuropore [Species: Mouse, approximate human age: 25 days, frontolateral view]

- At the beginning of fourth week, buccopharyngeal membrane ruptures to form communication between amniotic cavity and primitive gut.^{MCQ}
- Cloacal membrane divides into anterior urogenital membrane and posterior anal membrane (for details read Chapter 14).
- Surface ectoderm also forms the following structures:
  1. Epidermis, hair and nail
  2. Sebaceous glands and sweat glands
  3. Olfactory pit (Chapter 23)
  4. Optic vesicle and lens vesicle (Chapter 23)
  5. Otic vesicle (Chapter 24)
  6. Branchial clefts (Chapter 11)
  7. Rathke's pouch

Embryonic Period: Four to Eight Weeks of Development

8. Epithelial lining of cheek, gum, teeth enamel, root of mouth, nasal cavity and paranasal air sinuses
9. Salivary glands
10. Mammary glands
11. Pituitary glands

Some Interesting Facts
- All the muscles of the body are derived from the mesoderm except muscles of iris and arrectores pilorum of the skin are derived from ectoderm.

MESODERMAL DIFFERENTIATION

- By the end of third week, primitive streak starts regressing.
- Mesodermal cells that are migrated from primitive streak start forming rod-shaped on either side of notochord.
- Shallow longitudinal grooves separate condensed mesodermal rods into three parts (Fig. 8.4):

A. *Paraxial mesoderm*: Lies on either side of notochord underneath neural plate.
B. *Intermediate mesoderm*: Lies lateral to paraxial mesoderm.
C. *Lateral plate mesoderm*: The lateral most part of mesoderm.

- These components of mesoderm form specific structures in developing embryo.
- Mesoderm = paraxial mesoderm + intermediate mesoderm + lateral plate mesoderm.

Paraxial Mesoderm

- Paraxial mesoderm is situated on either side of notochord.
- *Extent*: It extends from prechordal plate to primitive streak.
- Paraxial mesoderm condenses to form a series of rounded, whorl-like mass called *somitomeres.*
- The somitomeres further develop a discrete block of segmental *paraxial mesoderm* called *somites* or *metameres.*^{Neet}

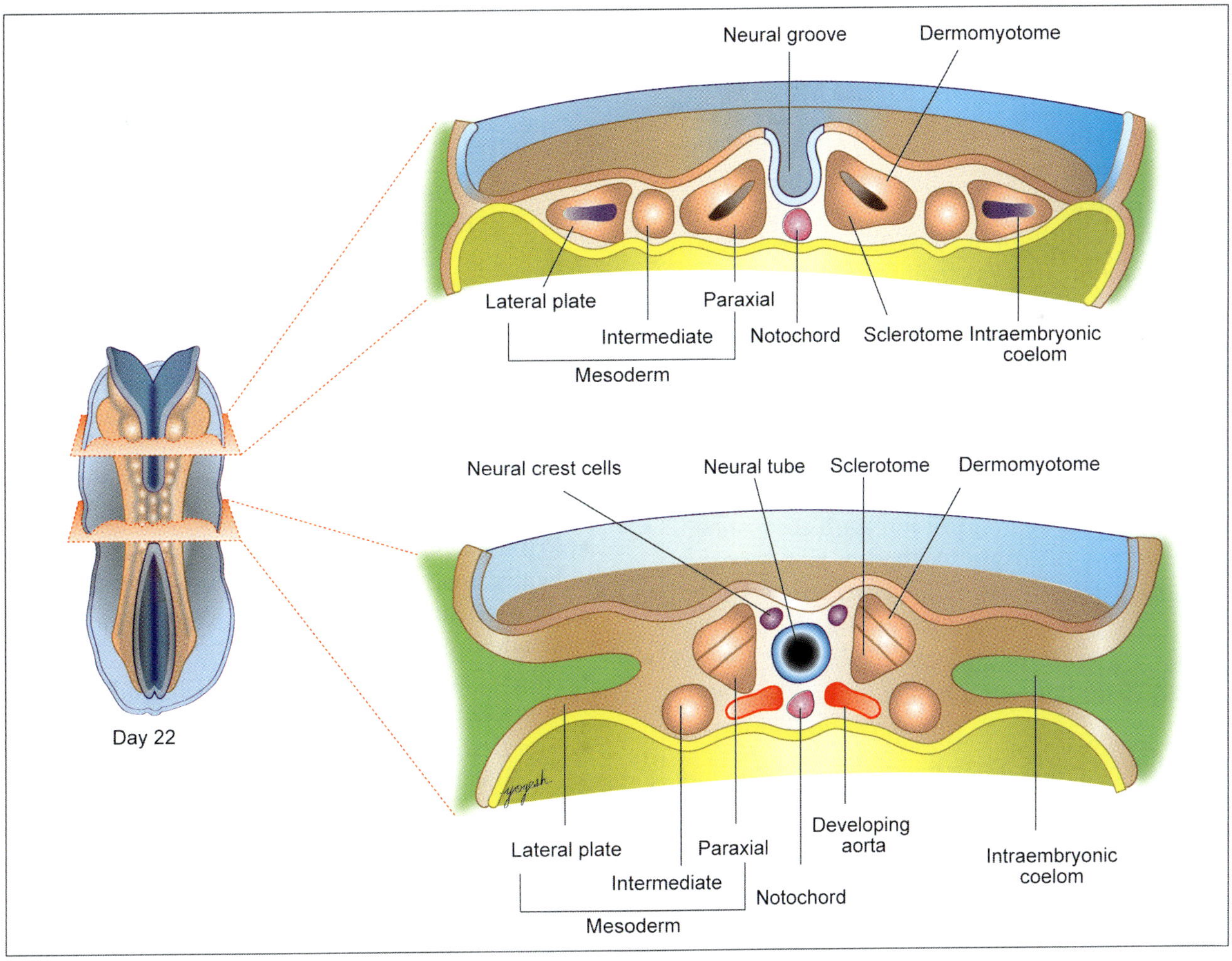

Fig. 8.4: Formation of somites

Intermediate Mesoderm

- It lies between the paraxial mesoderm and lateral plate mesoderm.
- On differentiation, intermediate mesoderm forms kidneys and sex glands (ovaries and testis).

Lateral Plate Mesoderm

- Lateral plate mesoderm extends from intermediate mesoderm to extraembryonic mesoderm.
- Cranially, lateral plate mesoderm is continued with pericardial bar. (*Pericardial bar* is mesodermal condensation cranial to the buccopharyngeal membrane.)
- Small cavities appear in the lateral plate mesoderm that fuse to form *intraembryonic coelom*.
- Similar cavity develops in pericardial bar called *pericardial sac*.

Formation of Coelomic Cavity

- Pericardial sac communicates with intraembryonic coelom to form inverted U-shaped tubular passage.
- Coelomic cavity forms pericardial, pleural and peritoneal cavities.[Neet]

Formation of Layers of Lateral Plate Mesoderm

- Intraembryonic coelom divides lateral plate mesoderm into two layers:
  A. *Somatopleuric layer*: It is a parietal layer that lies in contact with the ectoderm.
  B. *Splanchnopleuric layer*: It is a visceral layer that lies in contact with the endoderm.

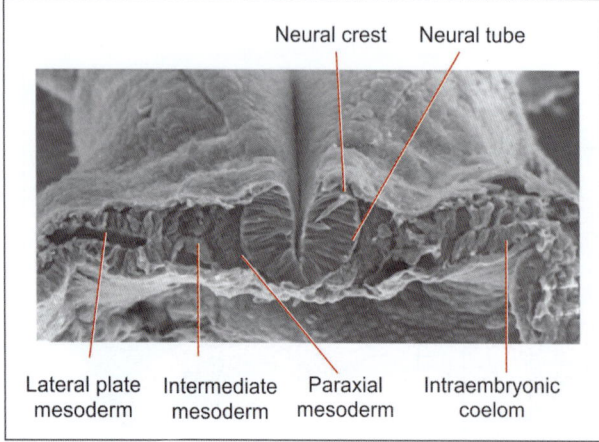

Scanning electron micrograph 8.2: Neural tube formation: SEM showing folding of neural plate and differentiation of intraembryonic mesoderm into paraxial, intermediate and lateral plate mesoderm [Species: Mouse, approximately human age: 22 days, transverse cut section]

- Continuously growing intraembryonic coelom separates somatopleuric and splanchnopleuric layers laterally and develop communication with extraembryonic coelom.
- Communication between intraembryonic and extraembryonic coelomic cavities provide nutrition till the complete development of uteroplacental circulation.
- A cranial mesodermal horseshoe-shaped bar connecting somatopleuric layer with splanchnopleuric layers is called *septum transversum*.
- Septum transversum later forms diaphragm and participate in formation of liver.

Fate of Lateral Plate Mesoderm

A. Somatopleuric layer
- It forms
  - Parietal layers of peritoneal, pericardial and pleural cavities
  - Dermis
  - Pectoral and pelvic girdles
  - Skeletal elements of limbs (muscles develop from migrating myotomes)

B. Splanchnopleuric layer
- It forms
  - Visceral layer of pericardial, peritoneal and pleural cavities
  - Musculature and connective tissue of gut, respiratory tract and heart

SOMITE

Q. Write short note on somites.

- From prechordal plate to primitive streak, the paraxial mesoderm undergoes condensation to form *somitomeres*.
- Later, somitomeres undergo segmentation to forms *somites*.
- Proximal somitomeres (underlying the developing brain, rostral to the otic vesicle) remains unsegmented and do not form somites. These forms striated muscles of face, jaw and throat.[MCQ]
- *Note*: Prechordal plate mesoderm form **preotic somites** that later forms extrinsic muscles of eye.
- The *first* pair of somites appears on day 20 on each side of the cranial end of the notochord in the occipital region (*cervical level*).[Neet, Viva]
- Somites continue to appear from day 20 to day 30 in cranio-caudal direction.
- In human, 42 to 44 pairs of somites form and they can be grouped as follows:

- Preoccipital   3 pairs
- Occipital   4 pairs
- Cervical   8 pairs
- Thoracic   12 pairs
- Sacral   5 pairs
- Coccygeal   8–10 pairs

- Many coccygeal pairs of somites eventually disappear till it reaches a final count of 37 pairs of somites.

Counting of Somites

- First somite pair appears on day 20 and further three pairs of somites get segmented each day until the end of the fifth week. Hence, somites give an idea about the foetal age (Table 8.1).[MCQ,Viva]

Table 8.1	The correlation between embryo age with a number of somites[MCQ]
Age in days (approximately)	Number of pairs of somites (approximately)
20	1–3
21	4–7
22	7–10
23	10–13
24	13–16
25	16–19
26	19–21
27	21–24
28	24–27
30	34–35
End of 5th week	42–44[Neet]

Structure of Somite

- A somite is a triangular mass of mesenchyme and it is differentiated into three parts as follows (Fig. 8.5):
    1. *Sclerotome*: It is ventromedial part and forms ribs and vertebrae.
    2. *Myotome*: It is the middle part and forms skeletal muscles. (Hence, paraxial mesoderm forms skeletal muscles through myotomes of somites.[Neet])
    3. *Dermatome*: It is dorsolateral part and it forms dermis of the skin.
- A small cavity (*myocele*) of somite is obliterated by proliferation of cells.
- Each somite is supplied by a single spinal nerve. Some authors consider **dermomyotome** instead of separate dermatome and myotome.
- *Note:* Occipital somites and preotic somites participate in the formation of skull base.
- The distribution of sites and their fate is listed in Table 8.2.

Table 8.2		Distribution and fate of somites	
Somites	Number (in pairs)	Muscular derivatives	Skeletal derivatives
Preoccipital	3	Extraocular muscles of eyeball	Base of skull
Occipital	4	Muscles of tongue except palatoglossus	
Cervical	8	Skeletal muscles of trunk, limbs and diaphragm	Vertebrae (ribs from thoracic somites)
Thoracic	12		
Lumbar	5		
Sacral	5		
Coccygeal	8–10		

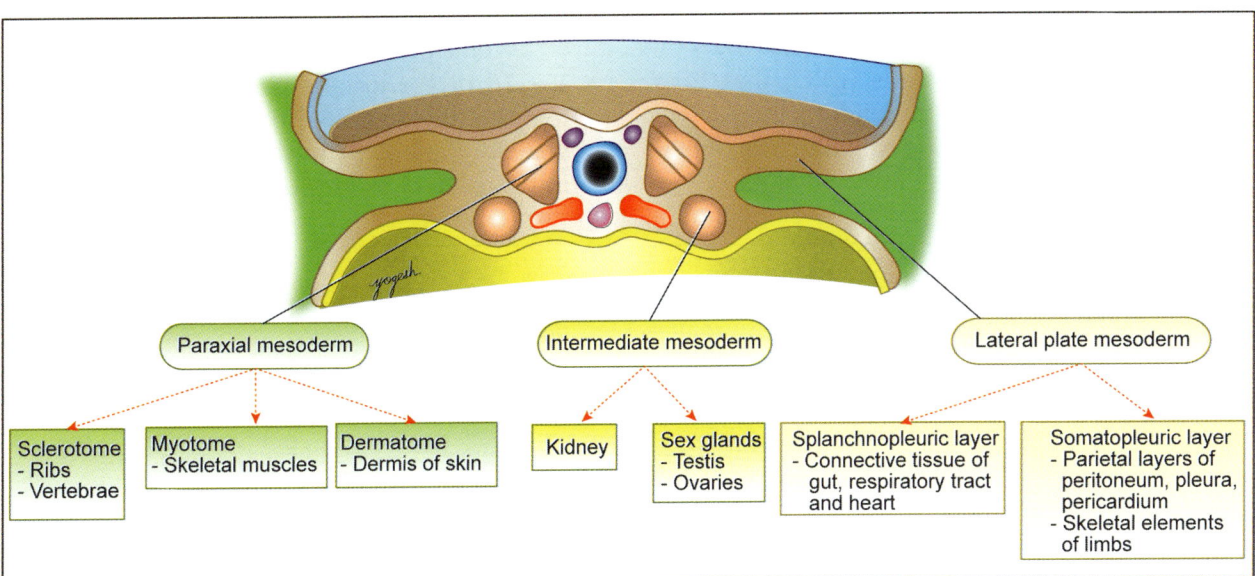

Fig. 8.5: Derivatives of the mesoderm. Intraembryonic mesoderm divides into paraxial, intermediate and lateral plate mesoderm that later give rise to various structures

Box 8.1: Midline structures of trilaminar germ disc

Q. Enlist the midline structures of germ disc.
- Trilaminar germ disc has the following structures in the midline from cranial to caudal direction:
  1. Septum transversum
  2. Pericardial sac
  3. Buccopharyngeal membrane
  4. Notochord, neural tube
  5. Primitive node
  6. Primitive streak
  7. Cloacal membrane

Box 8.2: Vasculogenesis and angiogenesis
- Vasculogenesis is formation of a new vessel from mesenchymal tissue in embryo.
- Angiogenesis is sprouting of vessel into adjacent area by endothelial budding.
- At beginning of the third week, formation of vasculature begins in extraembryonic mesoderm of yolk sac, connecting to stalk and chorion.^{MCQ}

Steps of formation of vasculature
- On day 17, mesenchymal cells differentiate into haemangioblasts (first in the splanchnic mesoderm of yolk sac and later in the mesoderm of the connecting stalk and the chorion) (Fig. 8.6).
- Haemangioblasts aggregate to form the cluster of cells called **blood island**.
- Haemangioblasts differentiate into two cell lineages as follows:
  A. Primitive haematopoietic stem cells (HSC) that on differentiation form erythropoietic cells, megakaryocytes and primitive macrophages.
  B. Endothelial precursor cells (EPC) that form epithelial lining of primitive endothelium.
- Small cavities appear in blood island to form lumen of primitive capillaries.
- Primitive haemangioblastic islands fuse to develop capillary networks (vasculogenesis).
- Endothelial precursor cells sprout into adjacent mesenchyme and fuse with adjacent haemangioblastic island and develop new capillaries (angiogenesis) to expand network.
- By the end of third week, yolk sac, connecting stalk and chorionic villi get completely vascularised.
- *Note*: Yolk sac is the first supplier of blood cells and it continues up to 60 days as haematopoietic organ. Later, liver, spleen, thymus and bone marrow take over the haematopoietic function.^{MCQ}

FOLDING OF EMBRYO
- In the third week, embryo is in the form of flat trilaminar germ disc.
- Reason for foldings of embryo: Cells in central part of germ disc multiply rapidly than that at periphery. Overgrown central part results in folding of germ disc and forms a primitive cylindrical embryo.
- Due to overgrowing tissue, the embryo shows folding in median plane (cephalocaudal folding) and lateral plane (*lateral folding*).
- Cephalocaudal folding can be studied as cranial **head fold** and caudal **tail fold**.
- Before embryonic folding, septum transversum lies at the cranial most part of the embryo.^{Neet}
- All folds converge on ventral surface of embryo to produce hourglass constriction of yolk sac.
- Amniotic cavity enlarges to enclose ventral surface of embryo and amniotic membrane forms a tubular covering around connecting stalk.
- Part of yolk sac trapped within embryo forms primitive gut and protruding part of yolk sac (extraembryonic part) forms an **umbilical vesicle**.
- **Vitellointestinal duct** (omphaloenteric duct) temporarily connects primitive gut with umbilical vesicle. Part of primitive gut cranial to vitellointestinal duct is **foregut** and caudal to it is **hindgut**,

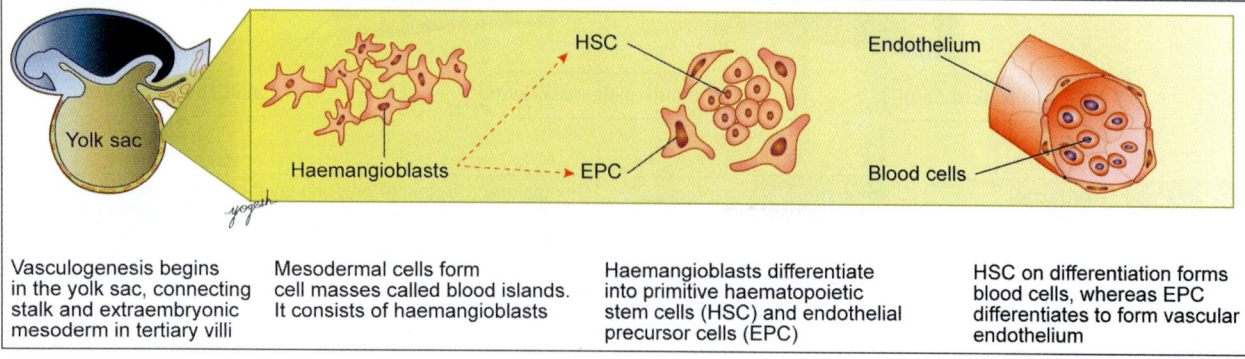

Fig. 8.6: Vasculogenesis

whereas part of gut communicating with vitellointestinal duct is called *midgut*.

Head Fold

- Overgrowing germ disc folds around cranial end of notochord to form a head fold (Figs 8.7 to 8.9, Practice Fig. 8.1).
- Head fold produces following changes:
  1. *Foregut*: Trapped part of yolk sac in head fold is called foregut.
  2. *Anterior intestinal portal*: It is a communication between foregut and midgut.
  3. *Ventral relations of foregut*: Buccopharyngeal membrane, pericardial sac and septum transversum come to lie ventral to foregut.
  4. *Dorsal relations of foregut*: Notochord and brain vesicles lie dorsal to the foregut.

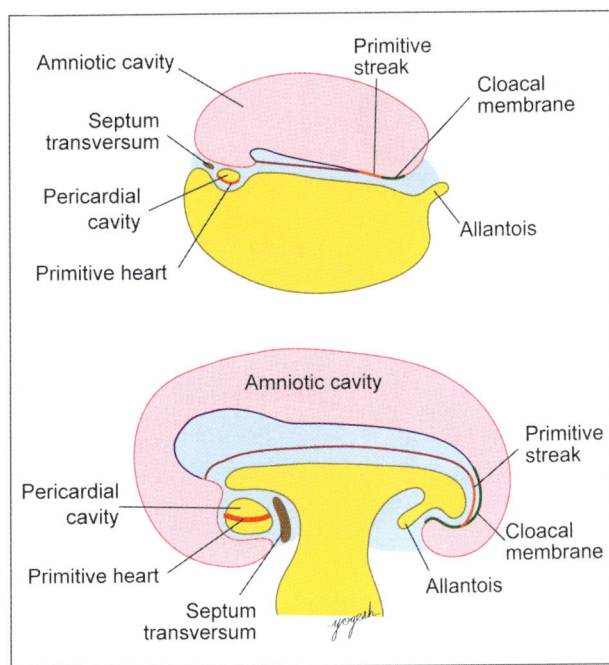

Practice Fig. 8.1: Head and tail folds of embryo

Some Interesting Facts

- Due to head fold, buccopharyngeal membrane comes to lie on ventral surface of embryo and becomes cranial to pericardial sac and septum transversum.
- During fourth week, buccopharyngeal membrane ruptures.
- Foregut is separated from pericardial sac by a cardiogenic plate (mesenchyme that forms a heart).
- Septum transversum is a mesenchymal tissue that lies caudal to the pericardial sac. Septum transversum form fibrous pericardium, part of diaphragm and part of ventral mesentery of foregut.
- Microglia and dura mater is mesodermal in origin.[Neet]

  5. *Cranial relation of foregut*: Rapidly growing forebrain vesicle lies cranial to foregut.

Tail Fold

- Overgrowing germ disc also fold ventrally around caudal end of notochord to form a *tail fold*.
- Tail fold produces the following changes:
  1. *Hindgut*: Trapped part of yolk sac in the tail fold is called *hindgut*.
  2. *Allantois*: Allantois communicates with hindgut and comes to lie ventral to hindgut in the form of *allantoenteric diverticulum*.
  3. *Cloacal membrane*: Bilaminar cloacal membrane later divides into urogenital and anal membrane and lies caudal to connecting stalk.
  4. Dorsal relations of hindgut: Notochord and neural tube lie dorsal to developing hindgut.
  5. Caudal relations of hindgut: Degenerating primitive node and streak lie caudal to developing hindgut.
  6. Allantoenteric diverticulum divides hindgut into pre-allantoic and post-allantoic parts.
  7. *Posterior intestinal portal*: It is a communication between midgut and pre-allantoic part of hindgut.

Lateral Folds

- Overgrowing central part of the germ disc forms two lateral folds (right and left) (Fig. 8.10).
- Lateral folds make the embryo cylindrical on fusion with head and tail fold at the primitive umbilical ring.

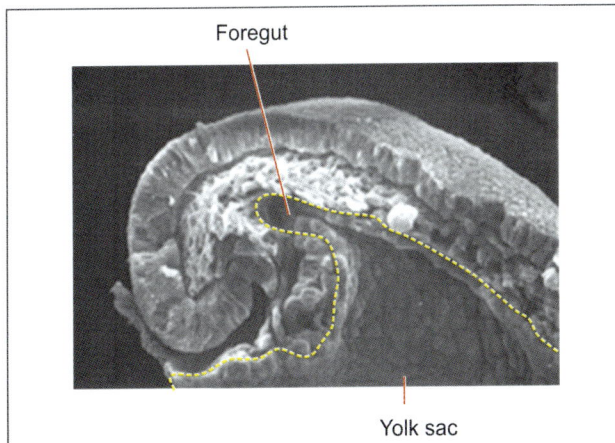

Scanning electron micrograph 8.3: SEM showing the formation of the head fold. Incorporated part of the yolk sac within the embryo can be seen [Species: mouse, approximate human age: 19 days, sagittal cut view]

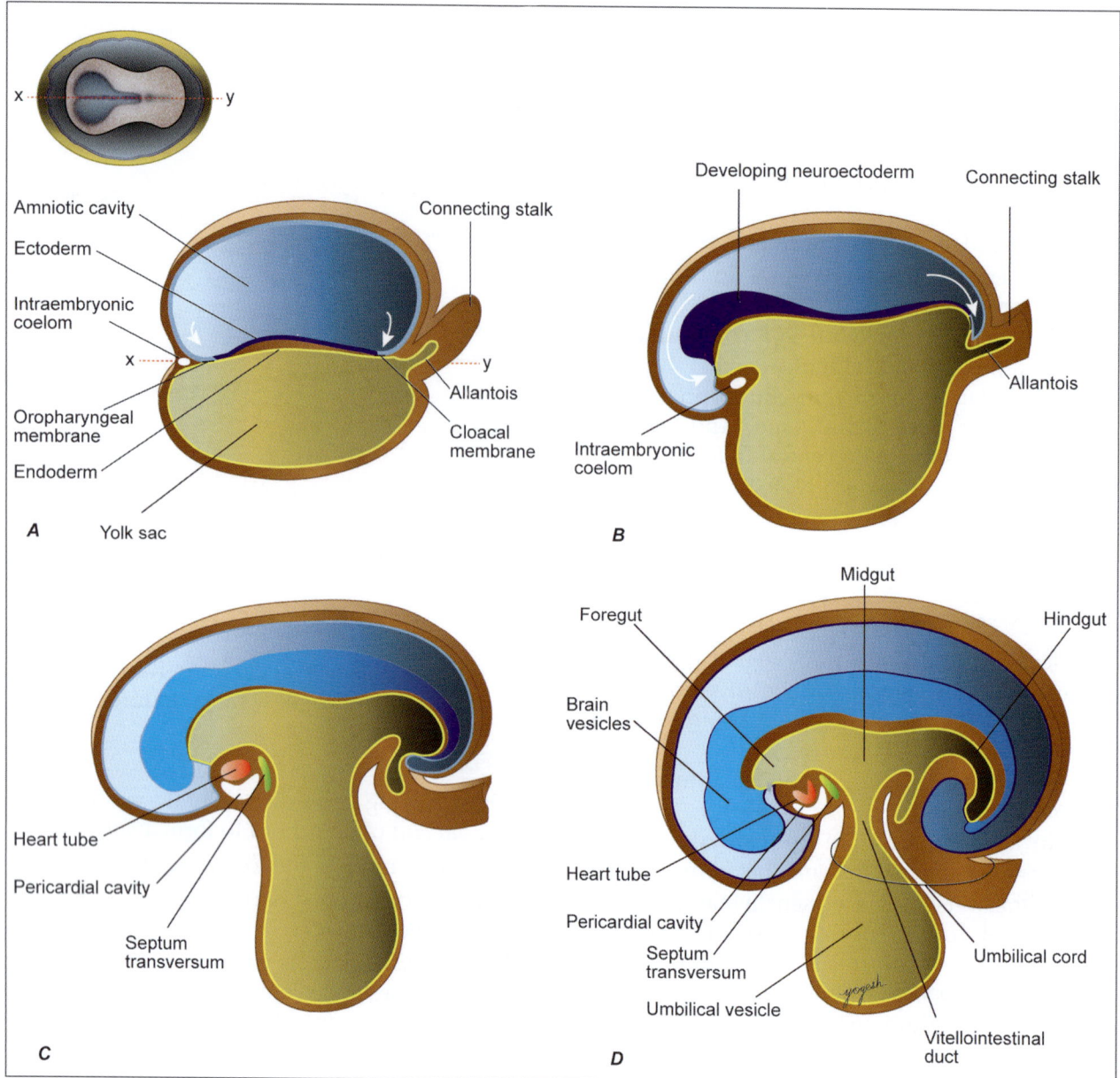

Fig. 8.7: Formation of craniocaudal (head and tail) foldings of the embryo. Progressive mid-sagittal sections of the developing embryo show craniocaudal foldings: (A) Day 18–19; (B) 22 days; (C) 24 days; (D) 28 days. Amnion is pulled ventrally. Yolk sac lining and endoderm form foregut, midgut, hindgut, vitellointestinal duct and umbilical vesicle

Changes Due to Formation of Lateral Fold (Fig. 8.10)

1. *Amnioectodermal junction*: Amnioectodermal junction comes to lie on umbilical cord (connecting stalk).
2. *Formation of midgut, vitellointestinal duct and umbilical vesicle*: Lateral fold trap part of yolk sac called *midgut*. Midgut communicates through a *vitellointestinal duct* with remaining small part of yolk sac called *umbilical vesicle*.
3. *Formation of dorsal mesentery of gut*: Lateral folds make splanchnopleuric intraembryonic mesodermal layer to cover ventrolateral surface of gut and to reflect dorsally on developing as dorsal mesentery.
4. *Peritoneal cavity*: Splanchnopleuric intraembryonic mesoderm (dorsal mesentery) continue with somatopleuric intraembryonic mesoderm via intermediate mesoderm. Somatopleuric intraembryonic mesoderm fuse ventrally in midline and converts intraembryonic coelom to *peritoneal cavity*.

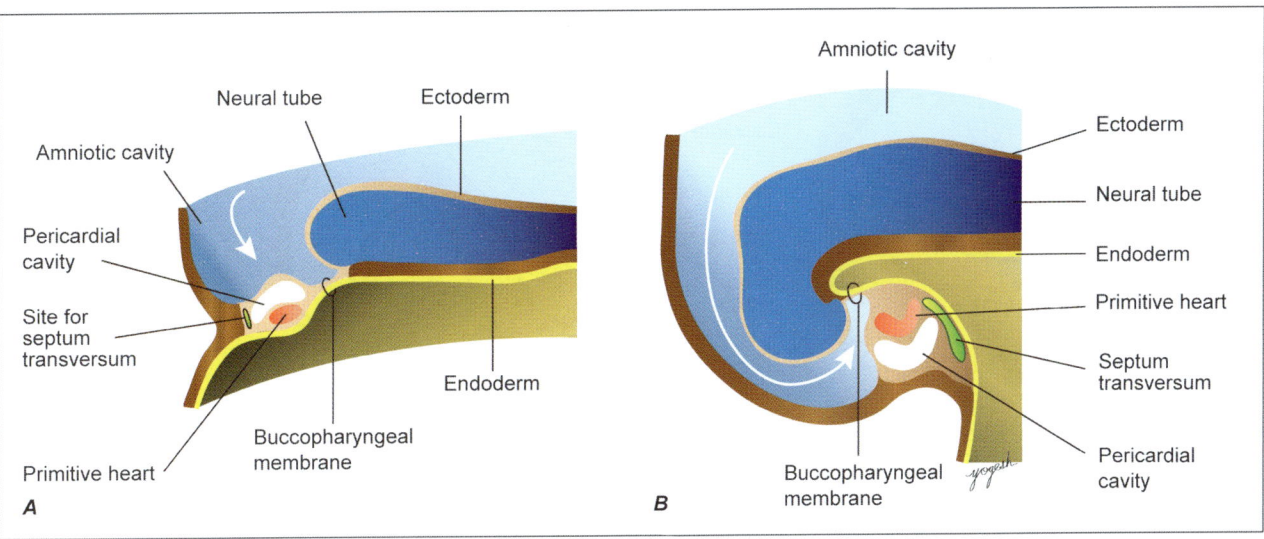

Fig. 8.8: Cranial folding of the embryo. Sagittal section of the embryo at the beginning (A) and at the end of the fourth week (B). Rapidly growing neural tube and change the positions of the buccopharyngeal membrane, pericardial cavity, primitive heart and septum transversum

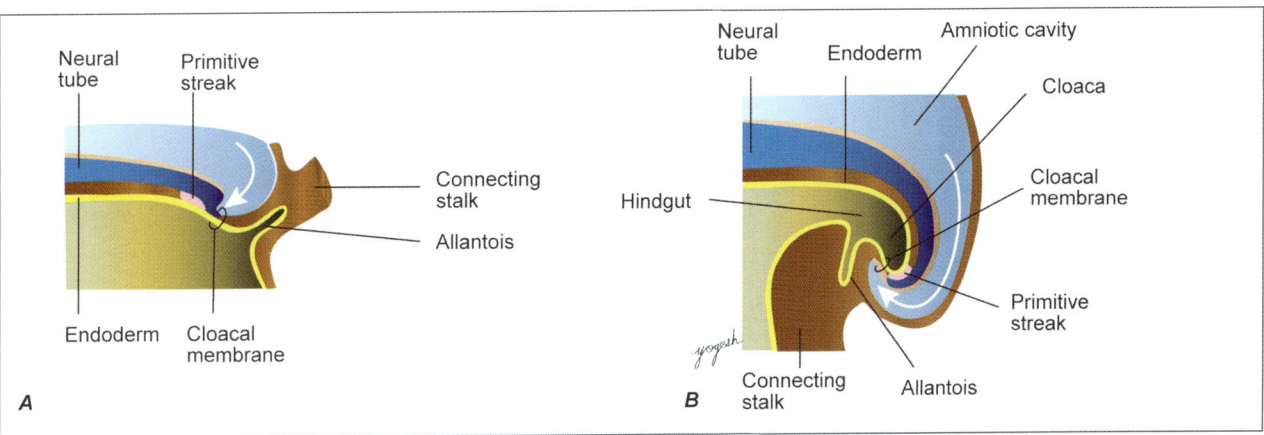

Fig. 8.9: Caudal folding of the embryo. Sagittal section of the embryo at the beginning (A) and at the end of the fourth week (B). Rapidly growing ectoderm and neural tube change the positions of the primitive streak, cloacal membrane, allantois and connecting stalk

Box 8.3: Connecting stalk

- Formation of tail fold moves attachment of connecting stalk form dorsal end of germ disc to ventral aspect of embryo and limit it at umbilical opening.
- Structure of connecting stalk in fifth week
- It contains following structures:
  1. Vitellointestinal duct
  2. Remnants of the yolk sac
  3. Extraembryonic mesodermal connective tissue that later forms Wharton's jelly (connective tissue of umbilical cord) and vessels of umbilical cord
- Connecting stalk is a site of amnioectodermal reflection and continuation of intraembryonic and extraembryonic coelom. This coelomic continuation persists up to 10th week.

DIFFERENTIATION OF ENDODERM

- Flat endoderm is converted into tubular structure due to formation of embryonic folding (head, tail and lateral folds).
- Endodermal tubular structure is divided into foregut, midgut and hindgut (Fig. 8.11).
- Derivatives of primitive gut are listed in Table 8.3. The detailed development of these structures is described in the Chapters on the development of the digestive tract.

CHANGES IN EMBRYONIC PERIOD

- Embryonic period extends from fourth week to eighth week.
- Changes of embryonic period are listed below.
- At the beginning of fourth week, embryonic disc is almost flat and has 4–12 somites.

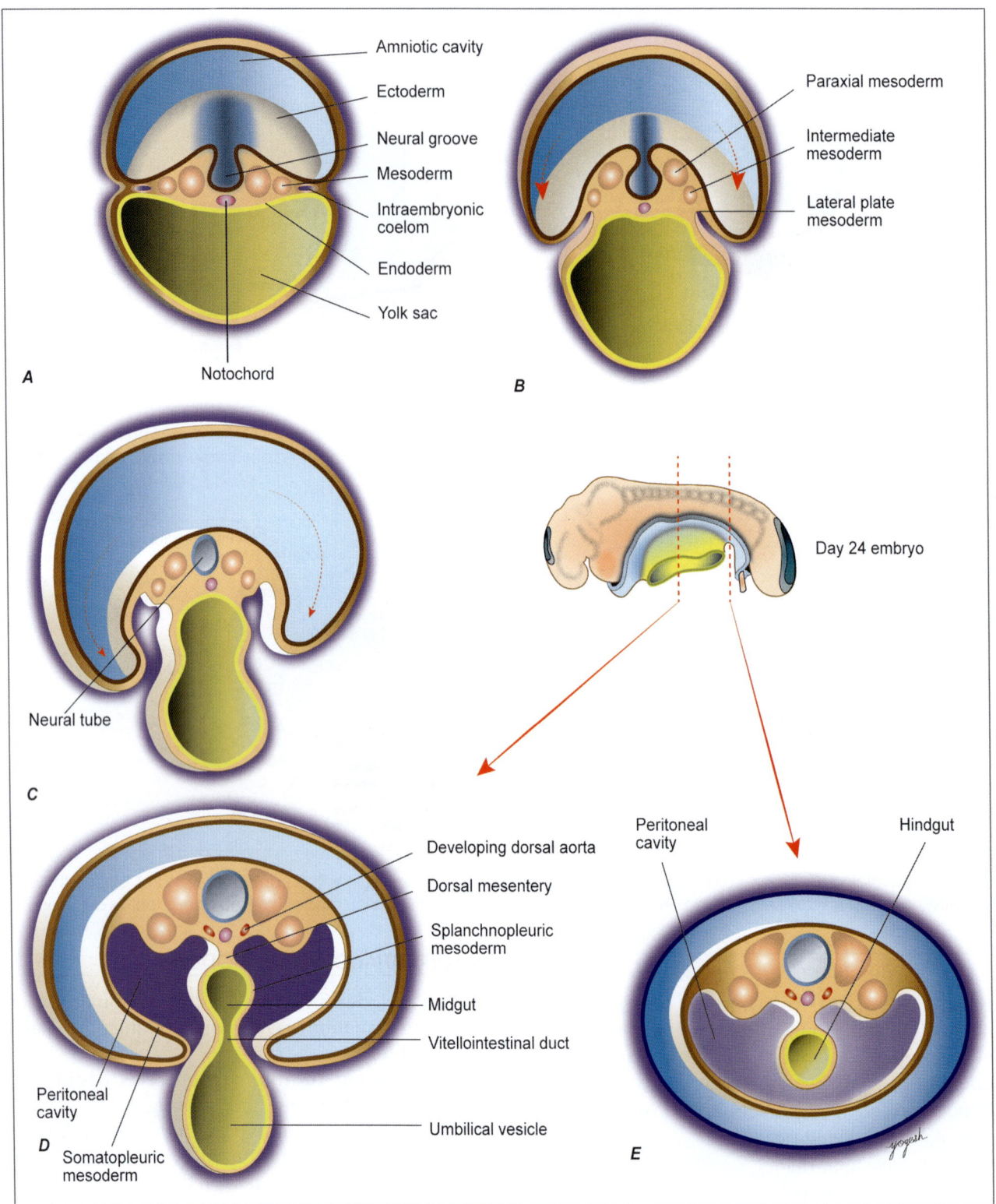

Fig. 8.10: Lateral folding of the developing embryo. Transverse sections through various stages of the embryo. Sections A, B, C, D pass through midway between craniocaudal axis, whereas E section passes through caudal part of embryo: (A) At the beginning of the third week, embryo shows neural folds; (B) By 20 days, intraembryonic coelom appears and divide lateral plate mesoderm into splanchnopleuric and somatopleuric layers; (C) By 21 days, intraembryonic coelom communicates with extraembryonic coelom; (D) By 24 days, lateral folds approach ventrally and make hourglass contracture of yolk sac. Midgut communicates with the yolk sac vesicle via vitellointestinal duct; (E) At the end of the fourth week, splanchnopleuric layer forms a double-layered membrane called dorsal mesentery. Dorsal mesentery connects developing gut with developing posterior wall of the embryo

Embryonic Period: Four to Eight Weeks of Development

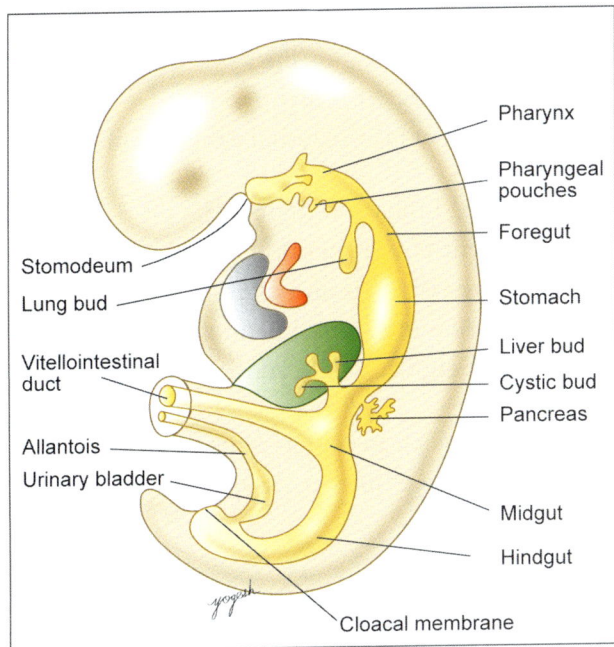

Fig. 8.11: Sagittal section of the embryo showing the derivatives of the endoderm. For understanding, other structures such as neural tube, dorsal aorta are not shown

Table 8.3	Derivatives of primitive gut^{MCQ,Viva}
Part of the gut	Derivatives
Foregut	• Lining of epithelium of pharynx, oesophagus, stomach, duodenum up to the ampulla of the Vater, tongue, floor of mouth • Lining epithelium of respiratory system, auditory tube, tympanic cavity • Parenchyma of tonsil, thyroid, parathyroid, thymus, liver and pancreas
Midgut	• Lining epithelium of distal part of duodenum, jejunum, ileum, caecum, appendix, ascending colon, right two-thirds of transverse colon
Hindgut	• Lining epithelium of left one-third of transverse colon, descending colon, sigmoid colon, rectum, anal canal up to mucocutaneous junction • Lining epithelium of urinary bladder except trigone, urethra (except posterior wall of prostatic part and terminal part of penile urethra), vagina[Neet] • Parenchyma of prostate (except glandular zone), bulbourethral gland[Neet]

Fourth Week

During fourth week of intrauterine life, the following changes occurs:
- Increase in the somite numbers
- Formation of three brain vesicles from the neural tube
- Formation of head and tail folds
- 21st days and later: Heart starts beating
- 24th day: First pharyngeal arch appears[MCQ]
- 26th day: Three pairs of pharyngeal arches
- 26th–27th day: Rudimentary forelimb bud
- 28th day: Rudimentary hind limb bud
- Formation of prominence of forebrain vesicle
- Otic pits, lens placodes (ectodermal thickening) appears

Fifth Week

During fifth week of intrauterine life, the following changes occur:
- Rapid growth of facial and head prominences
- Rapid growth of a second pharyngeal arch
- Growth of the limb buds
- Formation of alar and basal laminae of the neural tube
- Appearance of olfactory placodes, maxillary and frontonasal process.
- Appearance of gonadal ridges.

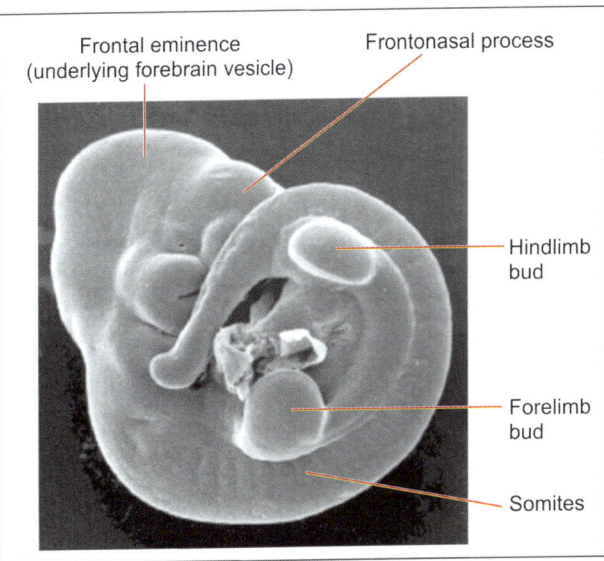

Scanning electron micrograph 8.4: SEM showing embryo of 5th week. Rapidly growing facial processes, head, and limb buds can be noted. The thickened ectoderm at the distal rim of the limb bud is termed the apical ectodermal ridge [Species: Mouse, approximate human age: 33 days, lateral view]

Sixth Week

During sixth week of intrauterine life, the following changes occur:
- Shows spontaneous movements
- Growth of brain vesicles

Human Embryology

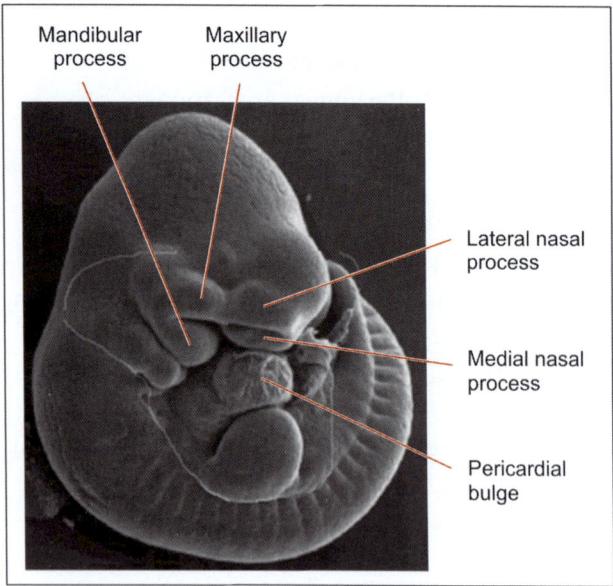

Scanning electron micrograph 8.5: SEM showing 6-week embryo with rapid growth of cranial and facial prominences [Species: Mouse, approximate human age: 6 weeks, lateral view]

- Appearance of nasal processes
- Buccopharyngeal membrane ruptures
- Development of appendix, caecum and spleen
- Differentiation of the limb digits begins. Differentiation in lower limb starts 4–5 later than upper limb.
- Umbilical herniation is common.

Seventh and Eight Weeks

During seventh and eight weeks of intrauterine life, the following changes occur:

- Development of face, external ear (auricular hillock) and eye
- Well-defined limbs and digits
- Development of metanephric kidney
- Development of testis and ovaries
- Differentiation of external genitalia
- During the eighth week, coordinated limb movements occur
- Primary ossification centers start appearing
- Caudal tail-like eminence disappears

Some Interesting Facts

- **Agenesis:** It is the absence of precursor cell of an organ with subsequent complete absence or non-development of the organ.[Neet]
- **Aplasia:** It is a partial failure of an organ to develop that result into rudimentary organ.
- **Atresia:** It is a closure or absence of a duct or passage or orifice that is usually present in the body.
- **Atrophy:** It is decrease in a size of an organ due to decrease in number of cells and size.

9
Placenta and Umbilical Cord

Chapter Outline

- Placenta
  - Gross features
  - Measurements
  - Structure
  - Development
  - Branching of villi
  - Placental barrier
  - Classification
  - Functions
- Umbilical cord
  - Measurements
  - Formation
  - Contents
- Amnion
  - Constituents of amniotic fluid
  - Functions of amniotic fluid
  - Volume of amniotic fluid
  - Clinical aspects
- Yolk sac
  - Formation and changes in yolk sac
  - Functions of yolk sac

PLACENTA

Q. Describe the placenta (Long-answer question for postgraduate students).

- Placenta is an organ that performs exchange of nutrients and gases between mother and foetus. Thus, the placenta is a foetomaternal organ.
- The placenta is a characteristic feature of eutherian mammals.
- Human placenta is discoid, chorio-deciduate organ.
- Placenta has two components
  A. *Maternal component* that is derived from uterine endometrium (decidua).
  B. *Foetal component* that develops from trophoblast and extraembryonic mesoderm (chorion).
- Placenta with foetal membrane is also expelled out of the uterus 30 minutes after childbirth.

Gross Features

Q. Draw a well-labelled diagram of the placenta showing maternal and foetal surfaces (Fig. 9.1).

- Full-term placenta is disc-shaped and shows two surfaces: Foetal and maternal (Fig. 9.1).

Foetal Surface

- Foetal surface of the placenta is shiny, grey and translucent.
- Foetal surface of the placenta is smooth and covered by amnion.^{Neet}
- It provides attachment to the umbilical cord.
- Radiating umbilical vessels can be easily seen under the translucent amnion.

Maternal Surface

- Maternal surface of the placenta is rough and dark maroon.
- It is divided into 15–30 polygonal lobules that are separated from each other by fissures (cobblestone appearance).
- These polygonal lobules are called *cotyledons*.
- Fissure separating cotyledons are occupied by *placental septae*.
- Each cotyledon mostly contains single stem villus and its branches.

Measurements

- The full-term placenta is discoid in shape, 15–20 cm in diameter.

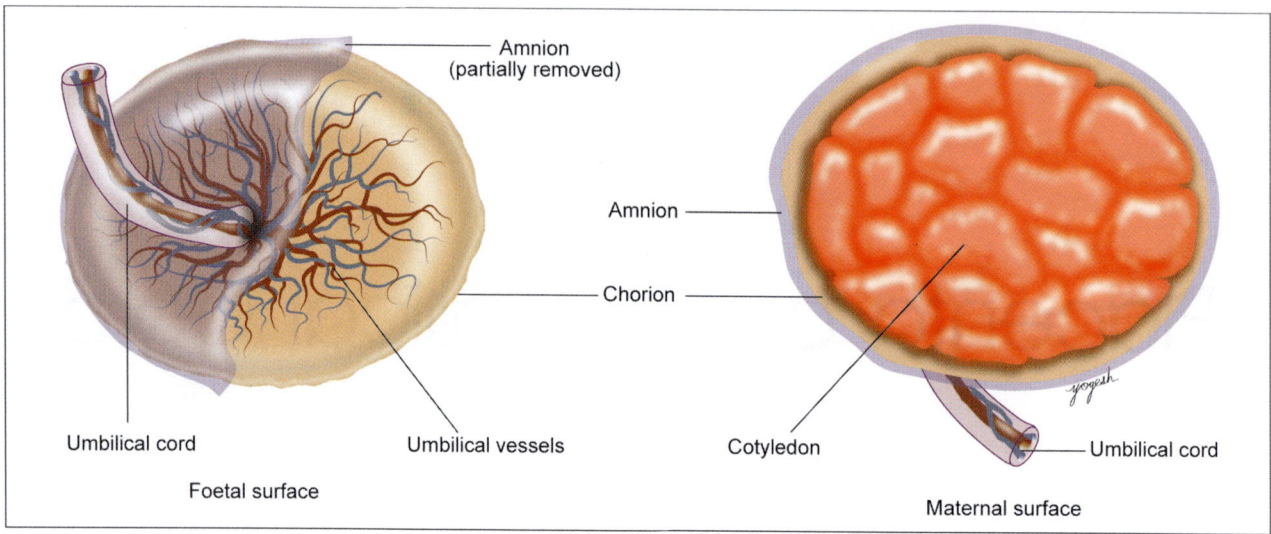

Fig. 9.1: Surfaces of placenta. Placenta has two surfaces: Foetal and placental. Foetal surface is smooth, covered by translucent layer of amnion and shows attachment of the umbilical cord. Maternal surface shows 15–30 polygonal cotyledons

- It is 3 cm thick in the centre.
- It weighs about 500–600 gm.

Structure of Placenta (Flowchart 9.1)

- Placenta consists of
  1. Chorionic plate
  2. Stem villi
  3. Intervillous space with maternal blood
  4. Basal plate
- Placenta shows basal plate on the maternal side and chorionic plate on the foetal side.

Basal Plate

- It consists of
  1. Stratum spongiosum of decidua basalis
  2. Cytotrophoblastic shell
  3. Syncytiotrophoblast layers

Chorionic Plate

- It consists of extraembryonic mesoderm, cytotrophoblast and syncytiotrophoblast (Box 9.1 and Box 9.2).

Development of Placenta

- Trophoblastic proliferation penetrates decidua (endometrium).
- On complete invasion of blastocyst, decidua can be divided into decidua basalis, decidua capsularis and decidua parietalis (Fig. 9.2).
- Trophoblastic layer differentiates into outer syncytiotrophoblast and inner cytotrophoblast (Fig. 9.3).
- Hypoblast cell forms an extraembryonic mesodermal layer.

Box 9.1: Decidua

- Uterine endometrium during pregnancy is called decidua (Fig. 9.2, Practice Fig. 9.1).^{Viva}
- Decidua forms maternal part of the placenta.
- Word *decidus* means *falling off* or *shedding* in the Latin.
- Decidua sheds off during parturition (childbirth).
- There are three regions of the decidua as follows:
  A. *Decidua basalis or serotina*: The part of decidua that lies deep to the blastocyst. Decidua basalis forms the placenta.^{Neet}
  B. *Decidua capsularis or reflexa*: The part of the decidua that covers the blastocyst.
  C. *Decidua parietalis or vera*: It is the remaining part of the decidua that lines uterine cavity.

Box 9.2: Decidual reaction

- The cellular and vascular changes in the decidua during pregnancy are called *decidual reaction* (Fig. 9.3).
- It includes glycogen and lipid deposition in decidual cells that produces enlarged pale-staining decidual cells.
- A high progesterone level in maternal blood is responsible for the decidual reaction.

- These syncytiotrophoblast, cytotrophoblast and extraembryonic mesoderm together form *chorion*.^{MCQ}
- Lacunar spaces appear in rapidly growing syncytiotrophoblast. These lacunar spaces occur more towards decidua basalis.

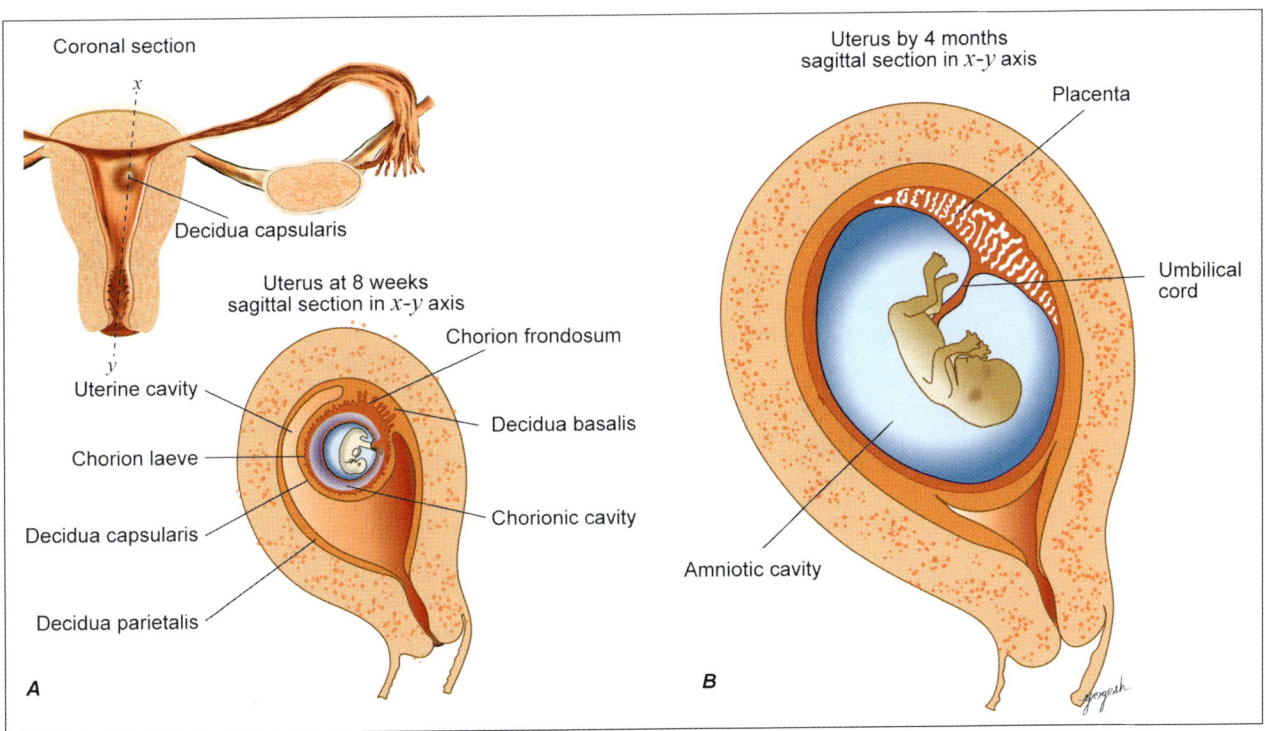

Fig. 9.2: Fusion of the decidua capsularis and parietalis: (A) By the end of the eighth week, decidua shows three zones as decidua basalis, capsularis and parietalis; (B) By beginning of the fourth month, decidua basalis is converted into placenta. Owing to the enlarging amniotic cavity, chorionic cavity and uterine cavity become obliterated and decidua capsularis fuses with decidua parietalis

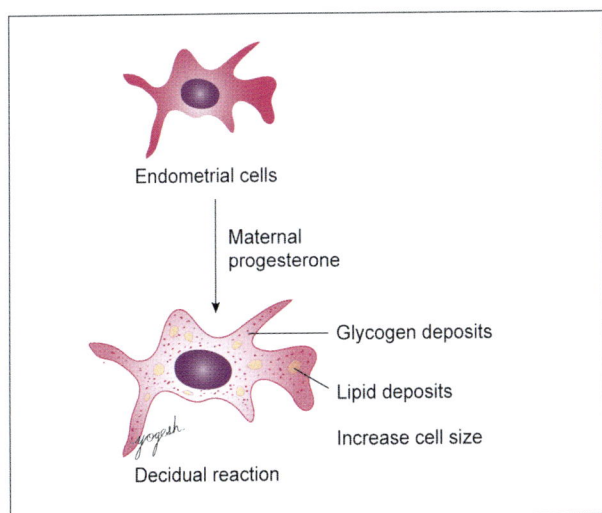

Fig. 9.3: Decidual reaction. During pregnancy, high level of progesterone enhances glycogen and lipid deposition in the decidual cells (cells of endometrium)

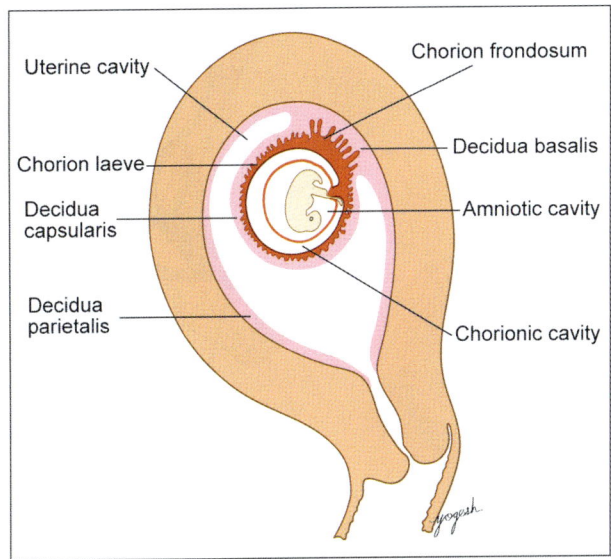

Practice Fig. 9.1: Zones of decidua (three zones: Decidua basalis, capsularis and parietalis)

- Enlarging spaces communicates with adjacent ones. In between adjacent lacunae, syncytiotrophoblast cells persist as columns called **trabeculae**.
- Expanding syncytiotrophoblast erodes maternal capillaries and maternal blood starts entering the lacunar spaces and induces **uteroplacental circulation** at 17–22 days (in 3rd week).[Neet]

- Columns of syncytiotrophoblastic trabeculae get penetrated by cytotrophoblast to form *primary villi*.
- Mesoderm enters the core of primary villi to form *secondary villi*.
- In third week, capillaries appear in the mesodermal core and the villi are then called *tertiary villi*.[Neet]

Human Embryology

Flowchart 9.1: Structure of the placenta

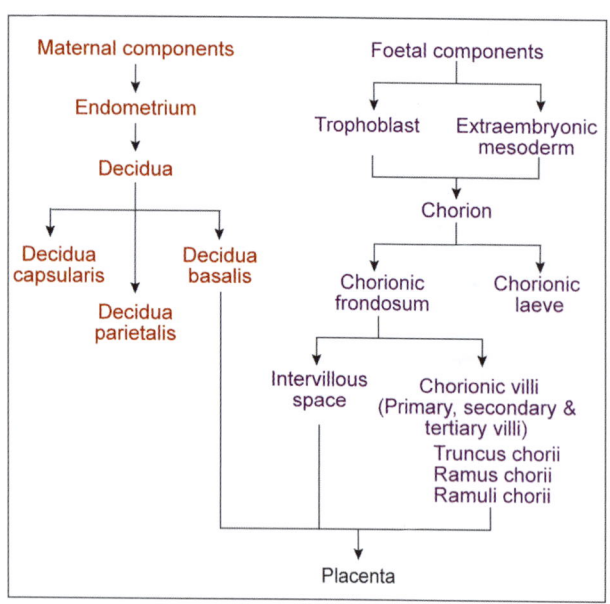

- On formation of villi, lacunar spaces are then termed *intervillous spaces* (Fig. 9.4).
- Cytotrophoblast penetrates the syncytiotrophoblast and forms an outer *cytotrophoblastic shell*.

Some Interesting Facts

- Foetal chorion frondosum and maternal decidua basalis together form the placenta.
- By the end of the third month, decidua capsularis fuses with decidua parietalis due to increased size of the foetus.
- Cytotrophoblast shell isolates syncytiotrophoblast from decidua basalis and helps in anchoring the placenta.
- Chorion = trophoblast + extraembryonic somatopleuric mesoderm.
- Decidua = stratum compactum of uterine endometrium during pregnancy.

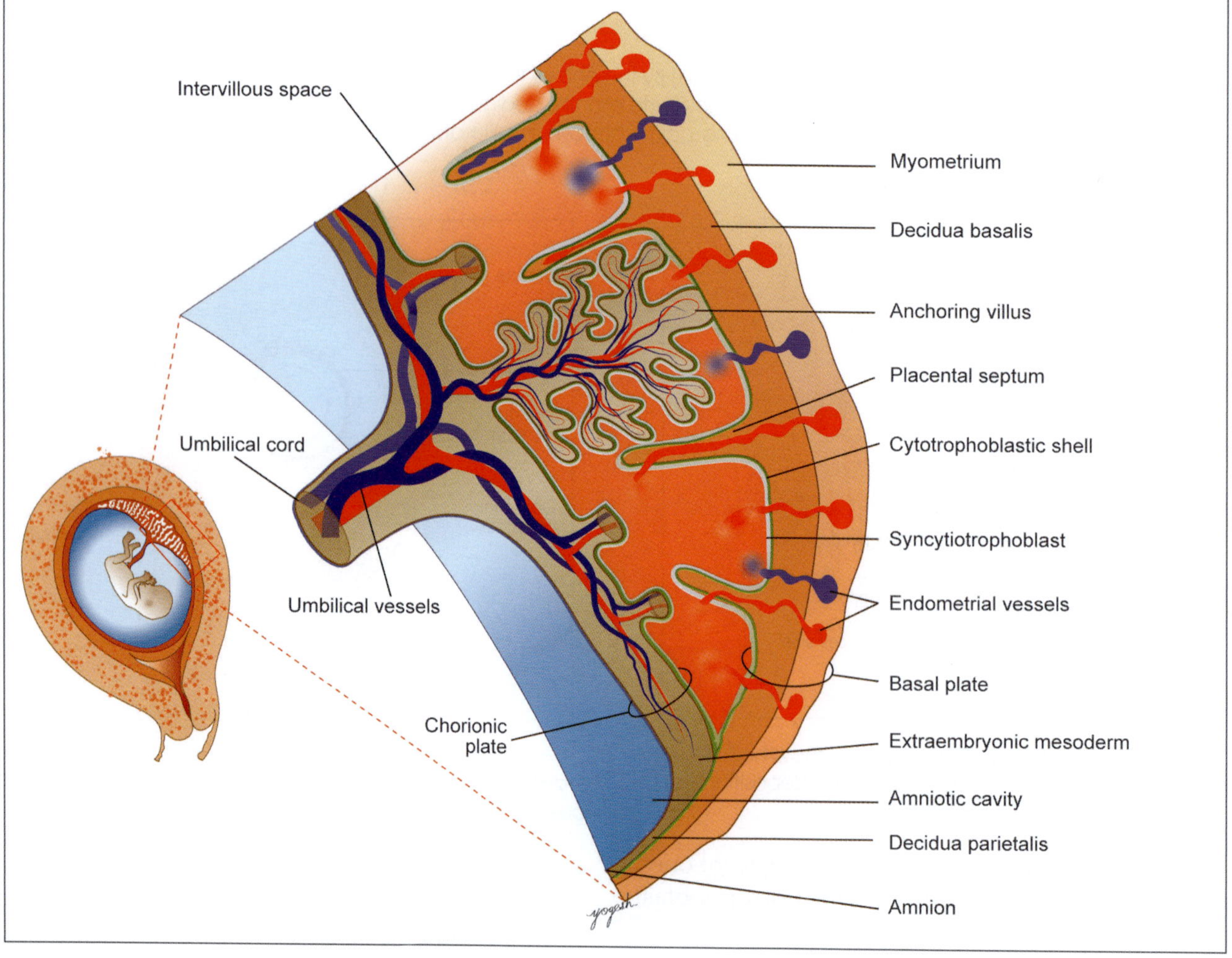

Fig. 9.4: Structure of the placenta. Intervillous spaces are filled with maternal blood. Cotyledons are partially separated by the decidual septa. Anchoring villi extend between basal plate and chorionic plate. Branches of the anchoring villus contain foetal blood vessels. Endometrial arteries bring oxygenated blood to intervillous space and drained by endometrial veins

Chorionic villi and their Branching Pattern

Q. Write short note on chorionic villi (Figs 9.4 and 9.5).

- Columns of syncytiotrophoblastic trabeculae get penetrated by cytotrophoblast to form *primary villi*. Mesoderm enters the core of primary villi to form *secondary villi*. Capillaries appear in the mesodermal core and the villi are then called *tertiary villi*.
- The villi towards decidua basalis proliferate rapidly to form **chorion frondosum**, whereas other villi degenerate and disappear. These villi are called *chorion laeve* (Fig. 9.2). Thus, placenta develops from decidua basalis (maternal component) and chorionic frondosum.^{Neet}
- The villi that extend from chorion (foetal side of the placenta) to the decidua basalis (maternal side of the placenta) are called *anchoring villi*.
- Several branches arise from the lateral side of anchoring villi that enter in the intervillous space. These branches are termed as follows (Fig. 9.5):
  A. *Truncus chorii* or stem villus that connects chorion with decidua basalis.
  B. *Rami chorii*: These are branches of stem villi.
  C. *Ramuli chorii*: These are finer branches of rami chorii.
  D. *Floating* or *free villi*: These are numerous villi that freely floats in the intervillous spaces.
- Microvilli of syncytiotrophoblast projects into the intervillous space and increases the surface area (up to 14 square metre) for absorption.^{MCQ}
- Zones of villi
  - Beta zone: In the beta zones, cytotrophoblast separates syncytiotrophoblast and foetal capillaries.
  - Alpha zone: On the disappearance of cytotrophoblast, syncytiotrophoblast fuse with foetal capillaries in some zones of villi. These zones are called *alpha zones*.
  - Exchange of nutrients takes place more rapidly through alpha zones than beta zones.

Some Interesting Facts

- Tips of the stem villi penetrate deeper in the endometrium (decidua basalis) than any other part of the chorion.
- The projecting stem villi are separated from each other by a portion of decidua. These decidual separation forms placental septa (decidual septa) and projecting stem villi form cotyledons.
- Size of placenta increases parallel to the developing foetus and uterus. Placenta covers approximately 15–30% of the internal surface of the uterus throughout the pregnancy.^{MCQ}

Box 9.3: Intervillous space

- Intervillous space is the placental space that is formed by fusion of lacunar spaces of syncytiotrophoblast.
- These intervillous spaces are partially separated from each other by placental septa as these septa do not reach chorionic plate (foetal surface).
- Maternal blood enters the intervillous space through spiral arteries of the decidua basalis. Intervillous space is drained by endometrial veins.
- The volume of intervillous space is about 140 ml.^{MCQ}
- About 500 ml/minute maternal blood flows through the intervillous space.^{MCQ}

Placental Barrier

Q. Write short note on placental barrier.

- In the placenta, maternal blood circulates through intervillous space, whereas foetal blood circulates through blood vessels of chorionic villi. Here, maternal blood is separated from foetal blood by a placental barrier.
- Placental barrier allows the exchange of gases, nutrients, foetal waste products between maternal blood and foetal blood.
- During the initial stages of the foetal development, the placental barrier consists of (Fig. 9.6, Practice Fig. 9.2):
  1. Endothelium of foetal blood vessels
  2. Basement membrane of endothelium of foetal blood vessels

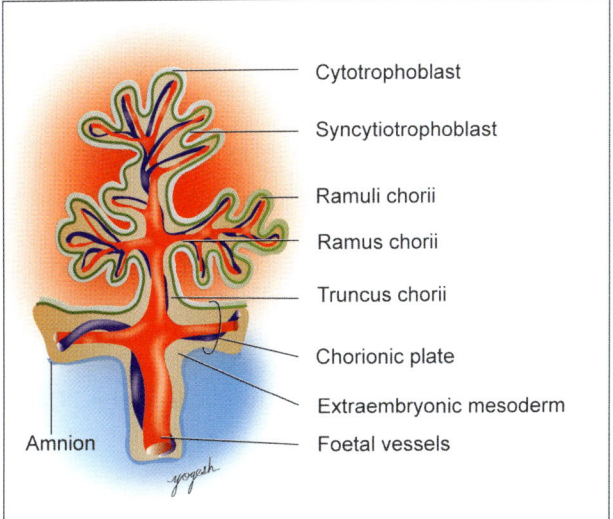

Fig. 9.5: Branching pattern of the villi. Villi are truncus chorii, ramus chorrii and ramuli chorii

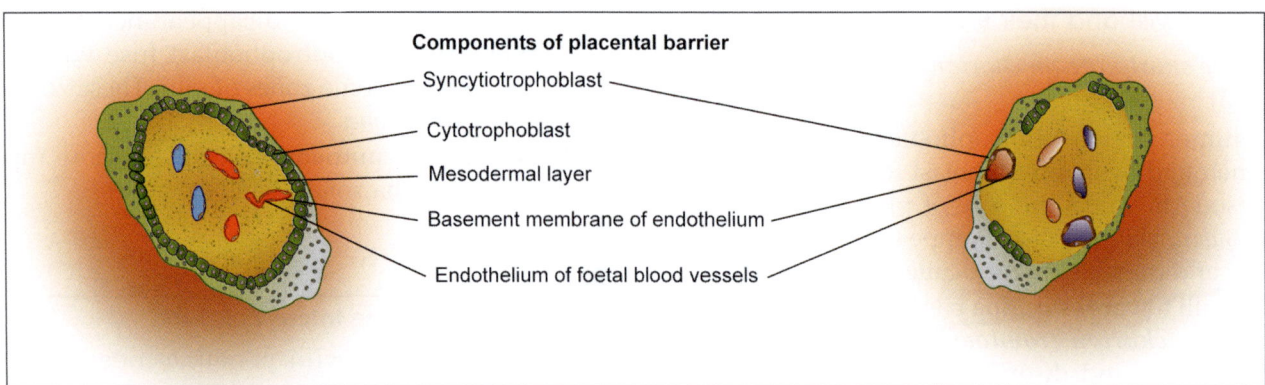

Fig. 9.6: Placental barrier. In early foetal life, placental barrier consists of endothelium of foetal blood vessels, its basement membrane, mesodermal layer, cytotrophoblast and syncytiotrophoblast. Fourth month onwards, cytotrophoblast and mesoderm thin out and thus, placental barrier is represented only by a thin layer of syncytiotrophoblast and foetal capillary endothelium

3. Mesodermal layer
4. Cytotrophoblast
5. Syncytiotrophoblast

- Fourth month onwards, cytotrophoblast and mesoderm thin out and thus, placental barrier is represented only by a thin layer of syncytiotrophoblast and foetal capillary endothelium (Fig. 9.6).

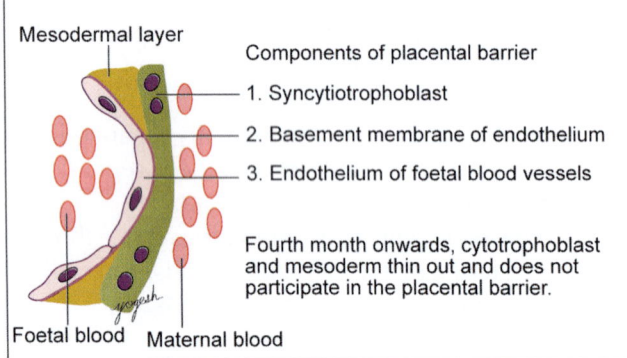

Practice Fig. 9.2: Placental barrier

Some Interesting Facts

Nitabuch's membrane
- Nitabuch's membrane is the fibrinoid deposition over the outer cytotrophoblast shell. It makes a demarcation between maternal and foetal tissue.

Rohr's Fibrinoid stria
- Rohr's fibrinoid stria is the fibrinoid deposition on the intervillous surface of the syncytiotrophoblast. It was first described by Wolska (1888).
- These membranes play a major role in an immunological separation of foetal tissue from maternal tissue.

Foetal cotyledons
- Chorionic plate shows 40–60 extensions that extend towards decidua basalis. These extensions are *foetal cotyledons*.

- Each foetal cotyledon consists of stem villus and its ramification.

Langhans layer
- Cytotrophoblast layer is also called *Langhans layer*. Some authors also refer the Langhans layer as a fibrinoid layer separating intervillous space from chorion.

Classification of Placenta

According to Shape

- According to the shape of the placenta, it can be classified as follows (Fig. 9.7):
  1. Discoid placenta: It is round or disc-shaped.
  2. Bidiscoid placenta: It consists of two discs.
  3. Lobed placenta: It consists of two or more lobes.
  4. Placenta succenturiata: It shows accessory lobe of the placenta.
  5. Placenta membranacea: It is diffuse and thin chorionic villi projecting around entire blastocyst.
  6. Circumvallate placenta: In the circumvallate placenta, peripheral edge of the placenta is covered by a circular fold of decidua.

According to the Attachment of the Umbilical Cord

- According to the attachment of the umbilical cord, placentae are classified as follows (Fig. 9.8):
  1. Normal placenta: Umbilical cord is attached to the centre of the placenta.^{MCQ}
  2. Battledore placenta: Umbilical cord is connected to the margin of the placenta.^{MCQ}
  3. Velamentous placenta: Umbilical cord is attached to foetal membranes near peripheral marginal of the placenta.^{MCQ}

According to Degree of Adhesion

- According to the degree of adhesion, the placentae are classified as follows (Fig. 9.9):

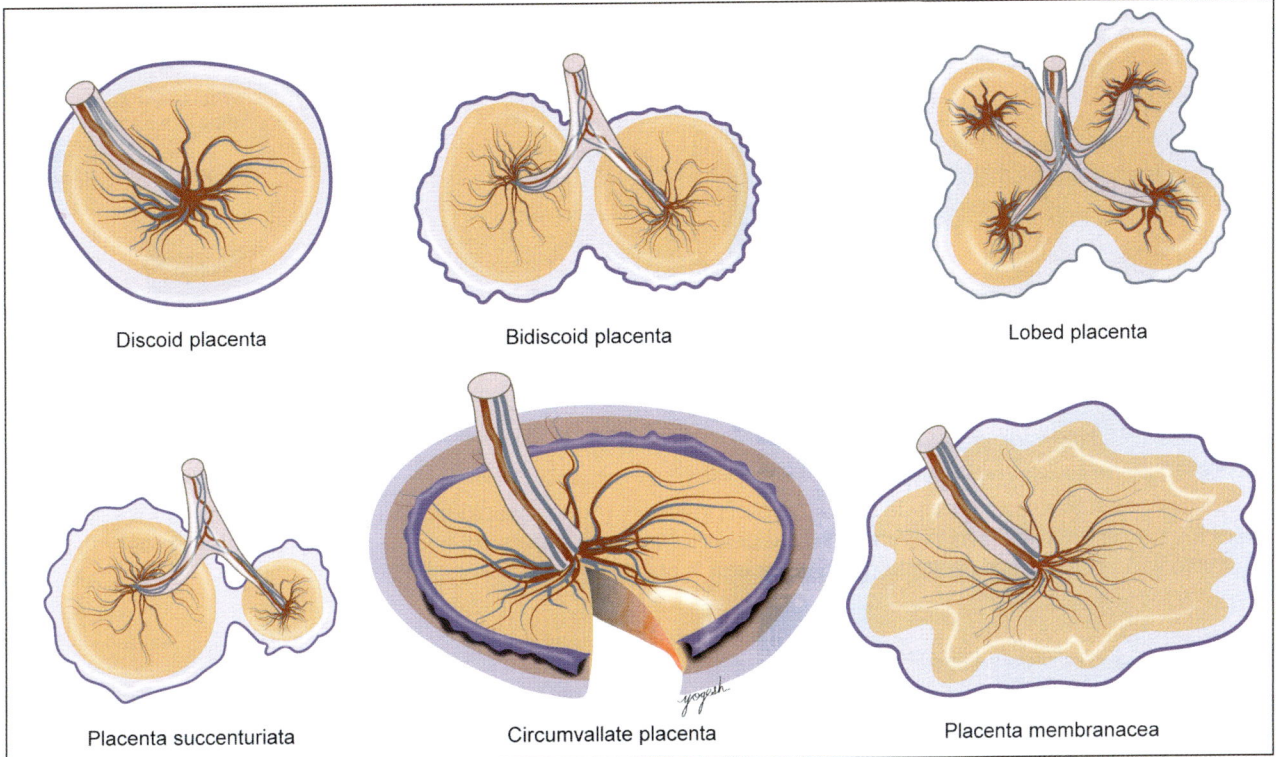

Fig. 9.7: Classification of the placenta according to its shape. Placenta can be classified as discoid placenta (round or disc-shaped), bidiscoid placenta (two discs), lobed placenta (two or more lobes), placenta succenturiata (accessory lobe), placenta membranacea (diffuse and thin), circumvallate placenta (peripheral edge of the placenta is covered by a circular fold of decidua)

1. Placenta accreta: It is pathologically adhered placenta with decidua basalis.
2. Placenta increta: This placenta penetrates the myometrium.
3. Placenta percreta: This placenta penetrates entire uterine wall.

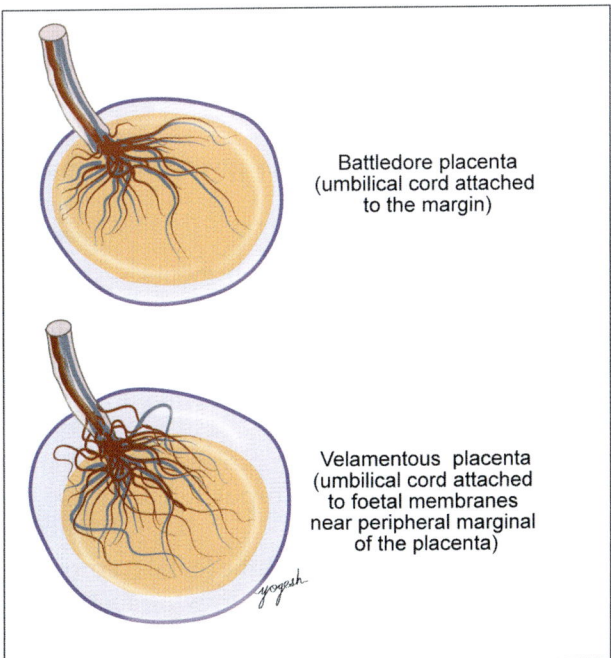

Fig. 9.8: Classification of the placenta according to the attachment of the umbilical cord. Placenta can be classified as battledore placenta and velamentous placenta. In normal placenta, umbilical cord is attached to the centre of the placenta

> **Box 9.4:** Phylogeny of placenta
> - Based on the retention of the maternal layers, placentae are classified as follows (Table 9.1):
>   A. Epithelio-chorial: Maternal endometrial epithelium remains intact. For example, pig.
>   B. Syndesmo-chorial: Endometrial epithelium disappears. For example, bovine placenta.
>   C. Endothelio-reticular: Endometrial epithelium and stroma is eroded. Maternal vessels come in direct contact with foetal placental (chorionic) vessels. For example, dog.
>   D. Haemo-chorial: Maternal blood vessels are eroded and maternal blood enters intervillous spaces of foetal chorion. For example, human.
>   E. Haemo-endothelial: Trophoblastic layers also degenerate and maternal blood makes direct contact with foetal placental (chorionic) blood vessels. For example, rabbit.

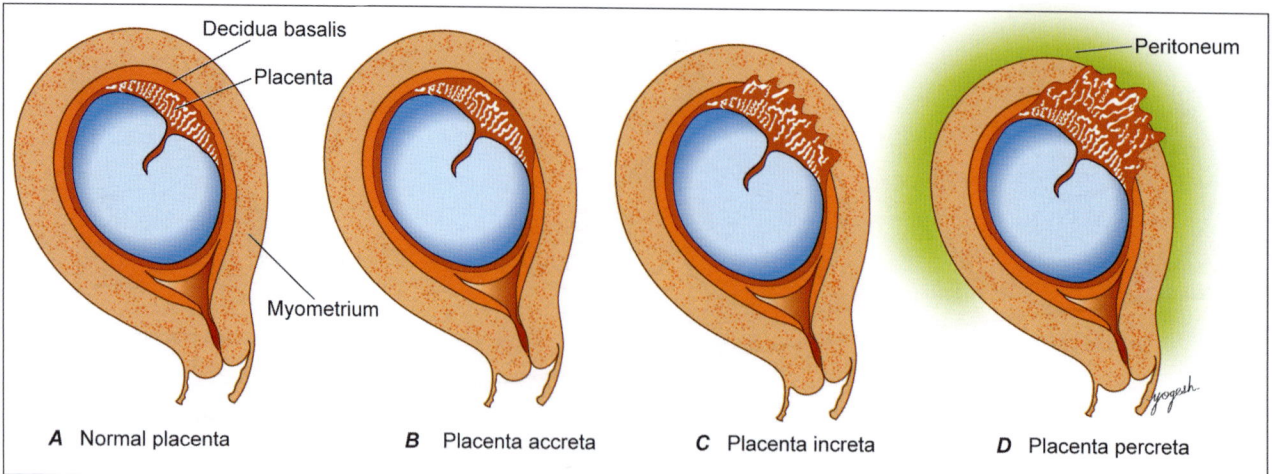

Fig. 9.9: Types of placenta according to the degree of adhesion: (A) Normal placenta; (B) Placenta accreta (placenta adhered with decidua basalis); (C) Placenta increta (placenta penetrates the myometrium) and (D) Placenta percreta (placenta penetrates entire uterine wall and reaches peritoneum). *Note*, foetus is not shown in the amniotic cavity

Table 9.1	Phylogeny of Placenta		
Type	Maternal component	Foetal component	Example
Epithelio-chorial	Intact endometrial epithelium	Trophoblast separates foetal blood vessels	Pig
Syndemso-chorial	Endometrial stroma		Bovine
Endothelio-chrorial	Endothelium of maternal vessels		Dog
Hemo-chorial	Erosion of endothelium of maternal vessels	Trophoblast separates maternal blood from foetal vessels	Human
Haemo-endothelial		Trophoblast disappears	Rabbit

Functions of Placenta (Fig. 9.10)

Q. Write short note on functions of placenta.

Q. Write short note on endocrine functions of placenta.

1. Gaseous exchange: O_2 and CO_2 exchange takes place across placenta through simple diffusion. Foetal haemoglobin has high affinity for the oxygen and high haemoglobin concentration in foetus facilitates the transfer of oxygen from mother to the foetus.
2. Transport of nutrients such as glucose, fatty acids, amino acids and electrolytes such as sodium, potassium and chloride.
3. Excretion of urea, uric acid and creatinine from the foetal blood into the maternal blood.
4. Passive immunity: Maternal antibodies (immunoglobulins) pass placental barrier by pinocytosis of syncytiotrophoblast. These antibodies provide passive immunity to the foetus against diphtheria, measles, smallpox and so on. Maternal antibodies do not protect from chickenpox and whooping cough.[MCQ]
5. Placental barrier: It prevents entry of many drugs and bacteria. But almost all viruses can cross the placental barrier. Some of the foetal blood cells may cross the placental barrier and circulate in the maternal blood.
6. Storage: The placenta stores glycogen, calcium and iron.
7. Endocrine function:
   Placenta secretes following hormones:
   – human chorionic gonadotropin
   – placental oestrogen
   – placental progesterone and
   – placental lactogen.

Human chorionic gonadotropin resembles luteinising hormone and maintains corpus luteum up to three months.[MCQ]

Placental oestrogen changes the female reproductive tract to make it suitable for growing foetus. These changes include growing size of uterus, relaxation of various pelvic ligaments and so on.

Human placental progesterone helps in growth of decidua (maternal endometrium).

Placental lactogen helps in growth of female breasts and makes it ready for lactation.

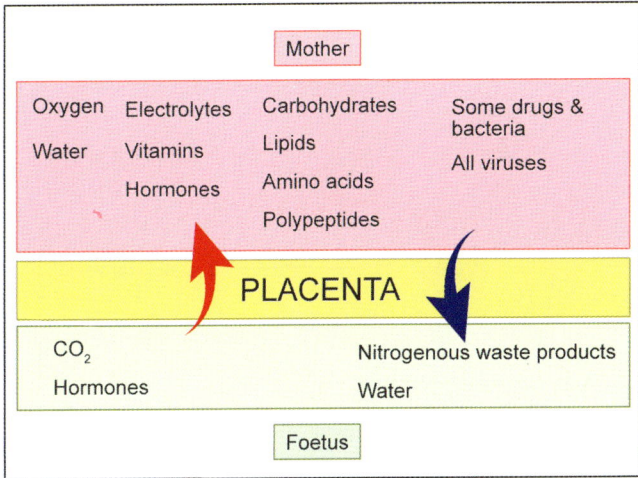

Fig. 9.10: Transport across placenta

Box 9.5: Hofbauer cells

- Hofbauer cells are small eosinophilic cells found in the placenta.
- These cells are named after J. Isfred Isidore Hofbauer (1878–1961).
- These cells are derived from mesoderm (extra-embryonic).
- Function: Hofbauer cells acts as *macrophage* and prevents transmission of an infectious agent from mother to foetus.

Box 9.6: Human chorionic gonadotropin (hCG)

Q. Write short note on human chorionic gonadotropin.

- The hCG is a hormone produced by syncytiotrophoblast of the placenta after implantation.
- The hCG is a polypeptide hormone (237 amino acids) identical to luteinising hormone (LH) of the anterior pituitary gland.
- It is excreted in the urine of the mother after one week of missed menstrual period.

Functions

1. It stimulates the corpus luteum to secrete progesterone for first three months of the pregnancy. Later, the placenta starts secretion of sufficient progesterone.
2. Through progesterone, hCG stimulates growth of decidua (uterine endometrium).
3. hCG repels maternal immune cells and protect foetus during the first trimester. hCG also induces maternal T cell apoptosis.

Clinical aspects

1. Owing to the similarity between hCG and LH, hCG is used for stimulating ovulation.
2. Chromatographic immunoassay or urine test is used for detection of hCG and confirmation of the pregnancy.
3. Positive immunoassay test can be seen after 6–12 days of ovulation.
4. Elevated hCG is seen in hydatidiform moles or molar pregnancy, germ cell tumours in males and teratomas (choriocarcinoma, seminoma).

UMBILICAL CORD

Q. Write short note on umbilical cord.

- Definition
  Umbilical cord is a tubular cord-like structure by which foetus is connected with the placenta.
- The umbilical cord is covered by an amniotic membrane.
- It has two ends:
  - Placental end: It is attached to the centre of the placenta.
  - Foetal end: It is attached to the umbilicus of the foetus.

Measurements Full-term Umbilical Cord

- Length: 50–55 cm
- Thickness: 2 cm

Formation of Umbilical Cord

- On the formation of embryonic folds, the yolk sac and connecting stalk come to lie on ventral surface of the foetus.
- Amnio-ectodermal junction comes to lie on ventral surface of the foetus and forms *umbilical ring* through which vitellointestinal duct and allantois protrude.
- Extraembryonic mesodermal tissue of the connecting stalk gets vascularised to form two umbilical arteries and two umbilical veins during third and fourth week of development. During later part of pregnancy, *right umbilical vein gets obliterated*.
- Mesodermal connective tissue of connecting stalk forms mucoid tissue called *Wharton's jelly*.

Contents of Umbilical Cord

Q. List the contents of umbilical cord.

Umbilical cord is made up of the following structures (Fig. 9.11, Practice Fig. 9.3, Table 9.2):

1. Umbilical vessels:
   - Umbilical cord has *two umbilical arteries and only one (left) umbilical vein*. **Right umbilical vein disappears.**[Neet]
   - Umbilical arteries carry deoxygenated blood from internal iliac arteries of foetus to the placenta.

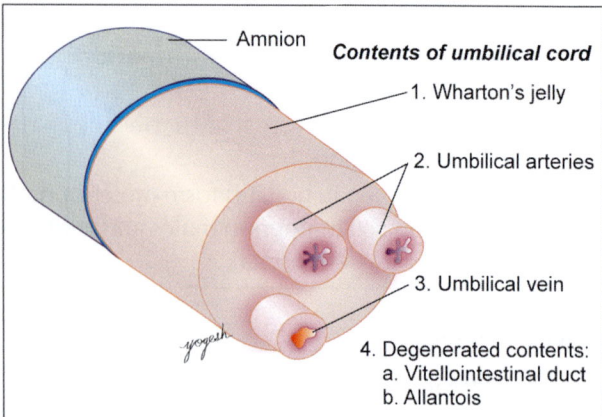

Fig. 9.11: Structure of the umbilical cord. It contains two umbilical arteries and one umbilical vein. Umbilical arteries carry deoxygenated blood from foetus to placenta (mother), whereas umbilical vein carries oxygenated blood from placenta to the foetus. Near the placental end, umbilical cord shows degenerating remnants of vitellointestinal duct and allantois

Table 9.2	Contents of umbilical cord[MCQ, Viva]
1. Two umbilical arteries	
2. One umbilical vein	
3. Wharton's jelly	
4. Part of allantois	
5. Vitellointestinal duct and umbilical vesicle	

- Umbilical veins are two in number, but the right umbilical vein disappears.[MCQ]
- Left umbilical vein convey oxygenated blood from placenta to the foetus.[Neet]
- Left umbilical vein joins the left branch of the portal vein that conveys blood to inferior vena cava via ductus venosus.[MCQ]
2. Wharton's jelly:
    - Mucoid connective tissue of the umbilical cord is called Wharton's jelly.
    - Twisting of the umbilical vessels produces beaded appearance of umbilical cord.
3. Part of allantoic diverticulum
    - Part of allantoic diverticulum enters in the umbilical cord (earlier connecting stalk) and it undergoes fibrosis to form urachus.
    - Remaining part of allantois forms part of urinary bladder.
4. Vitellointestinal duct and umbilical vesicle
    - Part of the yolk sac communicating with midgut forms vitellointestinal duct.
    - Unabsorbed part of the yolk sac forms umbilical vesicle.
    - In later part of pregnancy, vitellointestinal duct and umbilical vesicles disappears.

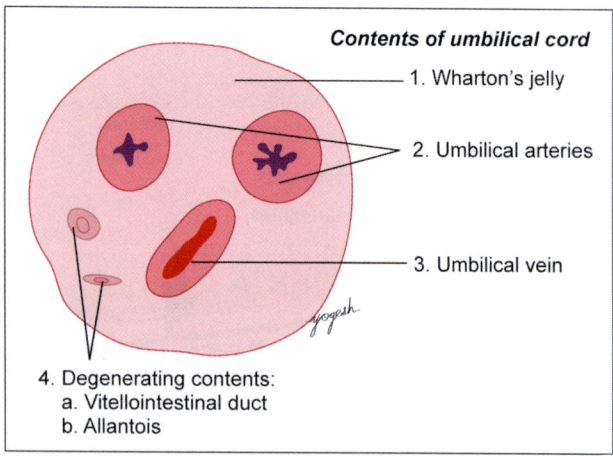

Practice Fig. 9.3: Structure of the umbilical cord

Some Interesting Facts
- Umbilical cord contains two umbilical arteries and only one (left) umbilical vein.[Neet]
- Close to the attachment of umbilical cord with placenta, two umbilical arteries are connected by transverse anastomosis called **Hyrtl's anastomosis**.[Neet]
- Left umbilical vein gets obliterated after birth and forms *ligamentum teres hepatis*.[MCQ]
- After the birth, umbilical arteries undergo muscle spasm earlier than umbilical vein and hence, newborn receives blood from placenta and does not give blood to placenta.

Box 9.7: Physiological umbilical hernia
- Midgut loop communicates with the yolk sac. The midgut loop elongates to form a U-shaped loop that projects into the proximal part of umbilical cord.
- Midgut loop projects from 6th to 10th week.
- This midgut herniation is called physiological hernia. It occurs due to smaller abdominal cavity that is not enough to accommodate enlarged elongated midgut loop.
- After 10th week, hernia decreases owing to increasing availability of the abdominal space.

AMNION
- Definition: Amnion is a thin membrane that lines the roof of the amniotic cavity.
- Inner cell mass (embryoblast) of the trophoblast form an amniotic cavity and get separated from a layer of amniotic cells.
- Amnion forms a roof and bilaminar germ disc forms floor of the amniotic cavity.

Placenta and Umbilical Cord

- Amnion consists of angiogenic cells covered by somatopleuric layers of extraembryonic mesoderm.
- By the end of the 8th week, on the formation of embryonic folding, amnion entirely covers embryo.
- The amniotic cavity contains amniotic fluid.
- Amniotic fluid is also called *liquor amnii* or *camerous fluid*.

Constituents of Amniotic Fluid

1. Water, electrolytes
2. Foetal waste including urine
3. Hormones: Human chorionic gonadotropin, human placental lactogen
4. Cells exfoliated from foetus

Functions of Amniotic Fluid

1. Shock absorption: Amniotic fluid provides *water-cushion* that absorbs jerks and protects the foetus.
2. Nutrition: Amniotic fluid provides nutrition to developing neuroectoderm as it passes through anterior and posterior neuropore.
3. Amniotic fluid allows free foetal movements.
4. Foetus excrete urine in amniotic fluid. Foetus swallow and absorb amniotic fluid through gut into foetal blood. Finally, foetal waste products reach maternal blood through foeto-placental circulation.

Volume of Amniotic Fluid

Amniotic fluid volume increases from 10th week to 28th week and then decreases (Table 9.3).

Clinical Aspects

1. Amniocentesis
    - It is a procedure to aspirate 20–30 ml of the amniotic fluid for the analysis.
    - The amniotic fluid analysis involves biochemical analysis (lecithin:sphingomyelin ratio for lung maturity), and chromosomal analysis by karyotyping for genetic disorders.

Table 9.3	Amniotic fluid volume
Gestational age	*Volume of the amniotic fluid*
10th week	25 ml
20th week	400 ml
28th week	800 ml
36th week	1000 ml (at birth)
42nd week	400 ml

- High level of α-fetoprotein in amniotic fluid is an indicator of neural tube defects.^{MCQ}

2. Oligohydramnios
    - It is a condition in pregnancy characterised by low volume of amniotic fluid (less than 400 ml).
    - It can be detected by ultrasonography when largest amniotic liquid pool size becomes less than 2 cm.
3. Amnion nodosum
    - It is a nodule on the foetal surface of amnion (mostly found in oligohydramnios).
    - It is composed of a squamous cell aggregate and is derived from vernix caseosa of the foetal skin.
4. Potter syndrome
    - It is a foetal condition produced by oligohydramnios.
    - It includes pulmonary hypoplasia, limb defects, cranial anomalies and renal defects.
    - Causes: Placental failure, renal agenesis, ruptured amnion leading to amniotic fluid leakage.
5. Polyhydramnios
    - It is the excessive amniotic fluid (more than 2000 ml).
    - Causes: Conditions causing defective swallowing in the foetus such as oesophageal atresia, foetal neurological disorders (anencephaly).
    - Due to defective swallowing, amniotic fluid cannot be absorbed by foetal gut.
    - Polyhydramnios is diagnosed by ultrasonography when amniotic fluid index is greater than 24 cm.

Box 9.8: Amniotic fluid index (AFI)

Q. Write short note on amniotic fluid index.

- AFI is an indicator of amniotic fluid quantity and foetal health.^{Viva}

Method of measurement

- Amniotic cavity is scanned ultrasonically.
- The cavity is divided into four imaginary quadrants.
- Vertical length of each quadrant is measured and added up.
- The quadrant containing loop of umbilical cord is excluded.

Interpretation^{MCQ}

AFI	Interpretation
8–18	Normal
< 5	Oligohydramnios
> 24	Polyhydramnios

YOLK SAC

Q. Write short note on yolk sac.

- Yolk sac is a cavity developed from the blastocystic cavity (Practice Fig. 9.4).

Formation and Changes in Yolk Sac

- The yolk sac is formed in the following three stages: Primary yolk sac → secondary yolk sac → definitive yolk sac → umbilical vesicle and vitellointestinal duct

Primary yolk sac

- Hypoblast cells multiply and forms a flat cellular lining of the blastocyst cavity. This lining layer is called Heuser membrane and then the blastocystic cavity is called primary yolk sac.

Secondary yolk sac

- On formation of the extra-embryonic coelom, part of yolk sac is pinched off and resultant reduced yolk sac cavity is termed *secondary yolk sac*.

Definitive yolk sac

- On formation of the embryonic folding, intra-embryonic part of yolk sac forms primitive gut and extraembryonic part forms *definitive yolk sac*.

Umbilical vesicle and vitellointestinal duct

- Extraembryonic part of the yolk sac or definitive yolk sac undergo hour-glass contraction due to embryonic folding and it form small umbilical vesicle that communicates with midgut through vitellointestinal duct.

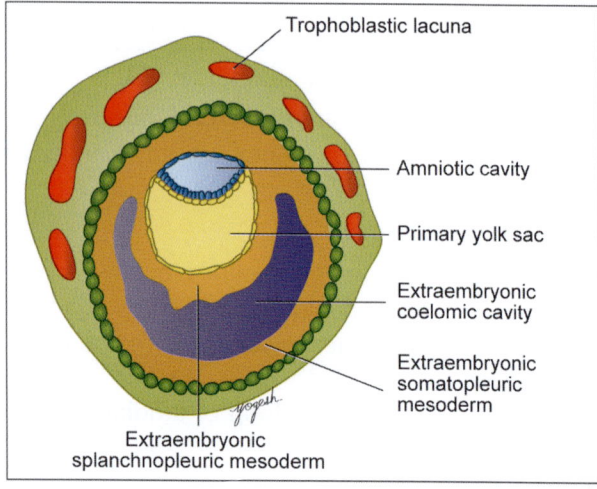

Practice Fig. 9.4: Yolk sac, amniotic cavity and extraembryonic coelomic cavity

Functions of Yolk Sac

- Haematopoiesis: Yolk sac produces blood cells up to sixth week of intrauterine life.
- Formation of primitive gut: Part of the yolk sac forms primitive gut.
- Formation of primordial germ cells: Primordial germ cells develop in the wall of the yolk sac. These cells migrate and forms gonads (ovary and testis) during fourth week.
- Allantois: A small diverticular extension of the yolk sac in the connecting stalk form allantois. Later allantois forms part of the urinary bladder.

Clinical Aspects

Meckel's diverticulum is the remnant of the vitellointestinal diverticulum.

CLINICAL EMBRYOLOGY

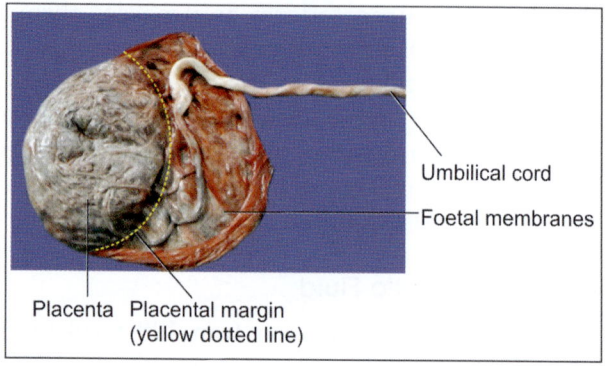

Clinical image 9.1: Velamentous placenta: Umbilical cord is attached to foetal membranes near peripheral marginal of the placenta. (Image courtesy: *Dr Haritha Sagili*)

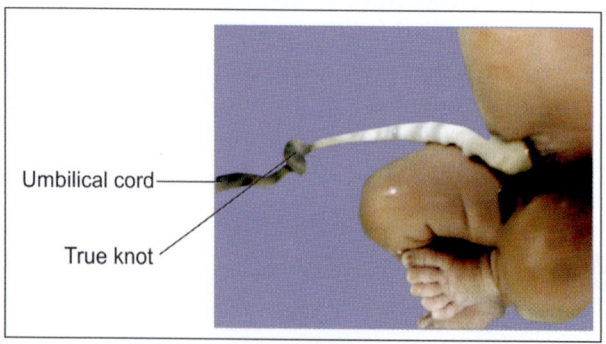

Clinical image 9.2: True knot of umbilical cord. Incidence: 0.3% to 2% of all births. (Image courtesy: *Dr Haritha Sagili*)

Placenta and Umbilical Cord

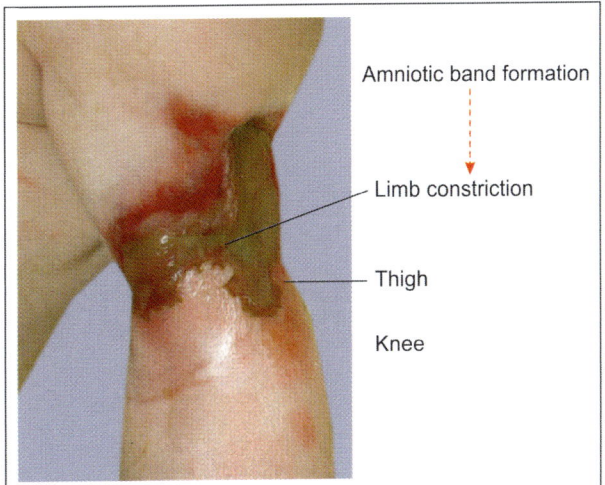

Clinical image 9.3: Limb constriction (soft tissue defect) probably secondary to amniotic band formation following domestic violence in pregnancy (Image courtesy: *Dr Haritha Sagili*)

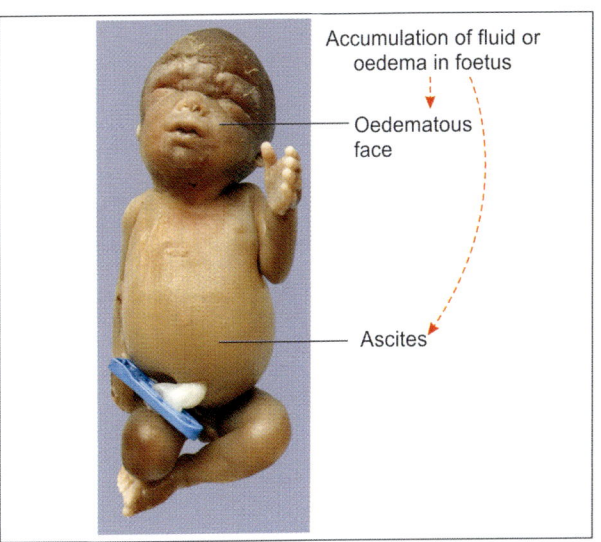

Clinical image 9.4: Hydrops fetalis. It is a condition characterised by an accumulation of fluid or oedema in foetus. Locations of hydrops foetalis include subcutaneous tissue (scalp), pleural cavity, pericardial cavity, peritoneal cavity. Foetal anemia is most common cause of hydrops foetalis. In the above image, protruding abdomen (due to ascites) and oedematous face are seen (Image courtesy: *Dr Haritha Sagili*)

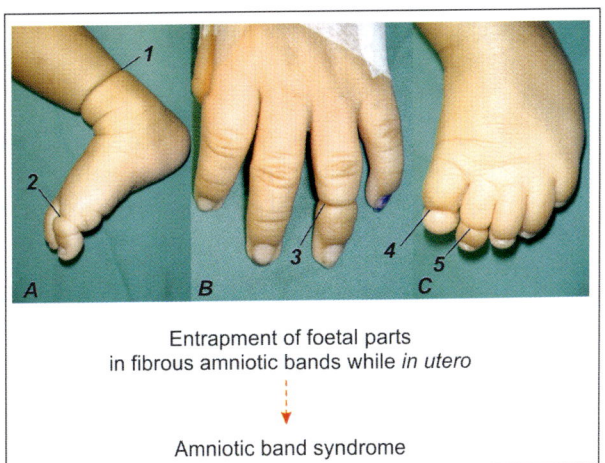

Clinical image 9.5: Amniotic band syndrome: (A) Right lower limb showing constriction rings in lower part of leg (1) and at proximal phalanx of great toe (2); (B) Left hand showing constriction ring at middle phalanx of ring finger (3); (C) Left foot showing constriction bands at distal phalanx of great toe with the absence of nail (4) and constriction band at middle phalanx of second toe (5) (Image courtesy: *Dr Kumaravel S*)

10
Integumentary System
Skin, its Appendages and Mammary Gland

Chapter Outline

- Development of skin
  - Stages of development
  - Developmental anomalies
- Development of hair
  - Stages of development
  - Anomalies related to hair
- Sweat glands
  - Eccrine sweat glands
  - Apocrine sweat glands
- Sebaceous glands
  - Development
  - Mode of secretion
- Nails
  - Structure of nail
  - Stages of development
  - Clinical aspects
- Mammary glands
  - Stages of development
  - Malformations

INTRODUCTION

Skin

- Skin and its appendages such as sebaceous glands, sweat glands, hairs and nails constitute integumentary system.
- Skin is the largest organ of body.
- It consists of two layers
  A. Epidermis—a superficial layer
  B. Dermis—a deep layer
- Epidermis consists of keratinocytes and has five layers as stratum basale (germinativum), stratum-spongiosum, stratum granulosum, stratum lucidum (only in palms and soles) and stratum corneum.
- Epidermis also contains a few melanocytes (produce melanin), Langerhans cells (antigen-presenting immune cells) and Merkel cells (mechanoreceptors for tactile/light-touch sensation).
- Dermis is a connective tissue layer that has a superficial papillary and a deep reticular layer.

DEVELOPMENT OF SKIN

Summary (Examination Guide)

- Epidermis develops from the surface ectoderm (Fig. 10.1, Table 10.1, Flowchart 10.1).
- Melanocytes and Merkel cells are derived from neural crest cells, whereas Langerhans cells from bone marrow (mesoderm).
- Dermis develops from the somatopleuric mesoderm.
- Appendages of skin (sebaceous glands, sweat glands and nails) are derived from the epidermis.

Table 10.1	Development of skin
Component of skin	Embryonic source
Epidermis	Surface ectoderm
Melanocyte (dendritic cells), Merkel cells	Neural crest cells
Langerhans cells	Mesoderm (bone marrow)
Dermis	Somatopleuric mesoderm
Sweat glands, sebaceous glands, nails, hairs	Surface ectoderm (epidermis)

Stages of Development

Epidermis

- Epidermis develops from the surface ectoderm (Fig. 10.1, Flowchart 10.1).
- Initially, surface ectoderm is a single cell-layer thick.
- In the second month (6th week), ectoderm differentiates into two layers.

Integumentary System: Skin, its Appendages and Mammary Gland

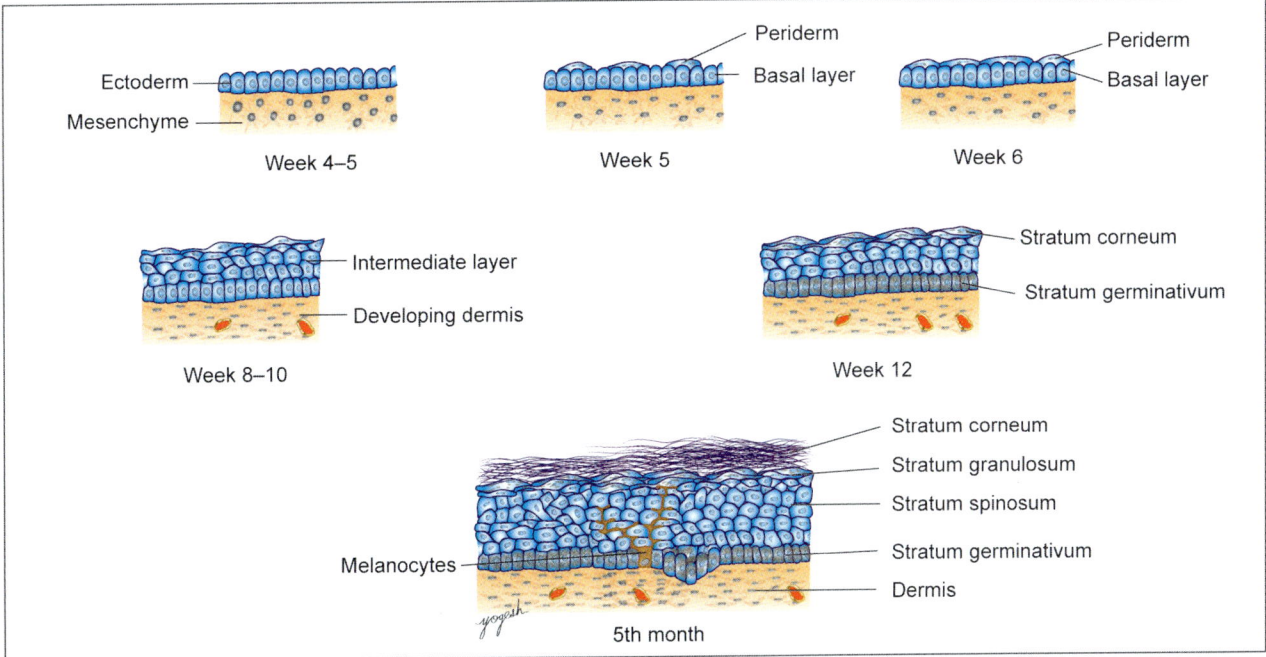

Fig. 10.1: Development of thin skin. Epidermis develops from surface ectoderm. Melanocytes are derived from neural crest cells. Dermis develops from somatopleuric mesoderm. Stratum lucidum is seen only in thick skin

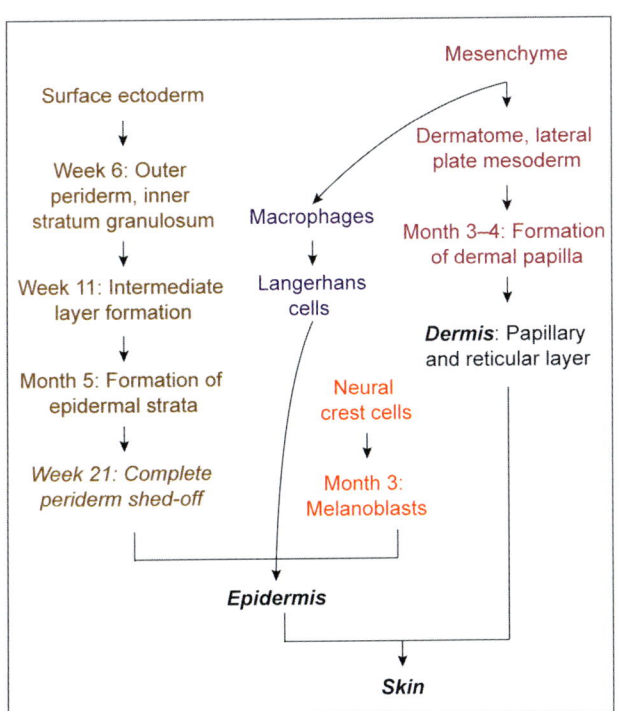

- Outer flattened cell layer as *periderm* or *epitrichium*.
- Inner cuboidal cell layer as *stratum germinativum* or *basal cell layer*.
- In 11th week, cells of the basal layer proliferate to form an intermediate layer.
- Cells of the intermediate layer produce keratin proteins.

- In 5th month, proliferating cells of stratum basale generate stratum spinosum, stratum granulosum and stratum corneum.
- Periderm layer gradually sloughed into the amniotic fluid. The **periderm shed off completely** by the 21st week.[MCQ]
- *Collodion babies* are the babies born with persistent periderm. This periderm usually shed during the first week of life spontaneously.[MCQ]
- *Vernix caseosa*: Cell of superficial layer of epidermis shed off slowly. These cells get mixed with secretions of sebaceous glands and hairs to form whitish sticky substance called *vernix caseosa*. It covers skin of the foetus and protects from maceration in amniotic fluid.[MCQ] Vernix caseosa is a whitish sticky coat on the skin of newborn.
- Formation of *epidermal ridges*: By 11th week, cells of the stratum basale proliferate and extend into the dermis to form epidermal ridges (become permanent by 18th week).[MCQ]
- Epidermal ridges form a specific pattern of fingerprints (also in palm and sole) that is genetically determined.
- At birth, all the layers of the adult epidermis are present.
- *Melanoblasts* (dendritic cells): Neural crest cells invade the epidermis during **3rd month** and become melanoblasts. These cells start producing melanin.[Neet]
- Merkel cells are pressure-detecting mechanoreceptors in the skin (palms and soles). Their origin is not clear. They appear in 4th–6th months.

- *Langerhans cells* are the tissue macrophages. They arise in bone marrow and migrate into the skin from 7th week onwards.^{MCQ}

Dermis

- Dermis is derived from the mesenchymal connective tissue underlying the epidermis (surface ectoderm) (Fig. 10.1, Flowchart 10.1).
- Sources of mesenchymal cells forming dermis:
  1. Dermatomes
  2. Lateral plate mesoderm
  3. Neural crest cells
- Dermatomes form dermis over the dorsal aspect of head and trunk.
- Lateral plate mesoderm forms dermis over lateral and ventral aspects of trunk.
- Neural crest cells form dermis over most of the part of head and anterior aspect of neck.
- *Dermal papillae*: During 3rd–4th month, the dermis shows regularly spaced thickenings that project into the overlying epidermis and form the dermal papillae.
- Later, the dermis differentiates into a superficial papillary layer and a deep reticular layer.

Anomalies of Skin and Appendages

1. *Aplasia of skin*: It is a failure of development of skin in some regions of body.
2. *Albinism*: Reduced or absent synthesis of melanin pigment produces depigmented zones in skin, hair and eyes. This condition is albinism. It is an autosomal recessive disorder.^{MCQ}
3. *Vitiligo*: It is a patchy loss of pigmentation in skin, hair and oral mucosa due to loss of melanocytes in an autoimmune disorder.^{MCQ}
4. *Piebaldism* is a rare autosomal dominant disorder. In this condition, melanocytes are absent in patchy areas of hairs and skin, mostly affects forehead.^{MCQ}
5. *Ichthyosis* (Gr. *Icthyos* means fish): It is an autosomal recessive or X-linked disease characterised by fish-like scaling of skin due to hyperkeratinisation.^{MCQ}
6. *Harlequin foetuses* have rigid, deeply cracked skin. Harlequin babies die shortly after birth. Harlequin foetus occurs due to failure of
   - maturation of keratinocytes
   - desquamation of keratinocytes (shed off property).^{MCQ}
7. *Gorlin syndrome*: It is also called *nevoid basal cell carcinoma syndrome* (NBCCS). It is an autosomal dominant disorder due to chromosome 9q22.3 gene defect. It is characterised by basal cell carcinoma, pathogenic dyskeratotic pitting of hands and feet.^{MCQ}

Some Interesting Facts
• Skin of the neonate contains 20 times more blood vessels than required for thermoregulation.

Box 10.1: Dermatoglyphics
• It is a study of specific pattern of *epidermal ridges*.
• In 11th week, epidermal ridges start appearing and they become permanent by 18th week.^{MCQ}
• The pattern of epidermal ridges is genetically determined and remains fixed throughout life.
• As epidermal ridge patterns are individual specific, they are commonly used for identification of genetic disorders.
• For details, read book *Principles of Clinical Genetics* by Dr Yogesh Sontakke.

DEVELOPMENT OF HAIR

Q. Write short note on development of hair.

Summary (Examination Guide)

- Shaft of hair follicle develops from the surface ectoderm (Fig. 10.2, Flowchart 10.2).
- Dermal papilla develops from the mesenchyme of dermis.
- *Arrector pili* muscles develop from the *mesodermal* sheath.^{Neet}

Stages of Development

- Hair follicles first appear at the end of the second month on eyebrows, eyelids, upper lip and chin.
- Hair follicles do not appear in other regions until the fourth month.

Phases of Development

1. *Formation of hair germ (hair bulb)*: It is a small concentration of ectodermal cells in the stratum basale of epidermis (Fig. 10.2, Flowchart 10.2).
2. *Formation of hair peg*: The hair bulb proliferates in the dermis to form a solid rod-like structure called *hair peg*. Later hair peg expands to form a bulbous peg.
3. *Formation of dermal papilla*: Underlying dermal cells of hair peg proliferate to form a small hillock called *dermal papilla*. Invagination of dermal papilla makes the hair bulb cup-shaped.

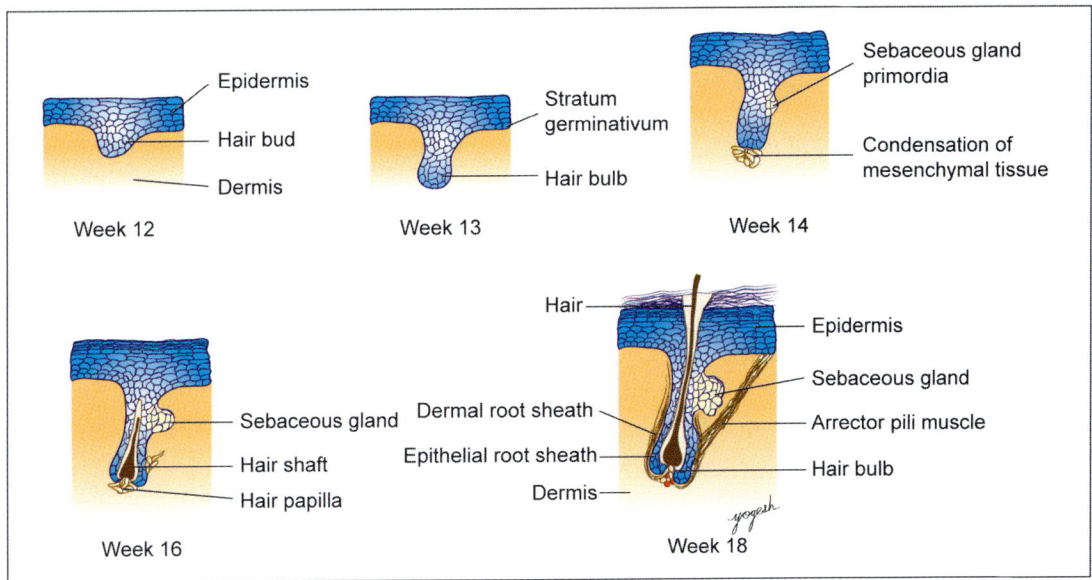

Fig. 10.2: Development of hair. Shaft of hair follicle develops form surface ectoderm. Dermal papilla develops from mesoderm of dermis. Arrector pili muscles develop from mesodermal sheath

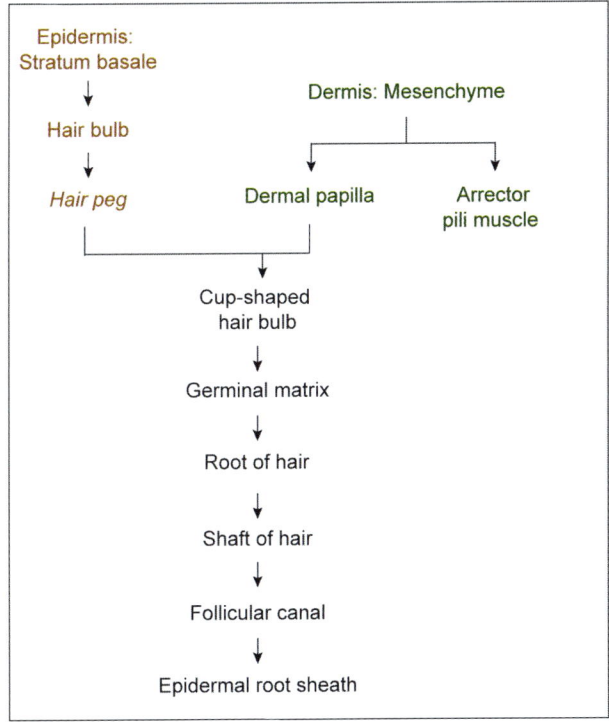

4. *Formation of germinal matrix*: Ectodermal cells covering dermal papilla become *germinal matrix* that produce root of hair.
5. *Formation of hair shaft*: Cells of hair root proliferate and get keratinised. These cells form hair shaft.
6. *Formation of follicular canal*: Growing hair shaft is pushed outwards by growth of hair root. Passage of hair shaft through the epidermis forms a *follicular canal*.
7. *Formation of epidermal root sheaths*: Cells lining follicular canal form inner and outer epidermal root sheaths.
8. *Development of arrector pili muscles*: Surrounding mesenchymal cells condense to form arrector pili muscles except for eyebrows and eyelashes. MCQ

Some Interesting Facts

- Melanocytes migrate into hair bulbs and transfer melanin to proliferating cells of germinal matrix. This is responsible for the colour of hair.
- *Lanugo*: These are fine, soft hairs that cover body and limbs of human foetus.
- Lanugo is replaced by coarser hairs during perinatal period.
- Terminal hair is more coarse and present in axilla and groin (moustache and beard only in males).
- *Definitive hair* once reaches to certain length, they cease to grow. Examples: Hairs of eyelashes and eyebrows, pubic hairs, axillary hairs.
- *Angora* is hairs that grow continuously. Examples: Hairs of scalp (hairs of moustache and beard only in males).

Anomalies Related to Hair (Clinical Facts)

1. **Hypertrichosis** is an excessive hair growth due to development of unusual abundance of hair follicles. It may be all over the body or may be patchy. It may

be persistence of Lanugo hairs that normally disappear after birth. *MCQ, Viva*
2. **Congenital alopecia** is a lack or loss of hairs due to the absence of hair follicles.
3. **Trichorrhexis nodosa** is a defect of the hair shaft due to metabolic disorder (argino-succinic aciduria and citrullinemia). In this disease, the hair shaft shows breaks. *MCQ*
4. **Menkes syndrome** is an X-linked recessive disorder of copper metabolism (ATPTA gene defect) having depigmented brittle hairs, neurological abnormalities and low serum calcium levels. *MCQ*
5. Curly hair is a result of asymmetrical hair follicles. It is an example of incomplete dominance. *MCQ*

SWEAT GLANDS

Q. Write short note on development of sweat glands.
- Sweat glands are also known as sudoriferous glands (*sudor* is sweat in Latin)
- Sweat glands are simple tubular exocrine glands that produce sweat on the surface of skin.
- There are two types of sweat glands: Eccrine and apocrine (Fig. 10.3).

Summary (Examination Guide)
- There are two types of sweat glands (Figs 10.3 and 10.4)
  - Eccrine sweat glands—open directly on skin surface and develop from invagination of surface ectoderm.
  - Apocrine sweat glands—open into hair follicles and develop from outgrowth of hair follicle.
  - Myoepithelial cells are derived from mesoderm (dermis).

Eccrine Sweat Glands
- They are distributed almost all over the human body (more in number in palms and soles) (Fig. 10.4).
- These glands open directly on surface of skin and pour secretions directly on the skin surface.
- These are **merocrine** in nature (secrete by exocytosis)
- Their secretions are watery and help in maintenance of body temperature.
- Eccrine sweat glands develop from surface epithelium before birth as follows:
  1. At 20th week, epidermis develops down growths in the dermis.
  2. Cells of stratum germinativum proliferate to form enlarging solid mass (bud) of epithelial cells in dermis.

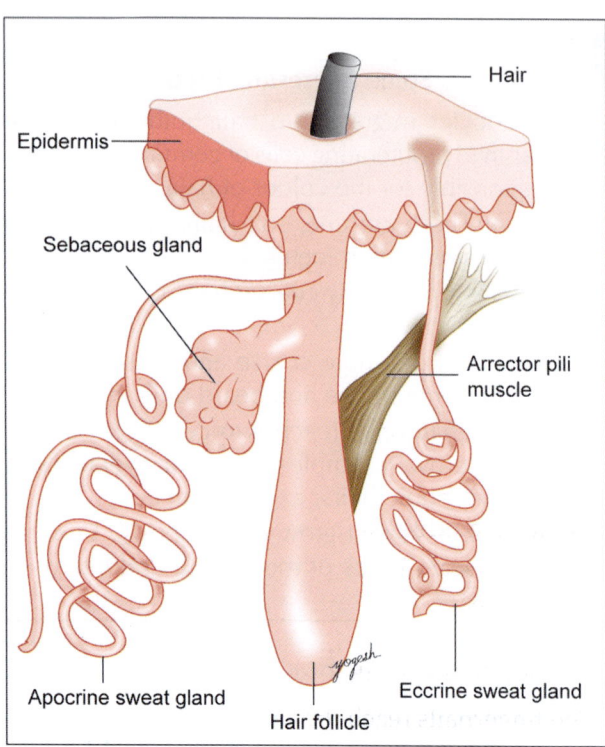

Fig. 10.3: Apocrine and eccrine sweat glands

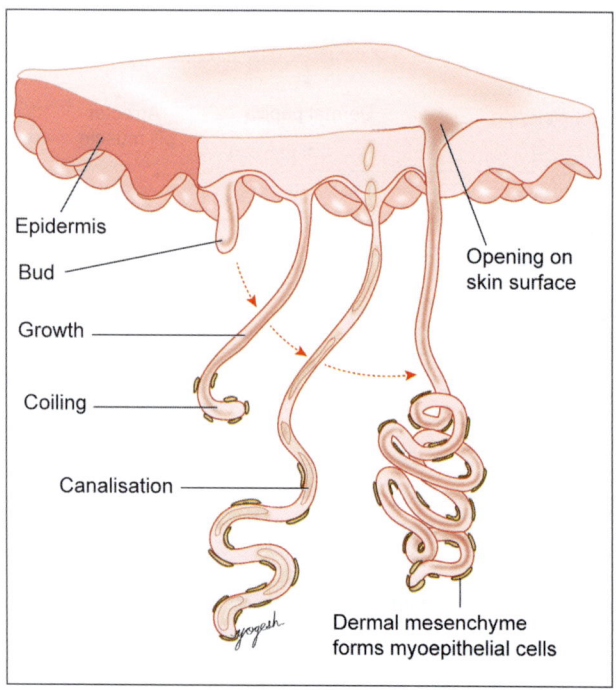

Fig. 10.4: Development of eccrine sweat gland. At 20th week, cells of stratum germinativum proliferate to form enlarging solid mass (bud) of epithelial cells in the dermis. Deeper end of bud continues to grow and becomes coiled and later, solid bud gets canalised to form lumen. Straight part of gland forms duct, whereas deeper coiled part forms secretory segment. Surrounding mesenchymal cells form myoepithelial cells. Arrow indicates advancing stages of gland development

3. Deeper end of bud continues to grow and becomes coiled.
4. Later, solid buds get canalised to form lumen.
5. Straight part of gland forms duct, whereas deeper coiled part forms secretory segment.
6. Surrounding mesenchymal cells modify to form myoepithelial cells.

Apocrine Sweat Glands

- They are confined to axilla, pubic and perianal regions, areola of the nipple, ear and eyelids.
- These glands open into hair follicles.
- These are *apocrine* in nature (shed off a portion of cell in the form of secretion).
- Their secretion is thick and produces odour.
- These glands develop at puberty as epidermal outgrowths from hair follicles.

SEBACEOUS GLANDS

- Sebaceous glands are exocrine glands that secrete an oily substance called *sebum*.
- Sebaceous glands are distributed in the skin of all parts of the body except palms and soles.
- Meibomian glands of eyelid (tarsal glands), Montgomery's areolar tubercles surrounding female nipples, preputial (Tyson's) glands in genitalia are modified sebaceous glands. *MCQ*

Development (Fig. 10.2)

- Sebaceous glands develop as a bud that arises from epithelial root sheath of hair follicle in 13th–16th week of IUL.
- The bud grows and divides into number of branches to form acini and their ducts.

Mode of Secretion

- Sebaceous gland is **holocrine** in nature (whole cell rupture to become secretion).
- Note: *Merocrine* by exocytosis and *apocrine* by membrane budding or loss of cytoplasm.

NAILS

Q. Write short note on development of nail.

- Nail is a horn-like covering at the tips of fingers and toes.
- Nails consist of a tough protein called *alphakeratin*.

Structure of nail

The nail shows the following parts (Fig. 10.5):
1. **Nail plate** (body) consists of keratinised cells. Nail plate grows over underlying nail bed.

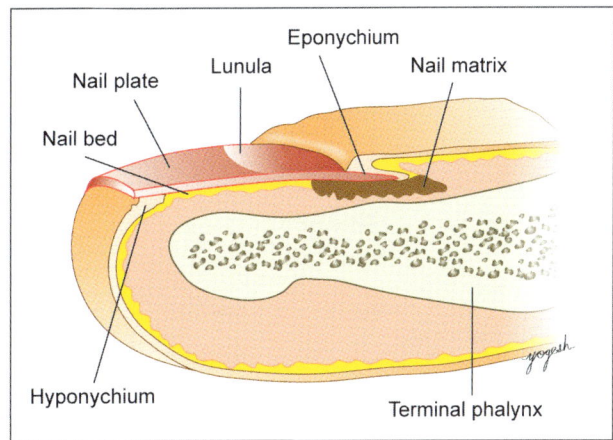

Fig. 10.5: Parts of nail

2. **Nail bed** is a highly vascular connective tissue layer that lies deep to the nail plate.
3. **Hyponychium** is a part of epidermis that lies under free edge of the nail plate (Greek, *onyx* is nail).
4. **Germinal matrix** (nail root) is a growing area of nail.
5. **Lunula** is a proximal soft, half-moon shaped part of nail plate that overlies nail bed.
6. **Cuticle** is an overlapping epidermis around the base of nail (overlies matrix).
7. **Nail walls** are folds of skin that overlap sides of nail.
8. **Perionychium** includes nail wall and cuticle area.
9. **Eponychium** is an extension of base of nail plate under that nail plate emerges from the matrix.

Stages of development

- *Nail field* appears by the end of 10th week as a thickened area at the tip and adjacent sides of fingers and toes (Fig. 10.6).
- At the base of nail field, U-shaped *epidermal nail folds* appear.
- Development of fingernails is followed by toenails.
- The underlayer of nailfold modifies to form a *germinal matrix*.
- In 5th month, a few cells of matrix get keratinised to form *nail plate*.
- Nail plate differentiates to form proximal lunula and remaining hard nail body.
- Adjacent epidermis forms *nailwall* and *cuticle*.
- Beneath the nail plate, surface epidermis pileup to form a mass called *hyponychium*.
- Nail plate reaches up to the tip of finger about 1 month before birth. *MCQ*
- The fingernails reach the fingertips by 32 weeks and toenails reach toe tips by 36 weeks. After birth, nails grow about 0.5 mm a week. *MCQ*

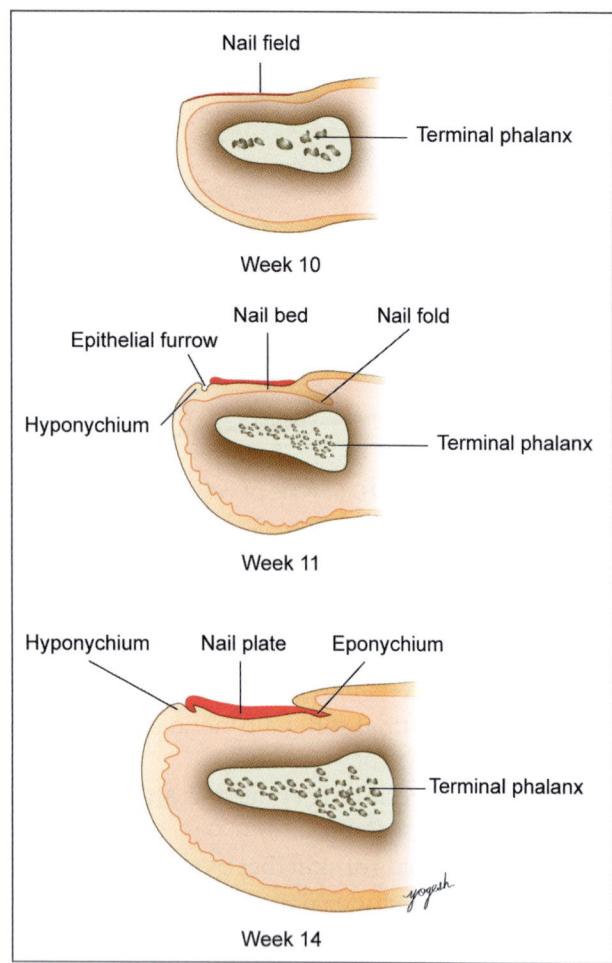

Fig. 10.6: Development of nail

Clinical Aspects

1. *Anonychia* is partial or complete absence of nails due to failure of germinal matrix to form nails.
2. *Dyskeratosis congenita* (DKC) (*Zinsser-Cole-Engman syndrome*): is a rare progressive congenital disorder due to short telomeres. It shows triad of abnormal skin pigmentation, nail dystrophy, and leukoplakia of the oral mucosa. *MCQ*

MAMMARY GLANDS

Q. *Write short note on development of mammary gland.*

Summary (Examination Guide)

- Mammary gland is a modified sweat gland (Figs 10.7 and 10.8, Practice Fig. 10.1, Flowchart 10.3, Table 10.2).
- Development of parenchyma: Parenchyma of mammary gland develops from ectodermal bud raising from the mammary ridge. Mammary bud forms solid cords that grow into surrounding mesoderm. Later, these cords get canalised to form

Table 10.2	Development of mammary gland
Structure	Embryonic source
Parenchyma (secretory part)	Mammary buds arising from ectodermal mammary ridge (extend from axillae to groins)
Myoepithelial cells	Surrounding mesenchyme
Fibrous stroma, suspensory ligaments and fat	Surrounding mesenchyme

lactiferous ducts, whereas their terminal parts form secretory acini.
- Fibrous stroma, fat and myoepithelial cells: Surrounding mesoderm forms fibrous stroma, suspensory ligaments and myoepithelial cells.

Stages of Development

Formation of mammary ridge (Fig. 10.7)

- In 6th week, surface ectoderm shows two thickened strips called *primitive mammary ridges* or *milk lines*.
- The ridges extend from axillae to inguinal regions. In humans, these ridges rapidly regress except in the thoracic region.

Formation of mammary buds (Fig. 10.8, Practice Fig. 10.1, Flowchart 10.3)

- Mammary buds arise from the persistent thoracic part of the mammary ridges.
- Mammary buds penetrate underlying mesenchyme and give rise to several secondary buds that later form lactiferous ducts and their branches.

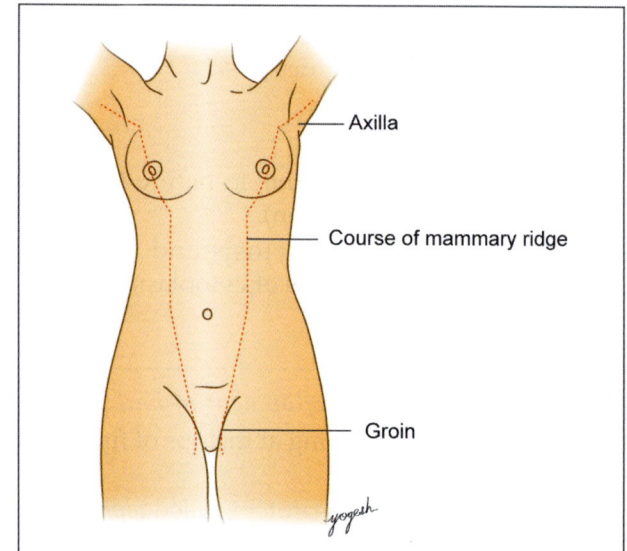

Fig. 10.7: Mammary ridge. In 6th week, surface ectoderm shows two thickened strips called primitive mammary ridges or milk lines. The ridges extend from axillae to inguinal regions. These ridges rapidly regress except in the thoracic region

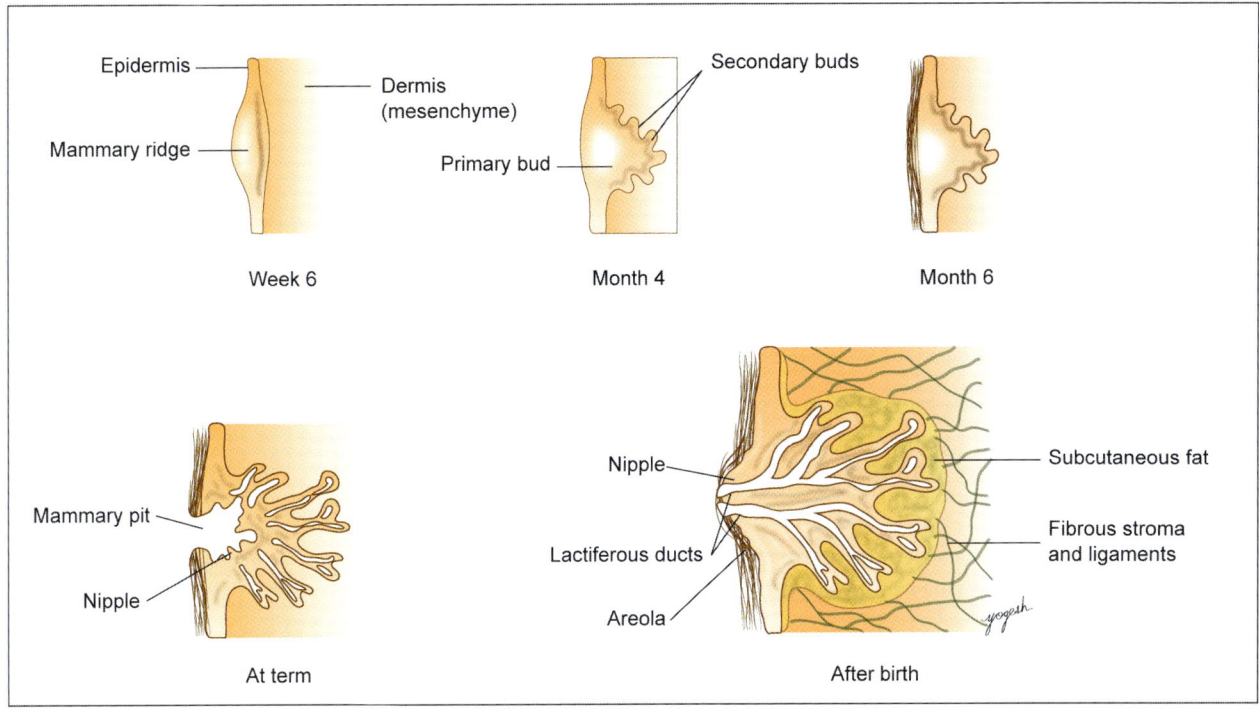

Fig. 10.8: Development of mammary gland

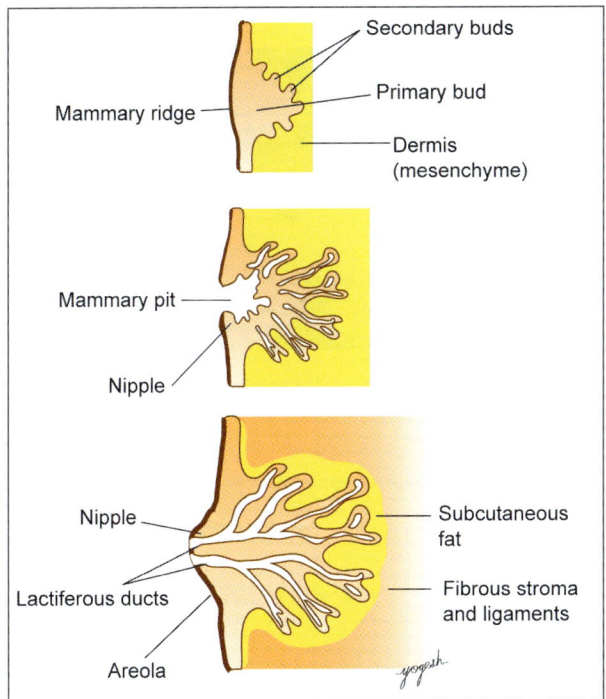

Practice Fig. 10.1: Development of mammary gland

- Lactiferous ducts canalise by the end of prenatal period.
- Only the main ducts are found at birth, and the gland remains undeveloped until puberty.

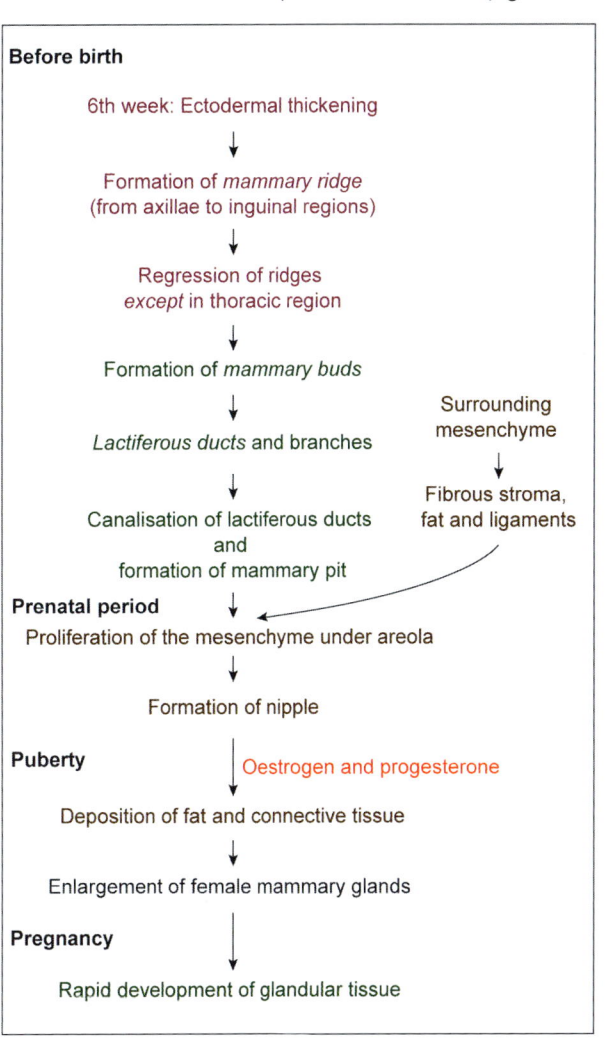

Flowchart 10.3: Development of mammary gland

Formation of fibrous stroma
- The fibrous connective tissue, suspensory ligaments and fat of mammary gland develop from surrounding mesenchyme.

Formation of mammary pit
- During the late foetal period, the epidermis becomes depressed to form a shallow mammary pit (epithelial pit).
- Lactiferous ducts open onto this epithelial pit.

Formation of nipple
- Nipple develops during the perinatal period due to proliferation of the mesenchyme under areola (circular area of skin around nipple).

Development at puberty
- At puberty, owing to the deposition of fat and connective tissue, female mammary glands enlarge rapidly.
- Under the influence of oestrogen and progesterone, duct system grows.

Development during pregnancy
- During pregnancy, the glandular tissue rapidly develops and form buds and alveoli.

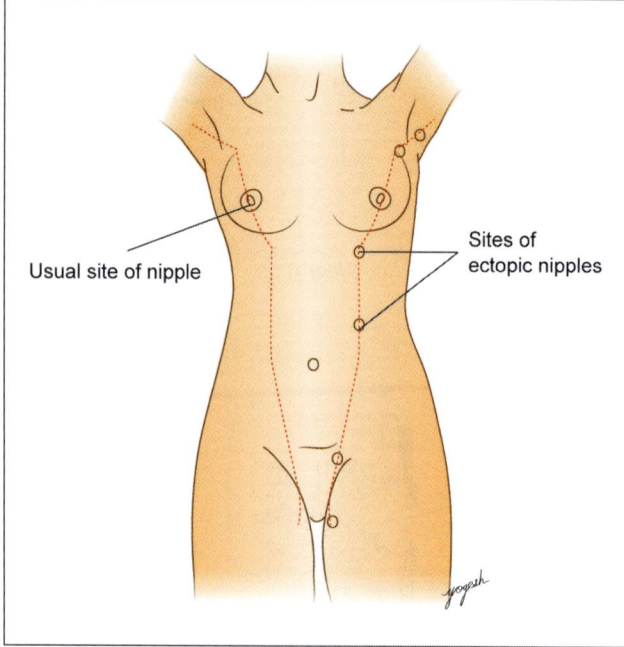

Fig. 10.9: Supernumerary nipples (polythelia)

Some Interesting Facts
- The male mammary glands undergo a little postnatal development
- *Witch's milk*: The mammary glands of both newborn males and females are often enlarged and may secrete a small quantity of milk called *witch's milk* or *neonatal milk*. It occurs due to the influence of maternal hormones passing into foetal circulation.

Malformations of Mammary Gland
- Athelia is an absence of nipple.[Neet]
- Amastia is an absence of mammary gland.[Neet]
- Polythelia is presence of supernumerary nipples (Fig. 10.9).[Neet]
- Polymastia is presence of supernumerary mammary glands. Polymastia is seen in about 1% of the female population.[Neet]
- Inverted or *crater* nipple: Due to a failure of the underlying mesenchyme to proliferate and push nipple out, the nipple fails to develop and evert after birth.
- *Gynecomastia* is unusual enlargement of male mammary glands.

CLINICAL EMBRYOLOGY

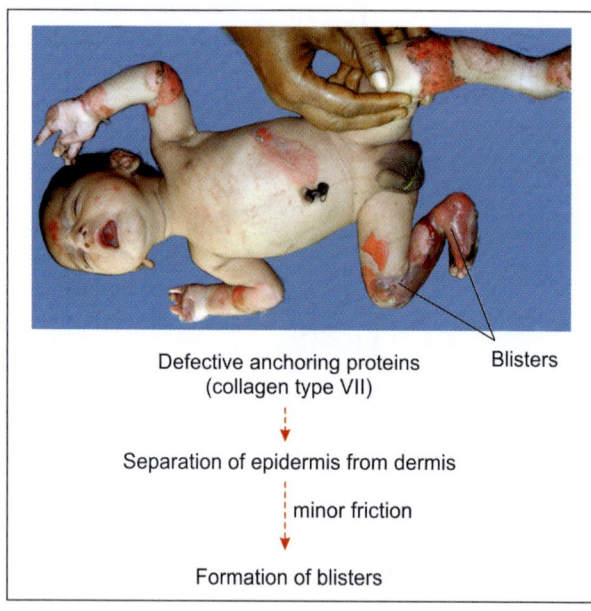

Clinical image 10.1: Epidermolysis bullosa (EB). It is a rare inherited connective tissue disorder that causes blisters on the skin and mucosal membranes. Its incidence is 20 per million newborns. It is a result of a defect in anchoring between the epidermis and dermis specifically type VII collagen. It results in skin fragility (even mild friction causes separation of epidermis from dermis). Hence, EB affected child is also called *butterfly children* (having fragile skin like butterfly) or *cotton wool babies*[MCQ] (Image courtesy: *Dr Kumaravel S*)

Integumentary System: Skin, its Appendages and Mammary Gland

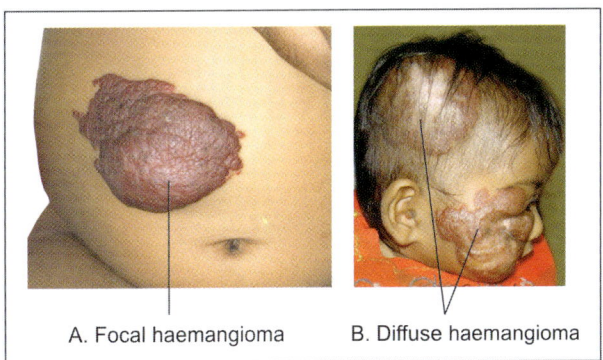

A. Focal haemangioma   B. Diffuse haemangioma

Clinical image 10.2: Infantile haemangioma: (A) Focal haemangioma; (B) Diffuse haemangioma. A haemangioma (infantile haemangioma) is a benign vascular tumour composed of collection of small blood vessels that form a lump under the skin (**strawberry mark**). It is one of the common benign tumours of infancy (occurs in 5–10% of infants). It appears during the first week of life and grows most rapidly during the first three to six months of life. Its involution commences by twelve months of age. Majority of infantile haemangioma regresses by five years of age. The cause of haemangiomas is not fully known. Probably it arises from placental tissue embolised to foetus. (Image courtesy: *Dr Kumaravel S*)

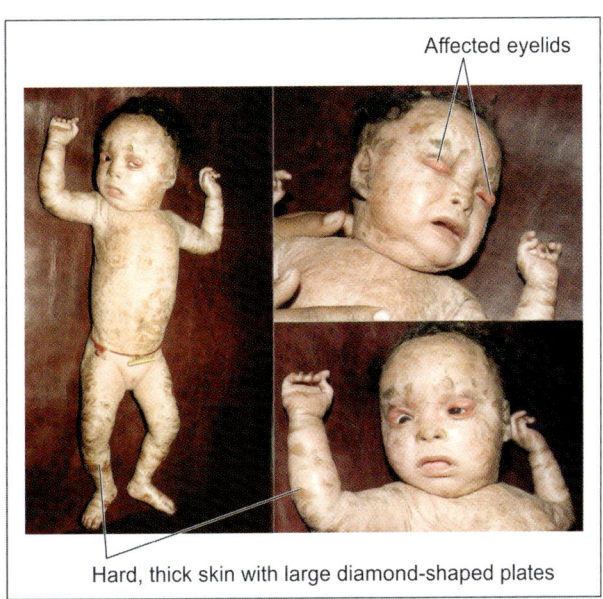

Affected eyelids

Hard, thick skin with large diamond-shaped plates

Clinical image 10.3: Harlequin ichthyosis. An infant with Harlequin ichthyosis has hard, thick skin with large diamond-shaped plates separated by deep cracks (fissures). It affects the shape of the eyelids, nose, mouth and ears. Restricted movement of the chest can lead to breathing difficulties. It occurs due to mutations of the ABCA12 genes that is inherited as an autosomal recessive disorder. ABCA12 gene product (protein) is essential for the normal development of skin cells and transport of lipids in the skin. This protein plays a major role in the transport of fats (lipids) in the outermost layer of skin. Its incidence is 1 in 300,000 births. (Image courtesy: *Dr Kumaravel S*)

11

Pharyngeal Apparatus

Chapter Outline

- Pharyngeal apparatus
- Pharyngeal arches
  - Skeletal elements
  - Muscular derivatives
  - Nerves of the pharyngeal arches
  - Arteries of arches
- Fate of pharyngeal clefts
- Branchial cyst
- Branchial fistula
- DiGeorge's Syndrome
- Pharyngeal pouches
- Caudal pharyngeal complex
- Development of palatine tonsil, thymus, parathyroid and thyroid glands
  - Development of palatine tonsil
  - Development of thymus
    - Involution
  - Development of parathyroid gland
  - Development of thyroid gland
    - Anomalies of thyroid gland
- Thyroglossal cyst and fistula
- Goldenhar syndrome

INTRODUCTION

- The pharynx is part of the throat behind the mouth and nose. It is a funnel-shaped tubular structure that develops from the foregut.
- On the formation of embryonic folds, foregut develops from the part of yolk sac that lies within the head fold.
- Overgrowing forebrain vesicle brings the buccopharyngeal membrane in the depression called *stomodeum* that lies cranial to the pericardial bulge.
- Primitive pharynx lies dorsal and caudal to the stomodeum.
- The primitive pharyngeal part has floor, roof and two lateral walls.
- *Relations of the primitive pharynx*
  - Cranial: Forebrain
  - Ventral (floor): Stomodeum, pericardial bulge, septum transversum
  - Dorsal (roof): Notochord and hindbrain vesicle
  - Lateral: Splanchnopleuric layer of the mesoderm, surface ectoderm
- In early developmental stages, the neck is not present. The neck is formed in between stomodeum and pericardial bulge due to mesodermal growth.
- In the neck zone, between stomodeum and pericardial bulge, mesoderm shows intermittent thickening. The thickened mesoderm forms bars (bulging) on the surface ectoderm. These bars extend ventrally and push and separate pericardial bulge from stomodeum (Fig. 11.1).
- Each mesodermal bar fuses with opposite bar in the midline to form arch-like, shoe-shaped structure called *pharyngeal arch or branchial arch* (Fig. 11.2).
- Subsequently, six arches appear, out of these, the fifth arch is small and rudimentary.*MCQ, Viva*
- When seen from the cavity of the foregut (primitive pharynx), endoderm of the foregut shows depressions between the adjacent pharyngeal arches. These six endodermal depressions in the floor and the lateral wall of the pharynx are called *pharyngeal pouches*.
- Surface ectoderm also shows depressions or groove in between adjacent arches. These four grooves are called *pharyngeal clefts*.

Pharyngeal Apparatus

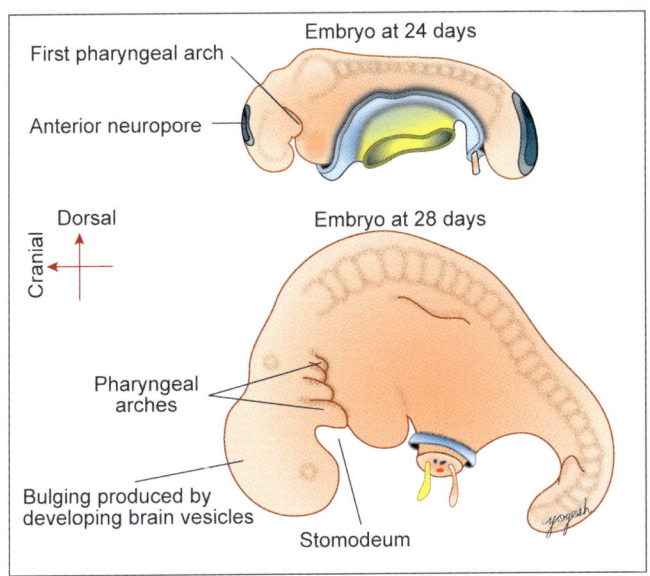

Fig. 11.1: Side view of the developing embryo with formation of pharyngeal arches. By 24th day, embryo shows the first pharyngeal arch. The number of arches increases to four by 28th day

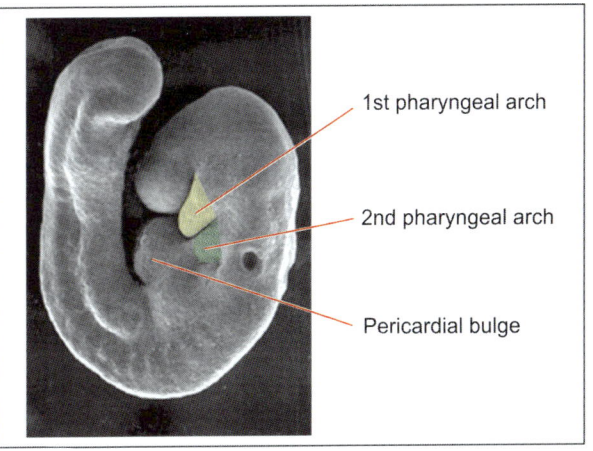

Scanning electron micrograph 11.1: SEM showing pharyngeal arches. On twenty-seventh day (by the time that anterior neuropore closes), the first and second pharyngeal arches are evident [Species: Mouse, approximate human age: 27 days, lateral view]

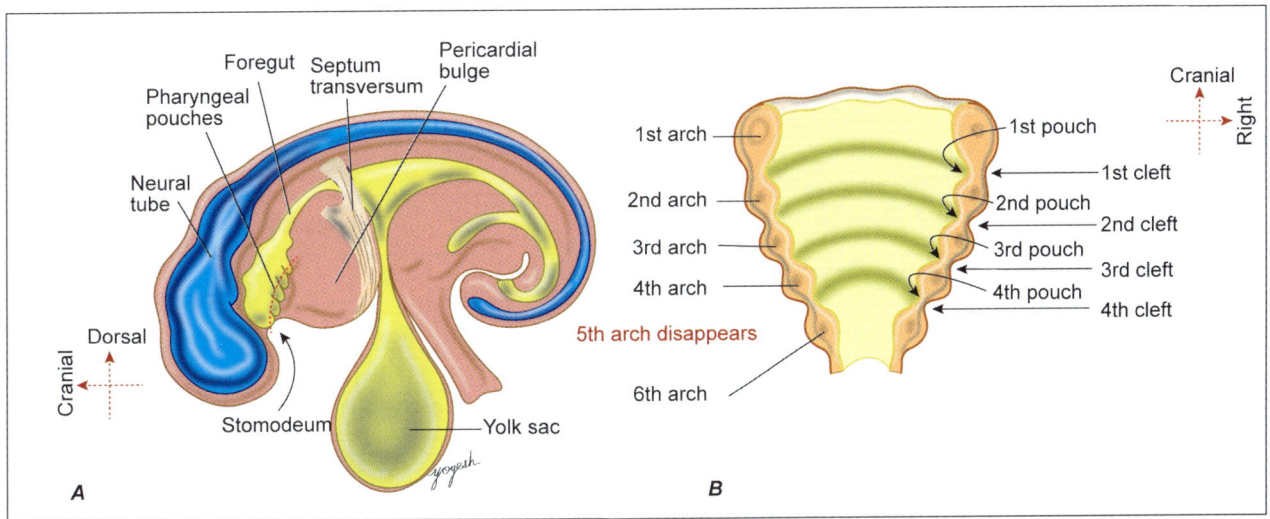

Fig. 11.2: (A) Section of the embryo showing the foregut and pharyngeal pouches; (B) Section of the embryo passing through the dotted red line shown in Fig. A. The mesodermal thickening forms six pharyngeal arches. Inner side of the foregut shows depressions in between adjacent pharyngeal arches. These depressions are called pharyngeal pouches. The surface ectoderm also shows depressions in between adjacent arches. These depressions are called pharyngeal clefts

- Pharyngeal arches appear in the fourth and fifth week of the development.^{MCQ}

PHARYNGEAL APPARATUS

Q. Define pharyngeal apparatus, pharyngeal arch, pharyngeal pouch and pharyngeal cleft.^{Viva}

- The pharyngeal apparatus consists of pharyngeal arches, pharyngeal pouches and pharyngeal clefts (Fig. 11.2).

Pharyngeal arches
- Thickened *mesodermal* bars present in the floor and lateral wall of the primitive pharynx are called pharyngeal arches.

Pharyngeal clefts
- Depressions (grooves) on the surface *ectoderm* in between adjacent arches are called pharyngeal clefts.

Pharyngeal pouches
- *Endodermal* depressions between adjacent pharyngeal arches in the floor and lateral wall of the primitive pharynx are called pharyngeal pouches.

- For study purpose, the derivatives of the pharyngeal apparatus are grouped into derivatives of pharyngeal arches, pharyngeal pouches and pharyngeal clefts.

Some Interesting Facts

- ***Pharyngeal membranes*** are the area of contact between pharyngeal pouches (endoderm) and pharyngeal clefts (ectoderm). ***Tympanic membrane*** is derived from 1st pharyngeal membrane (separates 1st pouch from 1st cleft) and represents all three derms.[Neet]
- In fishes and other aquatic vertebrates, the pharyngeal membranes rupture to form gill slits. Gill slits work as respiratory organ and help to take dissolved oxygen from water that flows from mouth and exits from gill slits.
- In the human embryo, a thin layer of mesenchyme appears between pharyngeal membranes and form fibro-areolar tissue of the neck. In human, pharyngeal membranes do not rupture.[MCQ]
- By the fourth week, buccopharyngeal membrane ruptures and foregut communicates with the amniotic cavity.[MCQ]
- By 4th week (22nd day) first and second pharyngeal arch appears.[MCQ] By 29th day (5th week), four pharyngeal arches appear.

PHARYNGEAL ARCHES

Q. Enlist the derivatives of first pharyngeal arch.

Definition
- Horseshoe shaped thickened mesodermal bars in lateral wall and the floor of the primitive pharynx is called *pharyngeal arch*.

Number
- There are *six* pharyngeal arches, but the fifth pharyngeal arch is rudimentary (small and disappears).

Components
- Each arch consists of splanchnopleuric mesoderm with invaded neural crest cells.
- These invading neural crest cells form skeletal elements and connective tissue of the head and neck region.[MCQ, Viva] Hence, facial skeleton or viscerocranium is derived from neural crest cells.[Neet]
- Each pharyngeal arch mesoderm differentiates to form muscle mass, pharyngeal arch artery and nerve (Fig. 11.3, Table 11.1, Flowchart 11.1).

Flowchart 11.1: Components of pharyngeal arch

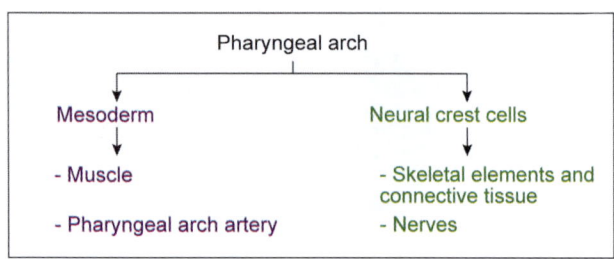

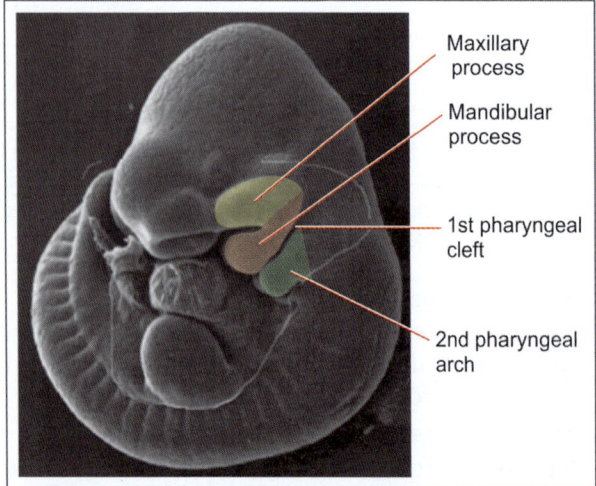

Scanning electron micrograph 11.2: SEM showing 6-week embryo with first and second pharyngeal arch. Maxillary and mandibular processes of first pharyngeal arch are also evident [Species: Mouse, approximate human age: 6 weeks, lateral view]

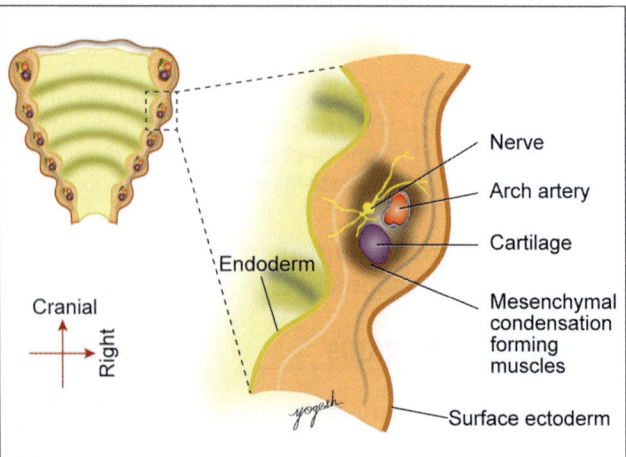

Fig. 11.3: Components of the pharyngeal arch. Each pharyngeal arch has one arch artery, cartilage, post-trematic nerve and muscles

Skeletal Elements

- Neural crest cells from the cartilaginous rod in the substance of the pharyngeal arch (Fig. 11.4, Practice Fig. 11.1, Flowchart 11.2).
- The fate of cartilages of the pharyngeal arches:
  - Some part of the cartilage persists
  - Some part disappears
  - Some part is converted into bone
  - Some part of perichondrium persists as ligament

First Arch

- The first arch is differentiated into smaller cranial maxillary process and larger caudal mandibular process (Fig. 11.4, Practice Fig. 11.1).
- Maxillary process form part of the upper lip, upper jaw and palate.
- Cartilage of mandibular part, the first arch, is called **Meckel's cartilage**.
- Meckel's cartilage forms –
  1. Malleus (ear ossicle) from dorsal part[MCQ]
  2. Incus (ear ossicle) from dorsal part[MCQ]
  3. Anterior ligament of malleus from perichondrium

Flowchart 11.2: Fate of neural crest cells in pharyngeal arches

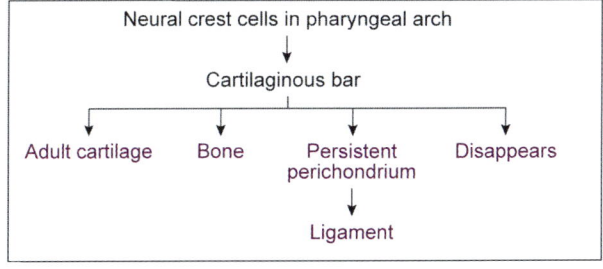

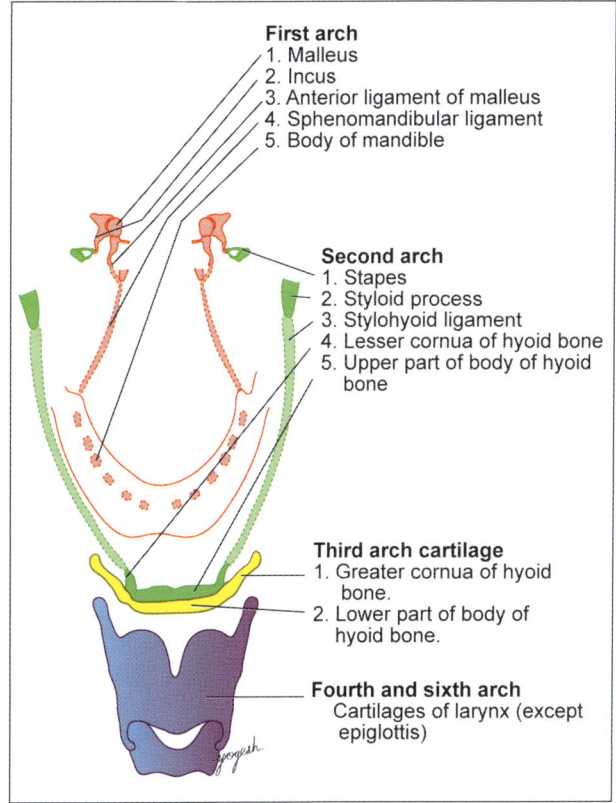

Practice Fig. 11.1: Structures derived from cartilages of the pharyngeal arches

  4. Sphenomandibular ligament
  5. Body of the mandible develops from fibrous surrounding of the Meckel's cartilage[MCQ]

Note: Meckel's cartilage does not form mandible. Maxillary part of the first arch forms pre-maxilla, maxilla, zygomatic bone, part of the temporal bone.

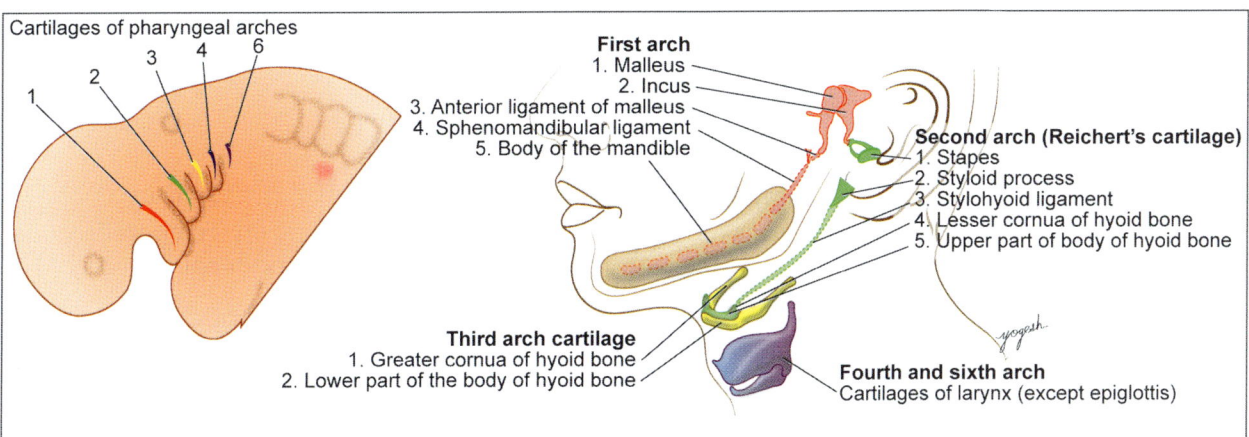

Fig. 11.4: Structures derived from cartilages of the pharyngeal arches. The first arch cartilage is Meckel's cartilage and the second one is Reichert's cartilage

Table 11.1	Derivatives of pharyngeal arches^{High yielding, Neet}			
Pharyngeal arch	Muscles ^{Neet}	Nerve ^{Neet}	Skeletal elements ^{Neet}	Ligament ^{Neet}
First arch (Meckel's cartilage)^{Neet}	Muscles of mastication (temporalis, masseter, medial and lateral pterygoid) Tensor veli palatini Tensor tympani Anterior belly of digastric Mylohyoid	Pre-trematic: Chorda tympani Post-trematic: Mandibular nerve^{Neet}	Premaxilla Maxilla Zygomatic bone Temporal bone Incus Malleus	Anterior ligament of malleolus Sphenomandibular ligament
Second arch (Reichert's cartilage)^{Neet}	Muscles of facial expression Posterior belly of digastric Stylohyoid Stapedius	Facial nerve^{Neet}	Stapes Styloid process Short (lesser) cornua of hyoid bone Superior part of body of hyoid bone	Stylohyoid ligament
Third arch	Stylopharyngeus ^{Neet}	Glossopharyngeal nerve ^{Neet}	Greater cornua of hyoid bone. Lower part of body of hyoid bone	—
Fourth arch	Cricothyroid, constrictors of pharynx, muscles of palate except tensor veli palatine ^{Neet}	Superior laryngeal nerve ^{Neet}	Laryngeal cartilages except epiglottis	—
Sixth arch	Intrinsic muscles of larynx except cricothyroid	Recurrent laryngeal nerve ^{Neet}		—

Second Arch Cartilage

Q. Enlist the skeletal derivatives of second pharyngeal arch.

- Cartilage of second (hyoid) arch is called **Reichert's cartilage** (Fig. 11.4, Practice Fig. 11.1).

Reichert's cartilage forms:
1. Stapes (ear ossicle) from dorsal part^{MCQ}
2. Styloid process of temporal bone from dorsal part^{MCQ}
3. Short (lesser) cornua of hyoid bone from ventral part
4. Superior (upper) part of body of hyoid bone from ventral part
5. Stylohyoid ligament from perichondrium of disappearing cartilage between styloid process and hyoid bone
   (Pneumonic: Note second arch derivatives starting from alphabet S.)

Third Arch Cartilage

- Dorsal part of the third arch cartilage disappears.
- Ventral part of the third arch cartilage forms –
  1. Greater cornua of hyoid bone
  2. Lower part of body of hyoid bone

Fourth and Sixth Arch

- Dorsal part of the fourth and sixth arch cartilage disappears.
- Ventral part of the fourth and sixth arch forms cartilages of larynx (except epiglottis) such as
  - Thyroid cartilage
  - Cricoid cartilage
  - Arytenoid cartilage
  - Corniculate cartilage
  - Cuneiform cartilage

Note: Epiglottic cartilage develops from hypobranchial eminence.^{MCQ}

Muscular Derivatives

- Mesodermal cells of arches differentiate to form striated muscles.
- These striated muscles migrate from their site of development. During migration, they carry their nerve.

First Arch

- Muscles derived from the first arch are as follows:^{MCQ}
  - 1–4. Muscles of mastication: Temporalis, masseter, lateral pterygoid and medial pterygoid
  - 5. Tensor tympani
  - 6. Tensor veli palatini
  - 7. Anterior belly of digastric
  - 8. Mylohyoid muscle
- Nerve supply: Mandibular nerve

Pharyngeal Apparatus

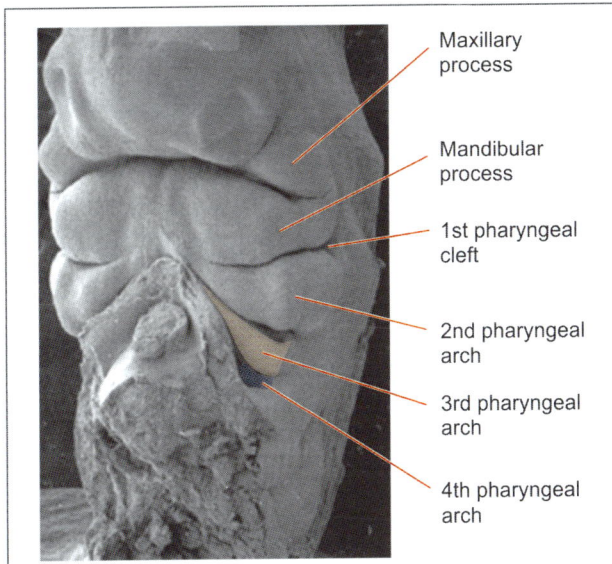

Scanning electron micrograph 11.3: SEM showing pharyngeal arches. The first, second, third and fourth arches are visible externally. The sixth arch does not form an external elevation. The heart has been removed in this specimen [Species: human, approximate age: fifth week]

Second Arch

- Muscles derived from second arch are as follows:
  1. Muscles of facial expression
  2. Posterior belly of digastric
  3. Stapedius
  4. Stylohyoid
- Nerve supply: Facial nerve

Third Arch

- The *stylopharyngeus* muscle develops from third arch.
- Nerve supply: Glossopharyngeal nerve

Fourth Arch

- Muscles derived from fourth arch are:
  1. Cricothyroid
  2. Constrictor muscles of pharynx
  3. Muscles of palate except tensor veli palatini
- Nerve supply: Superior laryngeal branch of vagus nerve

Sixth Arch

- Muscles derived from the sixth arch are: All the intrinsic muscles of the larynx except cricothyroid muscle.^{MCQ}
- Nerve supply: Recurrent laryngeal branch of vagus nerve

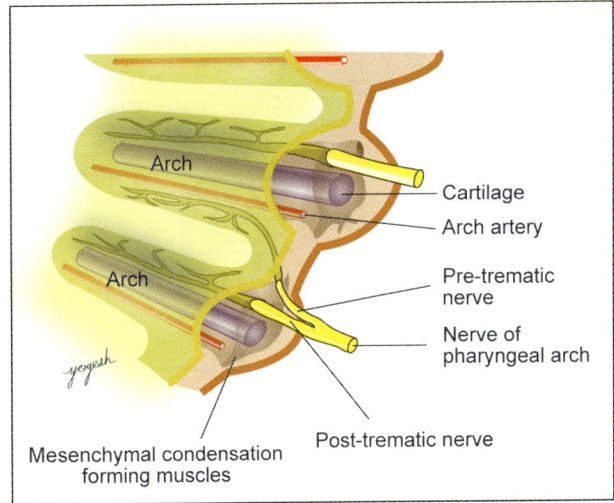

Fig. 11.5: Arrangement of nerves in the pharyngeal arch. The pre-trematic branch supplies the structures of the preceding arch, whereas nerve of the pharyngeal arch continues as post-trematic nerve and supplies the structures of the same arch

Some Interesting Facts

- Carotid body is derived from the third arch, whereas aortic body is derived from the fourth arch.^{MCQ}

Nerves of Pharyngeal Arches

Q. Name the nerves of pharyngeal arches.

- Pharyngeal arches receive nerve supply from hindbrain vesicle.
- Each nerve appears at the dorsal end of the cleft and divides into pre-trematic and post-trematic branches (Fig. 11.5).
- Pre-trematic branch supplies the arch cranial to the cleft, whereas post-trematic branch supplies caudal to the cleft.
- Pre-trematic nerve of all arches degenerate except the first arch. The pre-trematic nerve of the first arch forms chorda tympani nerve.^{MCQ}
- The nerve to the arch is mixed nerve as it supplies muscles and carry sensations from derivatives of pouches and clefts.
- Nerves of arches are as follows (Fig. 11.6):
  1. First arch: Mandibular nerve (pre-trematic) and chorda tympani branch of facial nerve (post-trematic)
  2. Second arch: Facial nerve
  3. Third arch: Glossopharyngeal nerve
  4. Fourth arch: Superior laryngeal nerve
  5. Sixth arch: Recurrent laryngeal nerve

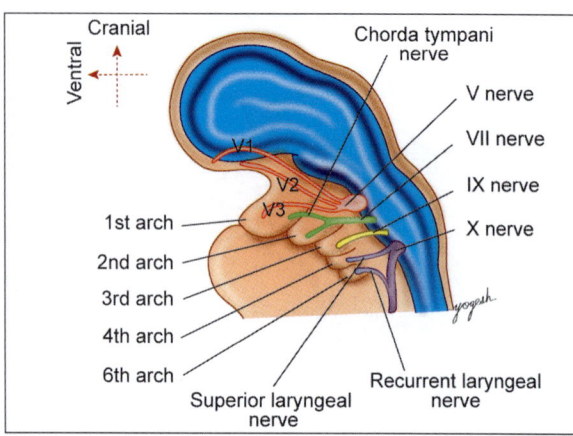

Fig. 11.6: Nerve supply of the pharyngeal arches. First arch is supplied by mandibular nerve (V3) and chorda tympani nerve. Second arch is supplied by facial nerve, third arch by glossopharyngeal nerve and fourth arch by superior laryngeal nerve, whereas sixth arch by recurrent laryngeal nerve. Sixth arch is not prominently visible on the surface. V1, ophthalmic nerve; V2, maxillary nerve; V3, mandibular nerve

Arteries of Arches

- Each arch contains one arch artery.
- These arch arteries connect dorsal aorta with aortic sac (that lies ventrally).
- Aortic arches modify and forms following structures:
  1. First aortic arch artery: A part of maxillary artery
  2. Second aortic arch artery: Stapedial artery, hyoid artery^Neet
  3. Third aortic arch artery:
     a. *Common carotid artery* from ventral part of third aortic arch and
     b. stem of internal carotid artery from dorsal part of third aortic arch^Neet
  4. Fourth aortic arch artery:
     a. On the right side—proximal part of right subclavian artery.
     b. On the left side—arch of aorta.
  5. Fifth aortic arch artery: Disappears completely
  6. Sixth aortic arch artery:
     a. On the right side—right pulmonary artery.
     b. On the left side—left pulmonary artery and ductus arteriosus (after birth, ligamentum arteriosum).

FATE OF PHARYNGEAL CLEFTS

Definition

- The groove of the surface ectoderm between adjacent pharyngeal arches is called *ectodermal cleft*.
- There are *four* pharyngeal clefts.
- Only dorsal part of the *first pharyngeal cleft* **persists** and forms the epithelial lining of the external acoustic meatus and acuticular layer of the tympanic membrane (Fig. 11.7).^MCQ

Cervical Sinus

Q. Write short note on cervical sinus.

- The mesenchymal tissue of second pharyngeal arch grows rapidly and covers second, third and fourth clefts. This growing tissue fuses with epicardial ridge. Thus, second to fourth clefts bury under the bulging second arch and form a slit-like cavity called *cervical sinus* (Fig. 11.7).
- Cervical sinus is lined with ectoderm.
- Gradually cervical sinus disappears and neck becomes smooth (devoid of grooves).

Some Interesting Facts

- Ectodermal cells proliferate at the dorsal ends of the first, second and fourth pharyngeal clefts before their regression and form epibranchial placodes.
- Later epibranchial placodes contribute to sensory ganglia of 5th, 7th, 9th and 10th cranial nerves.

Box 11.1: Branchial cyst or cervical cyst

Branchial Cyst (Branchia = gills in Greek)

- Branchial cyst is a congenital cyst in the skin of the lateral part of the neck (Fig. 11.8).
- *Location*: Located along the **anterior border of the sternocleidomastoid muscle**, mostly close to the angle of the mandible.
- *Cause*: Branchial cyst is a result of **failure of obliteration of the branchial cleft**, mostly second cleft.
- **Symptoms**
  - Cyst presents as a smooth, slowly enlarging lateral neck mass.
  - Cyst is usually not present at birth. Its size increases with advancing age.
  - Cyst usually increases in size with upper respiratory tract infection.
- **Pathology**
  - Cyst wall may be lined by
    A. Stratified squamous cells or
    B. Simple columnar cells
- **Treatment**
  - Branchial cysts can be **removed surgically**, but mostly incomplete surgical removal leads to recurrence of the cyst.

Branchial Fistula

- If the branchial cyst opens both in the pharynx and externally on the skin of the neck, it is called **complete branchial** or **cervical fistula**.

Contd.

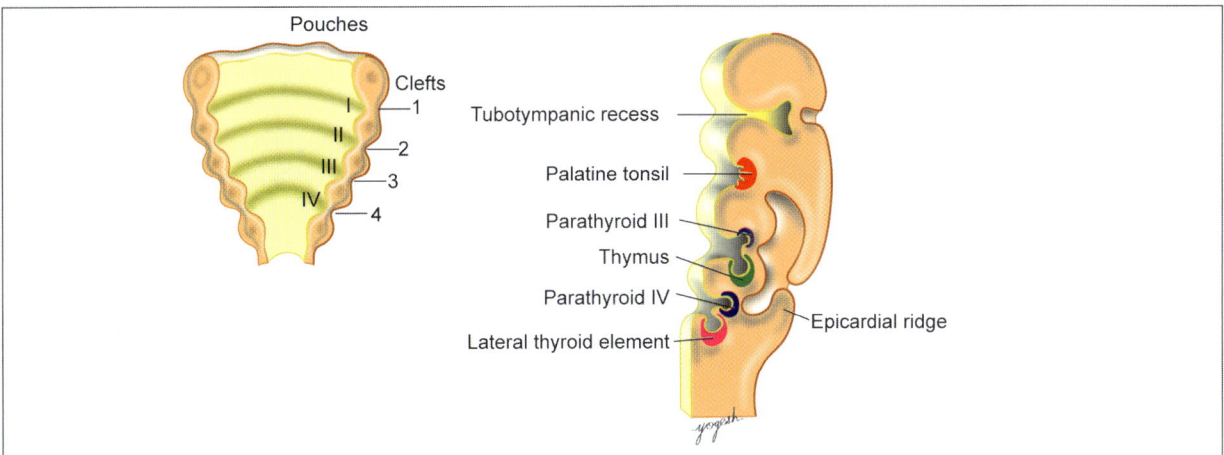

Fig. 11.7: Development of pharyngeal clefts and pouches. The second arch grows to cover the second, third and fourth clefts. Finally, fuses with the epicardial ridge. The trapped part of the second, third and fourth clefts forms the cervical sinus that later gets obliterated

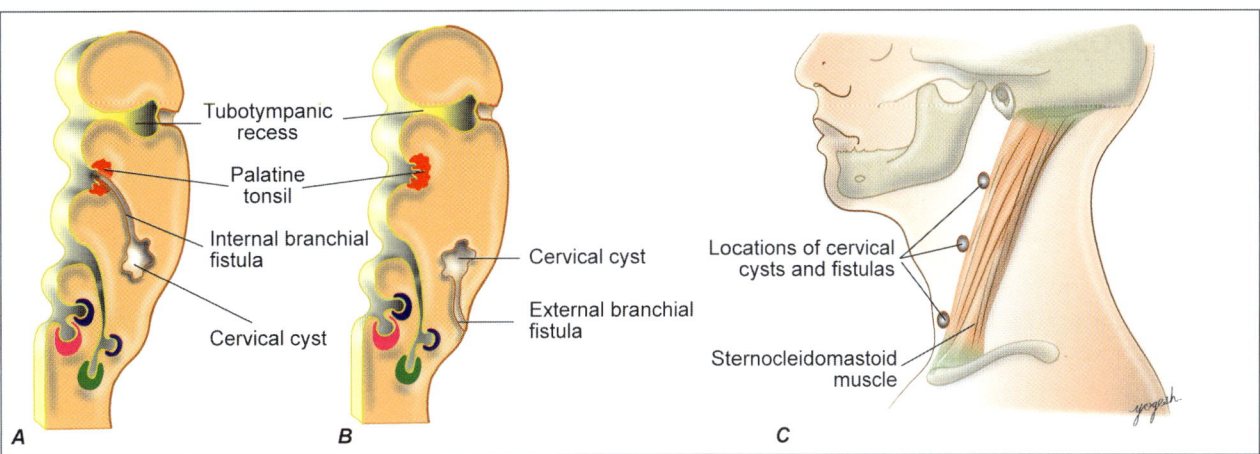

Fig. 11.8: (A and B) Cervical cysts and fistulas; (C) Locations of the openings of the cervical cysts in the neck

Contd.

- If the cyst shows only internal communication with pharynx, it is called **internal branchial fistula** or **sinus,** whereas if the cyst shows only external communication on the skin of the neck, it is called **external branchial sinus** or **fistula.**

Some Interesting Facts

DiGeorge's Syndrome (22q11.2 deletion syndrome)
- Also known as a **velocardiofacial syndrome** or **Shprintzen syndrome**.
- Cause: Microdeletion of chromosome 22.^{MCQ}
- Symptoms: It presents with congenital heart disease with fish mouth deformity (short philtrum), low sets of malformed ears, long face, small lower jaw bone.
- Incidence: 1 in 2000–4000 live births

Box 11.2: First arch syndromes

- First arch syndromes occur due to failure of migration of neural crest cells into the first arch.
- These neural crest cells form skeletal elements and connective tissue in the first arch.
- The first arch syndrome includes Treacher Collins syndrome and Pierre Robin syndrome.

A. Treacher Collins syndrome
- It is also called **mandibulofacial dystosis**.^{MCQ}
- Described first by Edward Treacher Collin in 1900.
- It is *autosomal dominant* disorder due to mutation in TCOF1 gene located on chromosome 5.^{MCQ}
- Incidence: 1:50,000 births
- Clinical presentation:
  – Underdeveloped lower jaw (mandibular hypoplasia)

Contd.

Contd.

- Underdeveloped zygomatic bone (malar hypoplasia)
- Down-slanting palpebral fissure
- External ear malformations (malformed pinna and meatal atresia)[Neet]

B. Pierre Robin Syndrome
- It has three main features:[MCQ]
  - Cleft palate
  - Retrognathia (small mandible) and
  - Glossoptosis (backward displacement of the tongue)
- Cause: Anomalies of chromosome 2, 11 and 17; mostly mutation in SOXG gene of chromosome 17.
- Incidence: 1 in 10,000 births

PHARYNGEAL POUCHES

Q. Draw a well-labelled diagram showing derivatives of pharyngeal pouches.

- There are *five* pairs of pharyngeal pouches (Fig. 11.9, Practice Fig. 11.2).
- Pharyngeal pouches are numbered craniocaudally.
- The fifth pharyngeal pouch is rudimentary.
- Ventrally right and left pouches fuse to form floor of the pharynx where tongue develops.
- The derivatives of pharyngeal pouches are listed in Table 11.2.

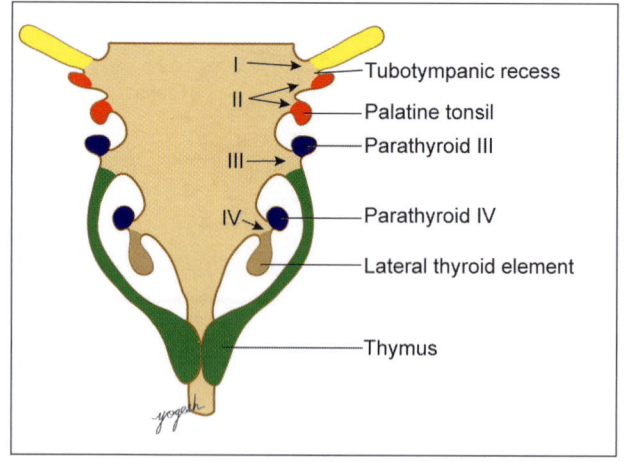

Practice Fig. 11.2: Derivatives of the pharyngeal pouches

Q. Enlist the derivatives of pharyngeal pouches.

Table 11.2	Derivatives of pharyngeal pouches[MCQ, Viva]
Pouch	Derivatives
First pouch	Auditory tube Tympanic cavity Inner surface of tympanic membrane
Second pouch	Palatine tonsil Tonsillar fossa, Intra-tonsillar cleft
Third pouch	Inferior parathyroid gland Thymus
Fourth pouch	Superior parathyroid gland
Caudal pharyngeal complex	Thymic element—part of thymus Lateral thyroid element—part of thyroid gland Ultimobranchial body—parafollicular cells of thyroid gland (neural crest cells)

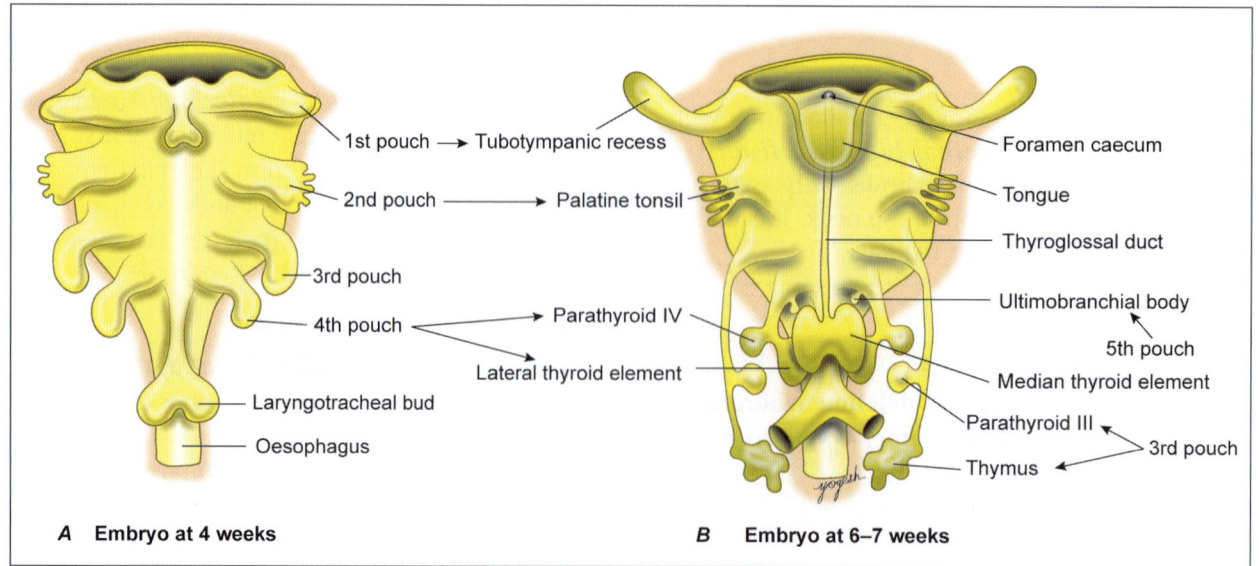

Fig. 11.9: Derivatives of the pharyngeal pouches: (A) In the fourth week, endoderm of the primitive pharynx outpouches to form pharyngeal pouches that later give rise to various structures as shown in this figure. (B) Inferior parathyroid develops from the third pharyngeal pouch, whereas superior parathyroid develops from the fourth pharyngeal pouch

Pharyngeal Apparatus

First Pouch

- Ventral part of first pouch is obliterated by the developing tongue.
- Dorsal part of the first pouch along with dorsal part of the second pouch form a diverticulum called **tubotympanic recess**.
- The proximal part of tubotympanic recess forms an *auditory (Eustachian) tube.*[Neet]
- Distal part of the recess forms middle ear cavity, mastoid antrum, mastoid air cells and inner lining epithelium of the tympanic membrane.

Second Pouch

- Dorsal part of second pouch fuses with dorsal part of the first pouch to form tubotympanic recess.
- Ventral part of the second pouch forms epithelial lining of **tonsil** and tonsillar crypts. Note: Lymphatic follicles of tonsil develop from mesoderm.
- *Intra-tonsillar cleft* (crypta magna) represents non-obliterated part of the second pouch.[MCQ]

Third Pouch

- Dorsal part (wing) of third pouch forms **inferior parathyroid gland** (parathyroid III).[MCQ]
- Ventral wing of the third pouch forms **thymus**.
- Both right and left wings lose their contact with pharynx and migrate caudally towards the developing heart.
- Finally, inferior parathyroid also lose its connection with thymus and gain permanent attachment with lower pole of the thyroid gland
- Thymus further continues caudal migration and come to lie within developing anterior mediastinum.

Note: Thymocytes develop in bone narrow (mesoderm) and migrate to the thymus, whereas *Hassall's corpuscles* are derived from the third pouch (endoderm).[MCQ]

Fourth Pouch

- Dorsal wing (part) of fourth pouch forms **superior parathyroid gland** (parathyroid IV).
- Dorsal wing loses contact with pharynx, migrate caudally and finally gain permanent attachment with posterior border of lateral lobe of the thyroid gland.

Fifth Pouch

- In some species, it forms the *ultimobranchial body*.
- In human, the fifth pouch is seen for a brief period.

> **Box 11.3:** Caudal pharyngeal complex
> - Ventral part of the fourth pouch fuses with a rudimentary fifth pouch to form caudal pharyngeal complex.
> - Caudal pharyngeal complex shows three components:
>   1. Thymic element: It gets incorporated in developing thymus.
>   2. Lateral thyroid element: It fuses with median thyroid element (that derives from thyroglossal duct) and arrests caudal migration of median thyroid element.
>   3. Ultimobranchial body: It forms parafollicular or C-cells of the thyroid gland.
>
> *Note:* Neural crest cells migrate to thyroid gland via ultimobranchial body and forms parafollicular cells.[MCQ]

DEVELOPMENT OF PALATINE TONSIL, THYMUS, PARATHYROID AND THYROID GLANDS

Development of Palatine Tonsil

Q. Write short note on development of palatine tonsil.

- Palatine tonsil develops from two sources
  - Endoderm of second pharyngeal pouch
  - Mesoderm (lymphocytes)

Stages of Development

- During the third month of development, ventral part of the second pouch proliferates outwards in surrounding mesoderm as several solid cords called **tonsillar buds**.
- On degeneration of central cells, tonsillar buds cannulate to form hollow **tonsillar crypts**.
- During 3rd to 5th month, lymphocytes aggregates on the mesoderm that surrounds crypts and form lymphatic follicles.
- Mesodermal cells condense to form a **capsule** of the tonsil.
- Lymphocyte proliferates and forms pharyngeal tonsillar bulging.
- The remnant of the pouch is represented by an intra-tonsillar cleft.[MCQ]

Development of Thymus

Q. Write short note on development of thymus.

- Thymus develops from the following two sources:
  - A. Endoderm of the third pharyngeal pouch
  - B. Mesoderm forms thymocytes and other connective tissue.

Stages of Development

- Ventral part of the third pharyngeal pouch descends caudally and form thymic rudiment.
- The thymic rudiment and inferior parathyroid gland (that develops from the dorsal part of the third pharyngeal pouch) descends caudally and lose contact with pharynx.
- Finally, thymic rudiment loses contact with inferior parathyroid and continue to decent caudally.
- Endodermal third pouch forms cytoreticulum and Hassell's corpuscles of thymus.^{MCQ}
- Thymocytes (lymphocytes) migrate from bone marrow and infiltrate the thymic rudiment.^{MCQ}

Involution

- Thymus continues to grow from birth till puberty and then undergo gradual atrophy called *thymic involution*.

Development of Parathyroid Gland

Q. Write short note on development of parathyroid gland.

- There are four parathyroid glands.
- *Two superior parathyroid glands are derived from fourth pharyngeal pouch, whereas two inferior parathyroid glands are derived from third pharyngeal pouch.*^{MCQ}

Stages of Development

- Dorsal part of the *third* pouch grows and lose contact with pharynx and then descend caudally along with thymus. Finally, it loses contact with thymus and forms *inferior parathyroid gland (parathyroid* III).
- Dorsal part of *fourth* pharyngeal pouch grows and lose contact with the pharynx. Later it descends caudally to form *superior parathyroid gland (parathyroid* III).

Development of Thyroid Gland

Q. Write a note on development of thyroid gland.

Summary (Examination Guide)

Thyroid gland develops from the following two sources (Fig. 11.10, Practice Fig. 11.3, Flowchart 11.3):
  A. *Follicles* from thyroglossal duct.
  B. *Parafollicular cells* from ultimobranchial body (a part of caudal pharyngeal complex).
- By the end of the third month (12th week) follicular cells start producing thyroid hormones.^{MCQ}
- The thyroid gland is the first gland that develops after fertilisation.^{MCQ}

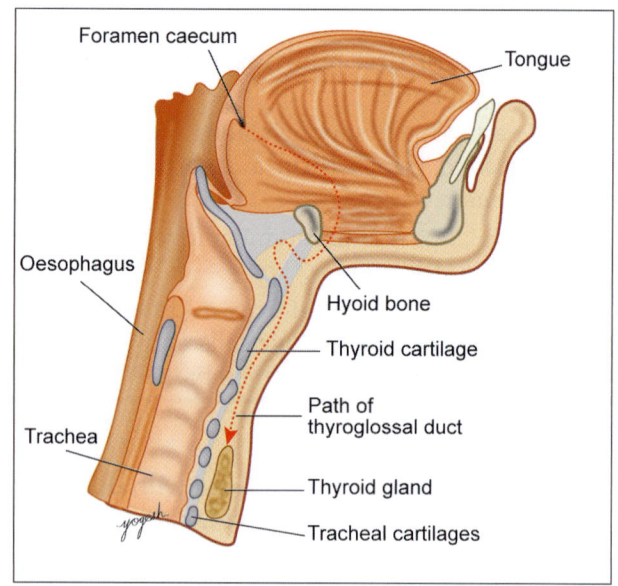

Fig. 11.10: Pathway of the thyroglossal duct. It extends from the foramen caecum to the neck

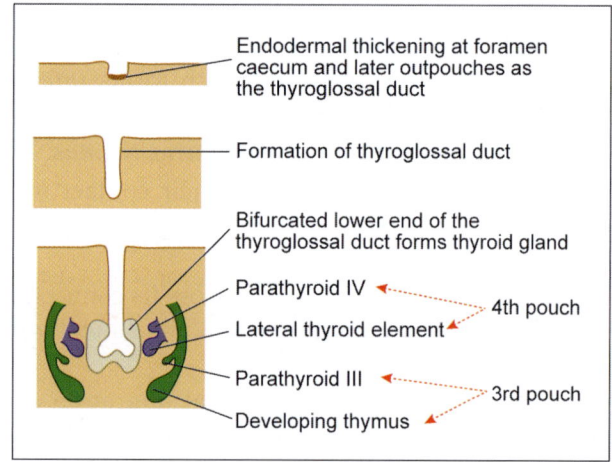

Practice Fig. 11.3: Development of thyroid gland

Flowchart 11.3: Development of palatine tonsil

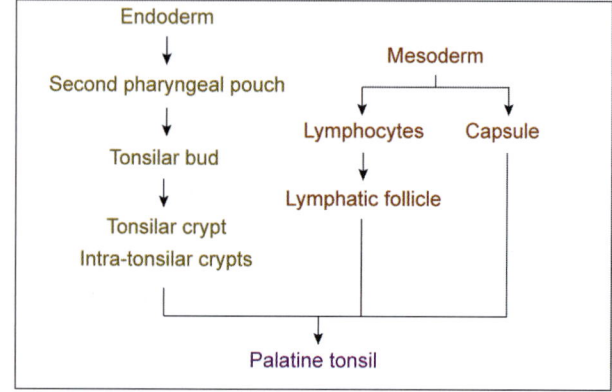

Stages of Development

- In the floor of the primitive pharynx, over the first arch in the midline, there is a swelling called **tuberculum impar**.
- By the 24th day, just behind tuberculum impar, pharyngeal epithelium forms a depression (diverticulum) called *thyroglossal duct*.
- The opening of thyroglossal duct in the pharynx is represented by the *foramen caecum*.
- Thyroglossal duct grows caudally (towards pericardial bulge) in the midline.
- Tip of the thyroglossal duct bifurcates to give rise to two lobes of the thyroid gland (by 7th week).
- Ultimobranchial body (a part of caudal pharyngeal complex meets thyroid gland and contribute as *parafollicular cells*).

Anomalies of the Thyroid Gland

1. *Pyramidal lobe*: It may arise from the isthmus or any one of the lobes. It is variable in the length. It is derived from thyroglossal duct.
2. Sometimes isthmus or one lobe of the thyroid gland may be absent or small.
3. Anomalies of location
   - The thyroid gland may lie at any position at the passage of thyroglossal duct.
   - Anomalies of the locations are listed in Table 11.3.
4. Ectopic thyroid tissue: Ectopic thyroid is the presence of thyroid tissue in locations other than usual (normal) thyroid gland locations. It is mostly found in larynx, trachea, oesophagus, pericardium and ovaries

Table 11.3	Anomalies of position of thyroid gland
Anomaly	Location
1. Lingual thyroid	Under mucosa of the dorsum of tongue.
2. Intra-lingual thyroid	Embedded in substance of tongue.
3. Suprahyoid thyroid	Lie in midline of the neck, above the hyoid bone.
4. Infrahyoid thyroid	Lie in the midline in the neck below the hyoid bone but superior to its usual position.
5. Infrahyoid thyroid	Lie in thorax.

Box 11.4: Thyroglossal cyst and fistula

- Thyroid gland develops from thyroglossal duct (parafollicular cells from ultimobranchial body).
- Usually, thyroglossal duct regresses. Remnant of the thyroglossal duct may form thyroglossal cyst or fistula anywhere along the course of thyroglossal duct (Fig. 11.11, Practice Fig. 11.4).
- Thyroglossal cyst is an irregular mass or lump in the midline of the neck.
- Occasionally thyroglossal cyst ruptures externally, resulting in a draining sinus called a **thyroglossal fistula**.
- Rarely it forms *thyroglossal cyst carcinoma*.

Box 11.5: Goldenhar syndrome

- Also called **oculo-auriculo-vertebral (OAV) syndrome**.
- It is a congenital anomaly characterised by hemifacial microsomia.
- Incidence: 1 in 5600 births
- Clinical presentation
  - Anotia or microtia (absent or small deformed ear)
  - Eye deformity
  - Fused hemivertebrae
  - Spina bifida
  - Heart defects

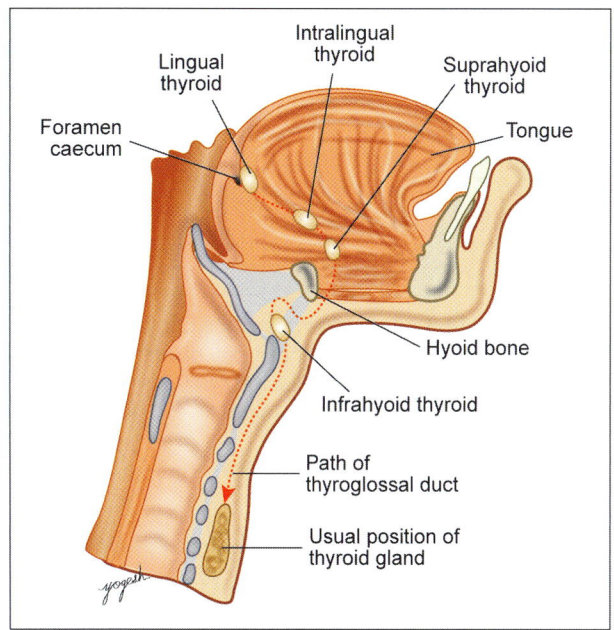

Fig. 11.11: Anomalies of the position of the thyroid gland and locations of the thyroglossal cyst. Thyroid gland may lie anywhere along the pathway of the thyroglossal duct. Thyroglossal cyst also may be present as the persistent pathway for the thyroglossal duct

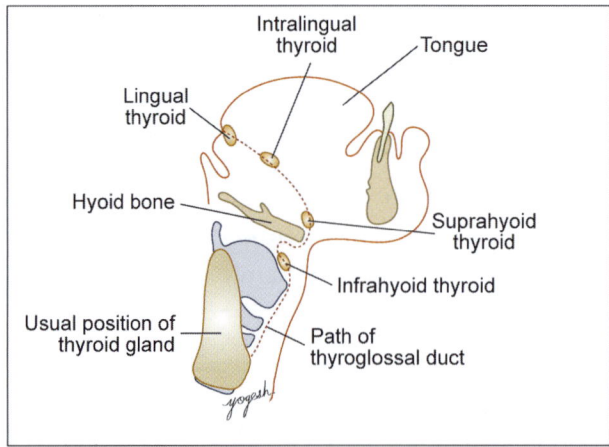

Practice Fig. 11.4: Anomalies of the position of the thyroid gland and locations of the thyroglossal cyst

CLINICAL EMBRYOLOGY

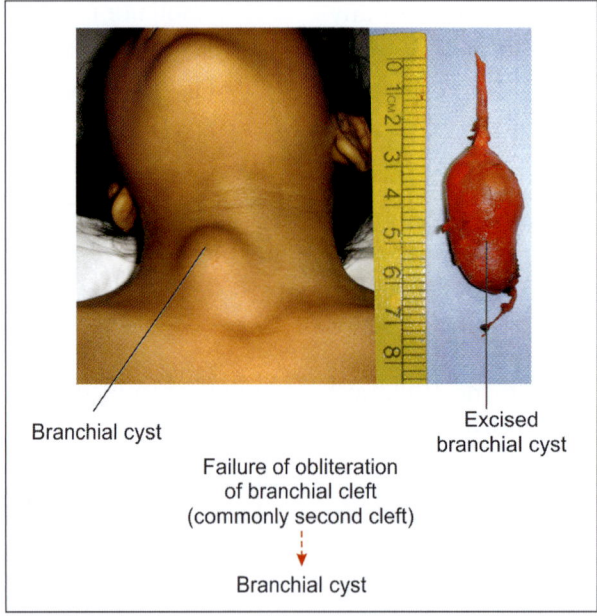

Clinical Image 11.1: (A) Unilateral branchial cleft cyst (right); (B) Excised branchial cyst from the same case. It is a cyst in the skin of the lateral part of the neck without any opening to the skin surface (In case of branchial fistula, there is opening on the surface of the skin) (Image courtesy: *Dr Kumaravel S*)

12

Alimentary Tract I
Development of Face, Nose, Palate

Chapter Outline

- Development of face
- Development of nasolacrimal duct
- Development of nose
- Development of paranasal air sinuses
- Intermaxillary segment
- Development of Palate
- Cleft lip
- Developmental anomalies of face
- Cleft palate

INTRODUCTION

- At the end of fourth week, embryo shows *stomodeum* as a depression in between bulging brain vesicle and pericardial bulge.
- *Buccopharyngeal membrane* lies in floor of the stomodeum.
- Mesoderm surrounding the stomodeum proliferates and forms elevations (processes) that later form face, palate and nose.

DEVELOPMENT OF FACE

- Face develops from **five mesodermal processes** that appears in 4th week surrounding the stomodeum[Neet] (Fig. 12.1, Practice Fig. 12.1). These processes are
  1. Frontonasal process (unpaired)
  2. Maxillary process (paired)
  3. Mandibular process (paired).
- The mesoderm surrounding the stomodeum thickens and produces above-mentioned processes (elevations) on the surface ectoderm.
- Facial development takes place between 4 and 8 weeks.[Neet] 7–8 weeks is the final period of facial development.[Neet]

Steps in Development of Face

- In the 4th week of IUL, the stomodeum is bounded cranially by the bulging *forebrain vesicle* and caudally by first pharyngeal (mandibular) arch.
- In the fifth week of IUL, mesoderm covering the bulging forebrain vesicle proliferates to form *frontonasal process* (Fig. 12.1).
- On the frontonasal process, bilateral localised thickening appears as *nasal placodes* or *olfactory placode* on either side of the median plane.
- On the olfactory placodes, depression called *nasal pit* or *olfactory pit* develops. Nasal pit later becomes continuous with roof of the stomodeum.
- Margins of the nasal pit form elevated ridges. Medial margin of the nasal pit forms *medial nasal prominence* (process), whereas lateral margin forms *lateral nasal prominence* (process).
- During the development of the nasal pit and nasal processes, the *maxillary process* develops from cranial side of dorsal part of the first pharyngeal arch.
- The maxillary process grows medially and finally fuses with the medial nasal process.
- *Note:* Lateral and cranial to the nasal placodes, a pair of lens placodes appears.
- Between 7th and 10th weeks, a fusion of the maxillary process with medial and lateral nasal processes separates the *nasal pit* from the stomodeum and thus, convert it into the *primitive anterior nares*.
- Continuous growth of the nasal process produces elevated bridge of the nose.
- Medial nasal process forms the *intermaxillary segment*. This segment forms philtrum (middle part) of the upper limb, pre-maxillary part of the maxilla and primitive palate.

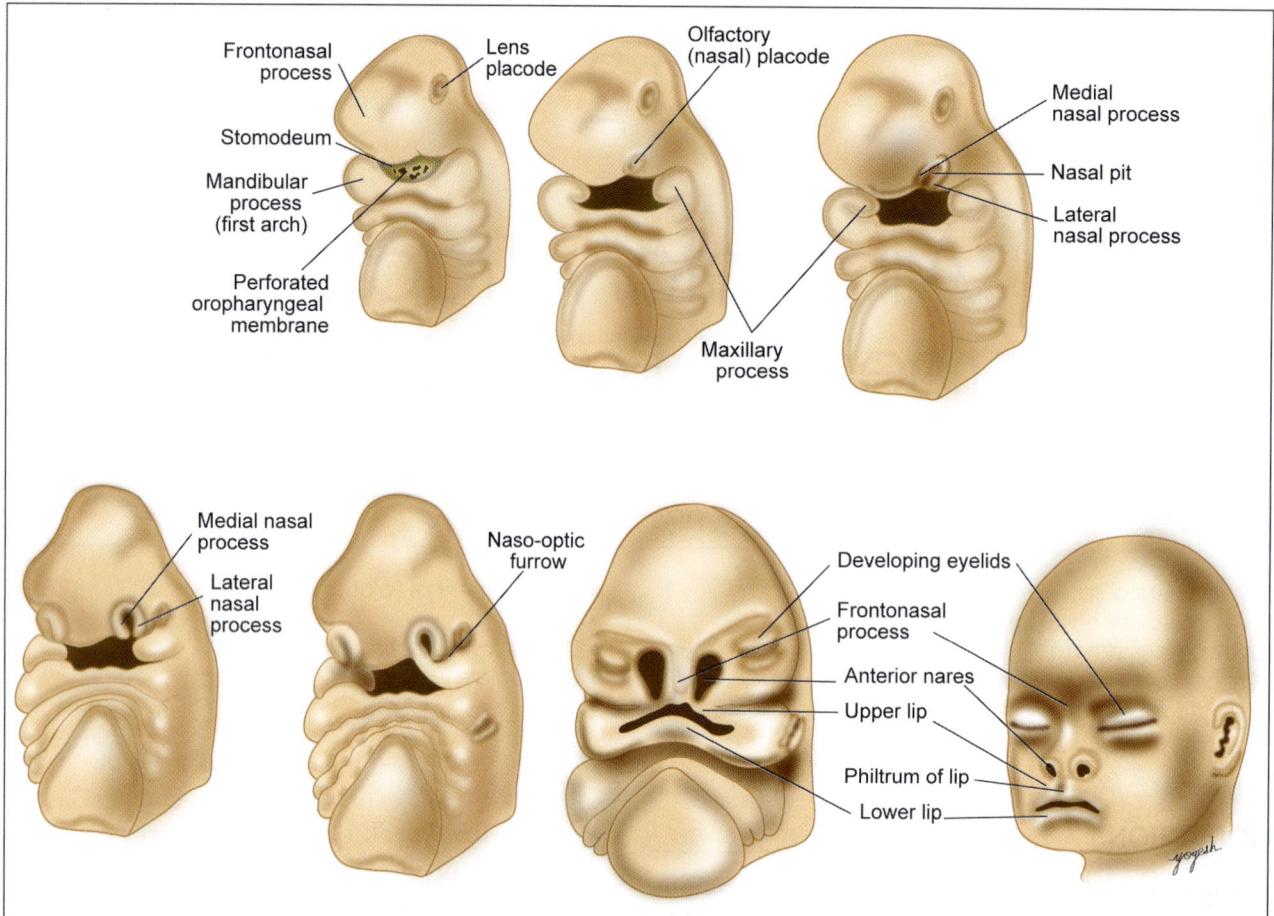

Fig. 12.1: Development of the face. Five facial primordia that appear as prominences around the stomodeum are: Single frontonasal process, paired maxillary process and paired mandibular processes. On appearance of the nasal placode and later nasal pit, the frontonasal process gives raise to medial and lateral nasal processes. The frontal nasal process forms the forehead and dorsum and apex of the nose. The lateral nasal processes form the alae of the nose. The medial nasal processes form the nasal septum. The maxillary processes form the upper cheek regions and the upper lip. The mandibular processes form chin, lower lip and lower cheek regions

- Lateral part of the upper lip is formed from maxillary processes. Lateral nasal processes do not form upper lips.^{MCQ}
- Stomodeum gets separated from pericardial bulge by first (mandibular) arch and later by the other arches.
- Mandibular arch develops the lower lip.
- *Note*: Both the maxillary process and mandibular process arise from the first pharyngeal arch and fusion of these processes forms lateral angles of mouth.
- Fusion of the maxillary process and the mandibular process continues on the lateral side, and reduces oral fissure (earlier stomodeum) and forms cheeks.
- Nerve supply: Derivatives of the frontonasal process are supplied by ophthalmic nerve, the maxillary process by maxillary nerve and the mandibular process by mandibular nerve.

Box 12.1: Development of nasolacrimal duct
- The maxillary process grows medially and fuses with lateral nasal process along *naso-optic furrow* (nasolacrimal groove).
- During fusion of maxillary process with the lateral nasal process, some ectodermal cells along naso-optic furrow get buried into mesenchyme and form a solid cellular cord. Later this cord forms the *nasolacrimal duct*.
- Upper part of the nasolacrimal duct dilates and forms the *lacrimal sac*.
- Failure of canalisation of nasolacrimal duct results into an atresia of the nasolacrimal duct.

Summary of Development of Face (Examination Guide) (Flowchart 12.1)

- Lower lip: Bilateral mandibular processes fuse in the midline to form a lower lip and jaw bone.

Alimentary Tract I: Development of Face, Nose, Palate

- Upper lip:
  - Central part (philtrum) of upper lip is derived from medial nasal process.
  - Lateral parts of upper lip are derived from bilateral maxillary processes.

  Note:
  - Lateral nasal process does not form upper lip.^{MCQ}
  - The ectoderm (skin) of maxillary process overgrows and cover central part (philtrum) of the upper lip; hence, skin of the upper lip is supplied by maxillary nerve (Fig. 12.2).^{MCQ, Viva}
  - Muscles of face are derived from second arch; hence supplied by facial nerve.^{MCQ}
- Cheeks:
  - Stomodeum is bounded by the maxillary, frontonasal and mandibular processes.
  - The maxillary and mandibular processes undergo fusion from the lateral side and form smaller stomodeum or normal oral fissure, whereas fused part forms cheek.
- For details of the development of eye and ear, read Chapters 23 and 24.

DEVELOPMENT OF NOSE

Summary (Examination Guide)

- External nose is derived as follows:
  1. Bridge of nose from frontonasal process.
  2. Dorsum and tip of the nose from fused medial nasal processes.

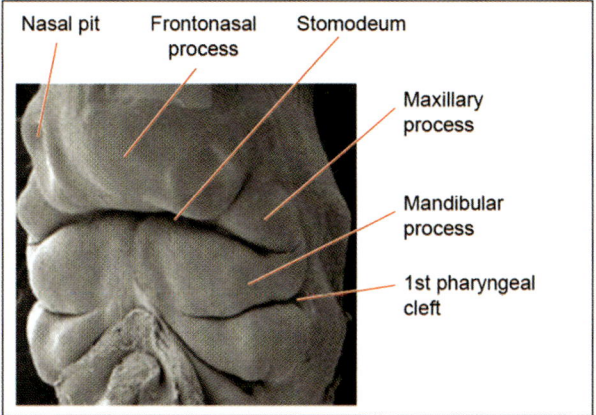

Scanning electron micrograph 12.1: SEM showing developing face. Frontonasal, maxillary and mandibular processes and nasal pits are visible. [Species: Human, approximate age: Fifth week]

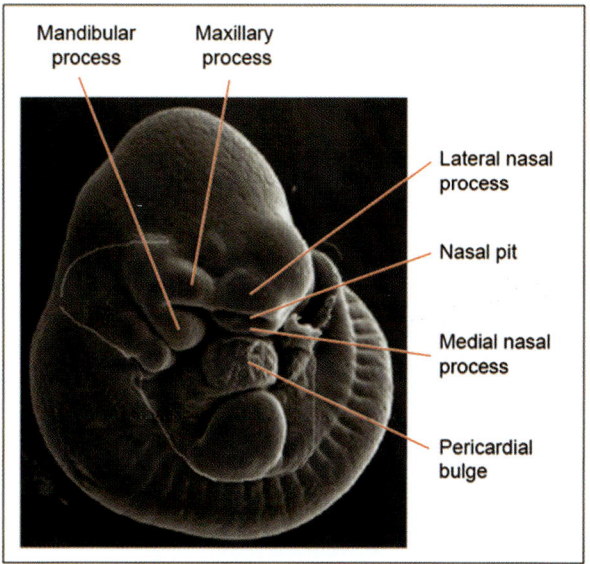

Scanning electron micrograph 12.2: SEM showing 6-week embryo with medial nasal, lateral nasal, maxillary and mandibular processes. [Species: Mouse, approximate human age: 6 weeks, lateral view]

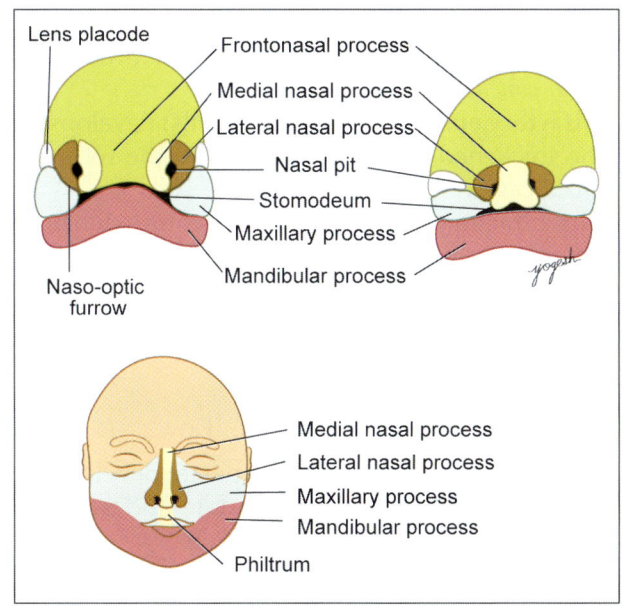

Practice Fig. 12.1: Development of the face

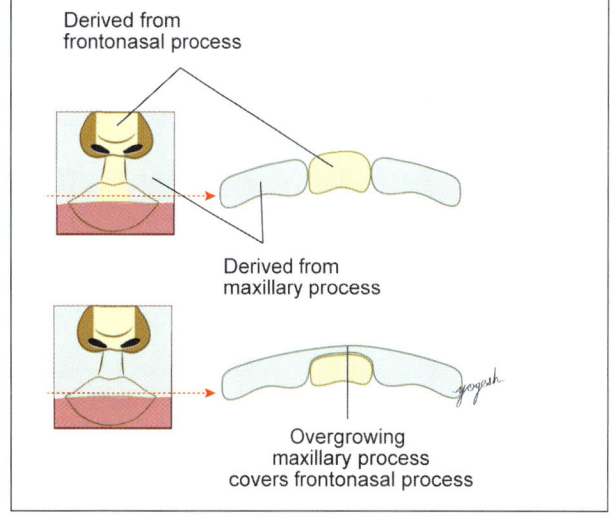

Fig. 12.2: Formation of the upper lip. The ectoderm of the maxillary process overgrows the frontonasal process. Hence, skin of the upper lip is supplied by the maxillary nerve

Flowchart 12.1: Development of face

```
Mesoderm over forebrain vesicle              First pharyngeal arch
              ↓                                        ↓
     Frontonasal process         Nasal placode    ┌─────┴─────┐
              ↓                        ↓          ↓           ↓
              ←──────────────── Nasal pit    Maxillary    Mandibular
        ┌─────┴─────┐                         process      process
        ↓           ↓                            ↓           ↓
     Medial      Lateral                    Angle of mouth
  nasal process  nasal process               and cheeks   Lower lip and
        │           │                                      lower jaw bone
        ↓           ↓
      Nose     Fusion site
        ↓           ↓
    Upper lip   Nasolacrimal furrow
                    ↓
              Nasolacrimal duct and sac
```

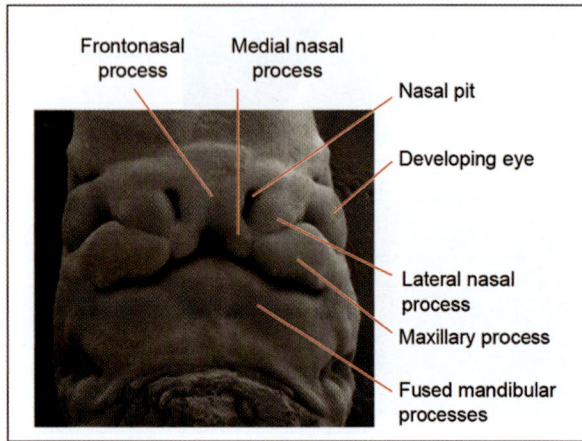

Scanning electron micrograph 12.3: SEM showing development of face, nose and upper lip. The medial nasal prominences merge in the midline to smooth the median furrow. [Species: Human, approximate age: Sixth week, frontal view].

3. Ala of nose from lateral nasal processes.
4. Anterior nares (nostrils) from nasal pit.
5. Nasal cavity from nasal sacs.
6. Posterior nares (choanae) from rupture of bucconasal membrane.

Stages of Development of Nose and Cavities

- During development of face, the *nasal pits* appear on the frontonasal process.
- Nasal pits sink deep and form communication with stomodeum.
- Elevated margins of nasal pits form *medial* and *lateral nasal processes*.
- Maxillary process first fuses with the lateral nasal process and later with medial nasal process.
- Lateral and medial nasal processes also fuse with each other and thus nasal pits get separated from stomodeum by *developing palate*.
- Nasal pit forms *anterior nares* (Fig. 12.3).
- Nasal pit sinks deep to develop *nasal sac*.
- Nasal sac enlarges dorsally and caudally. Dorsal to the primitive palate, the nasal sac is separated from stomodeum by a thin membrane called *bucconasal membrane* or *nasal fin*.
- Later bucconasal membrane rupture and develops communication between nasal sac and stomodeum that ultimately forms a *posterior nasal aperture*.
- Continuous narrowing of frontonasal process brings nasal sac close to each other and frontonasal process forms *nasal septum* and bridge of the nose.
- Medial nasal process forms dorsum and tip of the nose.
- Expanding lateral nasal process forms *lateral wall* of the nose.
- Inner elevated masses of lateral nasal process form *nasal conchae*.
- **Olfactory epithelium** (receptor cells) develops from the thickened ectodermal lining of the roof of the nasal cavity.
- The olfactory nerves develop from extension of neural processes of olfactory bulb of brain.

DEVELOPMENT OF PALATE

Q. Explain development of palate.

Summary (Examination Guide) (Flowchart 12.2)

- During the development, the palate develops from two components: Primary palate and secondary palate (Fig. 12.4, Practice Fig. 12.2).
- Frontonasal process forms *primary palate*, whereas maxillary process forms *secondary palate*.

Alimentary Tract I: Development of Face, Nose, Palate

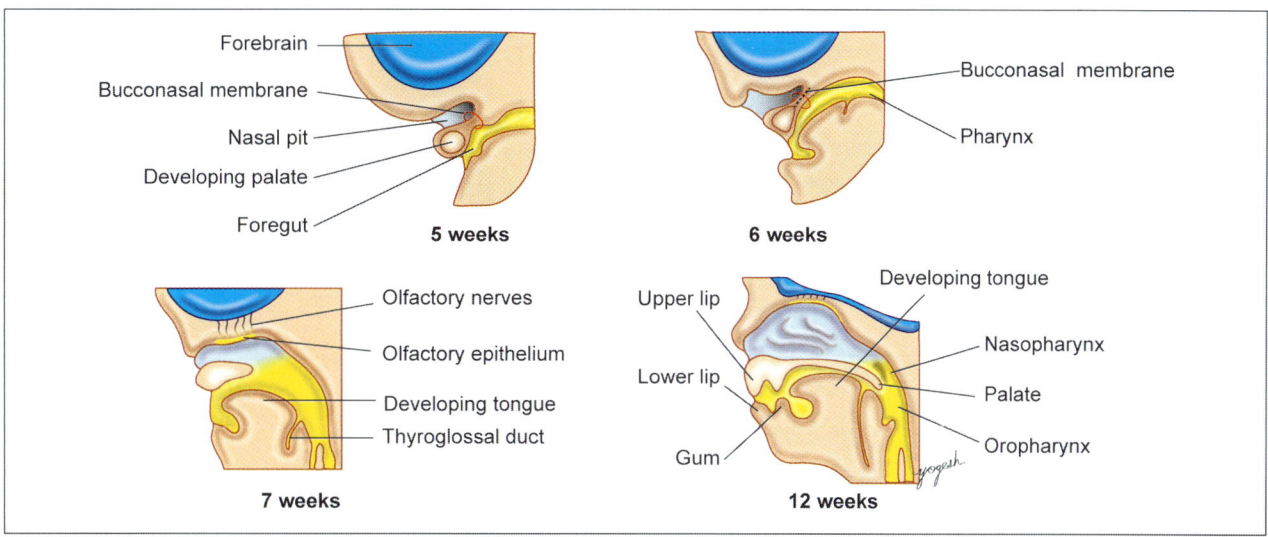

Fig. 12.3: Development of the nasal cavity. Nasal pits appear on the frontonasal process and it gets separated from stomodeum by the developing palate. Nasal pit forms anterior nares. Dorsal to the palate, the nasal sac is separated from stomodeum by bucconasal membrane. Later, the bucconasal membrane ruptures and forms posterior nasal aperture. Inner elevated masses of the lateral nasal process form nasal conchae. Olfactory epithelium develops from the thickened ectodermal lining of roof of the nasal cavity. The olfactory nerves develop from extension of neural processes of the olfactory bulb of the brain

---

Box 12.2: Development of paranasal air sinuses
- Paranasal sinuses are ectodermal in origin.
- Diverticulae (outpouching) develop from the nasal cavity. These diverticulae invade bones adjacent to the nasal cavity (frontal, sphenoid, ethmoid and maxilla) and enlarge to form paranasal air sinuses.
- Nasal opening of these diverticulae persists as orifices of the paranasal air sinuses in the nasal cavity.
- All paranasal air sinuses start developing before birth *except* frontal air sinus that develops after birth during 5th or 6th year of life.^{MCQ}
- The maxillary sinus is the first sinus to develop (in the third month of intrauterine life).^{MCQ, Viva}
- Paranasal air sinuses continue their growth till puberty.

Box 12.3: Intermaxillary segment
- In between maxillary processes, fused part of medial nasal processes forms the *intermaxillary segment*.
- The intermaxillary segment has the following parts:
  1. *Labial component*: Forms philtrum of upper lip.
  2. *Upper jaw component* is related to upper four incisor teeth.
  3. *Palatal component*: Forms triangular primary palate.

Stages of Palate Development
- Palatogenesis takes place between 5th week and 12th week of IUL.
- *Primary palate*
  - In sixth week, the *intermaxillary segment* forms a shelf-like projection (that later bear upper four incisor teeth) called *primary palate* or *median palatine process*.
  - Later primary palate forms *premaxillary part* of the maxilla.

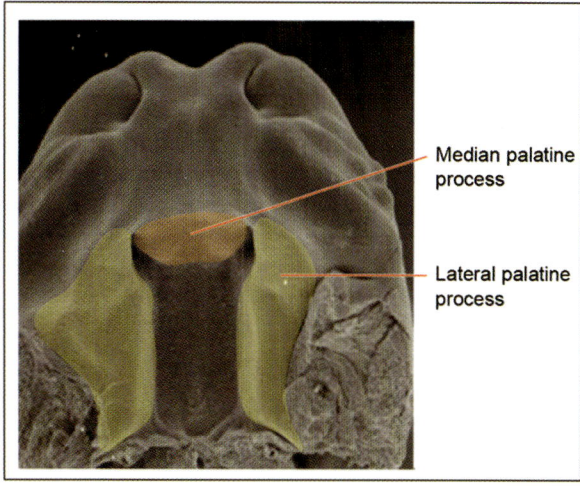

Scanning electron micrograph 12.4: Development of Palate. The secondary palatal shelves are considered to be part of the maxillary prominences. The medial nasal prominences contribute the tissues that will form the anterior part of palate, primary palate. [Species: Mouse, approximate human age: Seventh week]

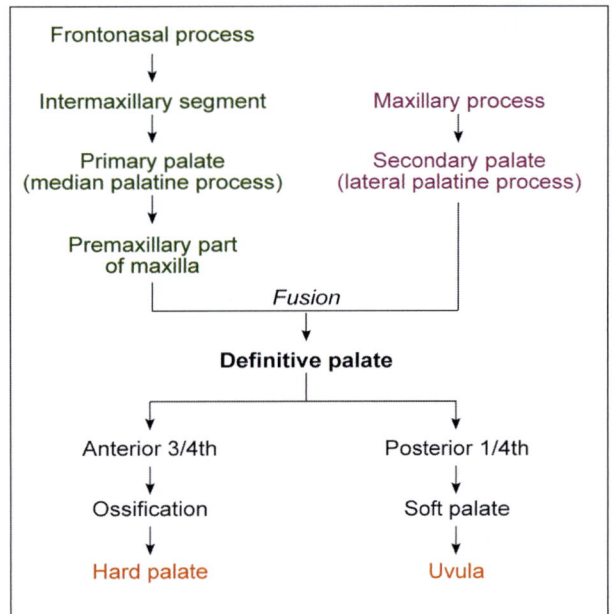

Flowchart 12.2: Development of palate

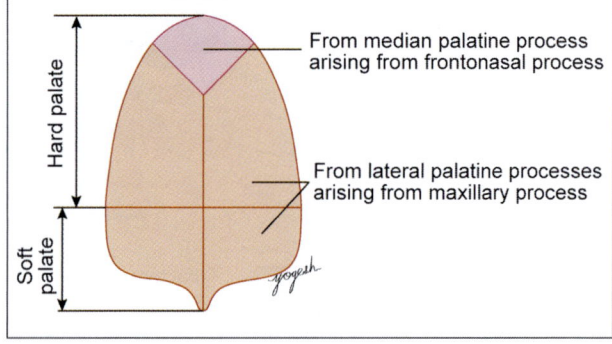

Practice Fig. 12.2: Development of palate

- Secondary palate
  - In sixth week, two mesenchymal projections extend from the inner aspects of maxillary processes. These projections are called *secondary palate* or *lateral palatine processes*.
- During 7th–8th weeks, the lateral palatine processes elongate and fuse:
  1. With each other in the midline.
  2. With nasal septum.
  3. With posterior part of the primary palate.
- Formation of definitive palate
- Primary palate fuse with secondary palate to form *definitive palate*. Incisive foramen divides primary and secondary palate.[Neet]

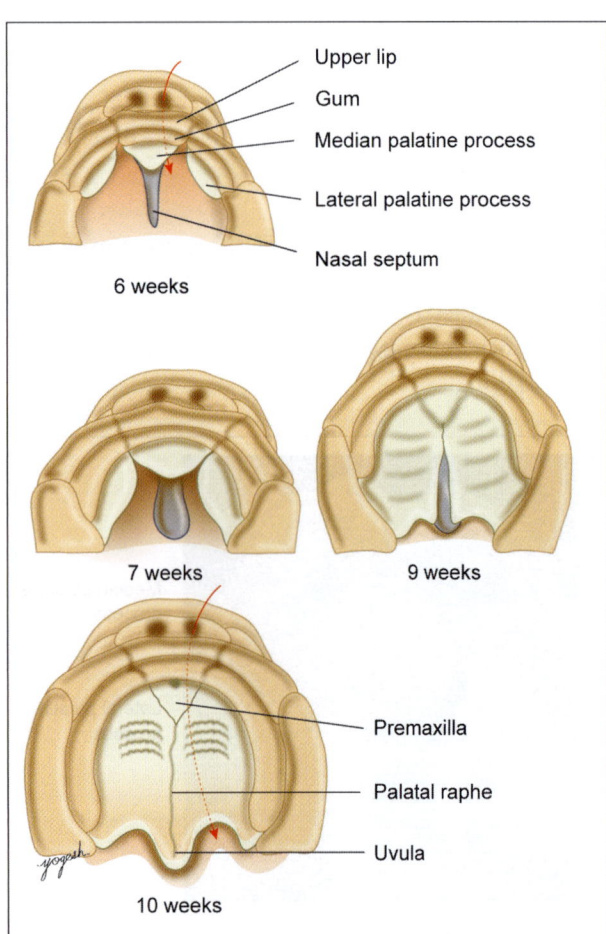

Fig. 12.4: Development of the palate. The intermaxillary segment forms median palatine process and later it forms premaxillary part of the maxilla. Two mesenchymal projections of the maxillary processes form lateral palatine processes. The lateral palatine processes elongate and fuse with each other in the midline, with the nasal septum and with posterior part of the primary palate

Box 12.4: Cleft lip (harelip)

Q. Write short note on cleft lip.
- **Definition:** Cleft lip is a congenital split in the upper lip of one or both sides of its centre (Fig. 12.5).
- Usually, upper lip of hare has cleft; hence, cleft lip is commonly called *harelip*.
- **Embryological basis:** Failure of fusion of the maxillary processes with the medial nasal process (part of frontonasal process) result in cleft lip. Midline cleft lip is due to failure of fusion of two medial nasal processes.[Neet]
- Harelip may be unilateral, bilateral or midline harelip.
- Cleft lip occurs more frequently (80%) in males than in females.
- Incidence of cleft lip is 1 in 1000 births.
- Incidence of cleft lip increases with increasing maternal age.
- If a couple has a cleft lip child, there are 4% chances that the next baby will have a cleft lip.[MCQ]
- If two babies of a couple are affected, then the chances of increases are up to 9%.[MCQ]
- **Treatment:** Cleft lip can be corrected surgically.

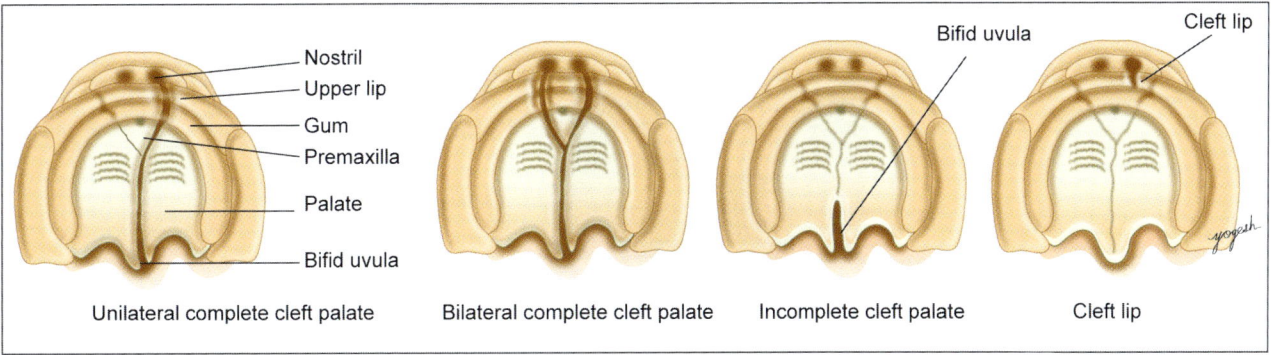

Fig. 12.5: Cleft lip and cleft palate. Non-fusion of the median and later palatine processes result in the cleft palate. It may be unilateral or bilateral complete cleft palate or incomplete cleft palate. Failure of fusion of the maxillary processes with medial nasal process results in the cleft lip

- Anterior three-fourths of the definitive palate ossifies and form *hard palate*.
- Posterior one-fourth of the definitive palate remains unossified and forms *soft palate* with *uvula*.
- Small persistent *nasopalatine canal* in the median plane of premaxilla forms the *incisive fossa*. In the incisive fossa, right and left incisive canals open.

Developmental Anomalies of Face

Q. Name the developmental anomalies of the face.

- *Oblique facial cleft* may result due to non-fusion of maxillary and lateral nasal process. It results in a cleft from medial angle of the eye to the mouth and non-formation of nasolacrimal duct.
- *Macrostomia* is a wide mouth due to incomplete fusion of mandibular and maxillary processes.
- *Microstomia* is a small mouth due to excessive fusion of mandibular and maxillary processes.
- *Proboscis* is an elongated cylindrical projecting nose. In some cases of proboscis, cyclops (fusion of both the eyes) is present.
- *Retrognathia* is a small mandible in that chin does not reach the rest of the face.
- *Agnathia* is the absence of jaw, may be due to failure of mandible development.
- *Hypertelorism* is widely placed eyes due to broad nasal bridge. It is caused by wide frontonasal process.
- Harelip or cleft lip. Refer to Box 12.4.

Box 12.5: Cleft palate

Q. Write short note on cleft palate.

- **Definition:** Cleft palate is a congenital split defect of palate that causes communication between oral and nasal cavities (Fig. 12.5).
- Patient with cleft palate usually has eating problems, speech, dental problems.
- The commonest cause of cleft lip with or without cleft palate is multifactorial inheritance.
- **Incidence**
  - 1 in 2500 births.
  - Cleft palate is more common in females (67%).
  - Incidence of cleft palate is not related to the maternal age.
  - If a couple has a child with cleft palate, there are 2% chances that another baby will have cleft palate. MCQ
  - Unilateral cleft of upper lip is the commonest congenital anomaly of face. MCQ

Embryological basis
  - Non-fusion of median and later palatine processes result in cleft palate.

Classification
- Cleft palate may be complete or incomplete (partial).
- *Complete cleft palate* may be unilateral or bilateral.
  - Unilateral complete cleft palate: It results due to non-fusion of one lateral palatine process of the maxilla with the median palatine process of premaxilla.
  - It is always associated with harelip on the same side of the defect.
  - *Bilateral complete cleft palate*: It results due to non-fusion of both the lateral palatine process of maxilla with the median palatine process of premaxilla.
- *Incomplete cleft palate* may be cleft of hard and soft palate or only the cleft of soft palate or uvula.

Treatment
- Cleft palate can be corrected surgically.

CLINICAL EMBRYOLOGY

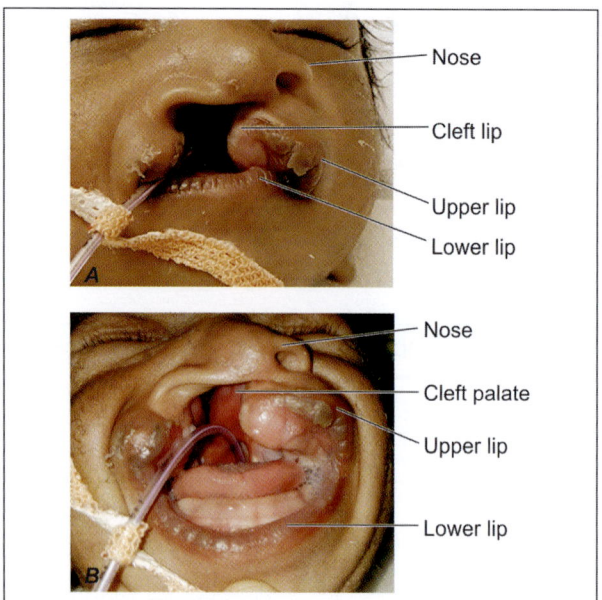

Clinical image 12.1: A 5-day-old baby with unilateral cleft lip and cleft palate (on the right side). Cleft lip is a congenital split in the upper lip that occurs due to failure of fusion of the maxillary processes with the medial nasal process (part of frontonasal process). Cleft palate is a congenital split defect of the palate that causes communication between oral and nasal cavities. Cleft palate occurs due to the non-fusion of the median and lateral palatine processes (Image courtesy: *Dr Prakhar Mohniya*)

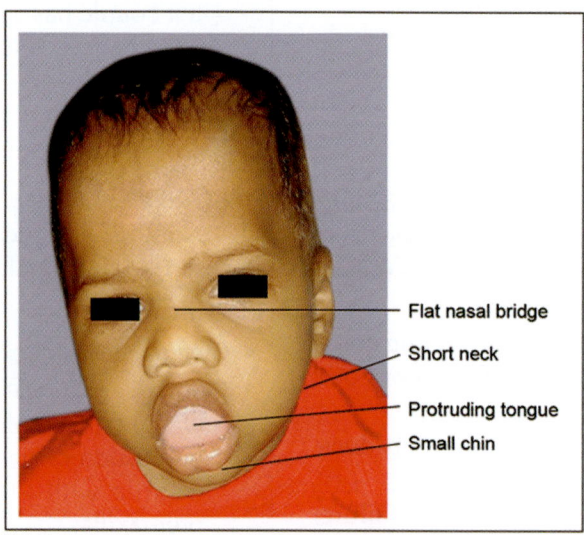

Clinical image 12.2: Facial features in a baby of Down syndrome showing flat and wide face, small chin, flat nasal bridge, protruding tongue due to small oral cavity and short neck (Image courtesy: *Dr Adhisivam B*)

13
Alimentary Tract II
Development of Teeth, Pharynx, Tongue and Salivary Glands

Chapter Outline

- Development of mouth cavity
  - Primitive oral cavity
  - Definitive oral cavity
- Development of teeth
  - Structure of tooth
  - Stages of teeth development
  - Development of permanent teeth
  - Anomalies of teeth
- Development of pharynx
- Development of tongue
  - Mucous membrane
  - Muscles of tongue
  - Nerve supply
  - Developmental anomalies
- Development of salivary glands
  - Parotid gland
  - Submandibular gland
  - Sublingual gland

DEVELOPMENT OF MOUTH CAVITY

- Mouth cavity develops from contribution of two derms:
  1. Ectoderm (stomodeum) forms the *primitive mouth cavity*.
  2. Endoderm (cephalic part of foregut) forms *definitive mouth cavity*.
- In the fourth week, *buccopharyngeal membrane* ruptures and endoderm becomes continuous with ectoderm (Fig. 13.1).

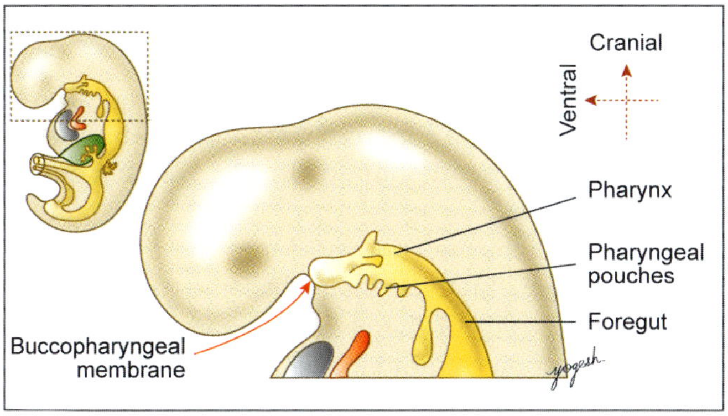

Fig. 13.1: Buccopharyngeal membrane

Primitive Oral Cavity

- *Primitive oral cavity* develops from stomodeum (ectoderm).
- *Stomodeum* is divided into nasal and oral part by the developing *palate*.
- Nasal part forms the mucous membrane of nasal cavity, nasal septum and palate.
- Oral part forms the mucous membrane of cheek, lips, gums and enamel of the teeth.

Definitive Oral Cavity

- The cephalic part of foregut (endoderm) forms definitive oral cavity.
- In the floor of oral cavity, the developing tongue gets separated from mandibular process by *linguo-gingival sulcus* (endodermal zone) (Fig. 13.2).
- Lateral to the linguo-gingival sulcus, in the ectodermal zone, a *labio-gingival sulcus* appears.
- Labio-gingival sulcus deepens. Expanding mandibular arch forms the lower lips, lower part of cheeks and lower jaw.
- The area between linguo-gingival sulcus and labio-gingival sulcus elevates and develops an alveolar process that later forms jaw and teeth.

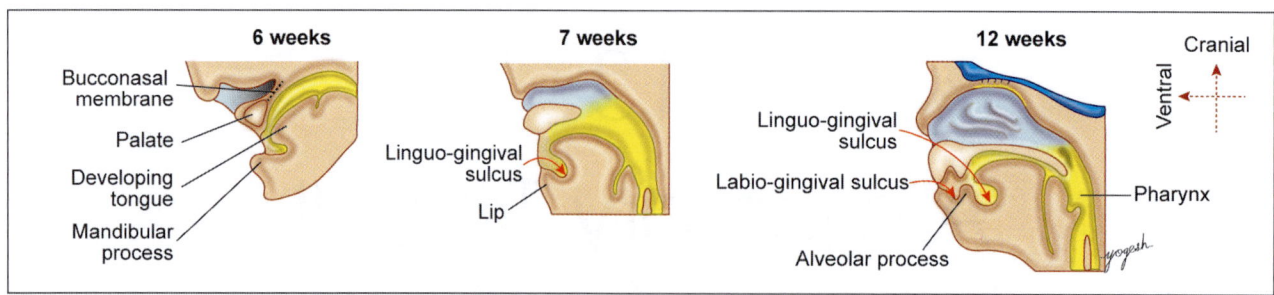

Fig. 13.2: Formation of oral cavity. The cephalic part of foregut forms definitive oral cavity. In the floor of oral cavity, the developing tongue gets separated from mandibular process by the linguo-gingival sulcus. Lateral to the linguo-gingival sulcus, in ectodermal zone, labio-gingival sulcus appears. Area between linguo-gingival sulcus and labio-gingival sulcus forms alveolar process

- Upper lip also gets separated from developing alveolar process by the labio-gingival furrow.

DEVELOPMENT OF TEETH

- Human have two sets of teeth
  A. Deciduous or milk teeth: Twenty in number.
  B. Permanent teeth: Thirty-two in number.
- *Successional teeth* are permanent incisors, canine and premolars as these teeth preceded by milk teeth.
- *Super-added teeth* are permanent molars as these do not precede by milk teeth.

Source of Development

Each tooth develops from:
- Surface ectoderm—that forms the enamel.
- Mesoderm that forms dentine, tooth pulp, cementum and periodontal ligament.

Structure of Tooth

Each tooth has the following parts:
- Enamel
- Dentine
- Cementum
- Pulp and periodontal ligament.

Stages of Teeth Development

Q. Describe the stages of development of tooth.

Tooth develops in the following stages (Figs 13.3 to 13.5, Flowchart 13.1, Practice Fig. 13.1):

1. Stages of dental lamina: During the 6th week of development, epithelium (ectoderm) in the region of developing an alveolar process (U-shaped zone) thickens to form *dental lamina* (Fig. 13.3).
2. Bud stage: In each alveolar process, the dental lamina thickens at ten places and form *tooth buds* (*enamel organ*) that grow towards underlying mesoderm.

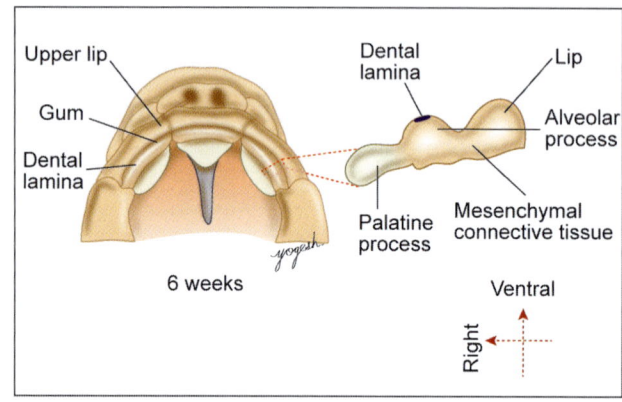

Fig. 13.3: Dental lamina

Flowchart 13.1: Formation of tooth

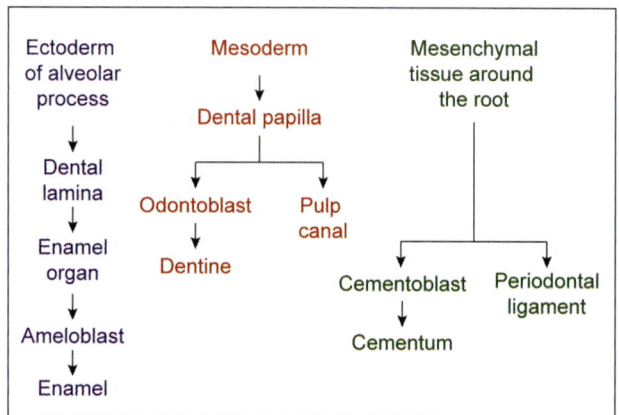

3. Cap stage: Mass of mesenchyme (mostly neural crest cells) occupies the core of enamel organ and makes enamel organ cap-shaped. In 8th week: Enamel organs appear.
   This mass of the mesenchyme forms the *dental papilla*. In 10th week: Enamel organs become cap-shaped.
4. Bell stage: Cells of the enamel organ facing dental papilla become columnar and form *ameloblasts*.
   Cells of the dental papilla facing ameloblasts, later form an epithelium-like layer called *odontoblasts*.

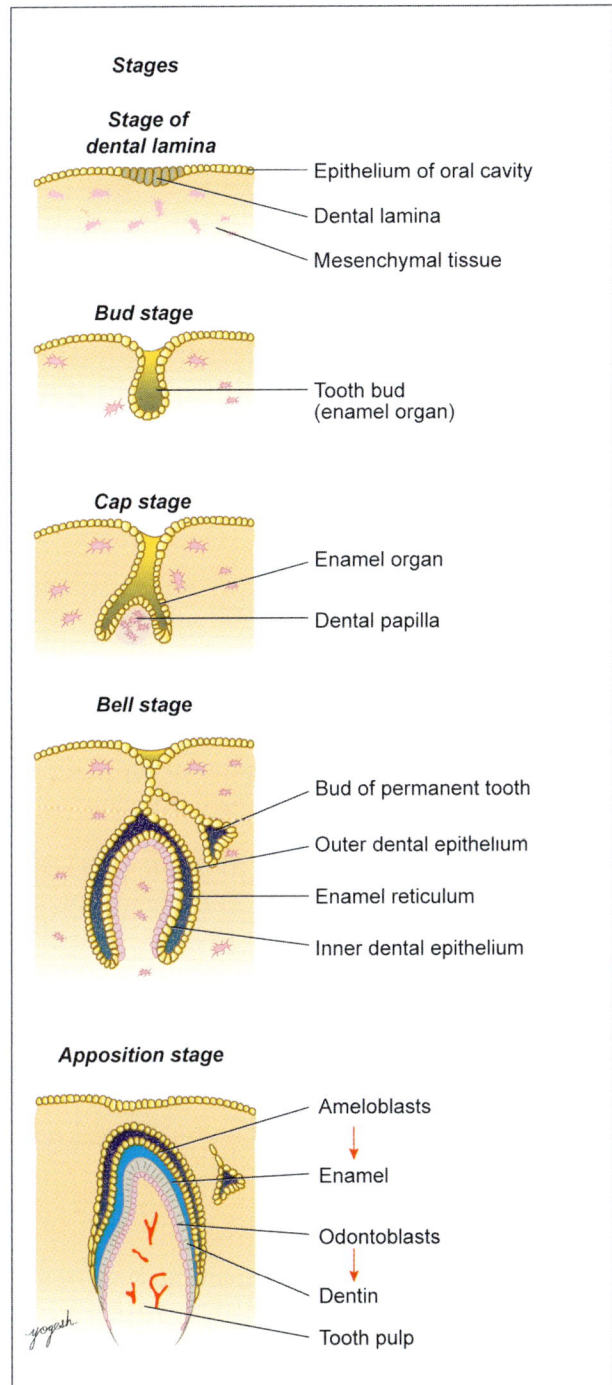

Fig. 13.4: Development of tooth: Stages of the dental lamina, bud stage, cap stage, bell stage and apposition stage

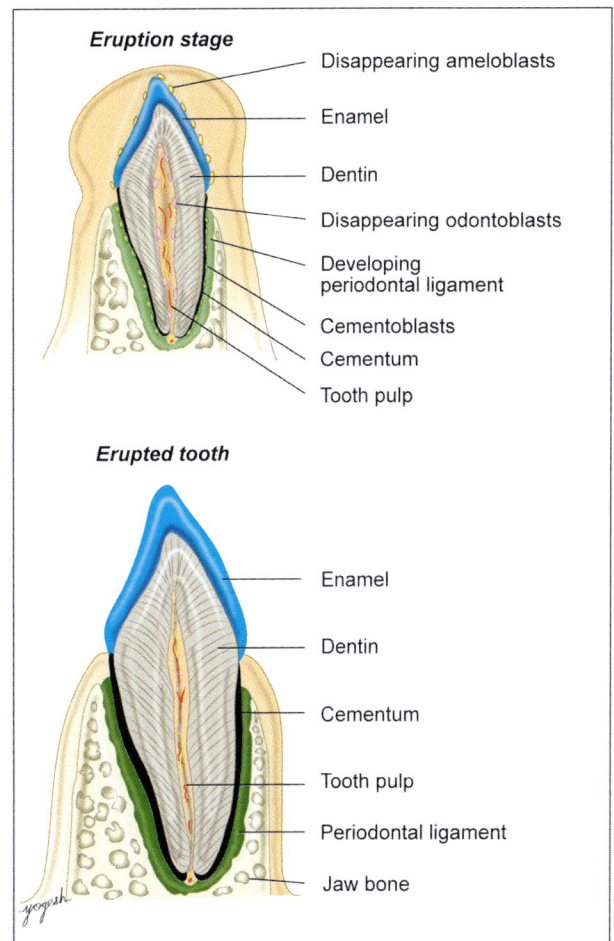

Fig. 13.5: Development of tooth: Stage of the eruption and structure of the erupted tooth

Enamel organ soon forms:
- outer cell layer as *outer dental epithelium*
- inner cell layer as *inner dental epithelium* (*ameloblasts*) and
- central core loose mesenchymal cells as *stellate reticulum* or *enamel reticulum*.

Growing dental cap forms a bell-shaped structure over underlying dental papilla; hence called *bell stage*.

5. Apposition stage: Ameloblasts lay down *enamel* on the outer surface of basement membrane separating ameloblasts and odontoblasts, whereas odontoblast laydown *dentine* on deeper surface of basement membrane.

The ameloblasts move towards outer dental epithelium through satellite reticulum. Finally, outer epithelium, reticulum and ameloblasts disappear, leaving behind *dental cuticle of Nasmyth* (a thin layer) over enamel.

On the formation of dentine, regressing odontoblast leaves behind their cytoplasmic processes (called odontoblastic processes or Tomes processes) that remains trapped in dentin.

Continuous deposition of dentine reduces pulp cavity to a narrow *pulp canal*. Blood vessels and nerves reach tooth through the pulp canal.

Mesenchymal cells covering the root of the tooth modifies to form *cementoblasts*.

The cementoblasts lay down a layer of dense bone called *cementum*. Cementum is produced just before the birth.

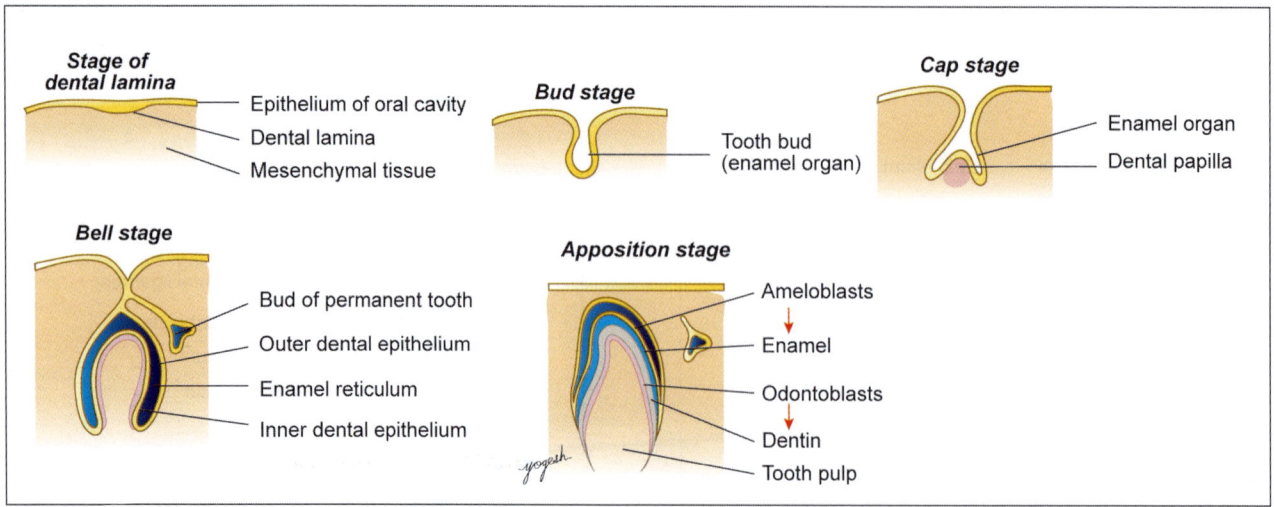

Practice Fig. 13.1: Development of tooth

Mesenchymal cells covering cementum form periodontal ligament that connects root of the tooth with jaw bone. After birth, before eruption of tooth, periodontal ligament appears.

6. Eruption stage: Growth of the root produces eruption of tooth. Eruption age of various teeth is listed in Table 13.1.

Q. Enlist the timings of eruption of temporary and permanent teeth.

Table 13.1	Time of eruption of teeth
Teeth	Time of eruption
Deciduous	
Lower central incisors	6–9 months
Upper incisors	8–10 months
Lower lateral incisors	10–11 years
First molar	11–12 years
Canines	11–12 years
Second molars	11–12 years
Permanent	
Central incisor	7–8 years
Laterl incisor	8–9 years
Canine	10–12 years
First premolar	10–11 years
Second premolar	11–12 years
First molar	6–7 years
Second molar	12 years
Third molar	18–25 years

Development of Permanent Teeth

- There are thirty-two permanent teeth.
- During the 3rd month of intrauterine life, a series of *tooth buds* arise from dental lamina from lingual side of milk tooth (Fig. 13.4).
- These buds remain dormant till six to seven years after birth and then forms permanent incisors, canines and premolars (Table 13.1).
- Developing permanent tooth pushes deciduous tooth outwards and finally, deciduous tooth shed off.
- For permanent molars, tooth buds arise from dental lamina and remain dormant till the age of eruption of permanent molars.
- Enamel is the hardest tissue of body, whereas dentin is the second hardest.

Anomalies of Teeth

1. *Anodontia*: Anodontia is a complete absence of teeth.
2. Supernumerary tooth (extra tooth) may be present that cause malocclusion (improper alignment of teeth).
3. *Natal teeth*: Occasionally teeth may be present at birth. These teeth are called natal teeth.
4. Germination is fusion of two or more teeth.
5. Impaction of tooth: It is the failure of a tooth to erupt. The third molar is most commonly impacted tooth.[MCQ]
6. *Amelogenesis imperfecta* is a condition due to hypocalcification of enamel in vitamin D deficiency (rickets). The enamel becomes soft, friable and yellowish–brown in colour.[MCQ]

7. *Dentinogenesis imperfecta* is an autosomal dominant disorder that involves long arm of chromosome 4 (4q). Enamel lose easily and dentine gets exposed.
8. *Dentigerous cyst* develops from unerupted permanent tooth.

Some Interesting Facts

- Development of tooth is a classic example of an epithelio-mesenchymal interaction.^{MCQ}
- Enamel is derived from ectoderm, whereas mesenchyme of dental papilla from neural crest cells.^{Neet}
- Teeth have *enamel knot* as a circumscribed region of the dental epithelium at the tooth buds. Enamel knot acts as a signalling center (organiser).^{MCQ}
- Humans are *diphyodont* (having only two successive sets of teeth). Many vertebrates (fishes, crocodiles) are *polyphyodont* (having continuously replacing teeth).
- Tooth regeneration from stem cell is new possibility developed in the field of tissue engineering and stem cell biology by Young et al. (2002).
- *Hertwig epithelial root sheath* (HERS) is a proliferation of epithelial cells of enamel organ. HERS stimulates differentiation of odontoblast in dental papilla and thus help in the formation of dentine. HERS cells completely disappear.
- *Epithelial cell rests of Malassez* (ERM) are residual cells of the HERS in the periodontal ligament. These residual cells may form odontogenic cysts.

DEVELOPMENT OF PHARYNX

- Pharynx develops from the cranial part of the foregut.
- In the lateral wall and floor of pharynx, the pharyngeal pouches form various structures (for details, refer to Chapter 11).

Box 13.1: Luschka

- Hubert von Luschka (1820–75) was a German anatomist.
- *Luschka's crypts* are mucous membrane indentation of the inner wall of the gallbladder.
- *Luschka's joint* (uncovertebral joint or neurocentral joint) is formed between uncinate process and uncus. These joints are present in the cervical region of vertebral column between C3 and C7 vertebrae.
- *Duct of Luschka* is an accessory bile duct.
- *Foramina of Luschka* are two lateral opening of the fourth ventricle of the brain.
- Pharyngeal bursa or *pouch of Luschka* is a cystic notochordal remnant in the posterior wall of nasopharynx at the lower end of pharyngeal tonsil.

- Laryngotracheal groove (furcula of His) develops in the floor of the pharynx caudal to the hypobranchial eminence. This groove deepens to form a diverticulum that gives rise to the respiratory system (For details, refer to Chapter 16).
- Formation of the nose, palate and respiratory diverticulum divide the pharynx into nasopharynx, oropharynx and laryngopharynx.
- *Pharyngeal bursa* or *pouch of Lushka* is a cystic notochordal remnant in the posterior wall of nasopharynx at the lower end of the pharyngeal tonsil.^{MCQ}

DEVELOPMENT OF TONGUE

Q. Write short note on development of tongue.

- Tongue develops in the floor of primitive pharynx and developing mouth.

Summary (Examination Guide)

- The tongue is derived from three different sources as follows (refer to Table 13.2, Fig. 13.6 and Practice Fig. 13.2):

Table 13.2	Development and nerve supply of tongue^{MCQ, Viva}	
Structure	Embryonic source	Nerve supply
Mucosa of tongue Anterior two-thirds of tongue	Endodermal lining of first arch Two lingual swellings Tuberculum impar	**General sensory:** Lingual nerve (branch of mandibular nerve) **Special sensory:** Chorda tympani branch of facial nerve
Posterior one-third of tongue and circumvallate papillae	Endodermal lining of third arch	**General and special sensory:** Glossopharyngeal nerve
Posterior most part	Endodermal lining of fourth arch	**General and special sensory:** Superior laryngeal branch of vagus nerve
Muscles All extrinsic and intrinsic muscles except palatoglossus	Occipital myotomes	Hypoglossal nerve (palatoglossus by vagus nerve)

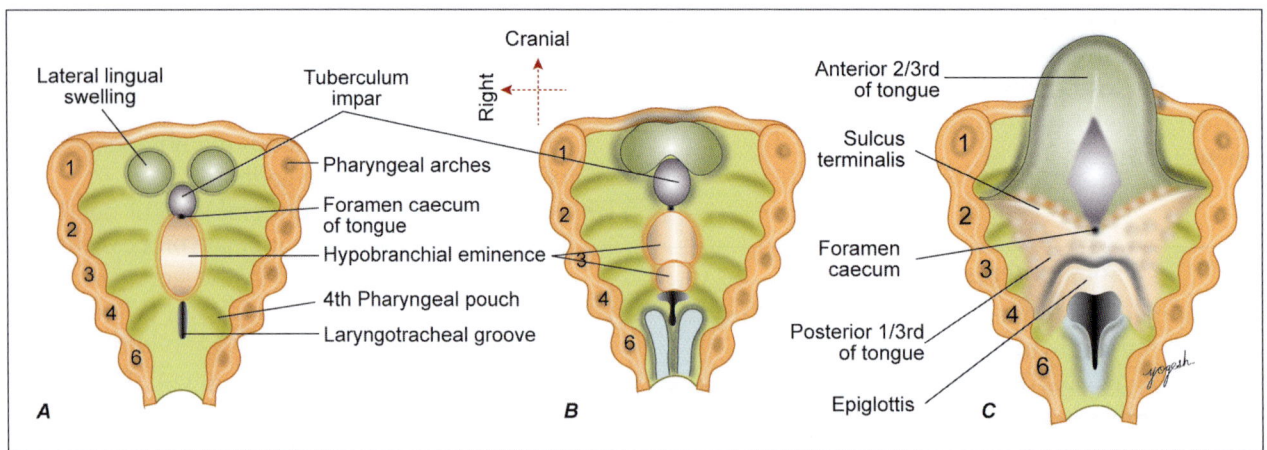

Fig. 13.6: Development of the tongue: (A) A section of pharynx of the embryo at 4th week. In the floor of pharynx two lateral lingual swellings, one median lingual swelling and more caudally hypobranchial eminence appear; (B) 6 weeks and; (C) 10 weeks: One medial and two lateral lingual swellings fuse to form anterior one-third of the tongue, whereas cranial part of the hypobranchial eminence forms posterior one-third of the tongue and circumvallate papillae

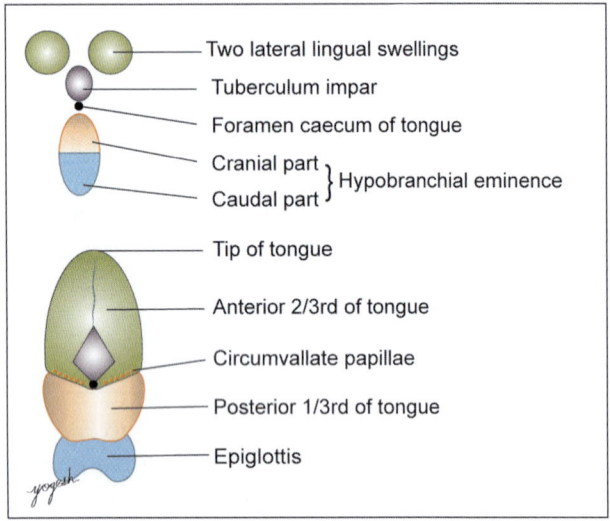

Practice Fig. 13.2: Development of tongue

1. Endoderm covering the pharyngeal arches form mucous membrane covering the tongue.
2. Mesenchyme of arches forms fibro-areolar stroma of the tongue.
3. Occipital myotomes form muscles of the tongue.

Mucous Membrane

- Mandibular arches show three swellings: Single midline swelling as **tuberculum impar** and two lateral **lingual swellings**. In 4th week, two lingual swellings and tuberculum impar become visible.
- Caudal to tuberculum impar, proliferating epithelium forms thyroglossal duct and its pharyngeal site is marked by a depression called *foramen caecum*.
- The lingual swellings grow and fuse with each other and with tuberculum impar. These combined swellings form ventral two-thirds of the tongue.
- Developing alveolo-lingual sulcus gradually separates tongue from floor of mouth.
- In relation to third and fourth arch, pharyngeal surface shows a midline swelling called *hypobranchial eminence* or *copula of His*. In 5th week, hypobranchial eminence becomes visible.
- The hypobranchial eminence is divided into ventral and dorsal parts. Ventral part expands to form posterior one-third of the tongue. Fusion of anterior and posterior part is represented by *sulcus terminalis*.
- Caudal part of the hypobranchial eminence forms *epiglottis*. Some cells migrate from posterior one-third of tongue and cross sulcus terminalis to form *circumvallate papillae*.

Muscles of Tongue

- 3–4 *occipital myotomes* migrate ventrally to the mesenchyme of the tongue and forms all extrinsic and intrinsic muscles of tongue.
- The occipital myotomes pull their nerve (hypoglossal nerve) during migration; hence hypoglossal nerve crosses both external and internal carotid arteries superficially.

Nerve Supply

- Mucosa of anterior two-thirds of tongue develops from mandibular (1st) pharyngeal arch. Hence, supplied by the mandibular branch of trigeminal nerve (post-trematic nerve of 1st arch) and for a taste sensation, supplied by chorda tympani branch of facial nerve (pre-trematic nerve of 1st arch).
- Mucosa of posterior one-third of tongue and circumvallate papillae develop from mucosa of the third arch by hypobranchial eminence; hence supplied by glossopharyngeal nerve (nerve of third arch).

- Mucosa of posterior part of the tongue (near vallecula) develops from mucosa of fourth arch by hypobranchial eminence; hence, supplied by vagus nerve (nerve of the fourth arch).
- Muscles of tongue *except* palatoglossus are derived from occipital myotomes; hence, supplied by hypoglossal nerve (Fig. 13.7).

Developmental Anomalies of Tongue

1. *Aglossia* is complete agenesis of tongue.
2. *Hemiglossia* is produced due to failure of one lingual swelling to form half part of the tongue.
3. *Bifid tongue* is split tongue in anterior two-thirds due to non-fusion of two lingual swellings.
4. *Tongue tie* or *ankyloglossia* occurs due to incomplete formation of alveolo-lingual sulcus. The tongue is connected with a floor of mouth by short frenulum.
5. *Microglossia* is a small tongue and *macroglossia* is a large tongue.
6. *Ankyloglossia superior* is a condition of adherent tongue with palate.
7. *Lingual thyroid* occurs due to failure of migration of the thyroid gland.

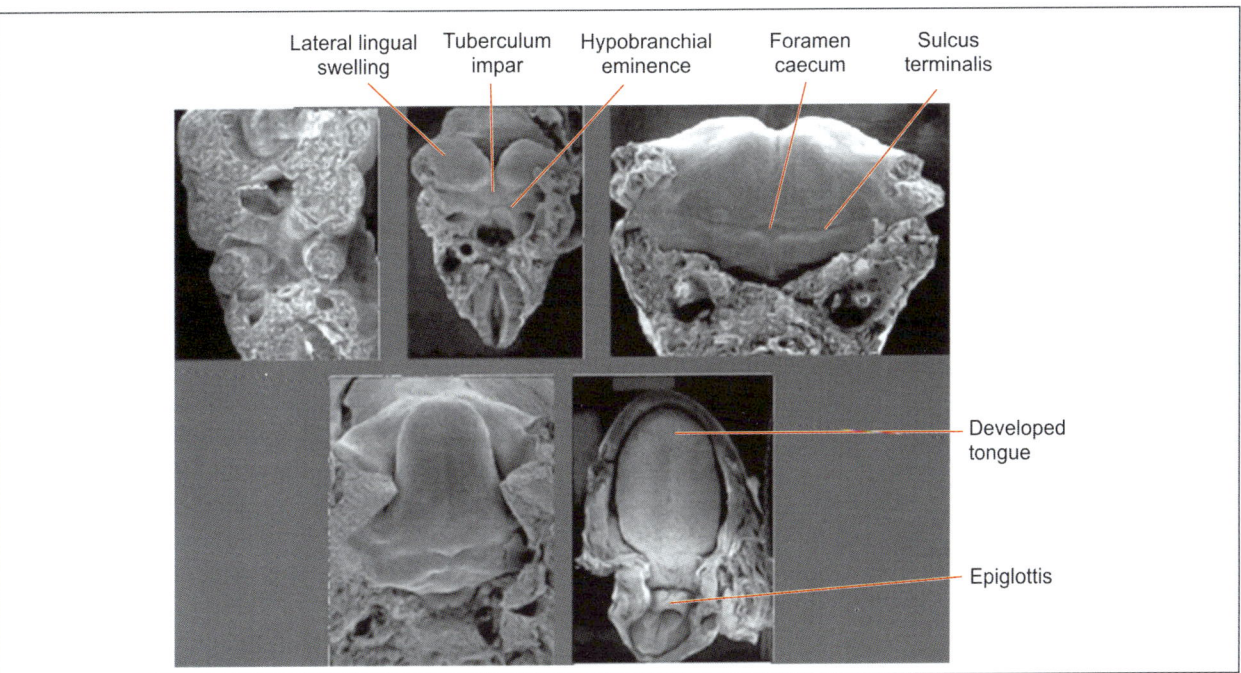

Scanning electron micrograph 13.1: SEM showing contribution of the pharyngeal arches to the developing tongue and epiglottis. A series of micrographs of sequentially older embryos also illustrate the contribution of arches to tongue. [Species: Mouse, approximate human age: Early 5th week, dorsal view]

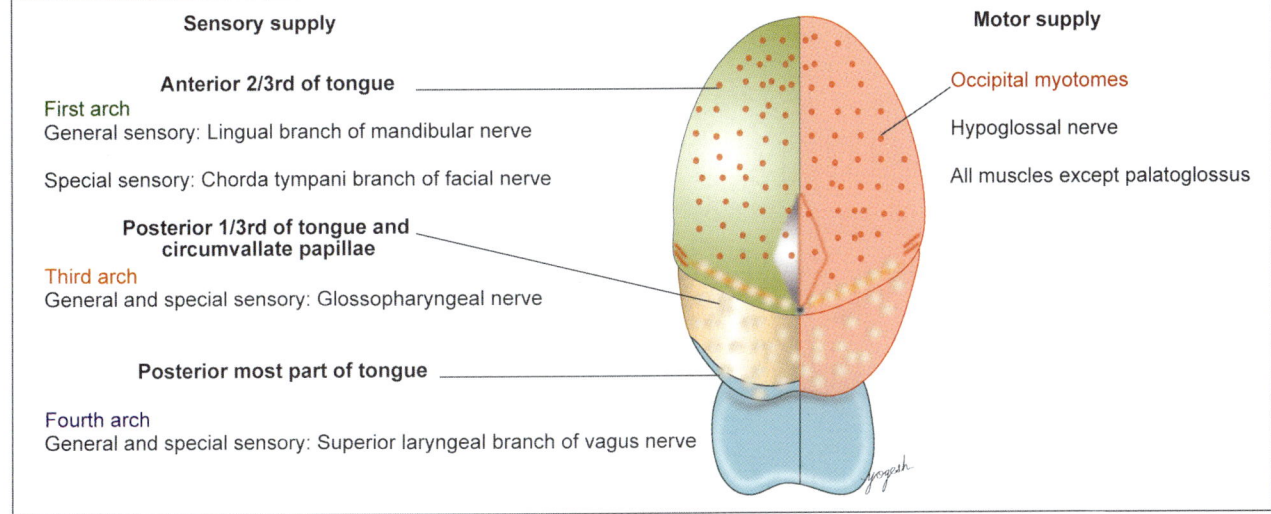

Fig. 13.7: Nerve supply of the tongue

DEVELOPMENT OF SALIVARY GLANDS

- There are three pairs of salivary glands, namely parotid, submandibular and sublingual.
- The parotid gland develops from ectoderm, whereas sublingual and submandibular salivary glands develop from endoderm.
- Each salivary gland develops as epithelial outgrowth that forms solid cords.
- Solid cords later get canalised and then they divide and redivide. Each cord at the end gets converted into acini.
- Main canalised cord form duct of salivary gland and its oral opening forms papilla of ductal opening of salivary gland (Fig. 13.8).

Parotid Gland

- The parotid gland develops during fifth week from an ectodermal outgrowth or furrow from cheek at the angle of stomodeum (between mandibular arch and maxillary process).
- Later the furrow gets canalised and forms parotid duct.
- Lateral end of duct proliferates and divide to form ductules and acini of parotid gland.
- Maxillary and mandibular processes fuse and reduce size of oral fissure. This fusion increases the length of parotid duct.
- Finally, the duct of parotid gland opens into vestibule of mouth (in adult opposite to upper second molar teeth).^MCQ
- Presence of myoepithelial cells surrounding parotid acini confirms its ectodermal origin.^MCQ

Submandibular Gland

- During sixth week, a solid endodermal outgrowth arises from floor of stomodeum, from floor of alveolo-lingual groove.
- Later furrow gets canalised and form submandibular duct.
- Lateral end of the duct proliferates and divides to form ductules and acini of submandibular gland.

Sublingual Gland

- During seventh week, multiple endodermal outgrowths arise from linguo-gingival sulcus and submandibular duct and finally these outgrowths form sublingual glands.

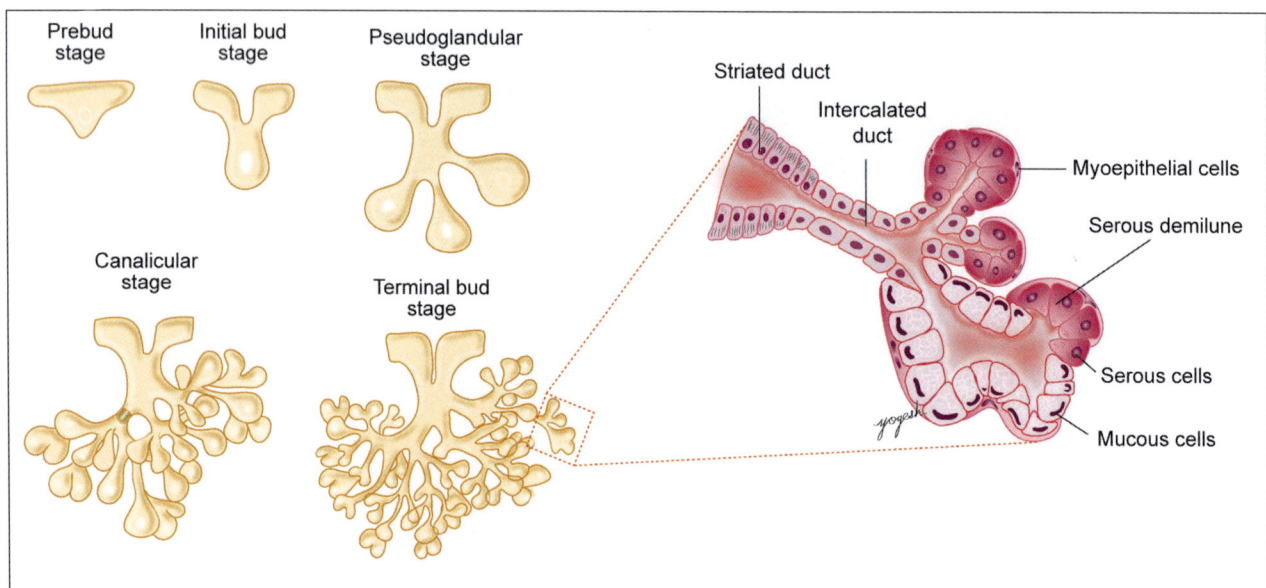

Fig. 13.8: Development of salivary gland

Alimentary Tract II: Development of Teeth, Pharynx, Tongue and Salivary Glands

CLINICAL EMBRYOLOGY

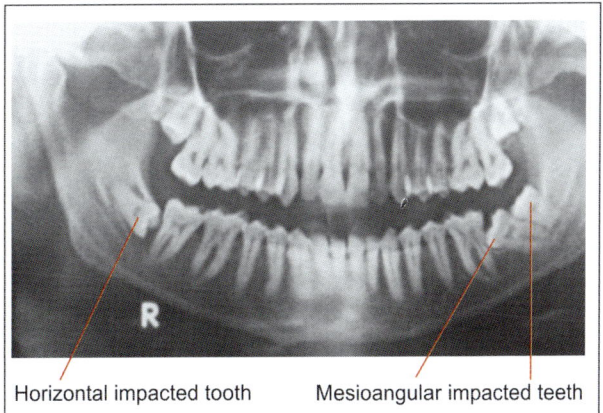

Horizontal impacted tooth   Mesioangular impacted teeth

Clinical image 13.1: Orthopantomogram (OPG) showing impacted teeth. Right lower third molar (48) tooth is horizontal impacted, whereas left lower second and third molar teeth (37, 38) are mesioangular impacted. Note OPG is a panoramic dental X-ray that produces a two-dimensional view of maxilla and mandible. While recording OPG, the machine rotates around patient's head. For reference purpose, dentition is divided into four quadrants: (1) upper right, (2) upper left, (3) lower left and (4) lower right. Hence, right lower third molar is referred to as tooth 48 (Image courtesy: *Dr Saikat Chakraborty*)

14

Alimentary Tract III
Development of Intestine

Chapter Outline

- Development of oesophagus
  - Stages of development
  - Congenital anomalies
- Development of stomach
  - Stages of development
  - Rotation of stomach
  - Changes in mesenteries
  - Histogenesis of stomach
- Congenital hypertrophic pyloric stenosis
- Development of duodenum
  - Stages of development
  - Anomalies of duodenum
- Development of midgut
- Physiological umbilical hernia
- Rotation of gut
  - Stages of rotation
  - Congenital anomalies of midgut
- Development of caecum and appendix
- Malrotation
- Meckel's diverticulum
- Development of hindgut
  - Development of urorectal septum
- Development of anal canal
- Meconium

INTRODUCTION

- The alimentary tract develops from *primitive gut*.
- On formation of head and tail folds, the part of *definitive yolk sac* gets trapped within the embryo. This trapped part forms *primitive gut*[Neet] (Fig. 14.1).
- The primitive gut extends from *buccopharyngeal membrane* cranially to *cloacal membrane* caudally. Oropharyngeal membrane and cloacal membrane are the regions where ectoderm and endoderm are opposed without intervening mesoderm.[Neet]
- Developing primitive gut communicates with
  1. Yolk sac through vitellointestinal duct.
  2. Allantoic diverticulum.
- Cranial part of the gut that lies in the head fold is *foregut*.
- Caudal part of gut that lies in the tail fold is *hindgut*.
- The part of gut that communicates with vitellointestinal duct is *midgut*.
- Vitellointestinal duct disappears by 5th week.[MCQ]

- *Anterior (cranial) intestinal portal* is the communication between foregut and midgut, whereas *posterior (caudal) intestinal portal* is the communication between midgut and hindgut.
- The *buccopharyngeal membrane* separates stomodeum form foregut, whereas *cloacal membrane* separates hindgut from proctodeum.
- Gut is attached to body wall by ventral and dorsal mesenteries.
- The primitive gut is supplied by coeliac artery for the foregut, superior mesenteric artery for the midgut and inferior mesenteric artery for the hindgut (Fig. 14.2).[Neet]
- During early development, *allantois* opens in caudal part of hindgut called **cloaca**.
- The **urorectal septum** divide cloaca in ventral *primitive urogenital sinus* and dorsal *primitive rectum* or *primitive anorectal canal*.[Neet]
- Attachment of urorectal septum also divides the cloacal membrane into ventral *urogenital membrane* and dorsal *anal membrane*.

Alimentary Tract III: Development of Intestine

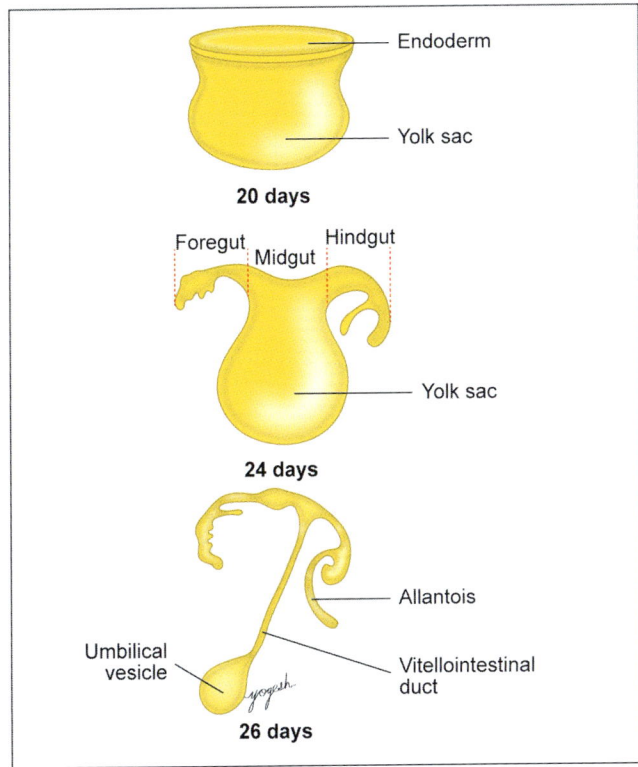

Fig. 14.1: Conversion of endoderm and yolk sac to gut

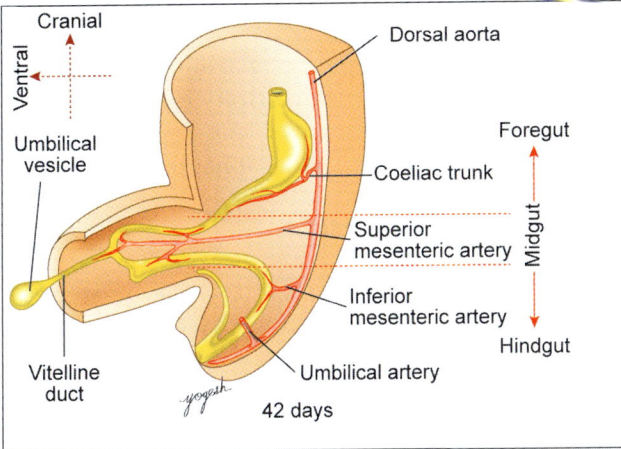

Fig. 14.2: Blood supply of developing gut. Foregut and its derivatives are supplied by the branches from coeliac trunk. Midgut is supplied by superior mesenteric artery, whereas hindgut by inferior mesenteric artery

DEVELOPMENT OF OESOPHAGUS

Q. Write short note on development of oesophagus.

- Oesophagus develops from the part of foregut between the pharynx and stomach.

Summary (Examination Guide)

- Derivation of the components of oesophagus:
  - Epithelium—from endoderm of foregut.

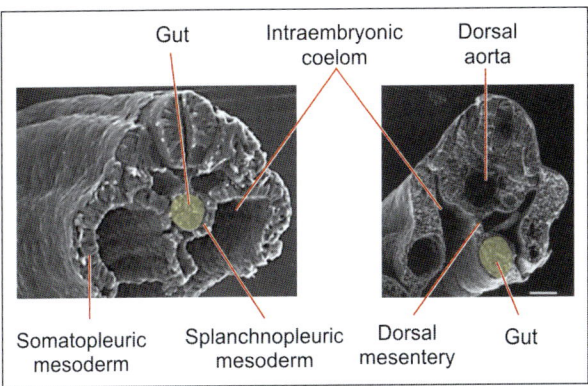

Scanning electron micrograph 14.1: Gut is suspended by dorsal mesentery. Intraembryonic coelom splits mesoderm into splanchnopleuric and somatopleuric mesoderm [Species: Mouse, approximate human age: 27–28. Transverse section]

- Muscles and connective tissue—from the splanchnopleuric mesoderm surrounding the foregut.
- Refer to Flowchart 14.1.

Stages of Development

- In lower part of the pharynx, a *laryngotracheal groove* appears that later form tracheobronchial (respiratory) diverticulum (Fig. 14.3).
- Tracheoesophageal septum divides the part of foregut caudal to tracheobronchial diverticulum in ventral trachea and dorsal oesophagus.
- Small oesophagus elongates due to formation of neck and descent of diaphragm, lungs and heart.

Flowchart 14.1: Development of oesophagus

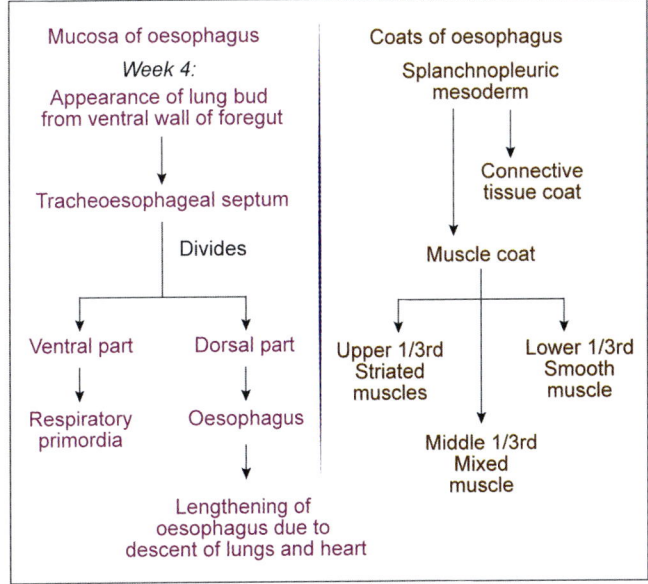

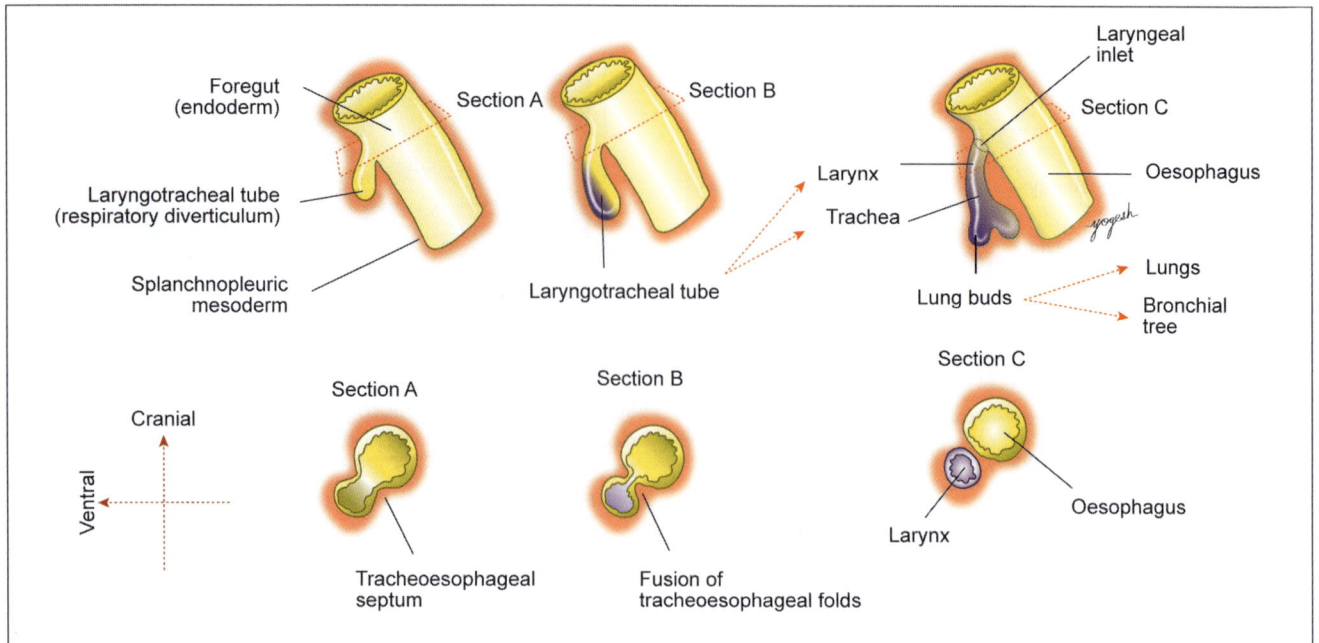

Fig. 14.3: Formation of tracheal bud and lung bud. Tracheoesophageal septum separates trachea from oesophagus

Some Interesting Facts

- Auerbach's and Meissner's plexus are derivatives of neural crest.^{Neet}
- Oesophagus has striated muscles in upper one-third, smooth muscles in lower one-third and mixed (both smooth and striated muscles) in middle one-third. ^{MCQ, Viva}
- Metaplasia of ciliated epithelium: Initially epithelium of oesophagus is ciliated, later it becomes simple columnar and finally it becomes stratified columnar.

Congenital Anomalies of Oesophagus

1. *Oesophageal stenosis*: Failure of canalisation of oesophagus results in oesophageal atresia (obliterated lumen). Oesophageal atresia results in *polyhydramnios* (excessive amniotic fluid) due to inability of ingestion of amniotic fluid by foetus.
2. *Oesophageal atresia*: It is a failure of development of part of the oesophagus. Continuous pouring of saliva from the mouth is the most important confirmatory sign of oesophageal atresia.^{MCQ}
3. *Tracheoesophageal fistula*: It is a communication of trachea with oesophagus due to the failure of proper development of tracheoesophageal septum. In this condition, proximal part of the oesophagus ends as blind pouch; whereas distal part of the oesophagus communicates with the trachea.

Q. Write short note on tracheoesophageal fistula.

4. *Achalasia cardia* or *cardiospasm*: Loss of the ganglionic cells in Auerbach's plexus of the oesophageal wall result in a failure of muscle relaxation in lower part of the oesophagus. This deformity is *achalasia cardia*. Barium swallow shows *bird-beak deformity* (pencil-shaped narrowing of the oesophagus).^{MCQ}

DEVELOPMENT OF STOMACH

Summary (Examination Guide)

- Stomach develops during 4th–5th week as a fusiform dilatation of the part of the foregut distal to the oesophagus.
- Refer to Flowchart 14.2 and Flowchart 14.3.

Stages of Development

- Adult stomach has anterior and posterior surfaces, lesser and greater curvature and fundus (Figs 14.4 and 14.5, Flowchart 14.2, Practice Fig. 14.1).
- Tubular foregut segment dilates and forms fusiform sac with ventral and dorsal borders.
- Dorsal border overgrows to form *greater curvature* of stomach.
- Ventral border grows slowly and forms *lesser curvature*.
- Ventral border is attached with septum transversum by *ventral mesogastrium,* whereas dorsal border is attached with dorsal body wall by *dorsal mesogas-*

Alimentary Tract III: Development of Intestine

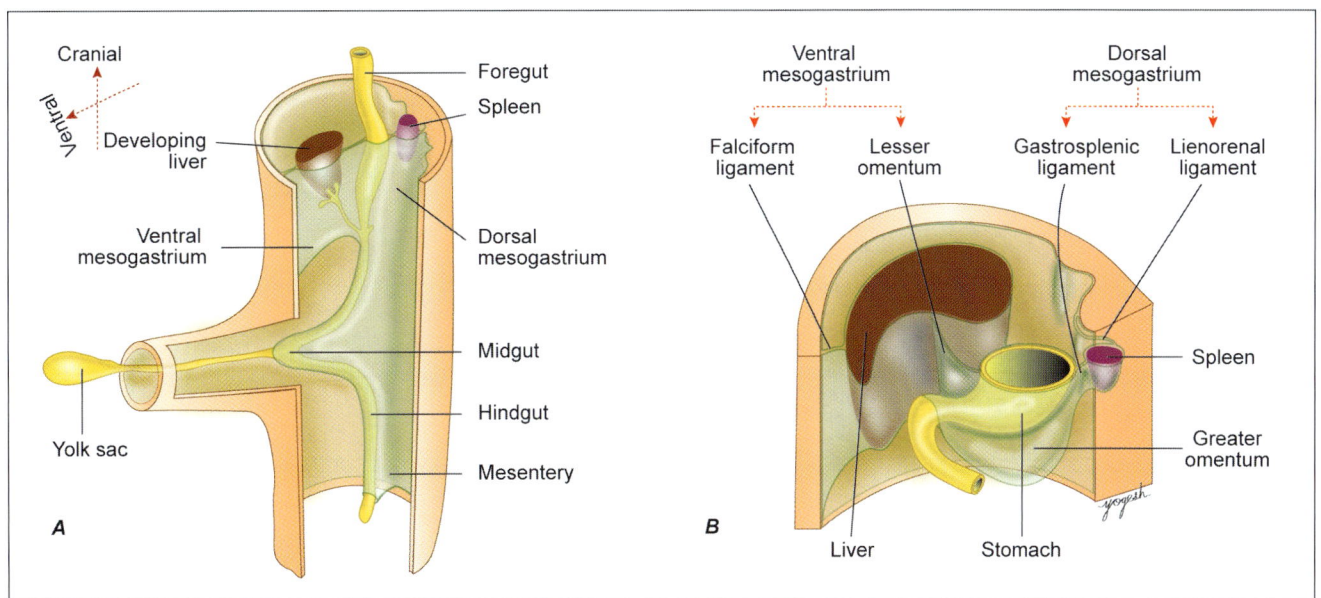

Fig.14.4: Transverse section through the region of stomach showing changes in the position of stomach, liver and spleen: (A) Positions at the end of fifth week; (B) Position at the end of 11th week. Ventral mesogastrium forms falciform ligament and lesser omentum, whereas dorsal mesogastrium forms gastrosplenic and lienorenal ligaments and greater omentum

Flowchart 14.2: Development of stomach

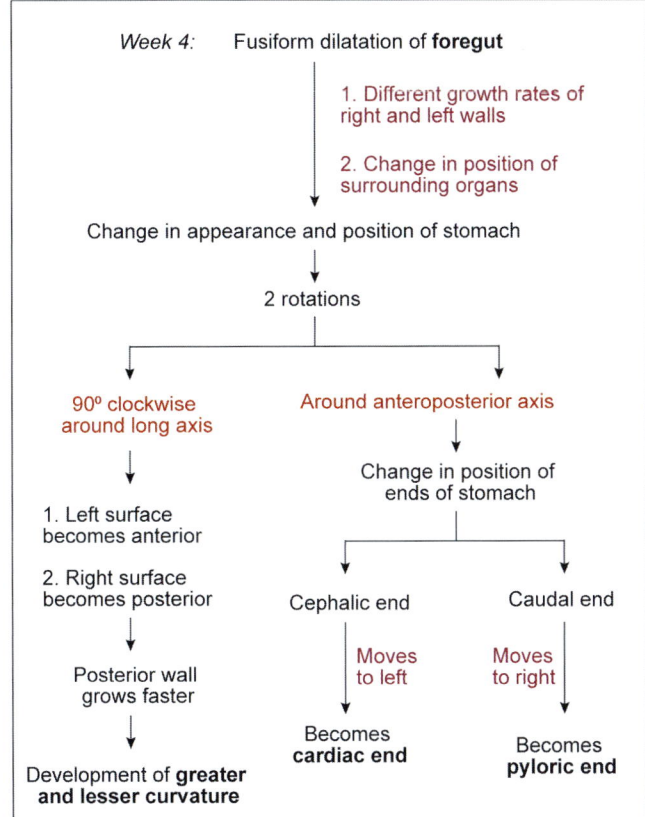

Flowchart 14.3: Development of mesogastrium

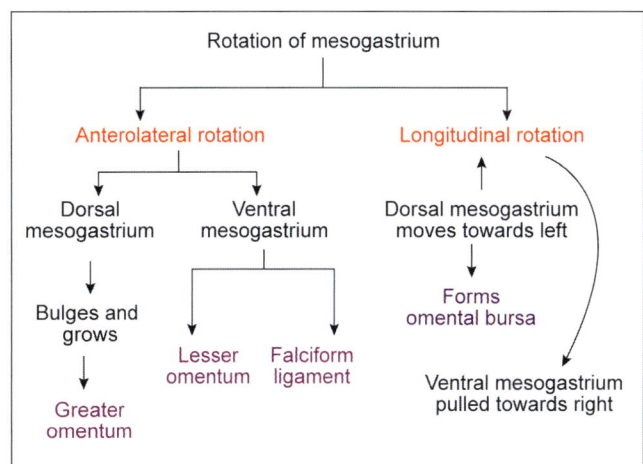

Rotation of Stomach

- Stomach rotates to the *right clockwise* (around 90°) along longitudinal axis and thus left surface of foregut forms anterior surface of adult stomach and right surface of foregut forms posterior surface of adult stomach.
- Hence, anterior surface of stomach is supplied by left vagus nerve, whereas posterior surface is by right vagus nerve.
- Stomach rotates along transverse (anteroposterior) axis and lower end rotates to the right. The right end forms pyloric end of stomach.

Changes in Mesenteries

- Liver develops in the ventral mesogastrium (Figs 14.4 and 14.5, Flowchart 14.3).

trium (mesentery). Spleen, coeliac trunk and dorsal pancreatic bud develop in dorsal mesogastrium, whereas ventral pancreatic bud, liver and gall bladder develop in ventral mesogastrium.

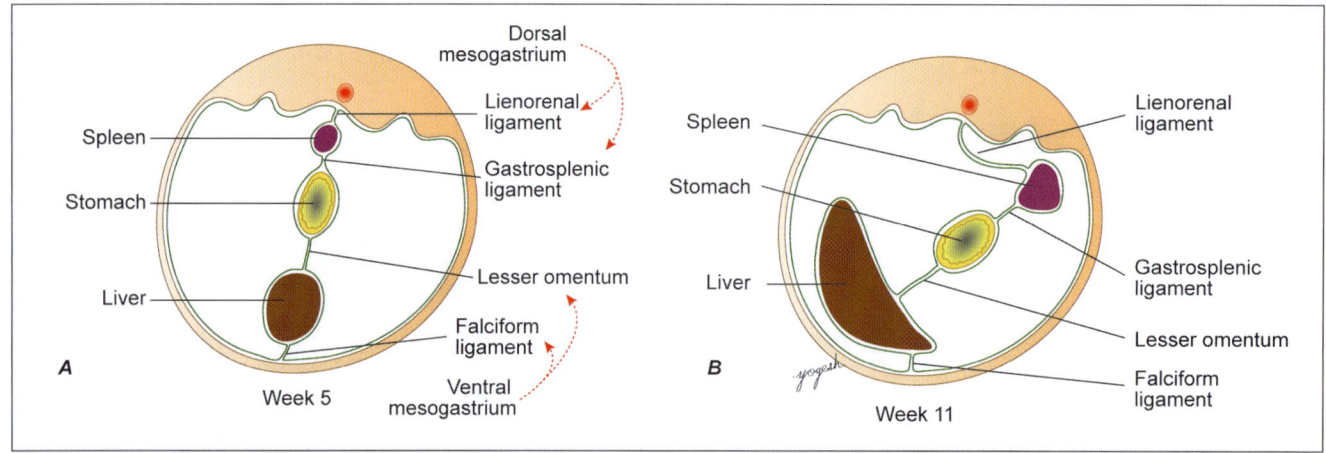

Practice Fig. 14.1: Development of transverse mesocolon and lesser sac (omental bursa)

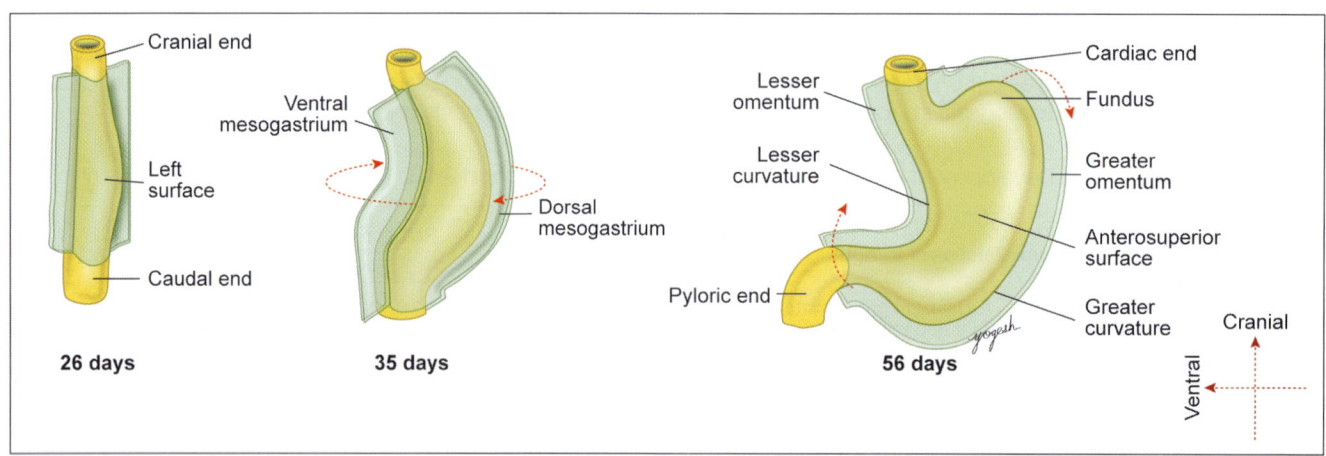

Fig. 14.5: Process of zygosis

- The developing liver divides ventral mesogastrium into two parts:
  - Falciform ligament—lies between liver and anterior abdominal wall.[Neet]
  - lesser omentum—lies between liver and stomach (lesser curvature). [Neet]
- Ventral mesogastrium also forms coronary and triangular ligaments.[Neet]
- Spleen develops in dorsal mesogastrium.[Neet]
- Developing spleen divides dorsal mesogastrium into two parts:
  - Gastrosplenic ligament—lies between greater curvature of stomach (fundus) and spleen (contains short gastric arteries)[Neet].
  - Lienorenal ligament—lies between the spleen and posterior body wall.
- Dorsal mesogastrium from rest of the greater curvature extends to form a *greater omentum*.

- Space behind lesser omentum, stomach and greater omentum form a *lesser sac* (lesser bursa).

Histogenesis of Stomach

- Epithelial lining and gastric gland—develop from endoderm of foregut.
- Muscles and connective tissue—develop from the splanchnopleuric mesoderm.
- Gastric glands appear in the third month, whereas oxyntic and zymogenic cells are differentiated in the fourth month of intrauterine life. [MCQ]

DEVELOPMENT OF DUODENUM

Summary (Examination Guide)
- Duodenum develops from two sources:[Neet]
  a. Foregut forms the part of duodenum proximal to the opening of common bile duct.
  b. Midgut forms the part of duodenum distal to the opening of bile duct.

Alimentary Tract III: Development of Intestine

> **Box 14.1:** Congenital hypertrophic pyloric stenosis
> - It is a congenital defect due to the hypertrophy of circular muscle layer at the pylorus. *Pyloric stenosis is one of the most common abnormalities of the stomach in infants.*
> - *Incidence*: 1 in every 150 male infants and 1 in every 750 female infants.
> - *Presentation*: Newborn is normal until first feed.
> - Newborn present projectile forceful vomiting after 2–3 hours of first feed. Vomitus does not contain bile.
> - *Treatment*: Surgical treatment of pyloric obstruction.

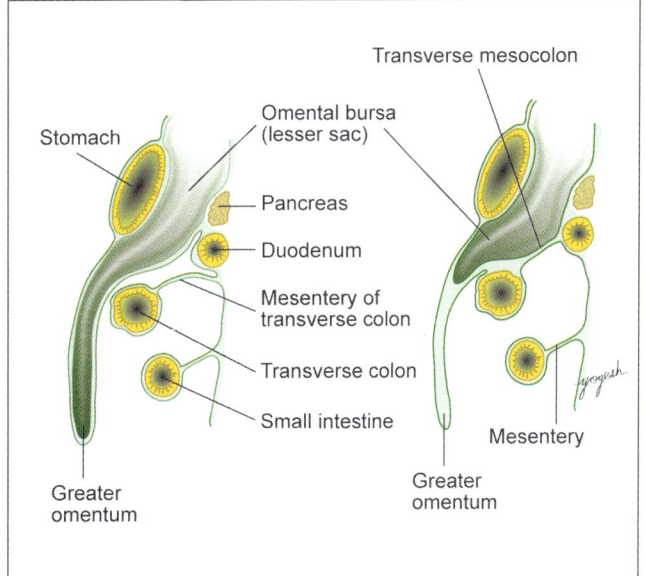

Fig. 14.6: Development of transverse mesocolon and lesser sac (omental bursa)

Stages of Development

1. Rotation of stomach brings midline duodenum to the right side.
2. Initially, duodenum is connected to posterior abdominal wall by dorsal mesentery (*mesoduodenum*).
   - Most of part of mesoduodenum undergo *zygosis* and duodenum becomes retroperitoneal organ except small proximal part of the duodenum near pylorus of stomach (Figs 14.6 and 14.7).
   - Blood supply:
     – Part of the duodenum derived from foregut is supplied by branches of *coeliac trunk*.
     – Part of the duodenum derived from midgut is supplied by branches of *superior mesenteric artery*.
   - Proliferation of the endodermal cells obliterates lumen by 8th week and it gets recanalised by 3rd month of intrauterine life (Fig. 14.8).^MCQ

Anomalies of Duodenum

1. *Duodenal stenosis*: Partial occlusion of duodenal lumen is *duodenal stenosis*. Incomplete recanalisation produces the duodenal stenosis. Newborn baby with duodenal stenosis vomits the feed that contains bile.^MCQ
2. *Duodenal atresia*: Complete occlusion of the duodenal lumen is *duodenal atresia*. It occurs mostly distal to the opening of hepatopancreatic ampulla. A newborn baby with duodenal atresia vomits the feed that always contains bile. *Duodenal atresia is most common intestinal atresia.* Duodenal atresia produces *polyhydramnios*. On ultrasonography, distended gas-filled stomach and duodenum produce *double-bubble sign*.^MCQ
3. *Duodenal diverticula*: Duodenal diverticulum usually arises from the second part of the duodenum.

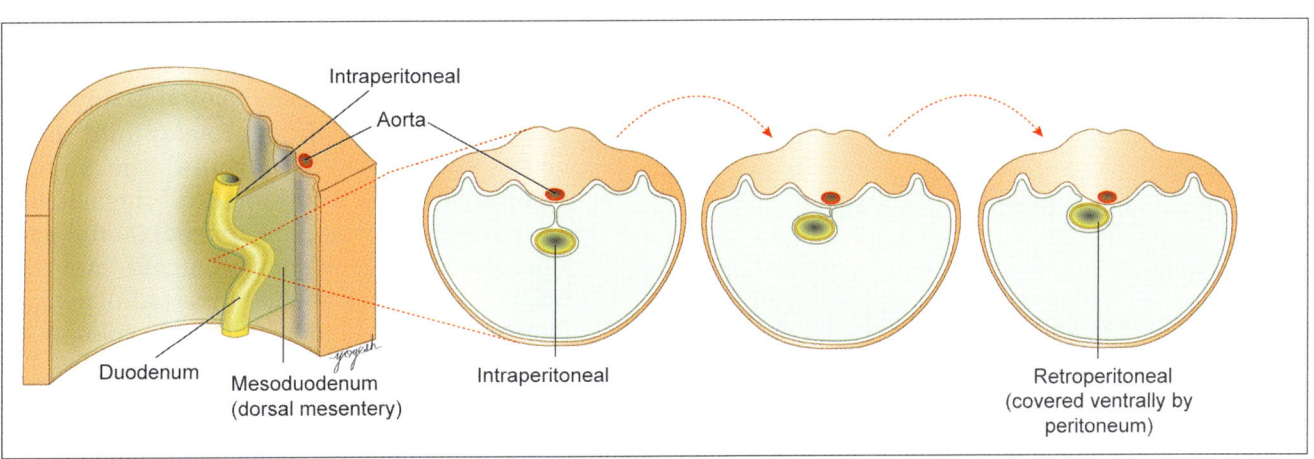

Fig. 14.7: Process of zygosis

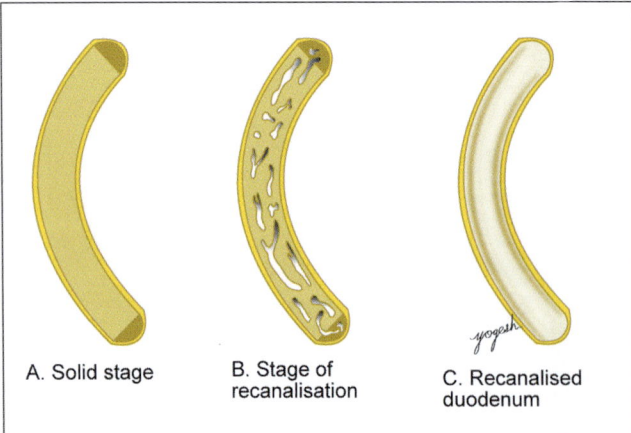

Fig. 14.8: Development of duodenum: (A) Solid stage: Endodermal cells proliferate to obliterate the lumen of the duodenum; (B, C) Stage of recanalisation: Small lacunae appear, enlarge and fuse to form the lumen of the duodenum

DEVELOPMENT OF MIDGUT

- Primitive midgut extends from *cranial intestinal portal* to *caudal intestinal portal*.
- Midgut is suspended with *dorsal mesentery* from posterior abdominal wall.
- Midgut communicates with a yolk sac through a *vitellointestinal duct* (vitelline duct or yolk stalk).
- Midgut is supplied by superior mesenteric artery.[MCQ]
- Superior mesenteric artery divides the midgut into
    - Pre-arterial (proximal) segment
    - Post-arterial (distal) segment
- Pre-arterial segment forms[Neet]
    - Distal part of duodenum
    - Jejunum
    - Ileum
- Post-arterial segment forms[Neet]
    - Terminal part of ileum
    - Caecum
    - Appendix
    - Ascending colon
    - Right two-thirds of transverse colon.

Rotation of Gut

Q. Write short note on rotation of gut.

- Midgut undergoes 270° counterclockwise rotation (Fig. 14.9, Practice Fig. 14.2).[MCQ]
- *Purpose of rotation*: To accommodate herniated midgut loop in the small abdominal cavity.

Box 14.2: Physiological umbilical hernia
Q. Write short note on physiological umbilical hernia.
- Physiological umbilical hernia is a natural, normal phenomenon.
- It is the protrusion of midgut loop (herniation) outside the abdominal cavity through umbilical opening.
- Duration: From 6th week to 12th week of intrauterine life. Reduction of physiological hernia occurs at ~10 weeks of embryonic period.[Neet]
- Physiology: Abdominal cavity is smaller to accommodate rapidly elongating gut. It results into the midgut loop herniation. The midgut rotation and increase in abdomen size accommodates midgut in the abdominal cavity.

Stages of Rotation

- Midgut is divided into pre-arterial and post arterial segment by centrally passing superior mesenteric artery.
- Midgut rotates 270° counterclockwise around the axis passing through the superior mesenteric artery.
- Before rotation, pre-arterial segment lies cranial to the superior mesenteric artery in the midline, whereas post-arterial segment lies caudal.
- Rotation of midgut can be divided into three stages, each stage consisting of 90° rotation.
- First 90° rotation brings back the midgut loop in the abdominal cavity, whereas remaining 180° rotation occurs within the abdominal cavity.
    1. First 90° rotation: Midgut rotates 90° counterclockwise around the superior mesenteric artery. This rotation brings pre-arterial segment on the right side and post-arterial segment on the left side in the horizontal plane.
    2. Second 90° rotation: Pre-arterial segment elongates to form coils of the jejunum and ileum. The midgut again undergoes second 90° counterclockwise rotation. Thus, pre-arterial segment (coils of jejunum and ileum) come to lie behind the superior mesenteric artery. This brings the superior mesenteric artery ventral to duodenum.
    3. Third 90° rotation: Midgut rotates third time by 90° counterclockwise around the superior mesenteric artery. Third rotation brings the post-arterial segment (caecum, appendix) on the right side. Post-arterial segment elongates and caecal bud come to lie in right iliac fossa (adult position). Due to the third rotation, transverse colon crosses the superior mesenteric artery.
- Initially, all parts of midgut are connected with the dorsal wall by dorsal mesentery. After intestinal rotations, dorsal mesentery of duodenum, ascending

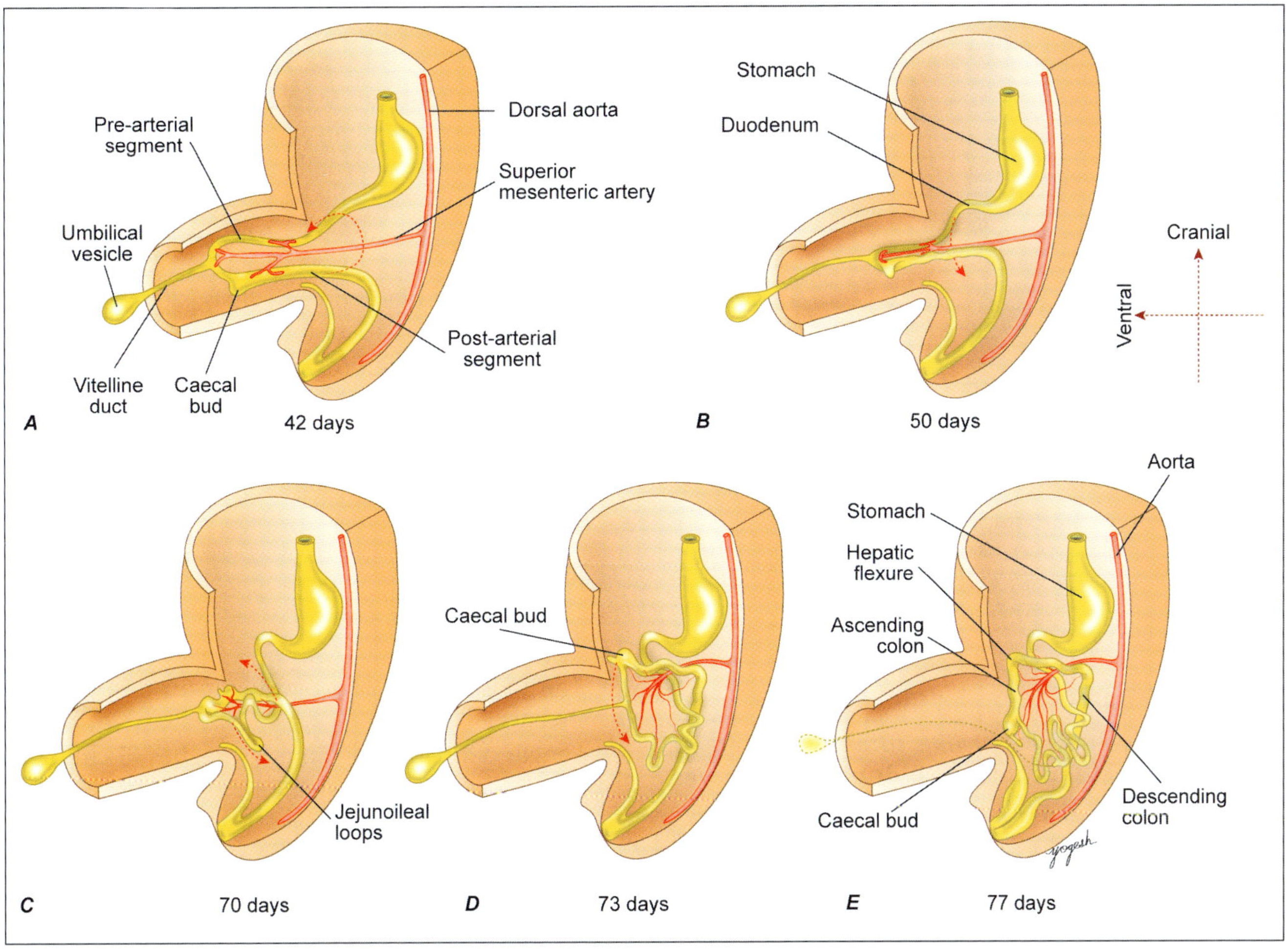

Alimentary Tract III: Development of Intestine

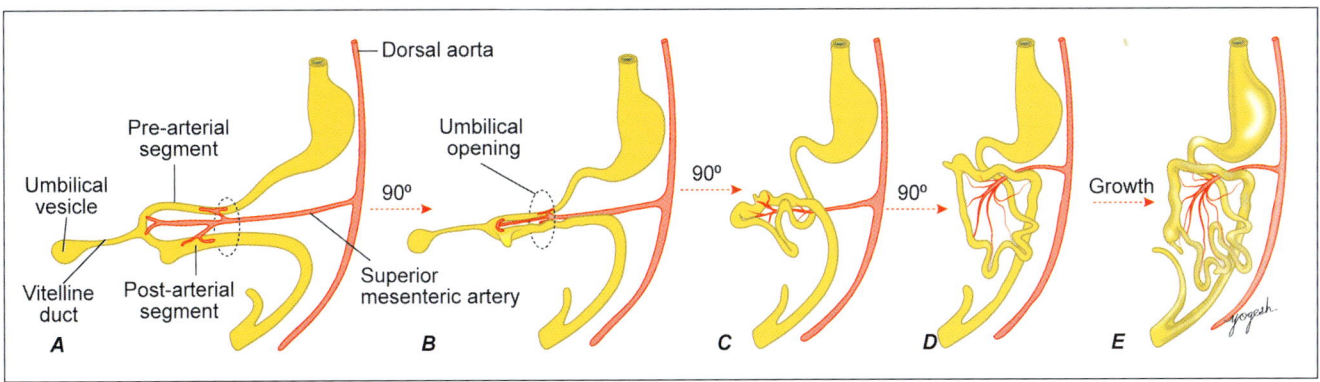

Fig. 14.9: Rotation of gut: (A) Position of the gut before rotation; (B) Position of the gut after first 90° counterclockwise rotation; (C) The position of the intestine after 180° counterclockwise rotation of gut; (D) The position of the intestine after 270° counterclockwise rotation of gut; (E) Caecal bud and appendix moves towards the right iliac fossa

Practice Fig. 14.2: Rotation of gut

colon and caecum, descending colon and rectum undergo zygosis and these organs become retroperitoneal (covered by peritoneum anteriorly).^{Neet}

- A persistent part of mesentery forms the mesentery of small intestine and mesocolon of transverse and sigmoid colon and mesoappendix for appendix.

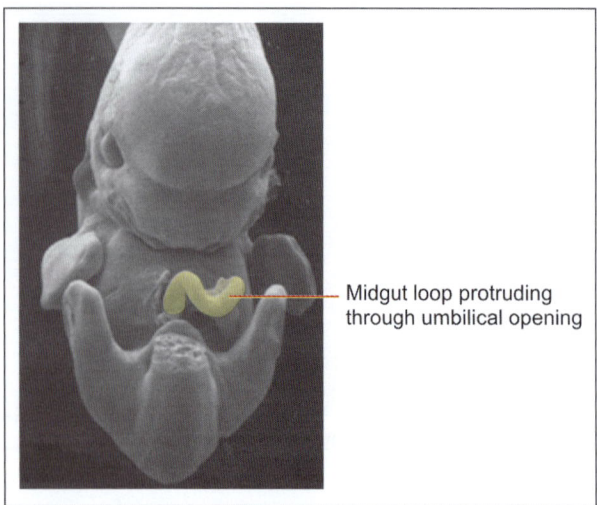

Scanning electron micrograph 14.2: Physiological hernia. Midgut elongates rapidly and during sixth week of development, it extends beyond body wall in umbilical cord (physiological umbilical herniation). [Species: Mouse, approximate human age: 40 days, ventral view]

Congenital Anomalies of Midgut

1. *Umbilical faecal fistula (vitelline fistula)*: It is caused by patent vitellointestinal duct. It involves communication of the small intestine with exterior and results in discharge of faecal matter (Fig. 14.10).
2. Meckel's diverticulum: Box 14.3 (Fig. 14.10).
3. *Enterocystoma (Vitelline cyst)*: It is the cyst of the vitellointestinal duct that occurs due to small persistent middle part of the duct (Fig. 14.10). Persistent vitellointestinal duct → Meckel's diverticulum, vitelline cyst (enterocystoma), umbilical fistula and umbilical (vitelline) sinus.^{Neet}
4. *Raspberry tumour* at umbilicus: Persistent distal part of the vitellointestinal duct (at the umbilicus) produces raspberry red tumour.

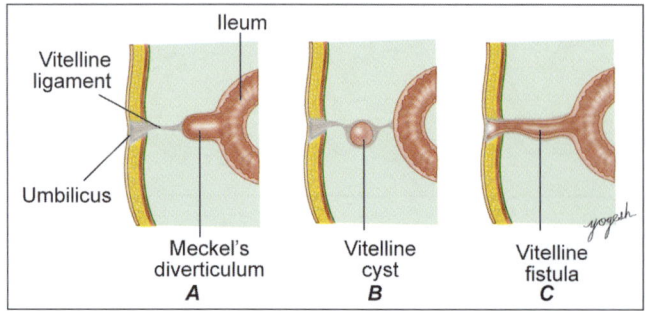

Fig. 14.10: Remnants of the vitellointestinal (vitelline) duct: (A) Meckel's diverticulum.; (B) Vitelline cyst; (C) Vitelline fistula that connects the lumen of the ileum with the umbilicus. Persistent part of vitelline duct may be present as vitelline ligament (omphalomesenteric ligament)

Box 14.3: Meckel's diverticulum (diverticulum ilei)^{High yielding, Neet}

Q. Write short note on Meckel's diverticulum.
- Meckel's diverticulum was first explained by GF Hildanus in the sixteenth century and later named after Johann Friedrich Meckel in 1809.
- Meckel's diverticulum is **true** congenital diverticulum of the *small intestine* as it consists of **all layers** of GIT.^{Neet} Meckel's diverticulum is the commonest congenital anomaly of intestine.^{MCQ}
- It is the persistent proximal part of *vitellointestinal duct* that is present in embryo (Fig. 14.10).
- Usually, vitellointestinal duct disappears during the 6th week of intrauterine life.
- Persistent part of vitelline duct may form vitelline cyst or vitelline fistula.

Features
- It occurs in 2% subjects.
- Male: female ratio is 2:1.
- The most common age at clinical presentation is 2 years.
- Length of the diverticulum is 2 inches (5 cm).^{Neet}
- Situation: About 2 feet or 60 cm proximal to ileocaecal valve.
- It shows 2 types of common ectopic tissues (gastric and pancreatic).
- Attachment: It is attached to the anti-mesenteric border of ileum.
- Its calibre is equal to that of ileum.
- The apex of diverticulum: Apex may be free or may be attached to umbilicus, to mesentery, or to any other abdominal structure by a fibrous band.

Clinical Anatomy
- Meckel's diverticulum may cause intestinal obstruction.
- It may have small regions of gastric mucosa.
- Acute inflammation of diverticulum (diverticulitis) may produce symptoms that resemble those of appendicitis.

Treatment
- Cases with complications can be treated with *surgical resection*, preferably laparoscopic resection.

5. *Exomphalos* or *omphalocele*: Usually physiological and reduces by 12th week of IUL. After birth, persistent gut loops at the closed umbilicus produces rounded mass called exomphalos.^{Neet}
6. *Congenital umbilical hernia*: It is the protrusion of the coils of intestine at umbilicus. The content is covered

by skin, connective tissue and peritoneum. Congenital umbilical hernia can be reduced by pushing back coils of intestine through umbilical opening, whereas it reappears on coughing or crying. It gets reduced, within 2–3 years on its own and if not reduced then can be treated surgically.

7. *Gastroschisis*: It is a congenital defect of the **anterior abdominal wall** through which the abdominal content protrudes outside. It occurs due to the **failure of complete lateral folding** of the embryo. Gastroschisis occurs in 1 in 10,000 births.[Neet]

8. *Errors of rotation*: Rotation of gut may fail partially or completely, even there may be reverse rotation. All these defects result in the change of usual positions of abdominal viscera. Suspensory ligament of duodenum (ligament of Treitz) is a key element for diagnosis of rotational anomalies of gut; usually it is on the left of body of first or second lumbar vertebrae.[Neet] Left-sided colon occurs if the midgut loop has not rotated at all.[Neet] Mixed rotation may result in the caecum lying inferior to the pylorus.[Neet] Nonrotation results in left-sided large intestine, right-sided small intestine, reversed rotation of duodenum (it lies anterior to transverse colon), transverse colon lies posterior to superior mesenteric artery.[Neet]

9. *Apple-peel atresia (Christmas tree intestinal atresia or type IIIb atresia)*: These are atresia of small intestine and accounts for 10% of all intestine atresias. In the apple-peel atresia, duodenum or proximal jejunum ends in a blind pouch and distal small intestine wraps around its vascular supply resembling an apple peel (spiral).[MCQ]

Box 14.4: Malrotation[Neet]

- It is a congenital anomaly of rotation of the gut that commonly causes intestinal obstruction.
- Ladd's band is present in malrotation. It is a fibrous stalk of peritoneal tissue that attach caecum to retroperitoneum in right lower abdominal quadrant.

Classical presentation

- Sudden onset of billious vomiting in newborn or
- Recurrent abdominal pain with billious vomiting in child due to obstruction.

Diagnosis

- S-shaped duodenum on barium follow through
- Abnormal position of ligament of Treitz
- Management: Ladd's pressure: It includes dissection of Ladd's band, broadening of mesentery base to reduce incidence of volvulus and appendectomy.

DEVELOPMENT OF CAECUM AND APPENDIX

- Caecum and appendix develop from a *caecal bud* that arises as dilatation of post-arterial segment of the midgut loop (Fig. 14.11).
- Caecal bud appears in the 6th week of intrauterine life.[MCQ]
- Proximal part of caecal bud dilates to form *caecum*, whereas distal part persists as narrow tube that forms a *vermiform appendix*.
- Caecal bud grows rapidly and forms two saccule one on either side. The right saccule grows faster than the left saccule, hence, attachment of appendix shift towards left (near iliocaecal junction).

DEVELOPMENT OF HINDGUT

- Hindgut gives rise to the following structures:
  1. Left one-third of the transverse colon
  2. Descending colon
  3. Sigmoid colon
  4. Rectum
  5. Upper part of the anal canal

Development of Urorectal Septum

- Distal part of hindgut that communicates with allantois is *cloaca*.
- Cloaca is divided into ventral broad *primitive urogenital sinus* and dorsal narrow *primitive rectum* by growing *urorectal septum* (Fig. 14.12).[Neet]
- Urorectal septum also divides the *cloacal membrane* into anterior *urogenital membrane* and posterior *anal membrane*. Cloacal membrane ruptures by seventh week.[Neet] Anal membrane lies at the proximal part of proctodeum.[Neet]
- Urogenital sinus forms urinary bladder and urethra, whereas primitive rectum forms rectum and upper part of the anal canal.
- Urorectal septum shows
  - *Tourneux fold* as vertical element that grows caudally between rectum and urogenital sinus.
  - *Folds of Rathke* project inwards from the lateral wall of cloaca.

DEVELOPMENT OF ANAL CANAL

Q. Write short note on development of anal canal.

Summary (Examination Guide)

- Anal canal is derived from two sources:
  1. *Endodermal cloaca* (distal part of primitive rectum) forms upper part of anal canal above the pectinate line.

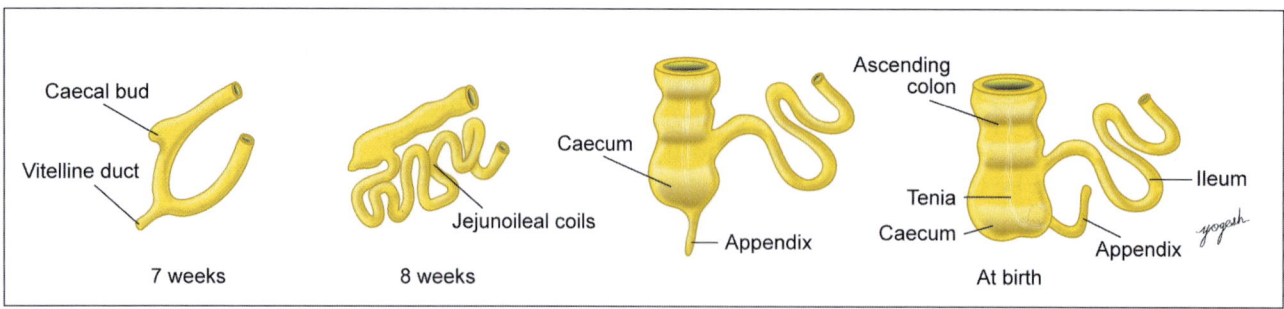

Fig. 14.11: Development of caecum and appendix

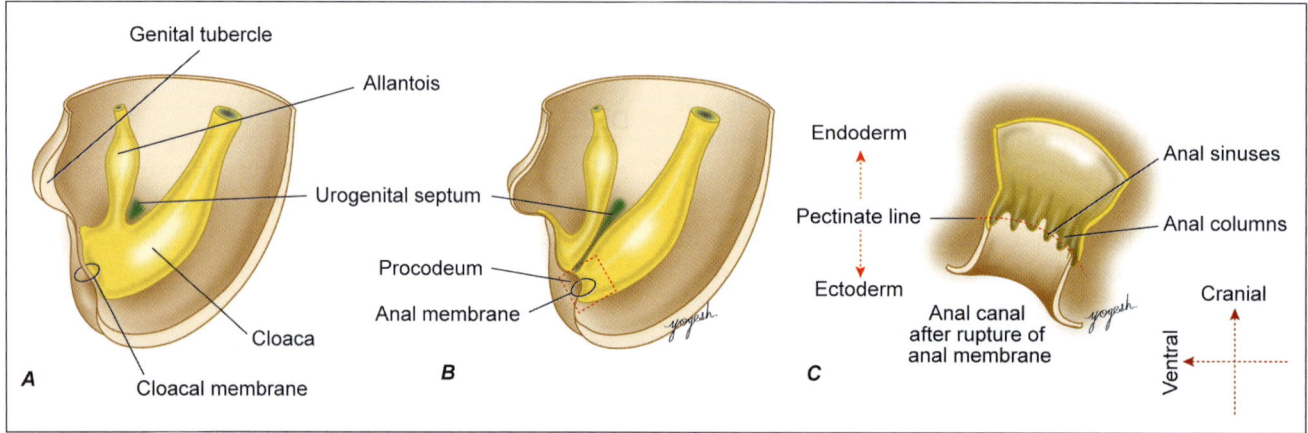

Fig. 14.12: Development of the anal canal. Urogenital septum divides cloaca into ventral primitive urogenital sinus and dorsal primitive rectum (A, B) and cloacal membrane into urogenital membrane and anal membrane. Surface ectoderm and lower part of primitive rectum (endoderm) forms the anal canal (C)

2. *Ectodermal anal pit* (proctodeum) forms lower part of anal canal below the pectinate line.
- Refer to Table 14.1 and Fig. 14.12.

Table 14.1	Development of anal canal	
	Above pectinate line (upper part of anal canal)	*Below pectinate line (lower part of anal canal)*
Origin	Endoderm	Ectoderm
Develops from	Endodermal cloaca (primitive rectum)	Proctodeum or anal pit
Arterial supply	Superior rectal artery	Inferior rectal artery
Venous drainage	Portal vein via superior rectal vein	Systemic vein (inferior vena cava) via inferior rectal vein
Nerve supply	Autonomic nerves	Somatic nerves

Stages of Development

- Proctodeum (anal pit) is a depression of the surface ectoderm. In the bottom of proctodeum, anal membrane and urogenital membranes are present (Fig. 14.12).
- The *anal membrane* perforates at 9 weeks and hindgut communicates with exterior. (In later life, anal membrane is represented by anal valves or pectinate line.)[Neet]
- Location of the anal membrane is represented by pectinate line of anal canal. Thus, part of anal canal above pectinate line is derived from endodermal cloaca, whereas part below pectinate line is derived from ectodermal proctodeum.[MCQ]
- Hence, the blood supply, lymphatic drainage and nerve supply above and below pectinate line are different (Table 14.1).

Congenital Anomalies

1. *Hirschsprung's disease* (congenital megacolon)[Neet]
    – It is a congenital anomaly of the large intestine.
    – It shows a dilated segment of a colon due to congenital absence of parasympathetic ganglia in the wall of gut (myenteric and submucous plexuses).

Alimentary Tract III: Development of Intestine

- It occurs due to failure of migration of neural crest cells before reaching anus.^{Neet}
- A segment without parasympathetic supply (aganglionated) shows constriction due to unopposed activity of sympathetic nerves and proximal part of colon to such constricted segment shows dilatation due to accumulated food.
- Incidence: 1 in 5,000 newborns.
- Treatment: Surgical resection of constricted segment.

2. **Imperforate anus**
   - The distal part of gut does not communicate with exterior.
   - Causes of imperforate anus
     a. Failure of rupture of anal membrane.
     b. Failure of development of ectodermal proctodeum.
     c. Failure of rectal development (rectal atresia).

3. **Ectopic anus**
   - Posterior growth of perineal body divides the cloacal membrane into ventral urogenital and dorsal anal membrane.
   - Failure or abnormality in this division may result into ectopic anal opening at the following sites:
     a. In female: Within vestibule.
     b. In male: At the base of scrotum, in intrabulbar fossa of spongy urethra.

4. **Rectal fistula**
   - A fistula is abnormal communicating tunnel between two organs.
   - Rectal fistulas are of the following types:
     a. Recto-vesical fistula (high fistula): Rectum communicates with urinary bladder.
     b. Recto-urethral fistula (low fistula): Rectum communicates with urethra.
     c. Recto-vaginal fistula (low fistula): Rectum communicates with vagina.

Box 14.5: Meconium

Q. Write short note on meconium.

- Meconium is the earliest *stool* of newborn.
- Meconium consists of material that is ingested by foetus during intrauterine life such as lanugo (very thin, soft foetal hairs), mucous, amniotic fluid, bile, intestinal epithelial cells and water.
- Meconium is viscous, sticky, dark olive green and odourless. Meconium (in Greek) means poppy (due to its appearance).
- *Meconium stained liquor*: If the foetus defecates before birth, the meconium stains amniotic fluid. This condition is *meconium stained liquor*.
- Aspiration of meconium by foetus result in *meconium aspiration syndrome*.
- In Hirschsprung's disease and cystic fibrosis, the newborn does not pass meconium.^{MCQ}
- *Meconium ileus*: Thickened and congested meconium in intestine is *meconium ileum*. It is first sign of the cystic fibrosis.^{MCQ}

DERIVATIVES OF GUT

- Derivatives of the gut are listed in Table 14.2.

Q. Enumerate derivatives of foregut, midgut and hindgut.

Table 14.2	Derivatives of the gut
Part of gut	Derivatives
Foregut	• Part of floor of mouth • Tongue • Pharynx • Oesophagus • Stomach • Proximal part of the duodenum up to major duodenal papilla • Pharyngeal pouches and their derivatives • Liver with intrahepatic biliary apparatus • Pancreas • Gallbladder with extrahepatic biliary apparatus • Respiratory system
Midgut	• Part of the duodenum distal to major duodenal papilla • Jejunum • Ileum • Caecum • Appendix • Ascending colon • Right two-thirds of transverse colon
Hindgut	• Left one-third of the transverse colon • Descending colon • Sigmoid colon • Rectum • Upper part of anal canal • Mucosal lining of urinary bladder and urethra

Human Embryology

CLINICAL EMBRYOLOGY

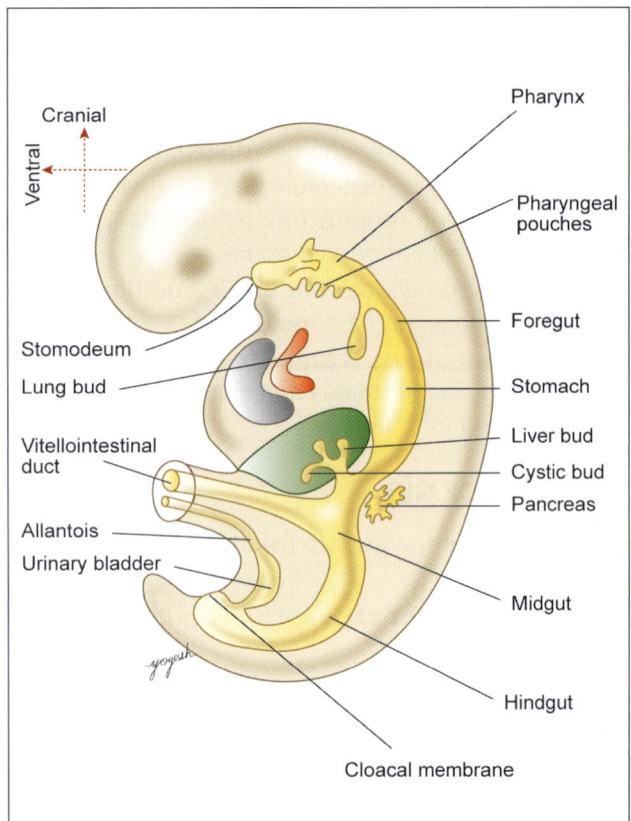

Fig. 14.13: Sagittal section of the embryo showing the derivatives of the endoderm. For understanding, other structures such as neural tube, dorsal aorta are not shown

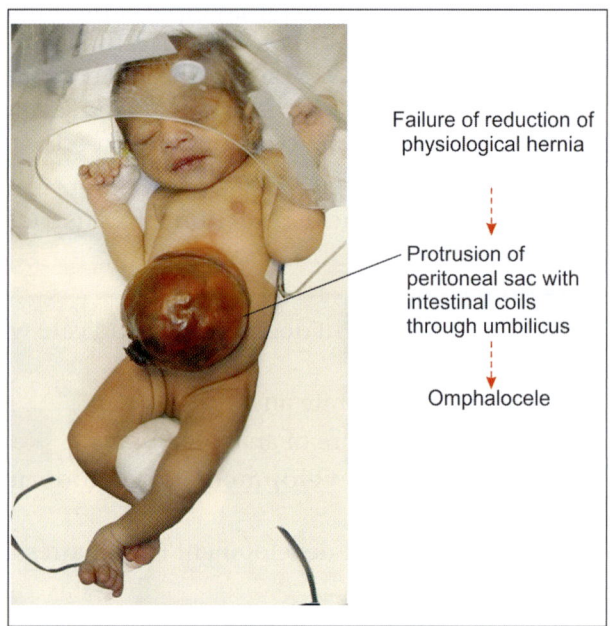

Clinical image 14.1: Omphalocele. It is a rare abdominal wall defect in that intestine (occasionally liver and other organs) remains outside of the abdomen in a sac because of failure of normal return of intestines and other contents back to abdominal cavity during around ninth week of intrauterine life. The sac is formed from an outpouching of peritoneum, protrudes in the midline, through the umbilicus (Image courtesy: *Dr Adhisivam B*)

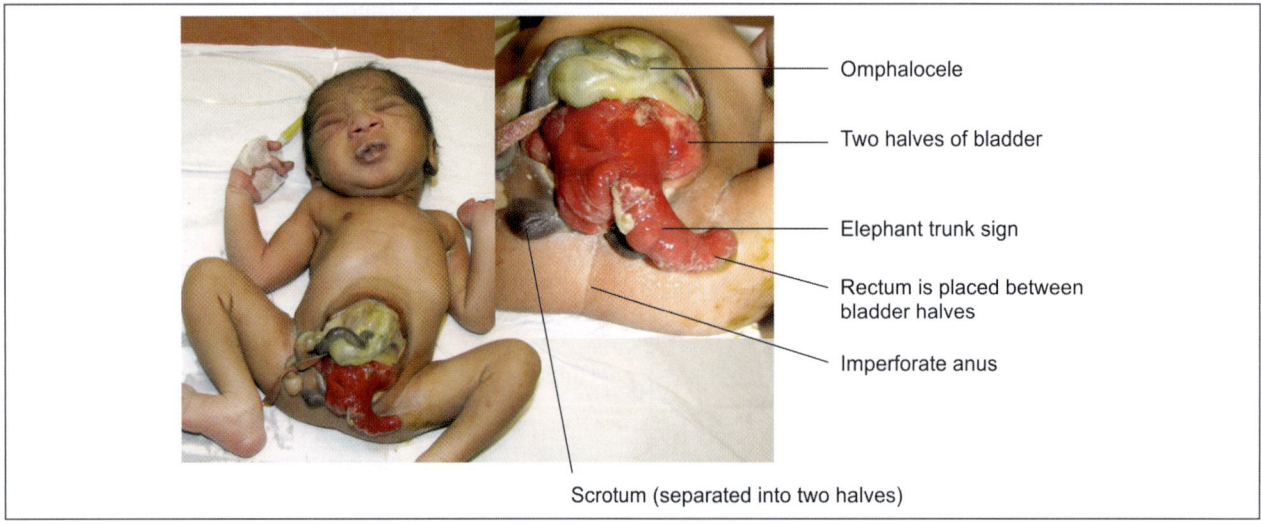

Clinical Image 14.2: Cloacal exstrophy. The case shows 'elephant trunk sign' representing the intussuscepted ileum. It is a rare condition having incidence of 1 in 200,000 pregnancies and 1 in 400,000 live births. It shows omphalocele (large intestine lies outside of the body), exstrophy of the bladder (bladder is open and separated into two halves) and rectum is placed between the bladder halves on the surface of the abdomen, imperforate anus (anus has not been formed or perforated) (Image courtesy: *Dr Kumaravel S*)

Alimentary Tract III: Development of Intestine

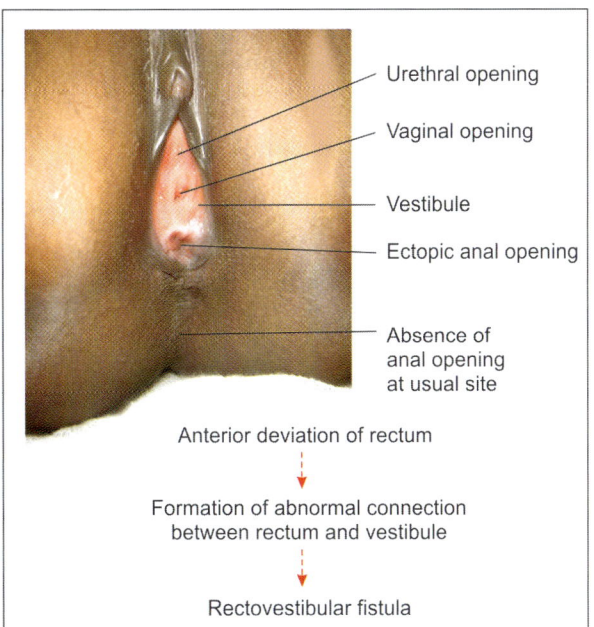

Clinical image 14.3: Rectovestibular fistula is an abnormal connection (fistula) between the rectum and vestibule of the female genitalia. It is the most common anorectal malformation in female patients. In the present case, vestibule has urethral, vaginal and rectal opening. There is no separate anal opening (in other cases, small anal opening may be present) (Image courtesy: *Dr Kumaravel S*)

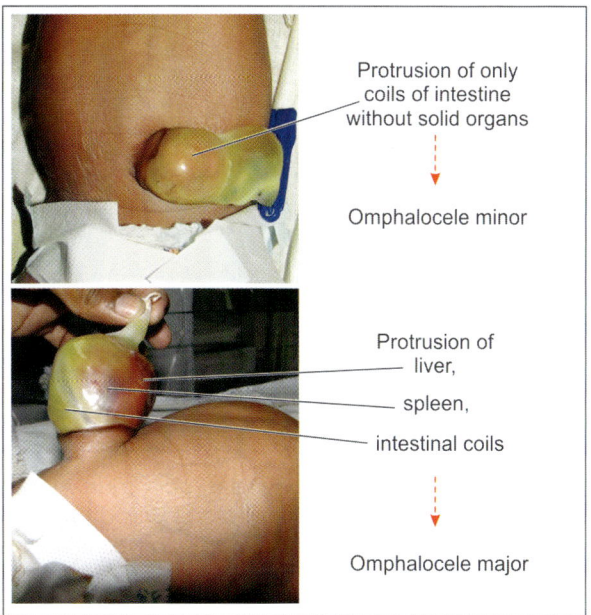

Clinical image 14.4: Omphalocele minor and major. Omphalocele is an abdominal wall defect in that abdominal contents are present in the cord outside the abdominal cavity. Omphalocele can be classified as *omphalocele minor* (only a few loops of gut in the sac) and *omphalocele major* (contain most of abdominal organs, including liver) (Image courtesy: *Dr Kumaravel S*)

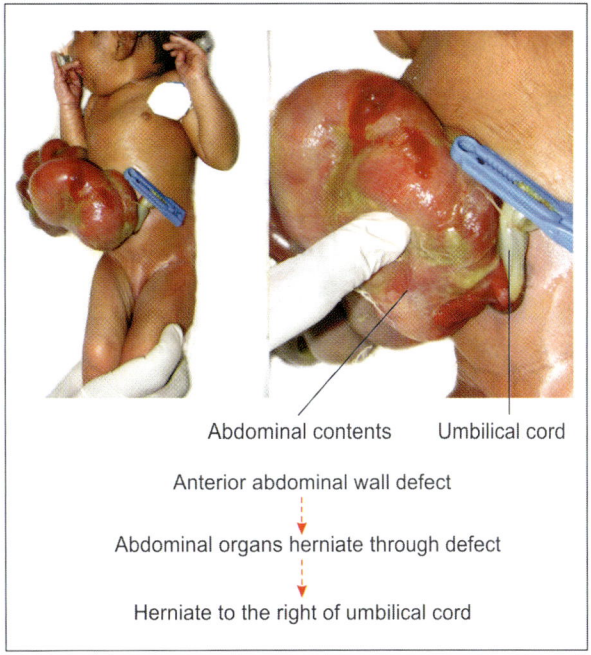

Clinical image 14.5: Gastroschisis. It is the condition of defective anterior abdominal wall. Through the defect coils of intestine and other abdominal viscera protrude outside. It differs from omphalocele in that there is the absence of parietal sac covering the contents and it lies on the right side of umbilical cord (in omphalocele, cord attaches to the herniated peritoneal sac) (Image courtesy: *Dr Kumaravel S*)

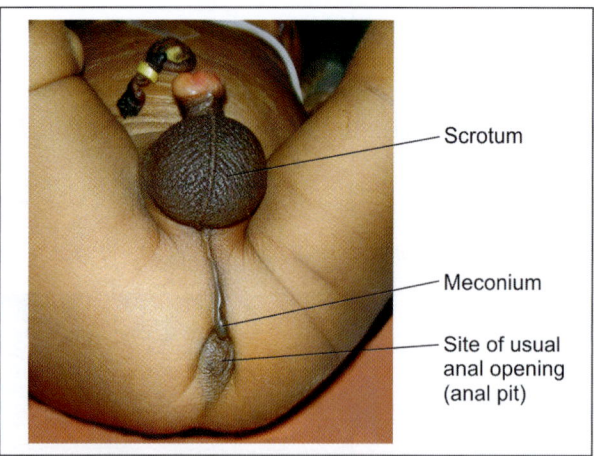

Clinical image 14.6: Male anorectal malformation. Anorectal malformation is a disorder in which anal canal does not open at its usual site. Anorectal malformations are classified based on location of the rectum in relation to the puborectalis sling into two types: High imperforate anus (rectum ends above the puborectalis sling) and low imperforate anus (rectum traverses the puborectalis sling). In high type, there is no external opening. In low type, there is a small opening covered by a layer of skin or other type of membrane through which meconium passes. The anorectal malformations also include *rectoperineal fistula* (slightly anterior, small anus), rectourethral fistula (rectum opening into urethra rather than its usual anal opening), rectovesical fistula (rectum opens into the urinary bladder), rectal/anal agenesis (no communication between genitourinary tract and rectum and no external anal opening), rectovaginal, rectouterine and rectovestibular fistula (rectum opens in vagina, uterus and vestibule respectively). Confirmation of anorectal fistula needs micturating cystourethrogram (radiograph) (Image courtesy: *Dr Kumaravel S*)

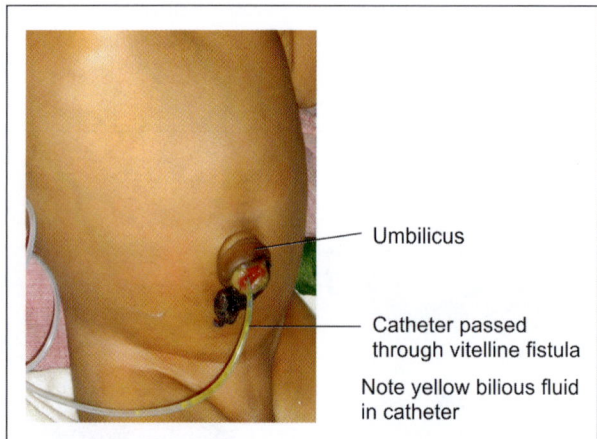

Clinical image 14.7: Patent vitellointestinal duct. The vitellointestinal duct connects midgut loop to the umbilical vesicle. Usually, vitellointestinal duct obliterates during 5th–6th weeks of IUL. Persistent vitellointestinal duct produces vitelline fistula causing discharge of yellow bilious fluid from the umbilicus (Image courtesy: *Dr Kumaravel S*)

15

Alimentary Tract IV
Development of Liver, Gallbladder, Pancreas and Spleen

Chapter Outline

- Development of liver
  - Stages of development
  - Molecular regulation of liver induction
  - Congenital anomalies of liver
- Histogenesis of liver
- Development of gallbladder and extrahepatic biliary apparatus
  - Stages of development
  - Anomalies of gallbladder
  - Anomalies of extrahepatic biliary ducts
- Development of pancreas
  - Stages of development of pancreas
  - Molecular regulation of pancreas development
  - Anomalies of pancreas
- Annular pancreas
- Development of spleen
  - Stages of development
  - Anomalies of spleen

INTRODUCTION

- Gastrointestinal tract develops to form foregut, midgut and hindgut.
- The liver, gallbladder, pancreas and spleen develop in relation to the foregut and midgut.
- This chapter includes development of liver, gallbladder, pancreas and spleen.

DEVELOPMENT OF LIVER

Q. Write short note of development of liver.

Summary (Examination Guide) (Table 15.1)

- Liver develops from the following sources:
  1. Endodermal bud forms the hepatocytes and intrahepatic biliary apparatus.
  2. Septum transversum (mesoderm) forms connective tissue of liver including fibrous capsule, Kupffer's cells and blood vessels.
  3. Vitelline and umbilical veins form sinusoids.

Table 15.1	Development of liver
Part of liver	Embryonic source
Lobes of liver – Liver parenchyma – Bile canaliculi – Bile ductules	Endoderm: Hepatic bud arising from the second part of the duodenum (that develops from foregut)
Connective tissue – Glisson's capsule – Connective tissue stroma – Kupffer's cells – Blood vessels	Mesoderm: Septum transversum
Liver sinusoids	Vitelline and umbilical veins
Ligaments of liver – Falciform ligament – Lesser omentum – Coronary ligaments – Triangular ligaments	Ventral mesogastrium
Ligamentum teres hepatis	Left umbilical vein
Ligamentum venosum	Ductus venosus

  4. Ventral mesentery forms lesser omentum, falciform, coronary and triangular ligaments.*Neet*

Stages of Development (Figs 15.1 and 15.2, Practice Fig. 15.1, Flowchart 15.1)

1. *Formation of hepatic bud*: During the 3rd week of IUL, *hepatic bud* arises from ventral border of terminal part of the foregut (developing second part of duodenum).
2. *Growth of hepatic bud*: The hepatic bud grows ventrally and cranially in the *ventral mesogastrium* and reaches the *septum transversum*.
3. *Division of hepatic bud*: The hepatic bud divides into cranial *pars hepatica* and smaller caudal *pars cystica* (forms gallbladder). The pars hepatica divides into *right* and *left hepatic ducts*. Each hepatic duct form solid cord of cells (interlacing columns) called *hepatic trabeculae*.
4. *Formation of hepatic sinusoids*: The hepatic trabeculae soon separate from each other to form *hepatic sinusoids*. The vitelline and umbilical veins that are passing through the septum transversum, breakup and establish a communication with the hepatic sinusoids.
5. *Formation of bile canaliculi*: The hepatic ducts branch to form intrahepatic biliary passages.
6. *Formation of peritoneal ligaments and liver capsule*: The mesenchyme of septum transversum form blood vessels, Kupffer's cells, haematopoietic cells and capsule of the liver.
7. Developing liver divides the *mesogastrium* into a *falciform ligament* and *lesser omentum*. Reflections of peritoneal covering (part of ventral mesogastrium) from liver to diaphragm form *triangular* and *coronary ligaments*.

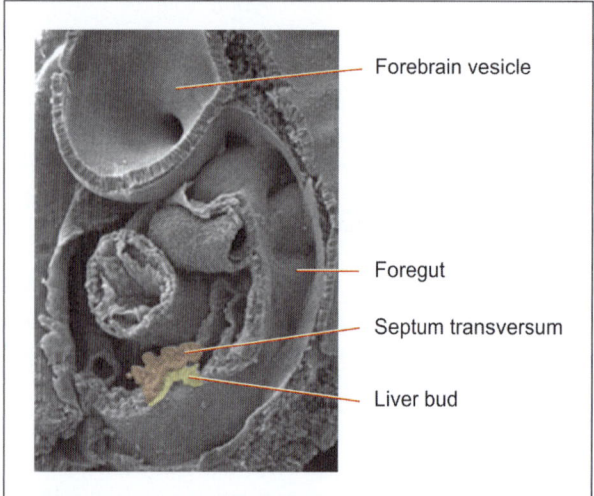

Scanning electron micrograph 15.1: SEM showing a midsagittal cut that illustrates endoderm-lined foregut and a diverticulum (liver bud) extending ventrally into tissue of the septum transversum. [Species: Mouse, approximate human age: 27 days, sagittal section]

Some Interesting Facts

- During early development, both the lobes (right and left) are of equal size.
- In 10th week, weight of liver is approximately 10% of the total body weight, whereas at birth it is 5% of the total body weight. By third month of IUL, the liver contributes one-tenth of the total body weight. By seventh month, it contributes one-fifth of the body weight.
- From the sixth week of IUL till birth, the liver also functions for haematopoiesis.^{MCQ}
- Liver starts bile secretion by 12th week of IUL.^{MCQ}

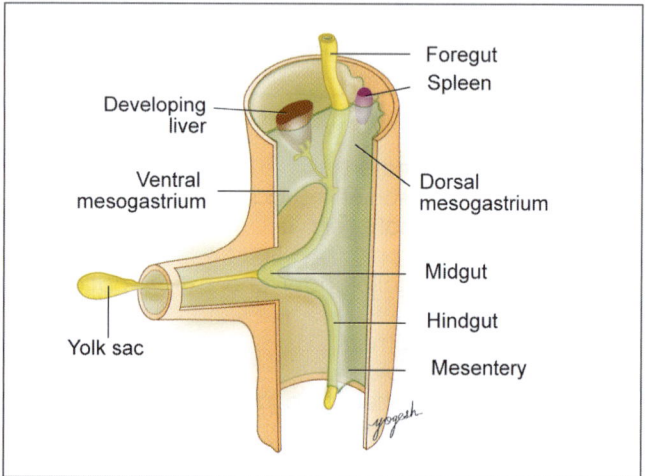

Fig. 15.1: Development of the liver and gall bladder. The liver develops in ventral mesogastrium with the contribution of the right and left hepatic buds (endoderm) and septum transversum (mesoderm). The gall bladder develops from cystic bud (endoderm)

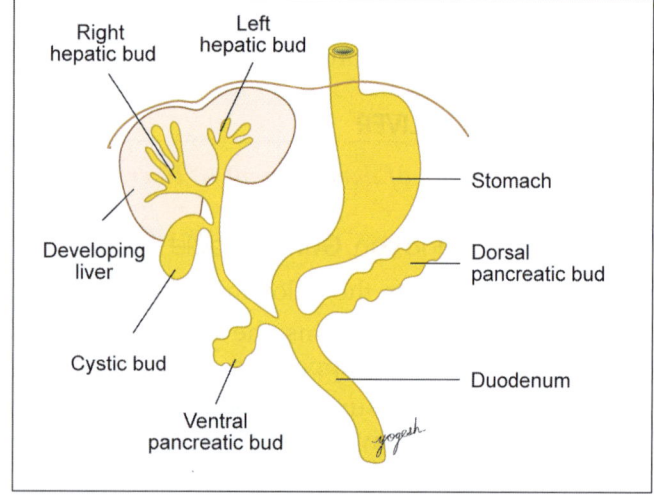

Practice Fig. 15.1: Development of liver and gall bladder

Alimentary Tract IV: Development of Liver, Gallbladder, Pancreas and Spleen

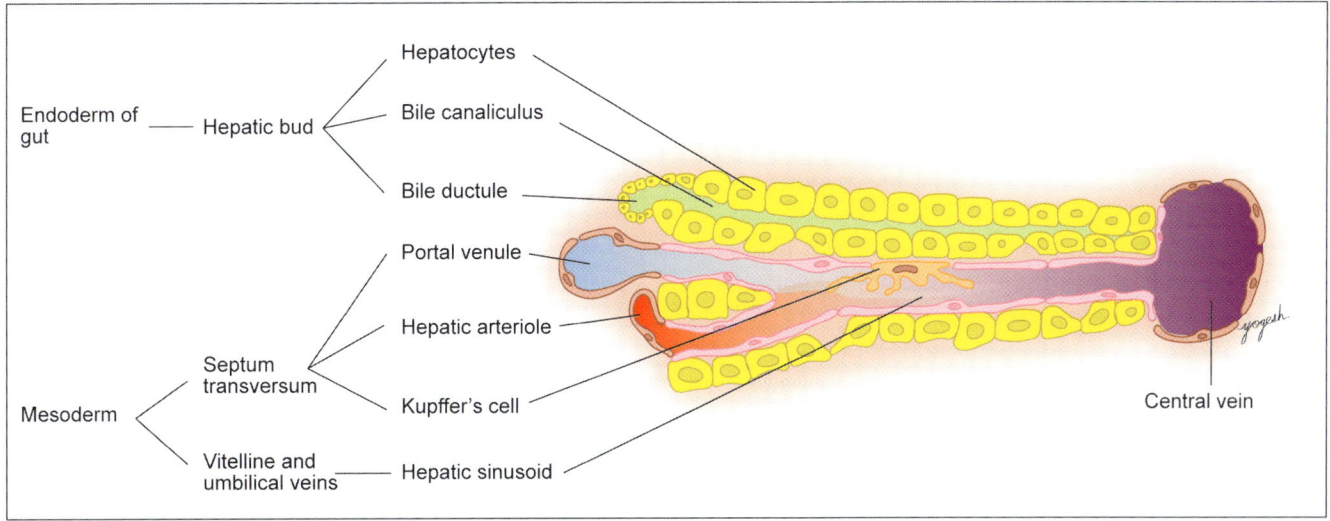

Fig. 15.2: Development of various components of liver

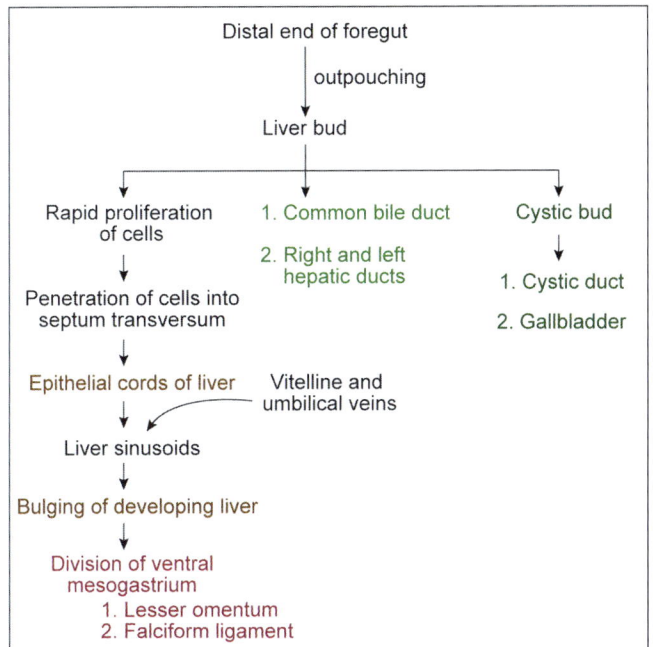

Flowchart 15.1: Development of liver

Molecular Regulation of Liver Induction

- The cardiac mesoderm secretes fibroblast growth factor 2 (FGF2) that induces expression of the liver-specific genes in gut tissue and form hepatic bud.
- Bone morphogenic proteins (BMPs) enhances action of FGF2 on the gut.
- Hepatocyte nuclear transcription factors (HNF3 and 4) controls differentiation of cells into hepatocytes and biliary cells.

Congenital Anomalies of Liver

1. *Riedel's lobe*: It is a downward tongue-like extension of the right lobe of the liver. Often, it is mistaken for abnormal abdominal mass and lead to surgery.

2. *Polycystic liver disease* (PLD): It is a rare condition that results due to failure of union of intra-hepatic biliary canaliculi and ductules with extra-hepatic bile ducts. It results in formation of cysts within the liver. PLD is frequently associated with polycystic kidney disease and cystic pancreas.^{MCQ} These are transmitted as autosomal dominant disorder.

3. *Intra-hepatic biliary atresia*: A failure of development of intra-hepatic biliary system (atresia) is a serious condition that can be treated only with liver transplantation.

4. *Caroli's disease*: It involves congenital cystic dilatation (extasia) of intra-hepatic biliary tree.^{MCQ}

5. *Congenital hepatic fibrosis* is the inherited fibrocystic liver disease. Hepatic fibrosis produces portal hypertension.

6. One lobe or part of a lobe of liver may be absent. An extra lobe may be present. Complete liver may be rudimentary. Ectopic liver tissue may be present in the lesser omentum or falciform ligament.

Box 15.1: Histogenesis of liver

- Hepatic bud is derived from endoderm of the gut.
- From this bud, solid extensions grow into mesentery and form trabeculae that break up vitelline and umbilical veins into smaller channels.
- Trabeculae latter anastomose freely with one another. Lumen begin to appear in the trabeculae at about the fourth week.
- The hepatic trabeculae later form cords of liver cells. Lumen appears in the cord to form bile capillary.

Contd.

Contd.

- Trabeculae are broken up into hepatic cords by the ingrowth of branches from the sinusoids.
- Initially, in primary hepatic lobules, the trabeculae are not arranged radially and there are several central veins in each lobule.
- Branches of the portal vein invade the primary lobules and divide them into several secondary lobules and simultaneously hepatocyte cords become arranged radially around the central veins in a characteristic manner.
- Hepatic artery grows in the liver secondarily and its branches follow the course of branches of the portal vein.

DEVELOPMENT OF GALLBLADDER AND EXTRA-HEPATIC BILIARY APPARATUS

Q. Write short note on development of gallbladder.
Q. Write short note on development of extrahepatic biliary apparatus.

Summary (Examination Guide)
- Refer to Table 15.2.

Stages of Development (Fig. 15.2, Practice Fig. 15.2)
- Extrahepatic biliary apparatus is endodermal in origin.
- Gallbladder develops from *cystic bud* that arises from the *hepatic bud*. Originally hepatic bud arises from terminal part of the foregut (later it forms second part of duodenum).
- The hepatic bud grows ventrally and cranially in the ventral mesogastrium. The hepatic bud divides into pars cystica (cystic bud) and pars hepatica (hepatic bud). The pars hepatica divides into right and left hepatic ducts.
- Cystic bud enlarges to form gallbladder and cystic duct.
- Common hepatic ducts and cystic duct join to form common bile duct.
- Differential growth of duodenal wall turns opening of the common bile duct from ventral aspects to dorsomedial aspects of duodenum along with ventral pancreatic bud.

Table 15.2	Development of extrahepatic biliary apparatus
Part	Embryological source
Gallbladder	Cystic bud
Cystic duct	Cystic bud
Right and left hepatic ducts	Primitive hepatic ducts
Common bile duct	Proximal part of hepatic bud

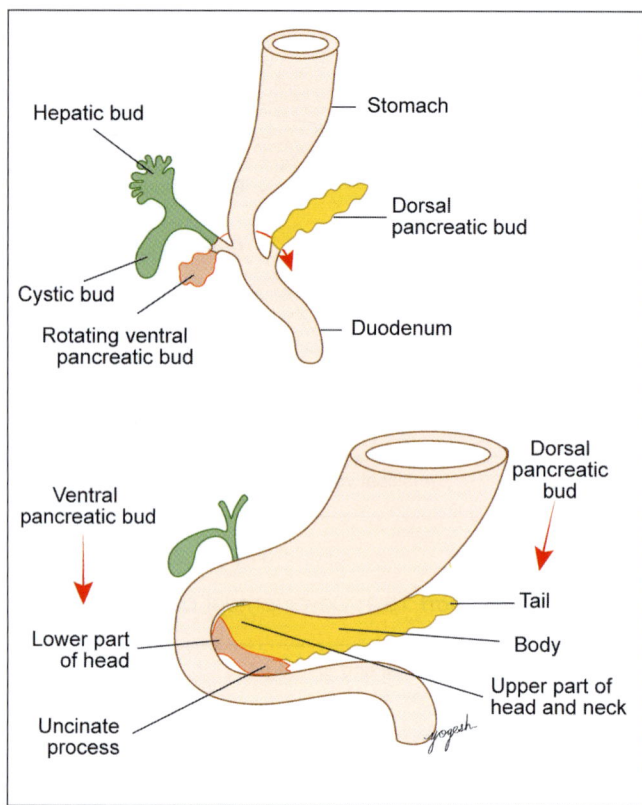

Practice Fig. 15.2: Development of pancreas

Anomalies of Gallbladder (Fig. 15.3)

1. *Agenesis of gallbladder* is an absence of gallbladder
2. *Sessile gallbladder* is an absence of cystic duct results in direct fusion of gallbladder with common bile duct.
3. *Phrygian cap*: It is a gallbladder with fundus folded on itself to form cap-like structure.
4. *Hartmann's pouch: It is an outpouching of neck* of the gallbladder.
5. *Septate gallbladder*: Lumen of the gallbladder is divided into several segments with partial septae.
6. *Double gallbladder*: In double gallbladder, two gallbladders are present that are connected with the cystic duct.
7. *Intra-hepatic gallbladder*: In this case, the gallbladder is embedded in the substance of liver.
8. *Floating gallbladder*: This gallbladder is lined by peritoneum on both surfaces and is free from liver.

Anomalies of Extrahepatic Biliary Ducts

1. *Atresia of ducts*: Ducts of extrahepatic biliary apparatus such as bile duct, common hepatic duct, hepatic ducts may be partially or completely absent.
2. *Accessory ducts*: Small accessory bile duct connecting liver with the gallbladder may be present.

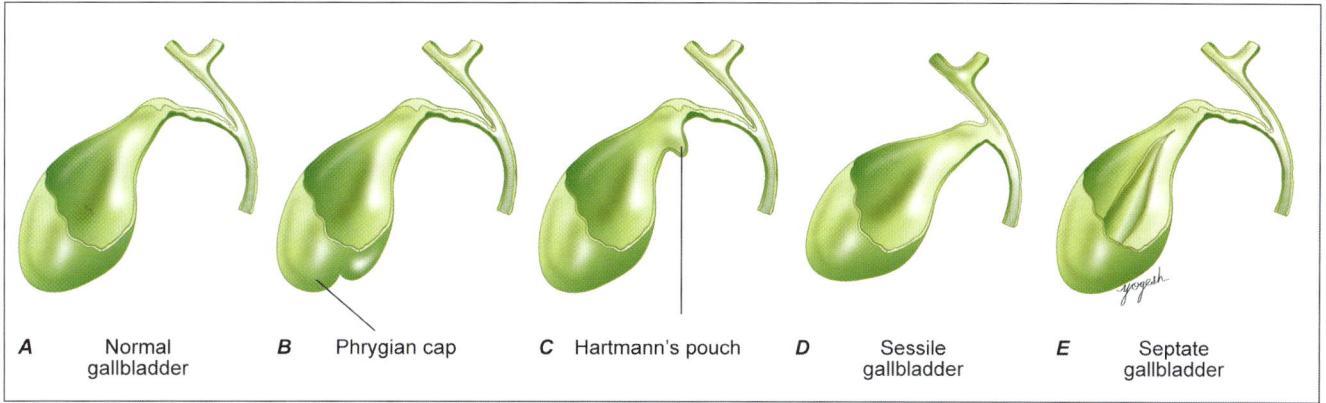

Fig. 15.3: Developmental anomalies of gallbladder

A. Normal gallbladder
B. Phrygian cap
C. Hartmann's pouch
D. Sessile gallbladder
E. Septate gallbladder

DEVELOPMENT OF PANCREAS

Q. Write short note on development of pancreas.

Summary (Examination Guide) (Table 15.3)

- Pancreas develops from endodermal ventral and dorsal pancreatic buds that arise from caudal part of the foregut (junctional zone of foregut and midgut).
- Proliferation of these endodermal buds form ducts, parenchyma (acini) and islets of Langerhans.
- Adjacent splanchnopleuric mesoderm condenses to form capsule, blood vessels and other connective tissue of pancreas.

Stages of Development of Pancreas (Figs 15.4 to 15.6, Flowchart 15.2, Practice Fig. 15.2)

1. *Formation of pancreatic bud*
   - By 3rd week, *ventral* and *dorsal pancreatic buds* arise from ventral and dorsal wall of terminal part of the foregut.[MCQ]

Table 15.3	Development of pancreas[High yielding, Neet]
Part	Embryological source
Lower part of head and uncinate process	Ventral pancreatic bud
Upper part of head and neck, body and tail	Dorsal pancreatic bud
Main pancreatic duct	Ventral pancreatic duct and distal part of dorsal pancreatic duct[Neet]
Accessory pancreatic duct	Proximal part of dorsal pancreatic duct[Neet]
Connective tissue	Mesoderm

Note: The pancreatic acini and islets of Langerhans are derived from endodermal pancreatic buds.[MCQ]
By 7th week, α-cells start secreting glucagon and by 10th week, β-cells start secreting insulin.[MCQ]

- Ventral pancreatic bud arises in combination of hepatic bud and they share a combined opening in the duodenum.
- Ventral pancreatic bud is larger and appears in the 4th week of IUL.
- Ventral pancreatic bud grows in ventral duodenal mesentery, whereas dorsal pancreatic bud grows in dorsal duodenal mesentery.

2. *Rotation of buds*
   - Differential growth wall of duodenum, and rotation of duodenum brings ventral pancreatic bud with common bile duct (arise from hepatic bud) to the right of duodenum and dorsal bud to the left of duodenum.
   - Continuous differential growth of duodenal wall brings the ventral pancreatic bud closer and proximal to the dorsal bud.
   - Finally, both the buds fuse with each other in 7th week of IUL.

3. *Formation of pancreatic ducts*
   - Ducts of dorsal and ventral pancreatic bud anastomose and derive the following ducts:
     a. *Main pancreatic duct*: It is formed by duct of ventral pancreatic bud and distal part of duct of dorsal pancreatic bud.
     b. *Accessory pancreatic duct*: It is formed by proximal part of duct of the dorsal pancreatic bud.

4. *Formation of acini and islet of Langerhans*:
   - Both ventral and dorsal pancreatic buds branch enormously.
   - At the end of each branch, pancreatic acini appear.
   - Some cells of pancreatic duct get separated and form islet of Langerhans by third week and start secretion of insulin by 10th week.[MCQ]

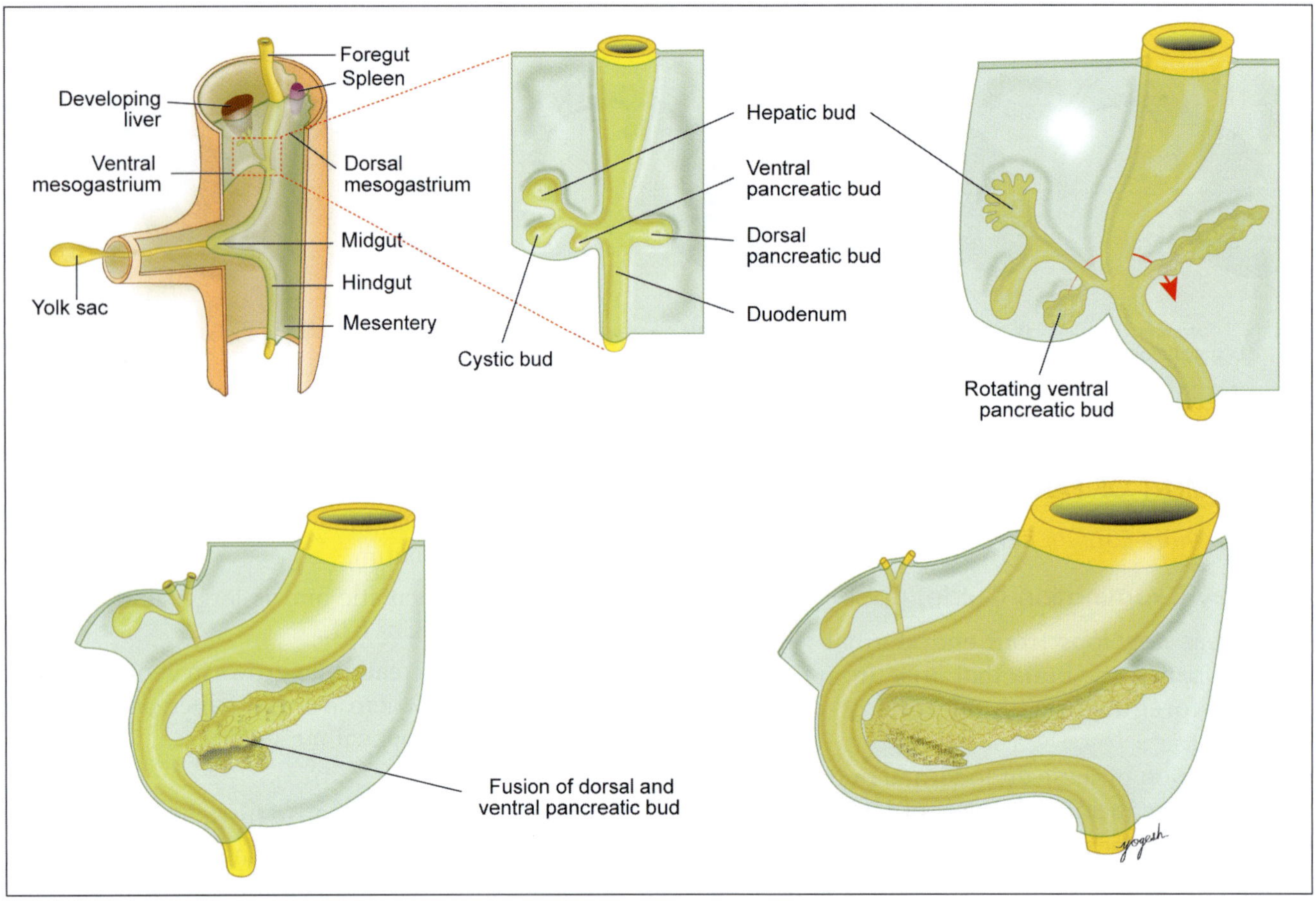

Fig. 15.4: Successive stages of development of pancreas. Pancreas develops by fusion of ventral and dorsal pancreatic bud

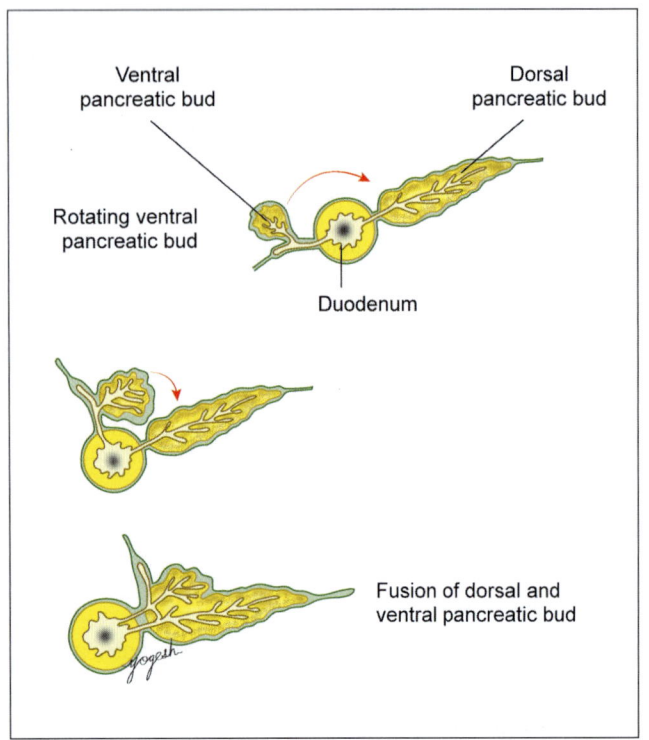

Fig. 15.5: Rotation of the ventral pancreatic bud during the development of the pancreas

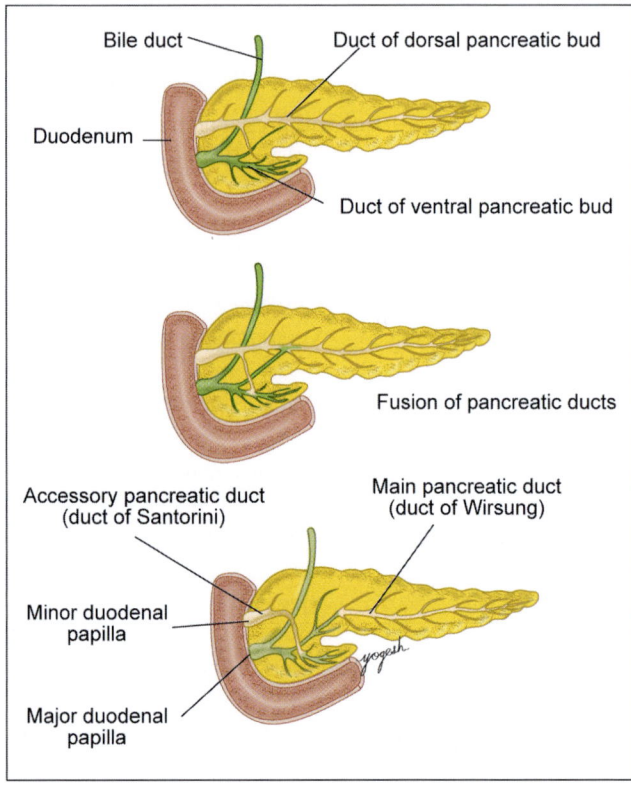

Fig. 15.6: Development of pancreatic duct system

Alimentary Tract IV: Development of Liver, Gallbladder, Pancreas and Spleen

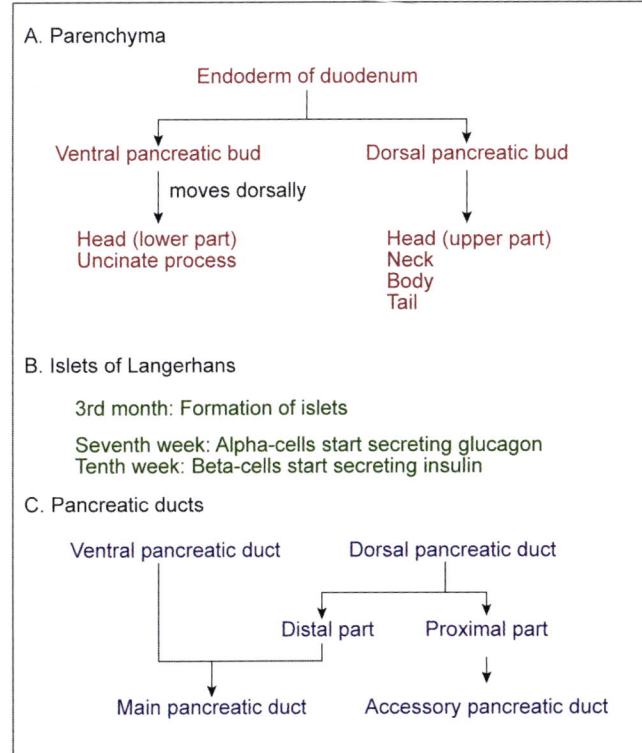

Flowchart 15.2: Development of pancreas

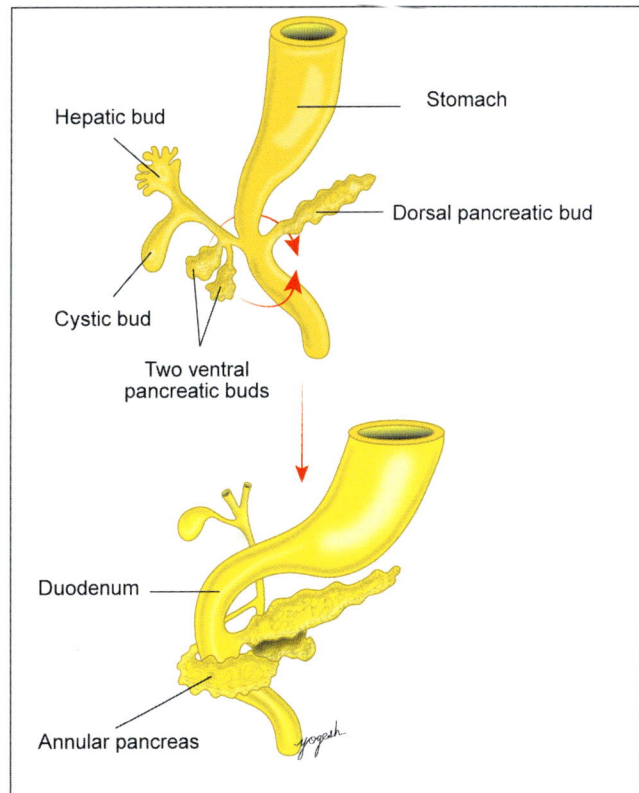

Box 15.2: Annular pancreas (Fig. 15.7)

Q. Write short note on annular pancreas.
- It is a congenital anomaly where second part of duodenum is surrounded by a ring of pancreatic tissue.
- Incidence: 1 in 12,000–15,000 newborns.
- Cause: Usually pancreas develops from ventral and dorsal pancreatic buds. Differential growth of duodenal wall and rotation of duodenum brings ventral and dorsal pancreatic bud together and they fuse. Failure of rotation of the ventral pancreatic bud may result in annular pancreas.
- Effect: Annular pancreas may cause duodenal obstruction. In intraembryonic life, it may result in polyhydramnios.
- Radiograph of abdomen shows *double bubble* appearance due to gas in stomach and proximal part of duodenum.
- Treatment: Surgical treatment to bypass the obstructed segment of duodenum by duodeno-jejunostomy is required.

5. Surrounding mesoderm form capsule, connective tissue, septae and blood vessels of the pancreas.
6. Along with duodenum, pancreas also becomes retroperitoneal except at its tail that lies in lienorenal ligament.

Molecular Regulation of Pancreas Development

- FGF2 and activin are produced by notochord and dorsal aorta upregulate pancreatic and duodenal homebox1 (PDX) genes.
- PDX6 expressing cells form *alpha cells* that secrete glucagon.
- PDX 4 and 6 expressing cells form *beta cells* that secrete insulin, *delta cells* that secrete somatostatin and *gamma cells* that secret pancreatic polypeptides.

Anomalies of Pancreas

1. Annular pancreas (Box 15.2).
2. *Divided pancreas (pancreatic divisum):* It occurs due to failure of fusion of dorsal and ventral pancreatic buds. Divided pancreas indicates failure of fusion of dorsal and ventral pancreatic buts. It is most common congenital anomaly of pancreas.[Neet]
3. *Accessory pancreatic tissue:* This ectopic pancreatic tissue that lies in the wall of duodenum, gallbladder, Meckel's diverticulum or stomach wall.[Neet]

Fig. 15.7: Formation of annular pancreas. There may be two ventral pancreatic buds that fuse with dorsal pancreatic bud surrounding duodenum to form annular pancreas

4. *Accessory pancreatic tissue*: This ectopic pancreatic tissue that lies in the wall of stomach, duodenum, gallbladder and Meckel's diverticulum.[Neet] Most common site of ectopic pancreatic tissue is stomach.[Neet]
5. *Inversion of pancreatic duct*: In this condition, the main pancreatic duct is formed by duct of dorsal pancreatic bud and opens at minor duodenal papilla, whereas duct of ventral pancreatic bud joins common bile duct and opens at the major duodenal papilla.

DEVELOPMENT OF SPLEEN

Q. Write short note on development of spleen.

- Spleen develops in the dorsal mesogastrium from mesoderm.[Neet]
- The dorsal mesogastrium is divided by developing spleen into ventral gastrosplenic ligament and dorsal lienorenal ligament.
- Mesoderm gives rise to capsule, septa, connective tissue network, reticular fibres, lymphocytes and haematopoietic cells.

Stages of Development (Fig. 15.8)

1. *Formation of splenculi*: During the 5th week of IUL, mesenchymal cells in dorsal mesogastrium form small mesenchymal masses called *splenculi* or *splenic lobules*.
2. *Fusion of spleniculi*: Spleniculi fuses to form a single splenic mass.
3. Lobulated development of spleen in an adult is indicated by splenic notches (usually lies along the superior border of spleen).[Neet]
4. *Formation of ligaments*: Developing spleen divides dorsal mesogastrium into *gastrosplenic* and *lienorenal ligaments*. Lienorenal (splenorenal) ligament contains splenic artery.[Neet]
5. *Change in splenic position*: The following factors bring the spleen to its usual position:
   - Rotation of stomach
   - Fusion of posterior layer of dorsal mesogastrium with posterior abdominal wall.

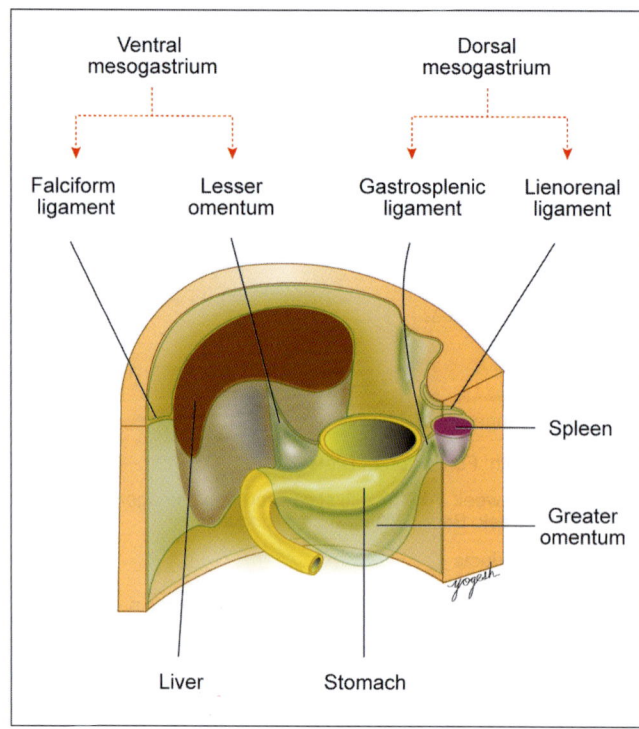

Fig. 15.8: Developing spleen in dorsal mesogastrium

6. Haematopoiesis: Spleen acts as haematopoietic organ in foetal life until birth.

Anomalies of Spleen

1. *Accessory spleen*: Failure of fusion of spleniculi with the main splenic tissue give rise to accessory spleen at the following sites:
   - Hilus of spleen
   - Gastrosplenic ligament
   - Lienorenal ligament
   - Tail of pancreas
   - Along the splenic artery
   - Left spermatic cord
2. *Lobulated spleen*: Incomplete fusion of spleneculi (persistent foetal spleen) produces lobulated spleen.
3. *Right-sided bilaterality or isomerism* is characterised by *asplenia* or *hypoplastic spleen*, whereas *left-sided bilaterality* is characterised by *polysplenia*.[Neet]

16
Respiratory System

Chapter Outline

- Introduction
  - Formation of lung bud
- Development of larynx
  - Stages of development
  - Anomalies of larynx
- Development of trachea
  - Anomalies of trachea
- Tracheoesophageal fistula
- Development of bronchi and lungs
  - Formation of pleural cavity and pleura
  - Formation of intrapulmonary bronchi
  - Parenchyma of lung
  - Maturation of lungs
  - Anomalies of lungs
- Hyaline membrane disease

INTRODUCTION

Formation of Lung Bud

- Respiratory system develops from
  - *Lung bud* that arises from foregut and
  - Connective tissue from *splanchnic mesoderm.*
- During 4th week, *laryngotracheal groove* appears caudal to the hypobranchial eminence in the floor of pharynx (Fig. 16.1, Flowchart 16.1).

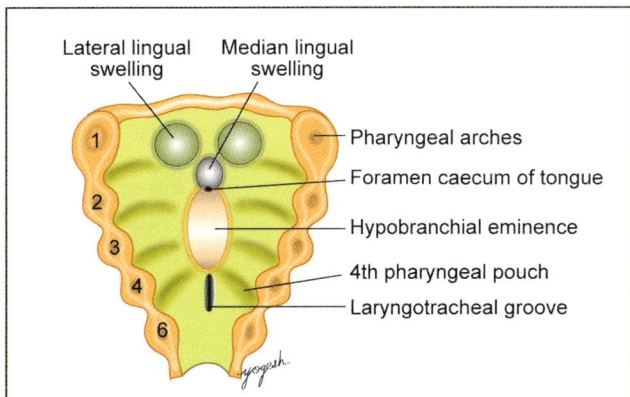

Fig. 16.1: A section of the pharynx of the embryo at 4th week. Laryngotracheal groove appears in the floor of the pharynx just caudal to the hypobranchial eminence

- The laryngotracheal groove deepens to form a *laryngotracheal tube (diverticulum)* that grows caudally.
- Laryngotracheal tube bifurcates to form **two (right and left) lung buds** (Fig. 16.2).
- Pharyngeal cells expressing **TBX4** factor forms lung buds.
- Fate of laryngotracheal tube and lung bud:
  - Proximal part of laryngotracheal tube forms *larynx*, whereas its distal part forms *trachea.*
  - Lung buds form primordium of *bronchial tree* and *lungs*.
  - Splanchnic mesoderm forms surrounding connective tissue.
- On either side of laryngotracheal tube (respiratory diverticulum), two *tracheoesophageal folds* arise.
- These folds fuse to form *tracheoesophageal septum* that separates laryngotracheal tube from the oesophagus.
- Cranial extension of tracheoesophageal septum is arrested by the inlet of larynx (*furcula of His*) through which the larynx communicates with pharynx.^{MCQ}
- Lung buds invaginate into *pericardio-peritoneal canals* that later form *pleural cavities*.

Flowchart 16.1: Development of respiratory system

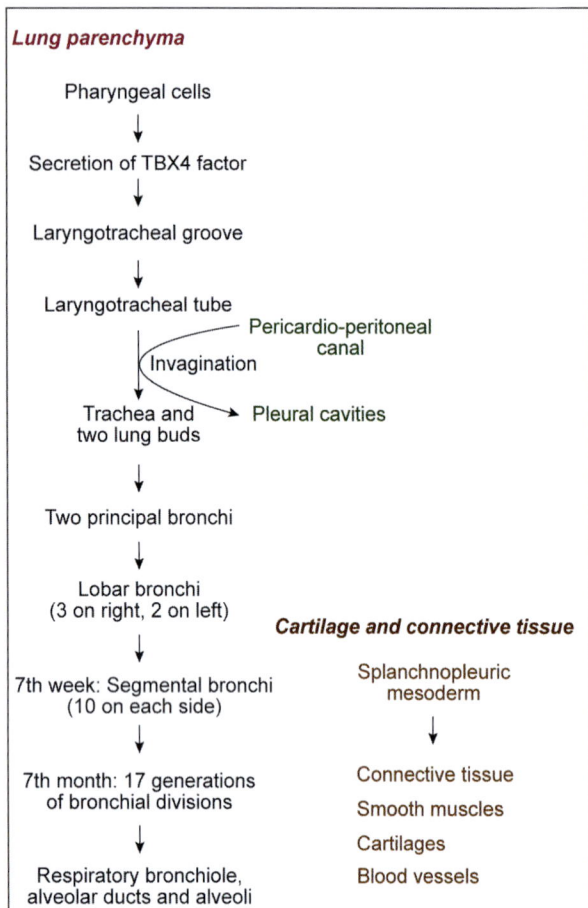

DEVELOPMENT OF LARYNX

Q. Write short note on development of larynx.

- The larynx is a voice box, a part of respiratory system that has a laryngeal inlet, vestibular and vocal folds, cartilages and muscles in the wall.

Summary (Examination Guide)

- Components of larynx are derived as follows (Table 16.1):
  1. *Lining epithelium* develops from endoderm of *laryngotracheal diverticulum.*

Table 16.1	Development of larynx
Part	Embryological source
Mucosa	Proximal part of laryngotracheal tube
Vestibular and vocal folds	Endodermal folds of laryngotracheal tube
Cartilages	All cartilages—fourth and sixth arch *except* epiglottis—hypobranchial eminence
Intrinsic muscles	All form sixth arch except cricothyroid from fourth arch.
Nerve supply	Motor All muscles by recurrent laryngeal nerve except cricothyroid by external laryngeal branch of superior laryngeal nerve Sensory Above vocal folds—internal laryngeal branch of superior laryngeal nerve Below vocal folds—recurrent laryngeal nerve

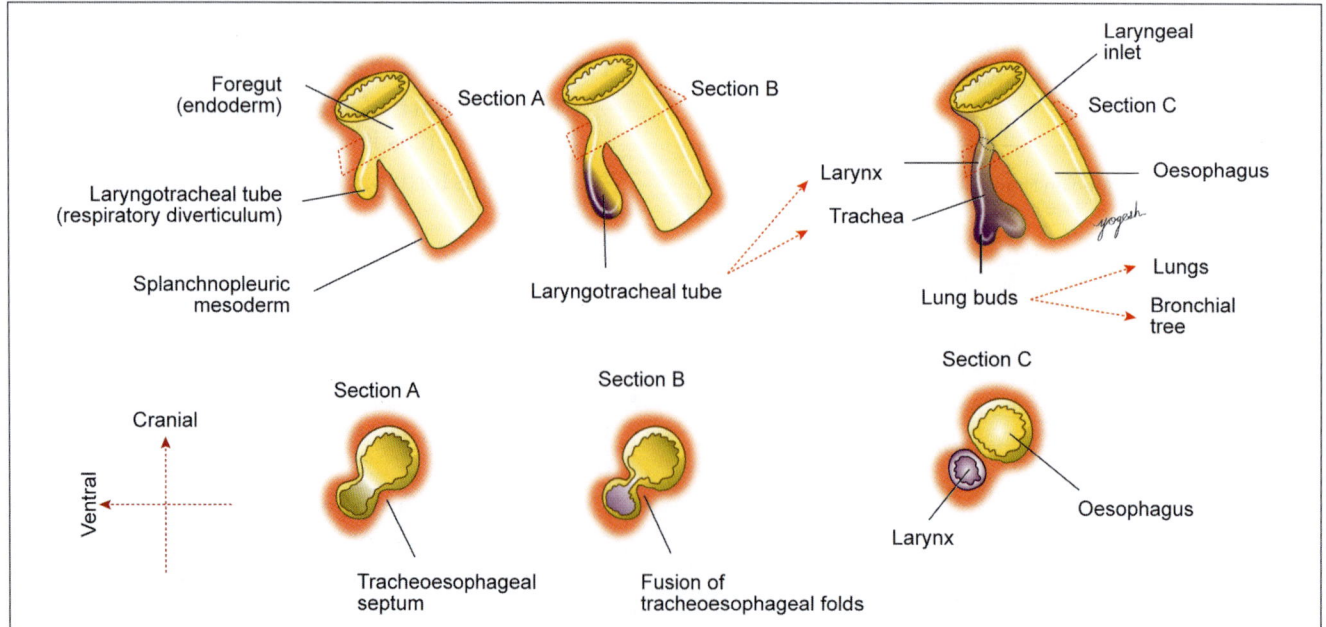

Fig. 16.2: Formation of tracheal bud and lung bud. Tracheoesophageal septum separates trachea from oesophagus

2. *Vestibular and vocal folds* develop from endodermal folds arising from a laryngotracheal diverticulum.
3. *Cartilages of larynx*: All the cartilages (thyroid, cricoid, cuneiform, corniculate, arytenoids) of larynx develop from the fourth and sixth arches, except epiglottis that develops from hypobranchial eminence.
4. *Muscles of larynx*: All muscles of larynx develop from fourth and sixth pharyngeal arches.
5. Nerve supply is derived from superior laryngeal nerve (fourth arch) and recurrent laryngeal nerve (sixth arch).

Stages of Development

- Larynx develops from cranial part of *laryngotracheal diverticulum* that arises from the floor of the pharynx.
- Communication between laryngotracheal diverticulum and pharynx forms the *inlet of larynx*.
- Due to differential growth of fourth and sixth arch, mesenchyme surrounding the larynx converts the laryngeal opening into a T-shaped orifice (Fig. 16.3).
- Endoderm of larynx proliferates to block the lumen. Later, the lumen gets recanalised.
- During luminal recanalisation, the endoderm form two pairs of folding, proximal vestibular and distal vocal pair of folds.
- *Vestibular fold* gives rise to false vocal cord and *vocal fold* to true vocal cord.
- The recess between vestibular fold and vocal fold forms *ventricle of larynx*.
- Mesenchyme of fourth and sixth arch forms all *cartilages of larynx* (thyroid, cricoid, arytenoids, corniculate and cuneiform) except epiglottis that derives from hypobranchial eminence.^{MCQ}

- All intrinsic muscles are derived from sixth arch except cricothyroid. Hence, all muscles of the larynx are supplied by recurrent laryngeal nerve except cricothyroid that is supplied by an external laryngeal branch of superior laryngeal nerve.^{MCQ}
- Vocal folds lie at the junction of fourth and sixth arches, hence mucosa above the vocal fold is innervated from an internal laryngeal branch of the vagus nerve (4th arch) and below the vocal fold is innervated by recurrent laryngeal nerve (6th arch).

Anomalies of Larynx

1. *Laryngocele*: It is congenital anomalous air sac in the neck communicating with the cavity of larynx.
2. *Congenital laryngeal atresia and stenosis*: It results from failure of the laryngeal recanalisation (atresia is blockage and stenosis means narrowing).
3. *Larygoptosis*: Larynx is localised in a lower position than its usual position, may be due to absence of some of laryngeal cartilages.
4. *Laryngeal web*: Lumen of larynx has membrane-like structure. It may result due to incomplete recanalisation of laryngeal lumen. It produces partial airway obstruction.

DEVELOPMENT OF TRACHEA

- Trachea develops from a part of *laryngotracheal tube* that lies between developing larynx and point of bifurcation of the tube (lung buds).

Summary (Examination Guide)

- Components of trachea develop as follows:
    1. Lining epithelium and glands develop from endoderm of *laryngotracheal tube*.

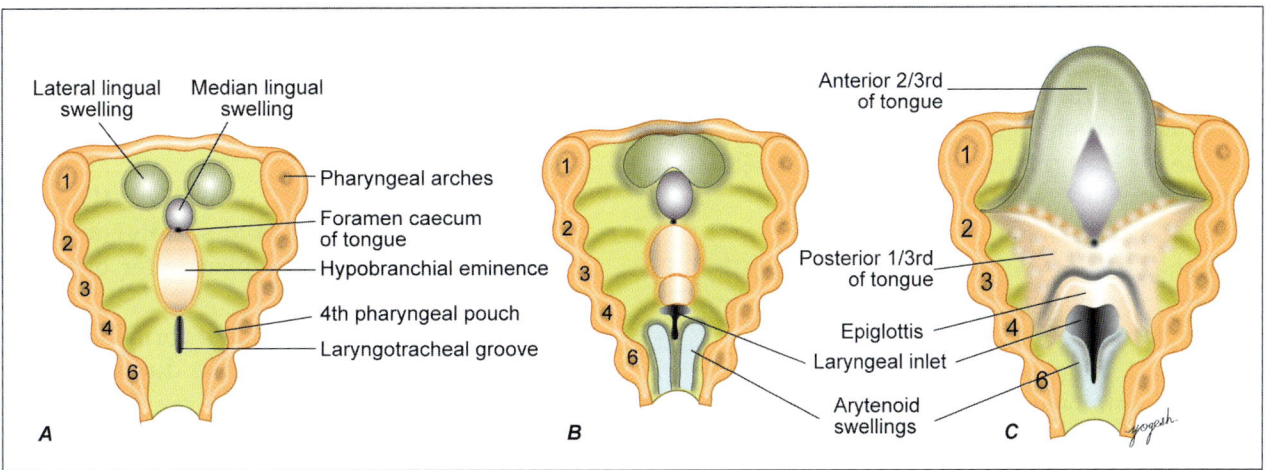

Fig. 16.3: (A) A section of pharynx of the embryo at 4th week. Slit-shaped laryngotracheal groove appears in the floor of pharynx just caudal to hypobranchial eminence; (B) 6 Weeks; and (C) 10 Weeks: On development of arytenoid swellings and epiglottis, laryngotracheal groove (later that forms inlet of the larynx) becomes T-shaped

2. Cartilages, connective tissue and trachealis muscle develop from *splanchnopleuric mesoderm* surrounding laryngotracheal tube.
- Trachea is separated from oesophagus by a *tracheoesophageal septum* that is derived from tracheoesophageal folds.

Anomalies of Trachea

1. *Agenesis of trachea*: Failure of formation of laryngotracheal tube results in agenesis of trachea.
2. *Tracheoesophageal fistula*: Box 16.1.
3. *Tracheal stenosis*: It occurs due to ventral deviation of the tracheoesophageal septum.
4. *Tracheal bronchus*: There may be a blind diverticulum (*tracheal bronchus*) arising from trachea.
5. *Tracheal lobe*: A separate bronchus may rise from trachea and supply an isolated lobe of lung called tracheal lobe.

DEVELOPMENT OF BRONCHI AND LUNGS

- During the 5th week of IUL, *laryngotracheal diverticulum* divides into right and left principal bronchus (initially *lung buds*).

Formation of Pleural Cavity and Pleura

- Lung buds grow in caudal and lateral direction and bulge into *pleuroperitoneal canals*.
- Soon small pleuroperitoneal canals get filled with the growing lungs. Later, the canals start enlarging to accommodate the growing lungs (Figs 16.5 to 16.7).
- Pleuropericardial and pleuroperitoneal folds separate the pleuroperitoneal canals from pericardial and peritoneal cavities respectively. Thus, isolated pleuroperitoneal canal forms pleural cavities (for details read Chapter 17).
- A layer of *splanchnopleuric mesoderm* in contact with lung bud form *visceral pleura* and *somatopleuric layer* form *parietal pleura* (Practice Fig. 16.1).

Formation of Intrapulmonary Bronchi

- *Left principal bronchus* divides into upper and lower secondary or lobar bronchi, whereas *right principal bronchus* divides into superior, middle and lower lobar bronchi (Fig. 16.7).
- Each *secondary bronchus* later supplies a lobe of lung that is separated by fissures.
- In the 7th week of IUL, the secondary bronchi divide to form *10 segmental bronchi*.
- Each segmental bronchus with surrounding splanchnopleuric mesoderm forms the *bronchopulmonary segments*.
- Up to the end of 7th month of IUL, about 17 generations of bronchial subdivisions occur. About 6–7 divisions take place after birth before formation of adult lung.^{MCQ}
- Distal bronchial subdivisions form bronchioles, respiratory bronchioles, alveolar ducts and alveoli.

Parenchyma of Lung

- Lining epithelium of bronchial tree and alveoli develop from *endoderm of respiratory diverticulum*.
- Cartilages, blood vessels and other connective tissue elements develop from *splanchnopleuric mesoderm*.

Box 16.1: Tracheoesophageal fistula (TEF or TOF)

Q. Write short note on tracheoesophageal fistula

- Definition: Tracheoesophageal fistula is an abnormal congenital communication between the trachea and oesophagus.
- Incidence: 1:3000–4500 births.
- Causes
  Right and left tracheoesophageal folds on fusion forms tracheoesophageal septum that separates the trachea from the oesophagus. Failure of fusion of tracheoesophageal septum results in TEF.
- Types (Fig. 16.4)
  TEF can be classified according to morphology and anatomical locations as follows:
  - *Type A*: It is not true TEF. Both proximal and distal oesophageal segments do not communicate with each other or with the trachea.
  - *Type B*: Proximal oesophageal segment communicates with lower tracheal segment and distal oesophageal segment form blind pouch.
  - *Type C*: Proximal oesophageal atresia (blind pouch) and distal oesophagus arise from the trachea.
  - *Type D*: Proximal and distal oesophageal segments communicates with the trachea.
  - *Type E*: Oesophagus communicates with the trachea without any atresia.
- Clinical presentation
- Oesophageal atresia and subsequent inability to swallow amniotic fluid results in *polyhydramnios* (excess accumulation of amniotic fluid).
- TEF present with coughing, vomiting, *cyanosis* in newborn with the onset of feeding (entry of milk in the lungs).
- Treatment: **Emergency surgical repair** is required to save the newborn. It involves surgical resection of fistula and anastomosis of proximal and distal oesophageal segments.

Respiratory System

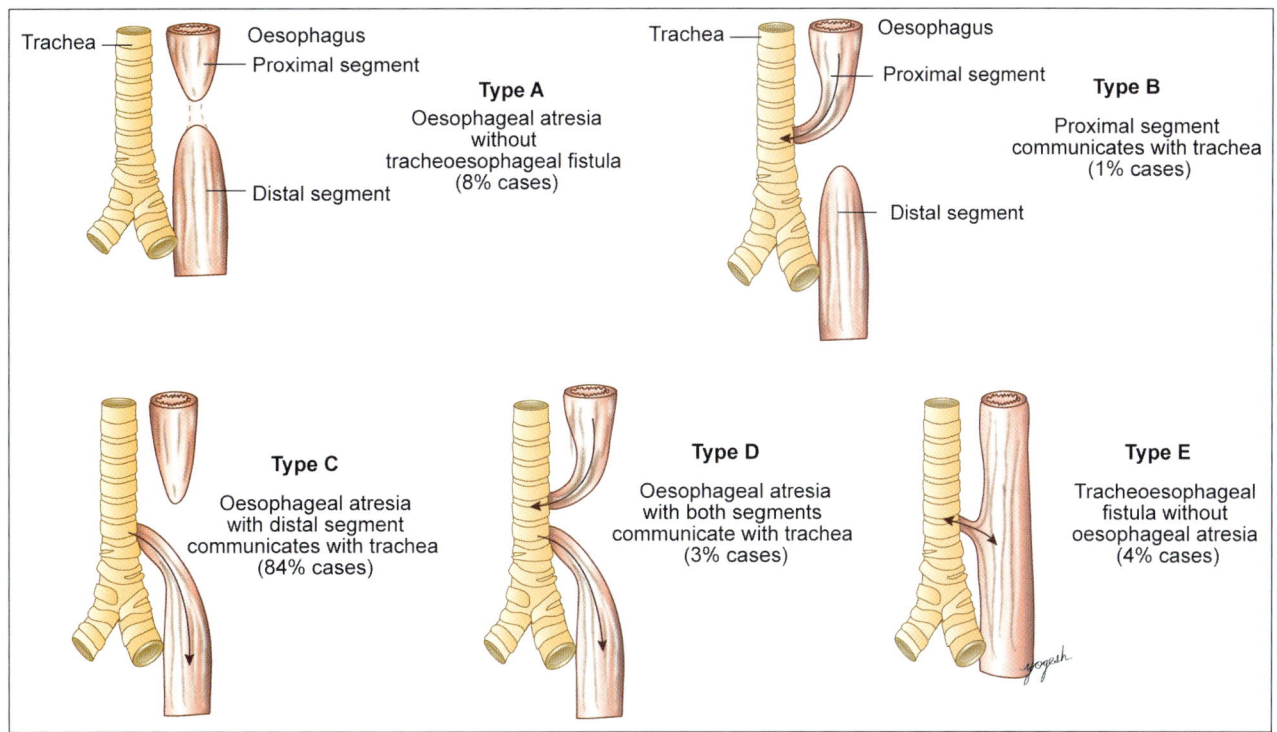

Fig. 16.4: Types of tracheoesophageal fistula

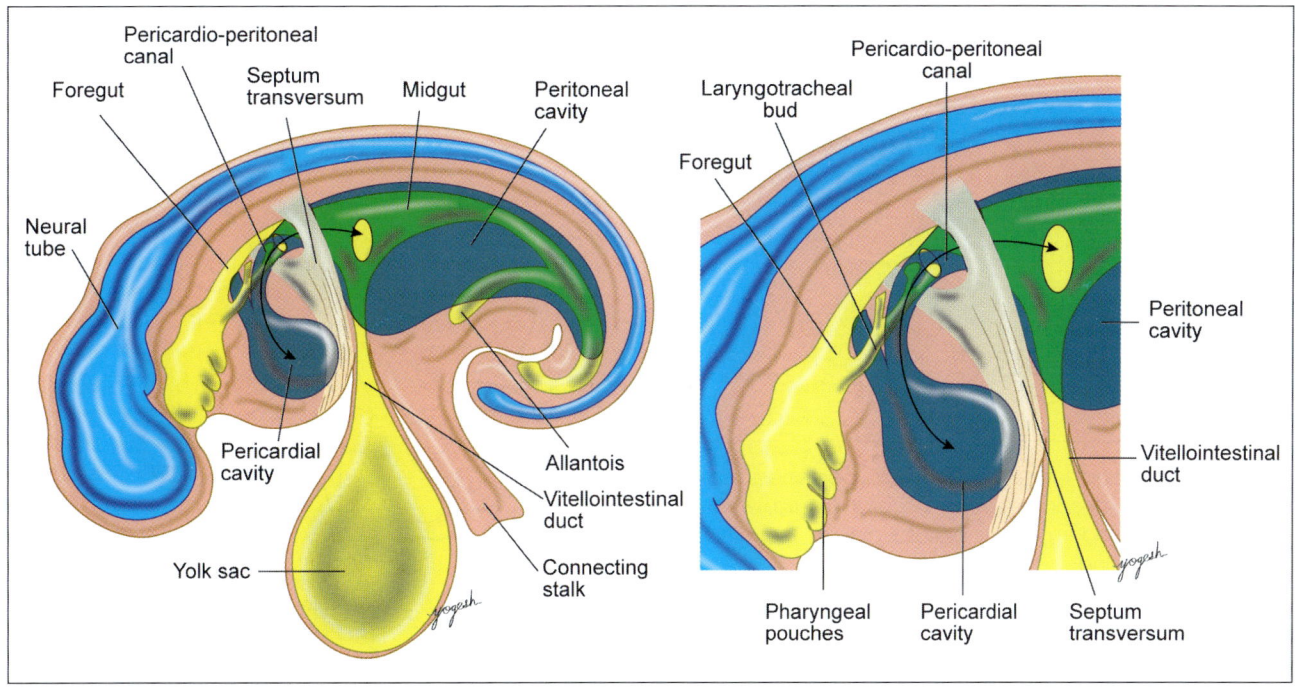

Fig. 16.5: Section of the embryo at 4th week. The laryngotracheal bud raises from the foregut and grows caudally. The laryngotracheal bud divides into two lung buds. Each one of the lung buds enter in the pericardio-peritoneal canal (shown by arrow) and enlarges to form lung. The pericardio-peritoneal canal communicates between the pericardial cavity cranially and peritoneal cavity caudally. Two pericardio-peritoneal canals run on either side of the foregut, behind the septum transversum

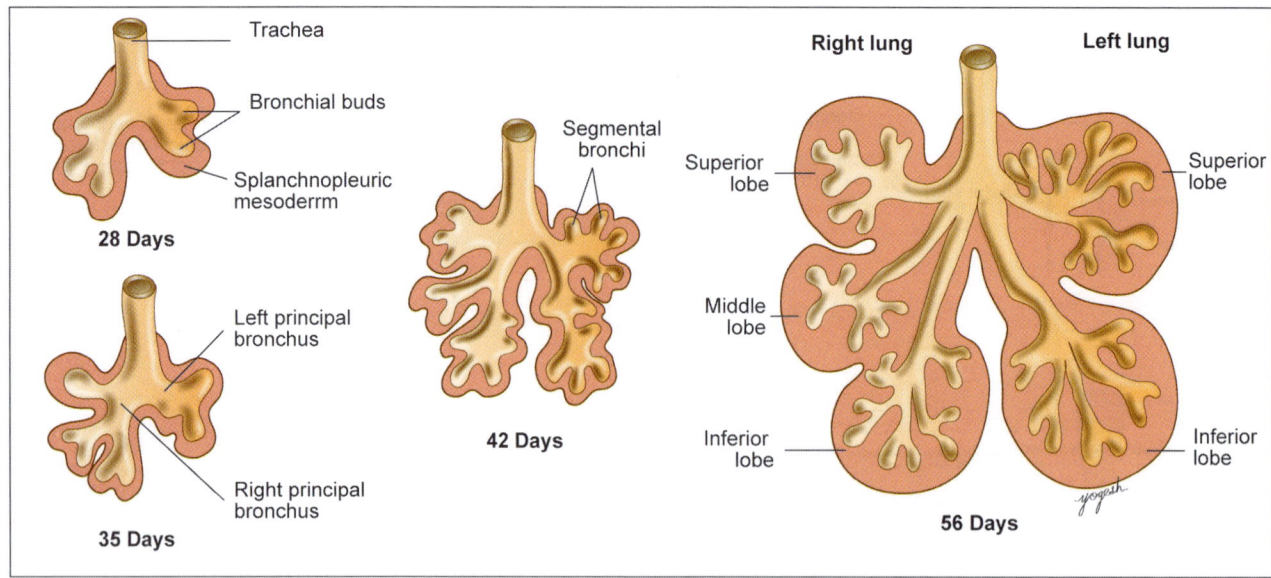

Fig. 16.6: Development of the lungs

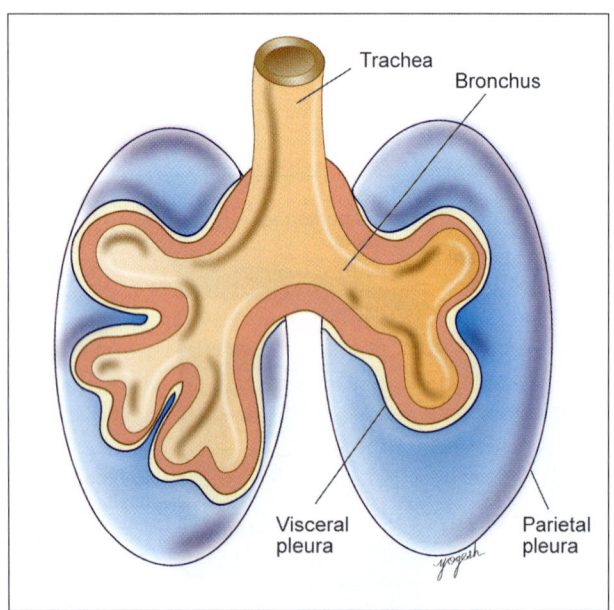

Fig. 16.7: Expanding lungs in pericardio-peritoneal canal. Splanchnopleuric mesoderm form visceral pleura, whereas somatopleuric mesoderm forms parietal pleura. The cavity of pleuroperitoneal canal forms pleural cavity

Some Interesting Facts

1. Foetal kidneys maintain amniotic fluid volume that helps in foetal lung development. Hence renal agenesis is associated with pulmonary hypoplasia (failure of lung development).
2. By the 7th month, pulmonary circulation becomes enough to provide adequate oxygen for sustaining the life. Hence, a newborn becomes viable at this age. *MCQ, Clinical fact*

3. TBX4 factor (T-box transcription factor) is a transcription factor that belongs to a T-box gene family that is involved in the regulation of embryonic developmental processes. This transcription factor is encoded by TBX4 gene located on human chromosome 17.

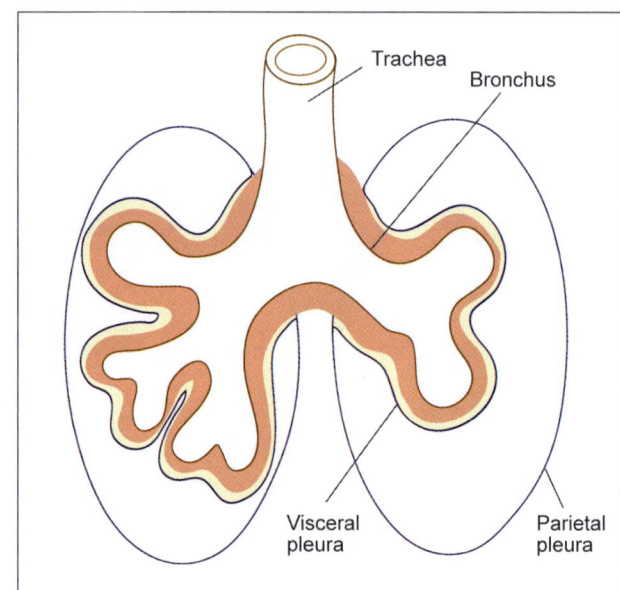

Practice Fig. 16.1: Formation of visceral pleura and parietal pleura

Maturation of Lungs

Q. Write short note on stages of maturation of lung.

- Maturation of lungs is divided into four phases or periods (Fig. 16.8, Practice Fig. 16.2)
  1. Pseudoglandular period (6–16 weeks)
  2. Canalicular period (16–26 weeks)

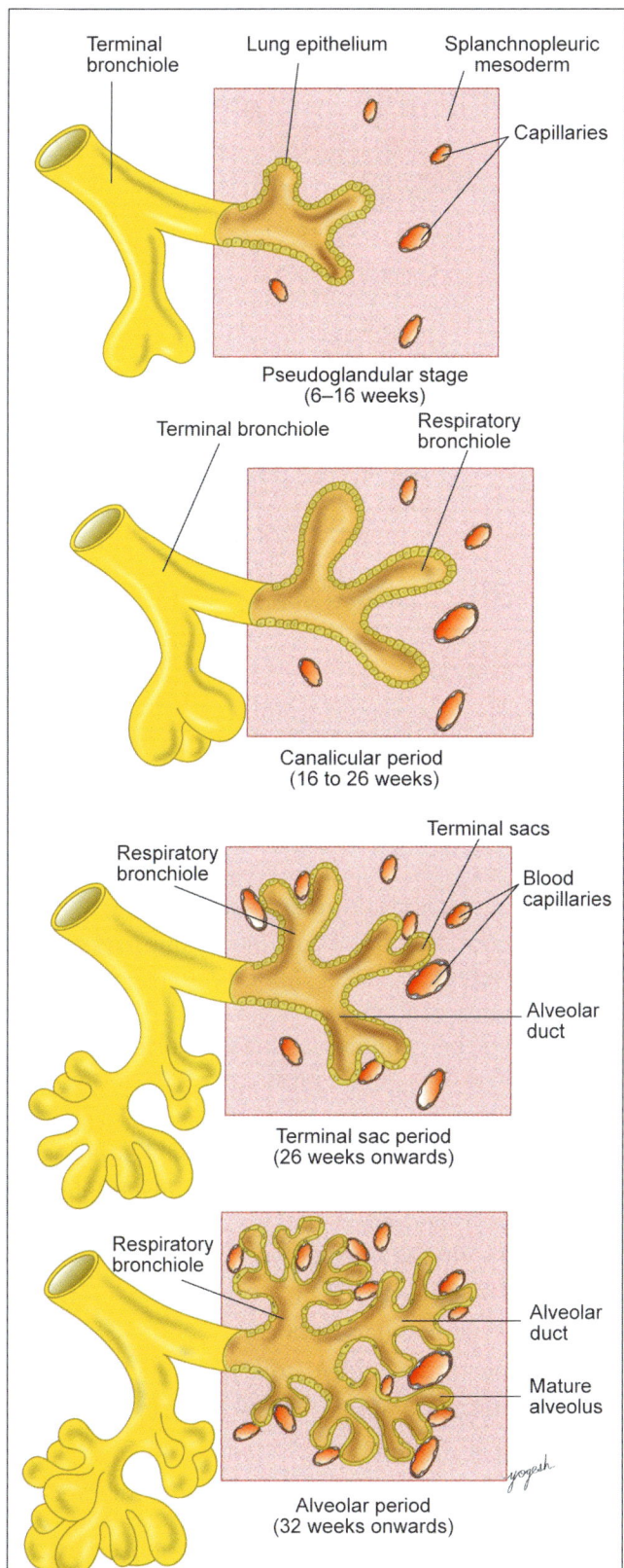

Fig. 16.8: Maturation of the lung. Alveoli are lined by simple squamous epithelium (type I pneumocytes) and some type II pneumocytes

3. Terminal saccular period (26 weeks to birth) and
4. Alveolar period (32 weeks to 8 years)

1. Pseudoglandular period
- Developing lung resembles an exocrine gland, hence called *pseudoglandular period*. At the end of this period, all the major elements of lung up to terminal bronchiole are formed.
- As respiratory bronchioles and alveoli are not yet developed, the foetus is not viable.

2. Canalicular period
- During this stage, respiratory bronchiole, alveolar ducts and primary alveoli are formed.
- Foetus born at the end of canalicular period can survive with intensive care. *Clinical Fact*

3. Terminal sac period
- During this stage, a substantial number of primary alveoli are formed.
- Blood–air barrier (endothelio-epithelial barrier) thin out.
- Alveoli are lined with type I and a few type II pneumocytes. Type II pneumocytes produce surfactant.
- The quantity of surfactant increases gradually towards the full-term.

4. Alveolar period
- During this period, definitive alveoli develop and increases in number.
- Type II pneumocytes continue production of more surfactant.
- Formation of definitive alveoli continues after the birth up to the age of 8th years.

Anomalies of Lungs

1. *Hyaline membrane disease* (Box 16.2).
2. *Agenesis and hypoplasia*: Part or complete lung on one side may be absent or underdeveloped.
3. *Abnormal lobulation*:
   - The absence of fissure results in a reduction of a number of lobes.
   - Extra fissure: It includes following cases:
     – A transverse fissure in left lung
     – A separate medial basal segment called *cardiac lobe*
     – A separate superior segment of lower lobe
4. *Azygous lobe (lobe of Wrisberg)*: Part of upper of lobe the right lung that lies medial to arch of azygous vein is called *azygous lobe* (Fig. 16.9). A vertical fissure separates azygous lobe from rest of the superior lobe

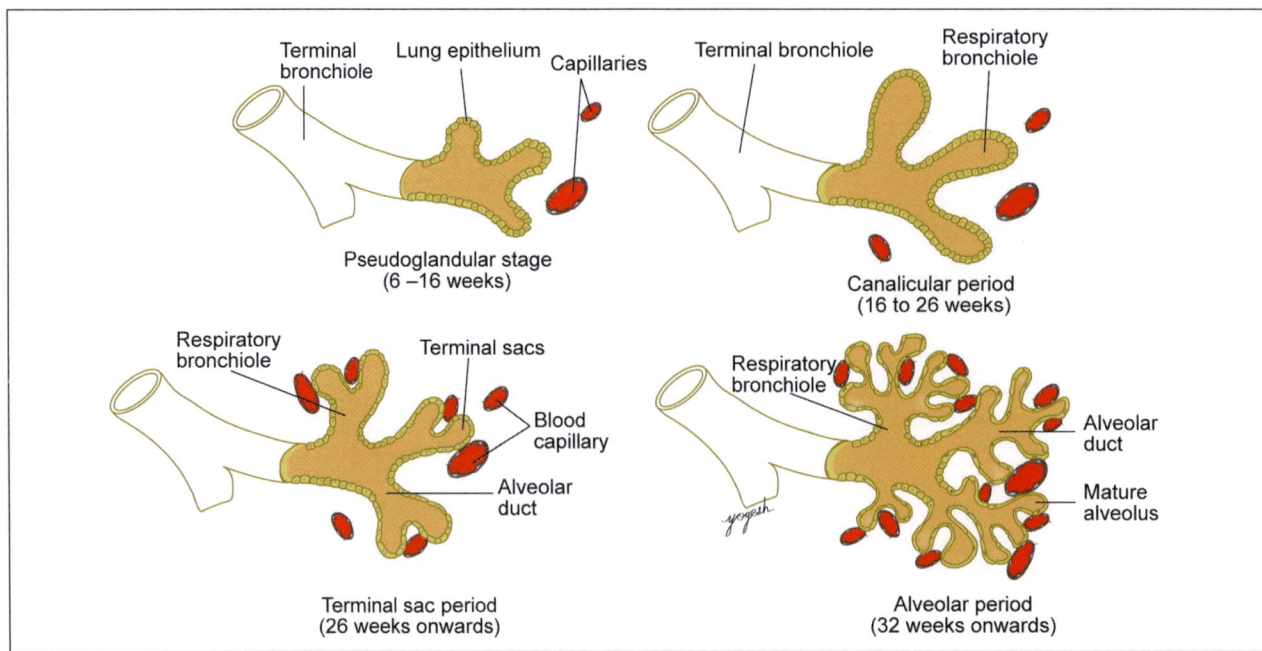

Practice Fig. 16.2: Maturation of the lung

of lung. Azygous vein lies on the floor of vertical fissure. Azygous lobe is commonest accessory lobe of the lung. *MCQ*

5. *Sequestration* of the lung tissue: A separation of area of embryonic lung tissue from tracheobronchial tree is called sequestration (means separation).
6. *Ectopic lung*: It occurs due to development of additional lung bud from oesophagus.
7. *Congenital polycystic lung*: The terminal bronchioles dilate to form multiple cysts and thus, produces honeycomb appearance on radiographs.
8. *Medicolegal aspect*: Lungs of newborn (live-born) contain air and hence float in water, whereas lungs of stillborn babies (dead born) do not contain air and

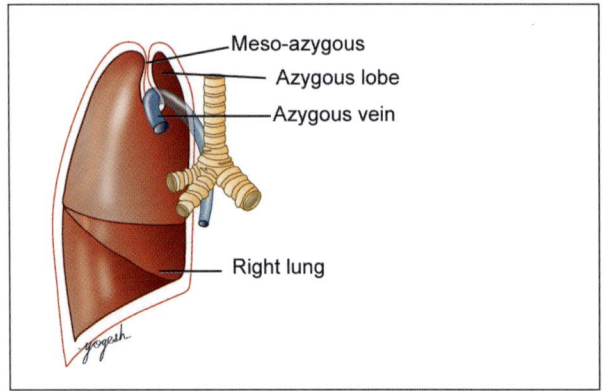

Fig. 16.9: Azygous lobe. Azygous lobe is separated from the apex of the right lung by meso-azygous. In the floor of the vertical fissure, the azygous vein is present

Box 16.2: Hyaline membrane disease or infant respiratory distress syndrome (IRDS)

Q. Write short note on hyaline membrane disease.
- It is also called *surfactant deficiency disorder or infant respiratory distress syndrome*.
- It is produced in premature infants due to deficiency of **surfactant**.
- Production of surfactant begins by the 20th week of IUL. *MCQ* The quantity of surfactant increases during last two weeks before birth.
- Incidence:
  – It affects about 1% of newborn infants and it is one of the leading causes of death in preterm infants.
  – Hyaline membrane disease accounts for 20% of deaths among newborns. *MCQ*

Signs and symptoms
  – rapid breathing (tachypnoea)
  – faster heart rate (tachycardia)
  – bluish discolouration of the skin (cyanosis).

Pathological finding
- Waxy appearing layers of hyaline membrane that line collapsed alveoli of lung.

Prevention
- To speed up production of surfactant, injectable *glucocorticoids* are given to the mother during last trimester (after the 7th month of pregnancy).

Contd.

Contd.

Diagnostic amniocentesis
- Lecithin sphingomyelin (L/S) ratio in amniotic fluid: L/S ratio less than 2:1 indicates insufficient surfactant.^{MCQ}
- Surfactant/albumin (S/A) ratio in amniotic fluid: The S/A ratio <35 indicates immature lungs, 35–55 indicates intermediate maturity and >55 indicates sufficient maturity of lungs.

Treatment
- A newborn can be supported with oxygen therapy, continuous positive airway pressure (CPAP). Exogenous surfactant can also be useful.

hence their lungs in the water. This fact can be used to differentiate between stillborn and killed live-born baby.

9. **Vacteral association** have the following components: *MCQ*

  – Vertebral anomalies
  – Anal atresia
  – Cardiac defects
  – Tracheoesophageal fistula
  – Esophageal atresia
  – Renal anomalies
  – Limb defect

17
Development of Body Cavities and Diaphragm

Chapter Outline

- Development of pericardial cavity
  - Stages of development
- Development of pleural cavity
  - Stages of development
- Development of peritoneal cavity
- Development of diaphragm
  - Stages of development
  - Descent of septum transversum
  - Factors producing descent of diaphragm
  - Congenital anomalies of diaphragm
- Congenital diaphragmatic hernia
- Formation of mesenteries
- Development of lesser sac
  - Stages of development

INTRODUCTION

- In the 3rd week, the small intercellular spaces appear in lateral plate mesoderm and pericardial bar. Later these spaces fuse to form U-shaped *primitive intraembryonic coelom* (Fig. 17.1).
- Central part of intraembryonic coelom forms the *pericardial sac*.
- Limbs of intraembryonic coelom are called *coelomic ducts*.
- Coelomic ducts communicate with extraembryonic coelom and thus, help in better nutrition.
- Pericardial, pleural and peritoneal cavities (serous sacs) are derived from the intraembryonic coelom.
- Intraembryonic coelom splits intraembryonic mesoderm into somatopleuric (parietal) layer and splanchnopleuric (visceral) layer.
- Somatopleuric intraembryonic layer lies in contact with ectoderm and laterally it is continuous with somatopleuric extraembryonic mesoderm layer.
- Splanchnopleuric intraembryonic mesoderm lies in contact with endoderm and laterally it is continuous with extraembryonic splanchnopleuric mesoderm.

Changes Due to Formation of Embryonic Folds

- Formation of embryonic folds changes the orientation of coelomic cavity.

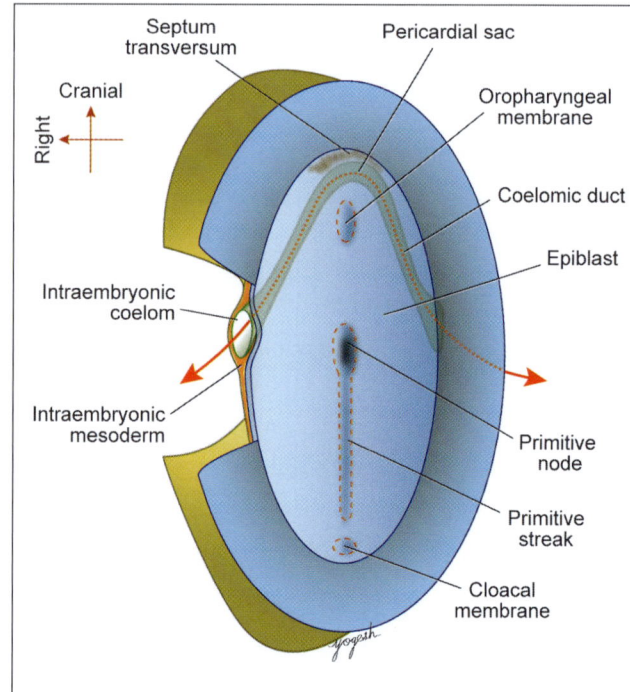

Fig. 17.1: Intraembryonic coelom. It lies in the lateral plate mesoderm and pericardial bar. In the figure red arrow is shown to be passing through the coelomic cavity. Pericardial bar lies between septum transversum and oropharyngeal membrane (not shown in this figure to maintain clarity)

Development of Body Cavities and Diaphragm

- On the formation of the head fold, the pericardial sac becomes ventral to foregut and it lies between stomodeum cranially and septum transversum caudally (*see* Figs 8.7 and 8.8, Chapter 8).
- On formation of lateral folds, ventrally coelomic ducts fuse with each other to form a peritoneal cavity.
- Part of coelomic ducts that communicates pericardial cavity with peritoneal cavity is called *pericardioperitoneal canals*. These canals lie on lateral sides of developing foregut.
- Lung buds arising from foregut invaginate pericardioperitoneal canals and convert (by expansion) these canals into *pleural cavities*.
- Later, pleuropericardial membranes, pleuroperitoneal membranes and diaphragm divide the coelomic cavity into peritoneal, pleural and pericardial cavities.

DEVELOPMENT OF PERICARDIAL CAVITY

A pericardial cavity develops from midline part of intraembryonic coelom that lies in pericardial bar.

Stages of Development

1. Before formation of headfold: Pericardial cavity lies between septum transversum cranially and prechordal plate caudally.
2. After formation of headfold: Pericardial cavity lies between stomodeum (cranially) and septum transversum (caudally). Dorsally pericardial cavity is related to cardiogenic area and foregut.
3. Formation of layers of pericardium:
   - Fibrous pericardium and parietal layer of serous pericardium develop from *somatopleuric layer* of intraembryonic mesoderm.
   - Visceral layer of serous pericardium develops from *splanchnopleuric layer* of intraembryonic mesoderm.

Further details of development pericardial cavity are included in Chapter 18.

DEVELOPMENT OF PLEURAL CAVITY

Pleural cavities develop from the right and left pericardioperitoneal canals that connect pericardial cavity with peritoneal cavities.

Stages of Development

1. *Invagination stage*: Lung buds invaginate pericardioperitoneal canals.
2. *Enlargement*: Pericardioperitoneal canals enlarge to accommodate enlarging lung buds.
3. *Separation*: Two folds of somatopleuric mesoderm appear in relation to invaginated lung buds as follows:
   - Cranial pleuropericardial fold (membrane) separates pericardial cavity from pleural cavity.
   - Caudal pleuroperitoneal fold (membrane) separates pleural cavity from the peritoneal cavity.
   - Both membranes become continuous with posterior border of septum transversum
4. *Closure of pleuropericardial opening*:
   - During the sixth week, pleuropericardial opening closes due to fusion of pleuropericardial membrane (pulmonary ridge of Mall) with the mesodermal tissue surrounding oesophagus.
   - Overgrowing lung bud turns pleuropericardial membrane and makes it vertical (initially oblique).
5. *Closure of pleuroperitoneal opening*:
   - Boundaries of pleuroperitoneal opening are as follows (Fig. 17.2):
     Ventral: Dorsal border of septum transversum
     Medial: Oesophagus, dorsal mesentery of oesophagus and dorsal aorta
     Dorsal: Mesonephric ridge with gonads
     Lateral: Pleuroperitoneal membrane
   - Pleuroperitoneal membranes grow ventrally and fuse with dorsal border of septum transversum and other structures forming boundaries of pleuroperitoneal openings.
6. *Expansion of pleural cavities*: Expanding lung buds cause expansion of pleural cavities and descent of septum transversum.
7. *Formation of pleuropericardial membrane*: Expanding pleural cavity splits mesoderm into two layers (Fig. 17.4):
   a. Outer layer forms wall of thorax
   b. Inner layer lines pericardial cavity. This layer is called pleuropericardial membrane and it later forms fibrous pericardium.

DEVELOPMENT OF PERITONEAL CAVITY

- Peritoneal cavity develops from horseshoe shaped limbs of intraembryonic coelom.
- Formation of lateral folds bring right and left intraembryonic coelomic ducts (limbs) closer and they fuse to form a peritoneal cavity.
- Peritoneal cavity initially communicates with pericardial cavity through pericardioperitoneal canals. On formation of pleural cavity from pericardioperitoneal canal, later peritoneal cavity separated from pleural cavity by septum transversum and pleuroperitoneal membranes.

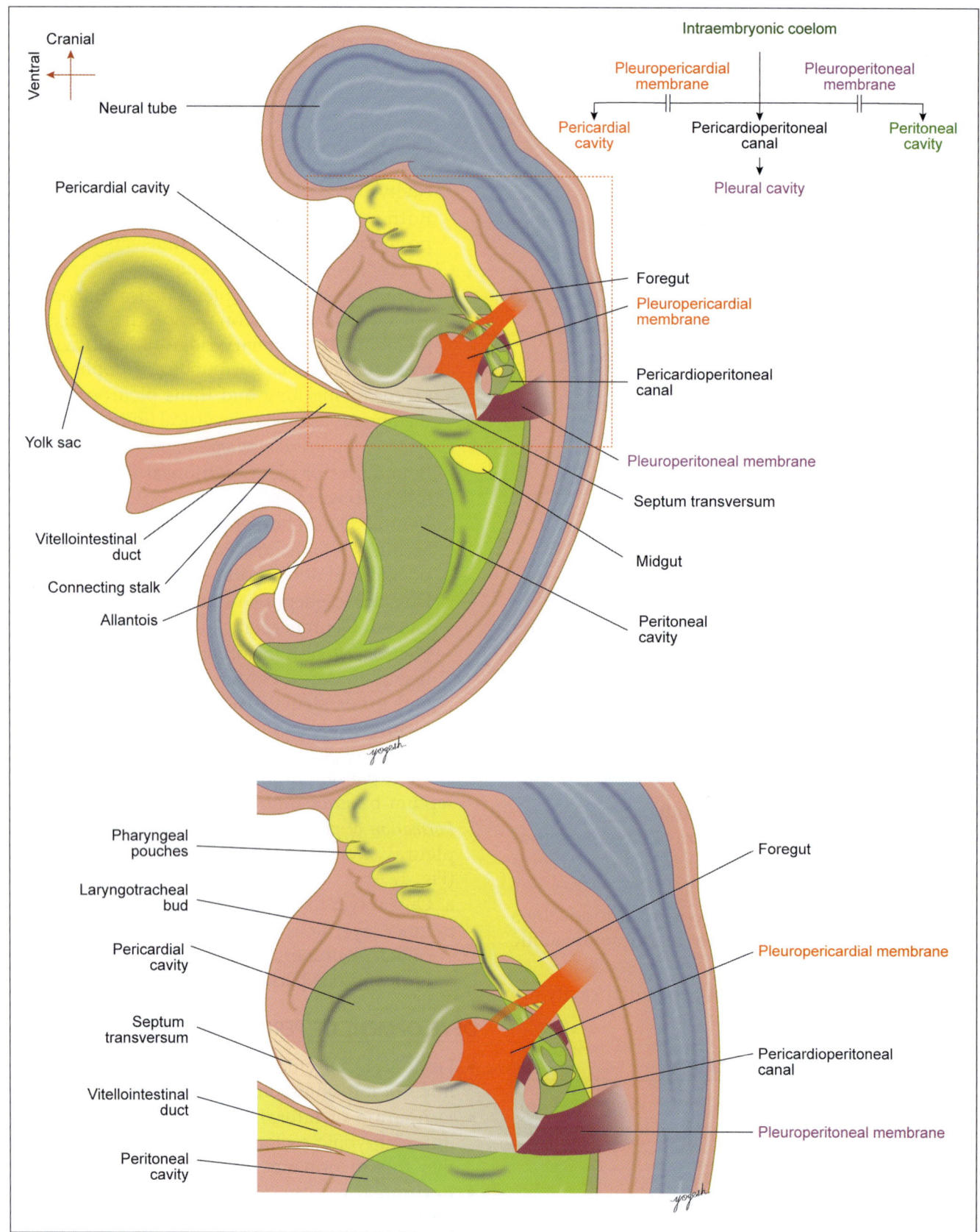

Fig. 17.2: Formation of coelomic cavities of body. Two folds of somatopleuric mesoderm, namely cranial pleuropericardial membrane (separates pericardial cavity from pleural cavity) and caudal pleuroperitoneal membrane (separates pleural cavity from peritoneal cavity) become continuous with the posterior border of the septum transversum

Development of Body Cavities and Diaphragm

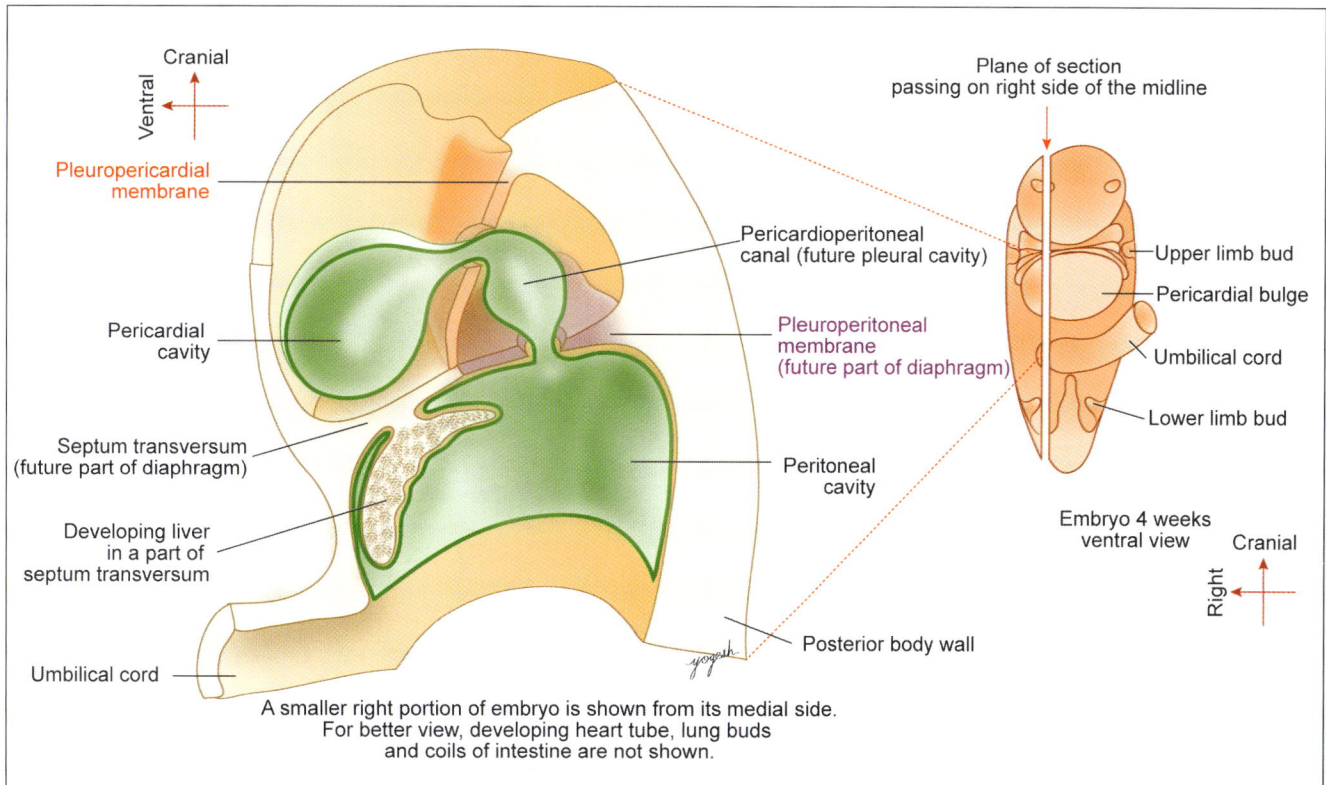

Fig. 17.3: Separations of pericardial, pleural and peritoneal cavities from each other. Cranial pericardiopleural membrane separates pericardial cavity from pleural cavity. Caudal pleuroperitoneal membrane separates pleural cavity from the peritoneal cavity. Both of these membranes become continuous with the posterior border of the septum transversum

- Up to 10th week, peritoneal cavity communicates with extraembryonic coelom at umbilicus (site for a physiological hernia).
- Layers of peritoneum: Parietal peritoneum develops from somatopleuric layer of mesoderm, whereas visceral peritoneum develops from splanchnopleuric layer of mesoderm.

DEVELOPMENT OF DIAPHRAGM

Q. Write note on development of diaphragm.

Summary (Examination Guide) (Table 17.1, Fig. 17.5 and Practice Fig. 17.1)

- Diaphragm is a musculotendinous partition between thoracic and abdominal cavities
- Diaphragm consists of central tendon and two crura.

Table 17.1	Development of diaphragm[MCQ]
Part of diaphragm	Embryonic source
1. Central tendon	Septum transversum
2. Small peripheral part	Pleuroperitoneal membranes
3. Large peripheral part (posterolateral)	Mesoderm of lateral body wall
4. Right and left crus	Dorsal mesentery of oesophagus

- Various parts of diaphragm develop as follows:
  1. Central tendon from septum transversum
  2. Crus of diaphragm from dorsal mesentery of oesophagus
  3. Small dorsal peripheral part from pleuroperitoneal membranes.
  4. Ventrolateral (large) peripheral part from mesoderm of lateral body wall.

Stages of Development

1. Septum transversum derivative: Septum transversum lies between thoracic and peritoneal cavities.
   Relations of septum transversum
   Cranial: Pleural and pericardial cavities
   Caudal: Peritoneal cavity
   Dorsal: Oesophagus and dorsal mesentery of oesophagus
   Dorsolateral: Pleuroperitoneal canals
   Note: Liver develops in caudal part of septum transversum, whereas central tendon of diaphragm develops from cranial part.
2. Derivative of pleuroperitoneal membranes: Right and left pleuroperitoneal membranes separate pleural cavities from peritoneal cavity and form a small part of diaphragm.

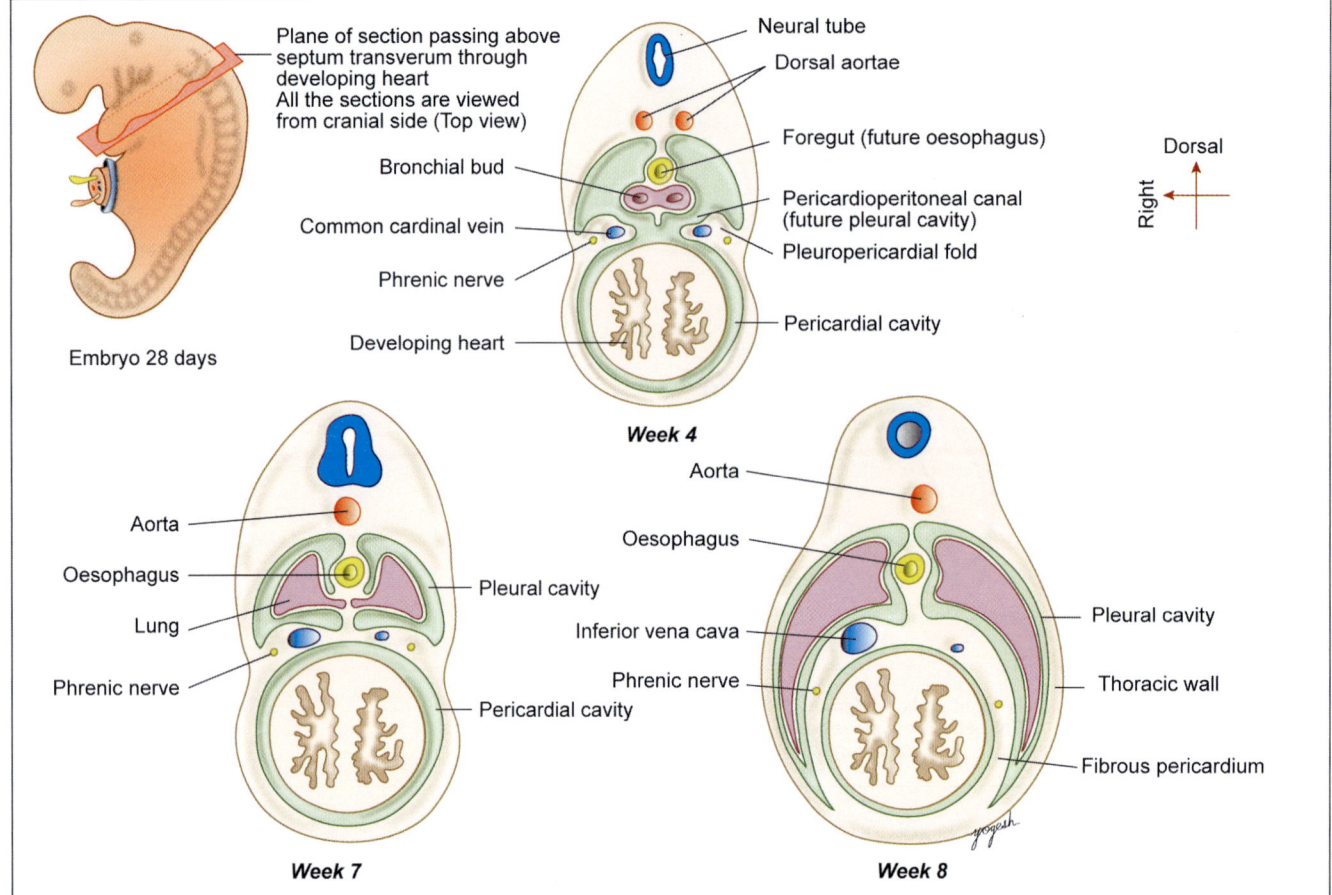

Fig. 17.4: Development of pleural cavities. Pleural cavities develop from right and left pericardioperitoneal canals that connect pericardial cavity with peritoneal cavities. Lung buds invaginates into pericardioperitoneal canals. These pericardioperitoneal canals enlarge to accommodate enlarging lung buds. Pericardiopleural folds (membrane) separate pericardial cavity from pleural cavity. Pleuroperitoneal fold (membrane) (not shown in this figure) separates pleural cavity from the peritoneal cavity. During the sixth week of IUL, pleuropericardial opening closes due to fusion of pleuropericardial membrane with mesodermal tissue surrounding oesophagus. Expanding lung buds cause expansion of pleural cavities anteroposteriorly and craniocaudally. Expanding pleural cavity splits mesoderm into two layers, outer layer forms wall of thorax and inner layer forms fibrous pericardium

3. Derivative of dorsal mesentery of oesophagus: It forms crura of the diaphragm.
4. Derivative of lateral thoracic wall: Developing pleural cavity divides lateral body wall into external and internal layers. External layer forms definitive body wall, whereas internal layer forms ventrolateral part of the diaphragm, peripheral to pleuroperitoneal membrane derivative.

Descent of Septum Transversum

- In 4th week, septum transversum lies in cervical region at the level of third, fourth and fifth cervical somitic nerves (later it develops phrenic nerve, C3-5 root value).
- Due to growth of lung buds in pericardio-peritoneal canals and heart development, diaphragm reaches to its definitive position by sixth week (opposite to T7 to T12 spinal segments).MCQ
- Descending diaphragm pulls its original nerve supply (phrenic nerve) with it.

Factors Producing Descent of Diaphragm

The following factors causes descent of diaphragm:
1. Elongation of neck (developing pharyngeal arches)
2. Enlarging pleural cavities
3. Development of heart

Congenital Anomalies

1. Congenital diaphragmatic hernia (CDH): Box 17.1 and Fig. 17.6
2. Congenital hiatal hernia
   - It is herniation of abdominal contents (mostly stomach) through oesophageal opening of the diaphragm.

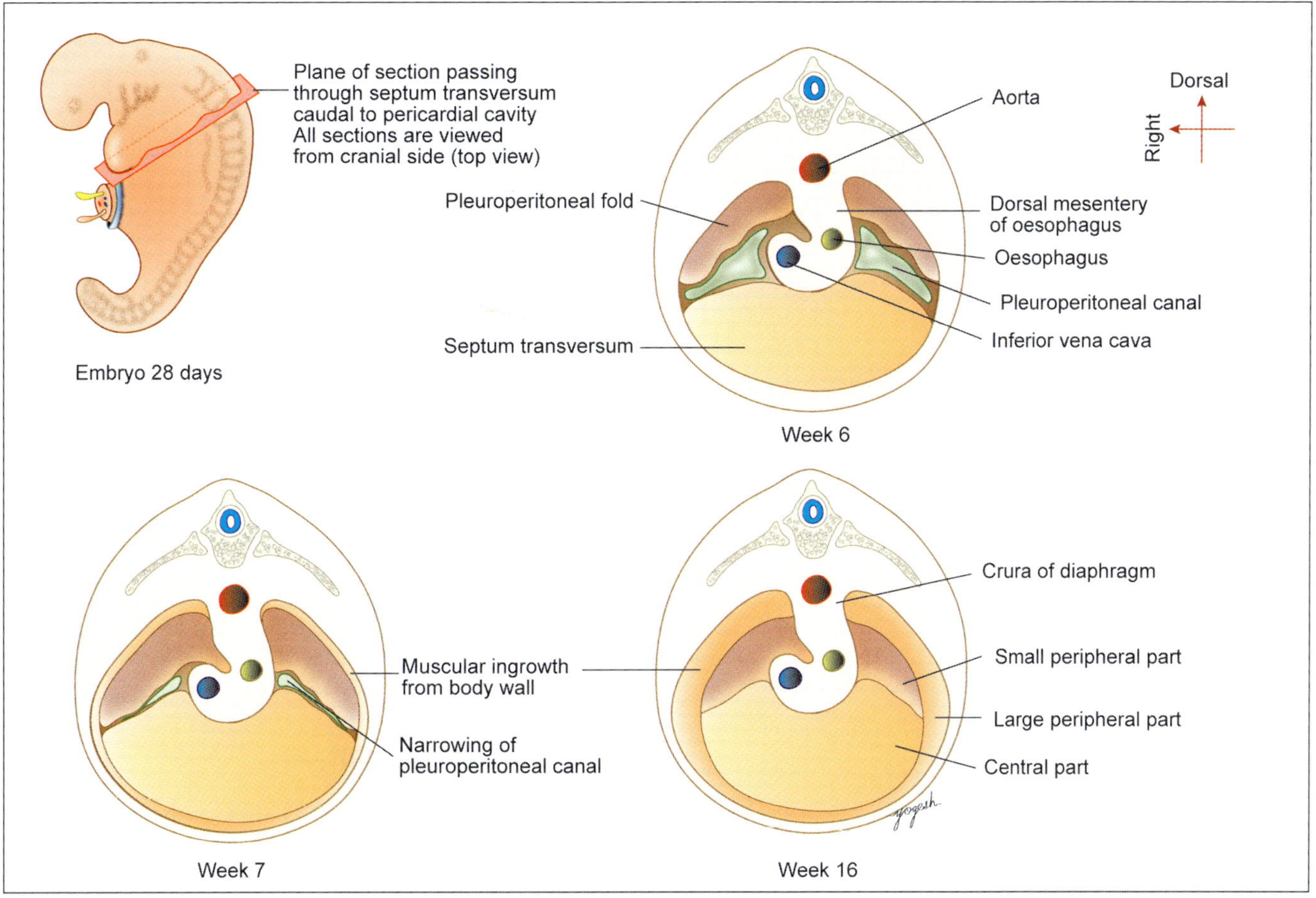

Development of Body Cavities and Diaphragm

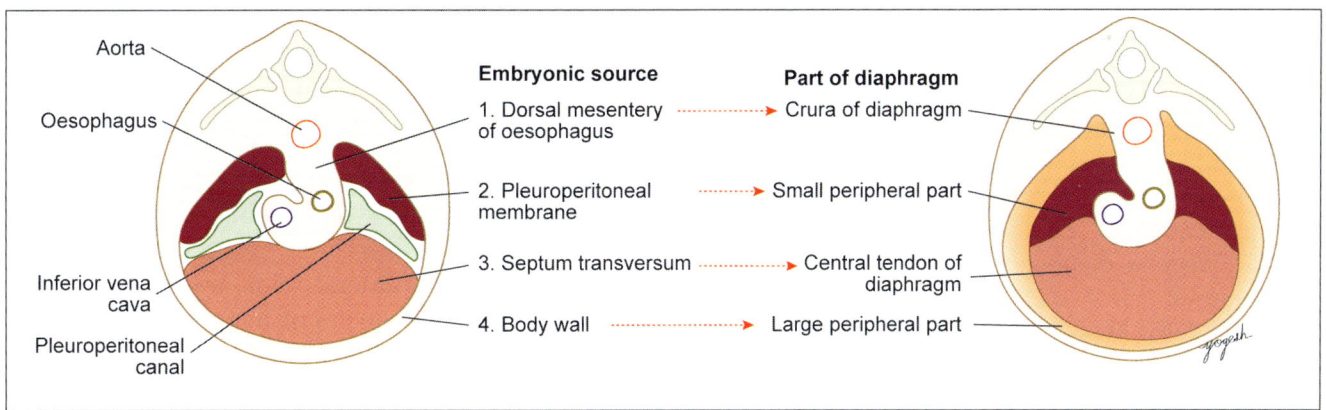

Fig. 17.5: Development of abdominothoracic diaphragm. Central tendon of diaphragm develops from septum transversum, crus of diaphragm from dorsal mesentery of oesophagus, small dorsal peripheral part from pleuro-peritoneal membranes, ventrolateral (large) peripheral part from mesoderm of the lateral body wall

Practice Fig. 17.1: Development of diaphragm

3. **Retrosternal (parasternal) hernia:** It is herniation of abdominal contents through enlarged foramen of Morgagni (gap between sternal and costal slips of diaphragm).

4. **Eventration of diaphragm:** It is an abnormal contour of diaphragmatic dome due to underdeveloped musculature of anyone dome of the diaphragm. Thin diaphragmatic zone outpouches with abdominal contents in thoracic cavity.

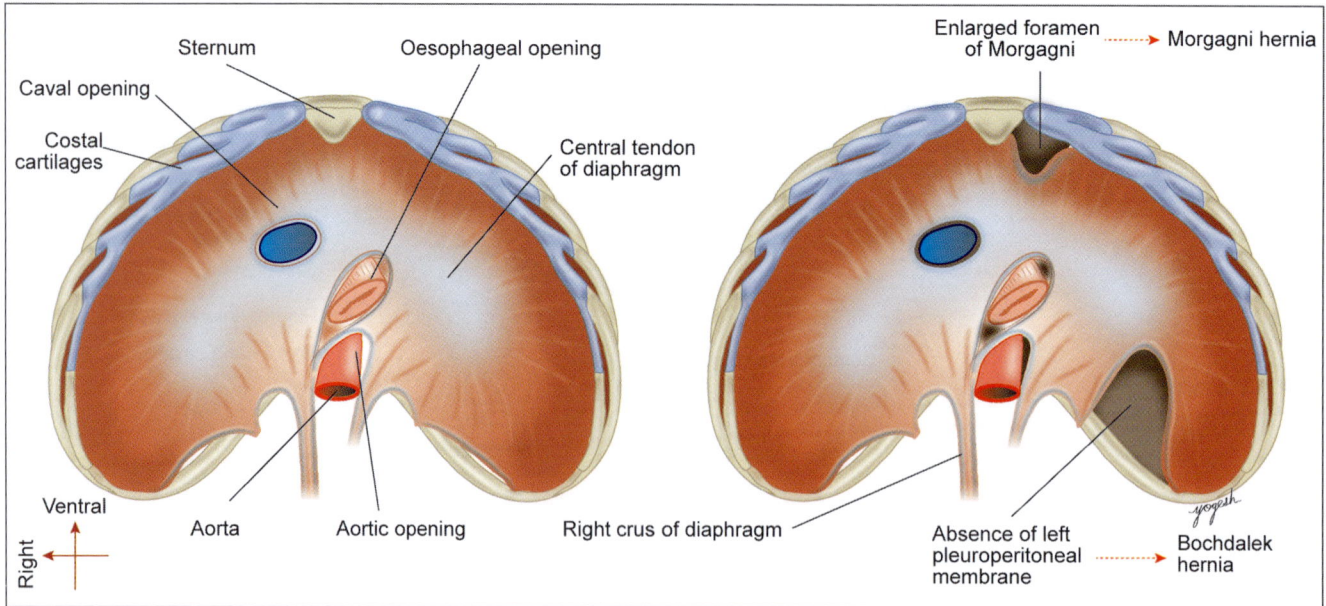

Fig. 17.6: Congenital diaphragmatic hernia. It is herniation of abdominal content into thoracic cavity due to failure of proper formation of the diaphragm. Bochdalek hernia occurs due to failure of pleuroperitoneal membrane contribution to the diaphragm, whereas Morgagni hernia involves protrusion of abdominal contents through enlarged foramen of Morgagni

Box 17.1: Congenital diaphragmatic hernia (CDH)

Q. *Write short note on congenital diaphragmatic hernia.*
- It is herniation of abdominal content into thoracic cavity due to failure of proper formation of the diaphragm.
- CDH is a life-threatening condition in infants as it may result in pulmonary hypoplasia.
- Incidence: 1:2000 births
- Most common cause of pulmonary hypoplasia is CDH. Respiratory distress is the commonest cause of death in CDH.^MCQ
- There are *three cardinal signs* of CDH: Breathlessness, cyanosis, unusual flat abdomen.^MCQ
- Genetic cause: Microdeletion of chromosome 15 in the region 15q26.^MCQ
- Classification:
  The congenital diaphragmatic hernia has three types as follows:
  A. Bochdalek hernia: It is also called posterolateral hernia. About 95% case of CDH are Bochdalek hernia.^MCQ It occurs due to the failure of pleuroperitoneal membrane contribution to the diaphragm. It is more common on left side (85–90% cases).
  B. Morgagni hernia (retrosternal or parasternal hernia): It is CDH that involves protrusion of abdominal contents through foramen of Morgagni.
  C. Diaphragmatic eventration: It refers to abnormal contour of diaphragmatic dome because of paralysis, aplasia, or atrophy to varying degrees of muscle fibres.

FORMATION OF MESENTERIES

- Mesentery is a connective tissue fold formed by two layers of peritoneum, that connects abdominal viscera (intestine) with abdominal walls.
- There are two mesenteries (Fig. 17.7)
  – Ventral mesentery—connects gut with anterior body wall.
  – Dorsal mesentery—connects gut with posterior body wall.
- Ventral mesentery disappears except for the following parts:
  a. Caudal part of oesophagus
  b. Stomach
  c. Proximal part of duodenum
- Ventral mesentery of stomach is called *ventral mesogastrium*.
- On formation of lateral folds, owing to fusion of splanchnopleuric layers of mesoderm, the midgut and hindgut have only dorsal mesentery.
- Rotation of gut and zygosis converts the dorsal mesentery into mesentery of jejunum and ileum, mesoappendix, transverse and sigmoid mesocolons (Fig. 17.8).

DEVELOPMENT OF LESSER SAC

Q. *Write short note on development of lesser sac.*
- Lesser sac is also called *omental bursa*. It is a part of peritoneal cavity.
- Lesser sac lies behind stomach and lesser omentum.

Development of Body Cavities and Diaphragm

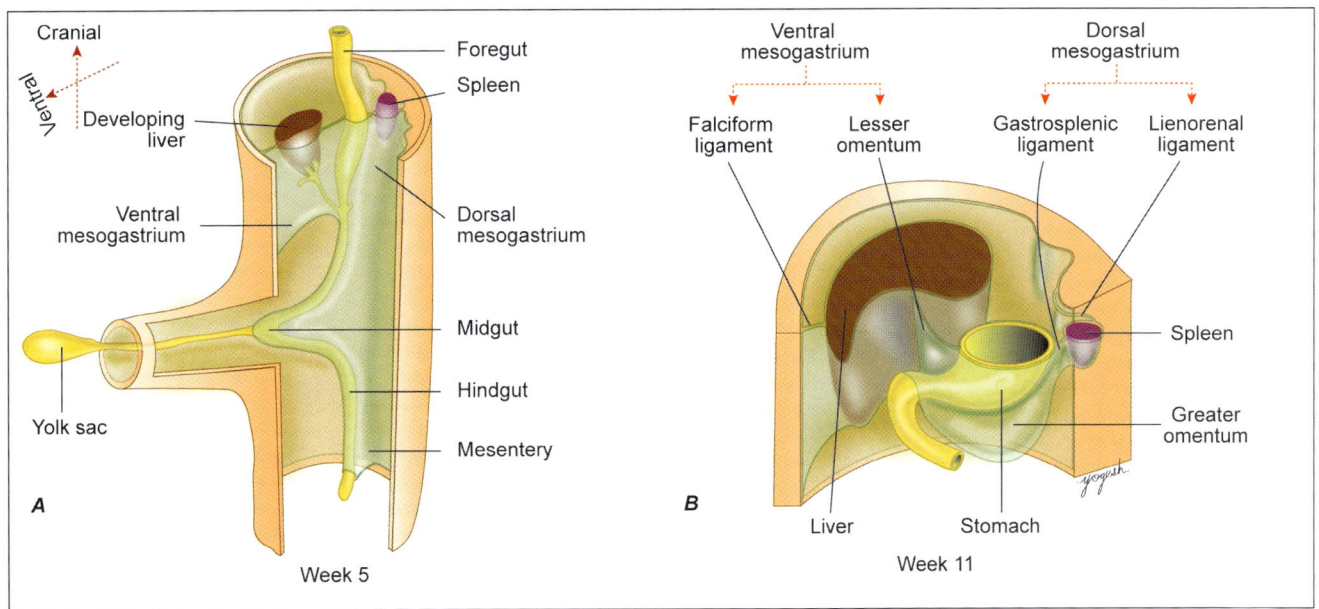

Fig. 17.7: Dorsal and ventral mesenteries of the gut. Transverse section through the region of the stomach showing the changes in the position of stomach, liver and spleen and mesogastrium: (A) Positions at the end of the fifth week; (B) Positions at the end of the 11th week. Ventral mesogastrium forms falciform ligament and lesser omentum, whereas dorsal mesogastrium forms gastrosplenic and lienorenal ligaments and greater omentum

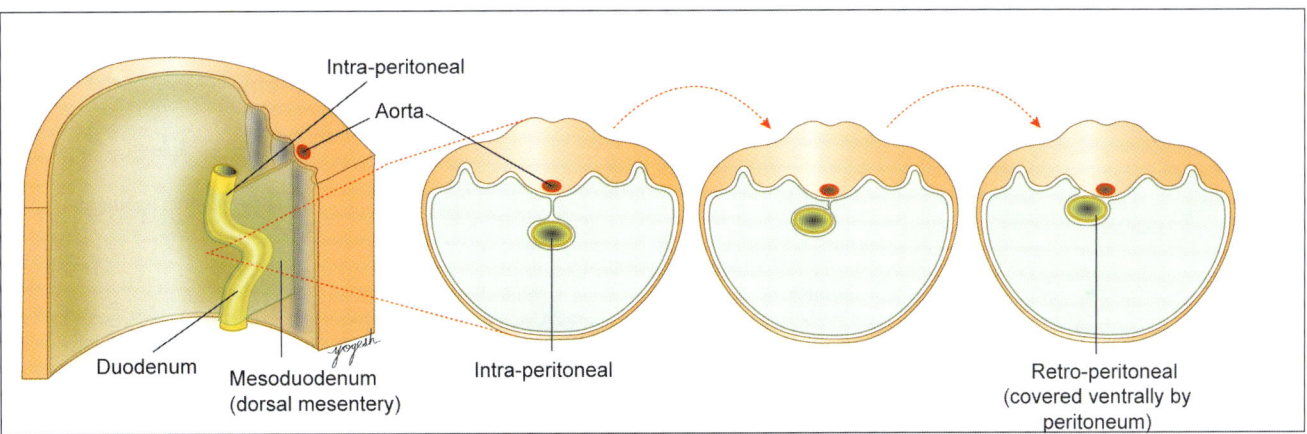

Fig. 17.8: Process of zygosis

Stages of Development

1. Formation of pneumoenteric recess in dorsal mesogastrium (Figs 17.9, 17.10 and Table 17.2).
   - Right and left pneumoenteric recess (small cavities) appear in dorsal mesogastrium.
   - Left one disappears soon.
   - Right recess fuse with peritoneal cavity and later expands on left side to form a major part of lesser sac behind the stomach.
   - Cavity of right recess expands cranially behind liver and forms superior recess of lesser sac.
   - Cranial extension of right pneumoenteric bursa above the diaphragm forms *infracardiac bursa*.

2. Formation of part of lesser sac behind lesser omentum:
   - Due to rotation of stomach and development of liver, the part of peritoneal cavity (forms vestibule of lesser sac) comes to lie behind the lesser omentum (derived from ventral mesogastrium).

3. Formation of lower part of lesser sac:
   - Developing spleen and stomach rotation (counter-clockwise) divide dorsal mesogastrium into gastrosplenic and lienorenal ligaments (that lies on left side of lesser sac).
   - Part of lesser sac extending between gastrosplenic and lienorenal ligaments is *splenic recess*.

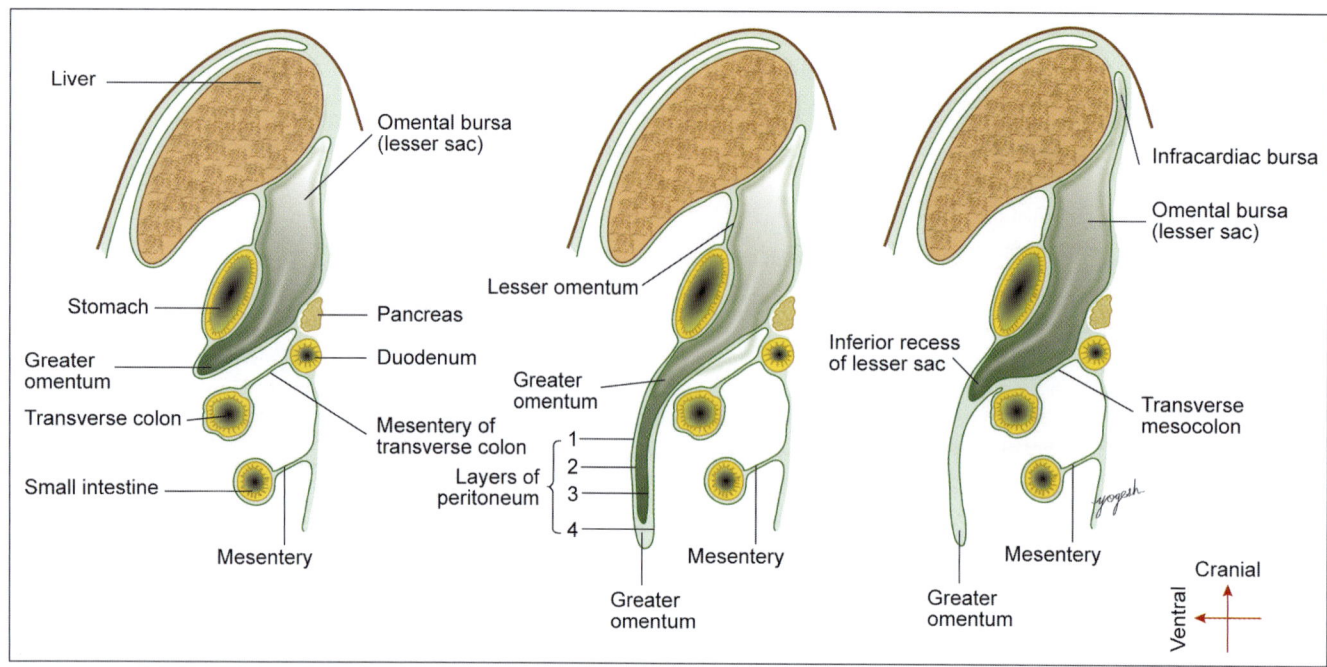

Fig. 17.9: Development of lesser sac and greater and lesser omentum

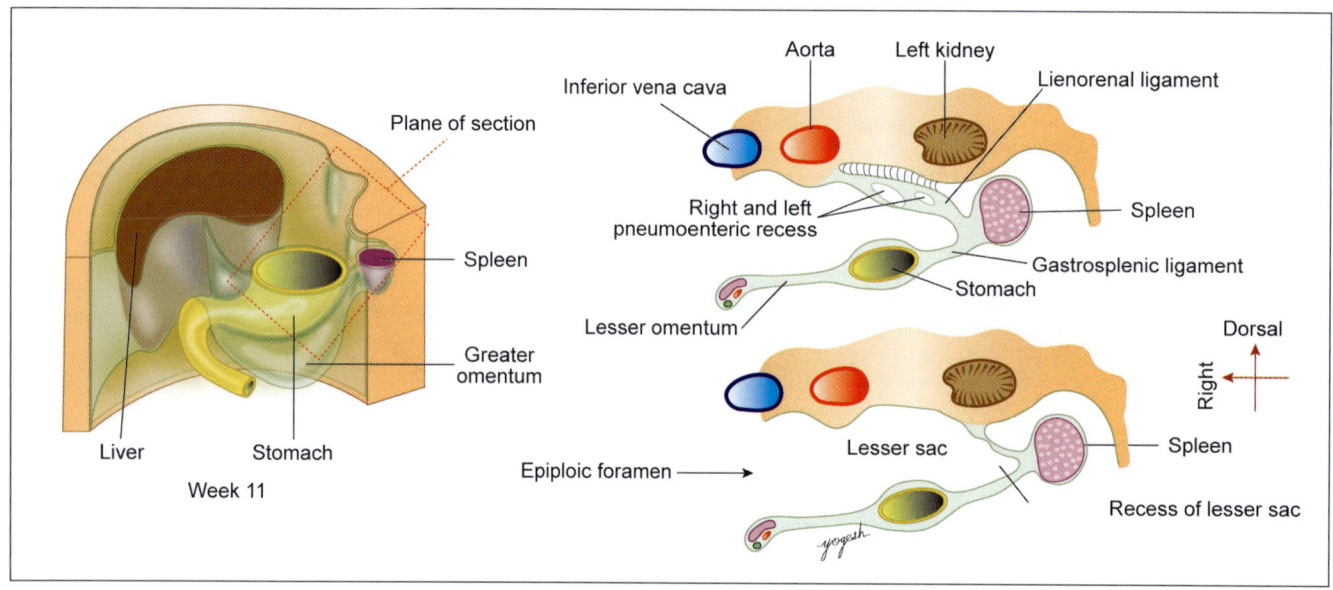

Fig. 17.10: Development of lesser sac

- The part of dorsal mesogastrium attached to greater curvature of stomach extends and forms greater omentum. Part of the lesser sac that lies within greater omentum is *inferior recess of lesser sac*.
- Cavity of the lesser sac communicates with rest of the peritoneal cavity through epiploic foramen of Winslow, that lies behind right free margin of the lesser omentum.

Table 17.2	Development of lesser sac
Part	Source
Vestibule	On rotation of stomach, a part of peritoneal cavity that lies behind ventral mesogastrium
Superior recess	Cranial extension of right pneumoenteric recess below diaphragm
Inferior recess	Caudal extension of cavity in elongating greater omentum
Splenic recess	Part of lesser sac extending between gastrosplenic and lienorenal ligaments

CLINICAL EMBRYOLOGY

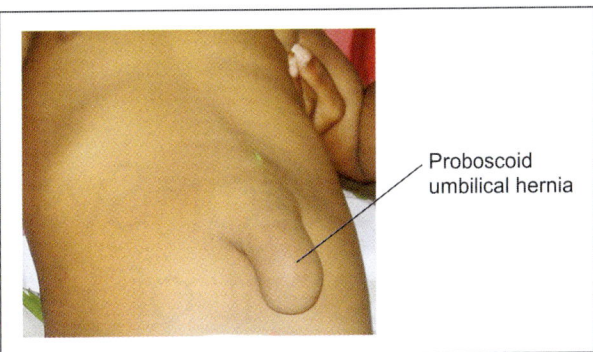

Clinical image 17.1: Proboscoid umbilical hernia. Umbilical hernia is the protrusion of abdominal contents through a defective anterior abdominal wall at the umbilicus. If the umbilical hernia is elongated, it is called proboscoid umbilical hernia (like elephant trunk). Usually, umbilical hernia regresses spontaneously by 2–3 years of age, but proboscoid umbilical hernia often requires surgical correction (Image courtesy: *Dr Kumaravel S*)

18
Cardiovascular System I
Development of Heart

Chapter Outline

- Fate of heart tube
- Acquisition of external features of the adult heart
- Development of atria
  - Right atrium
  - Left atrium
  - Sinus venosus
  - Atrioventricular canal
  - Interatrial septum
  - Foramen ovale
- Probe patency of foramen ovale
- Dextrocardia
- Atrial septal defects
- Development of ventricles
  - Bulbus cordis
  - Interventricular septum
  - Aorticopulmonary septum
- Development of valves of heart
  - Atrioventricular valves
  - Pulmonary and aortic valves
- Development of conducting system of heart
- Development of pericardial cavity
- Ventricular septal defects
- Tetralogy of Fallot
- Timing of embryologic heart formation

INTRODUCTION

- The nutritional supply of embryo changes according to development as follows:
  - During the first week, before implantation, deutoplasm (accumulated cytoplasmic nutrients) of oocyte supplies nutrition.
  - During the second week, breakdown products of endometrium (due to implantation) nourishes the embryo by simple diffusion.
  - After the third week, maternal blood nourish embryo through uteroplacental circulation.
- Increasing nutritional demand of growing embryo initiates development of cardiovascular system in the third week of intrauterine life.
- All components of cardiovascular system develop from mesoderm.
- The components of cardiovascular system can be studied as
  1. Development of heart
  2. Development of blood vessels
- This chapter deals with development of the heart.

Establishment of Cardiogenic Area (field)

- During the third week, *cardiac progenitor cells* develop just lateral to the primitive streak.
- These cells migrate through primitive streak cranially and forms horseshoe shaped *primitive heart field* in the splanchnopleuric mesoderm by end of the third week (Fig. 18.1).
- On formation of head fold, primary heart field come to lie on dorsal side of pericardial sac.
- Endoderm of primitive pharynx induces vasculogenesis (formation of blood cells and vessels) in the primary heart field.
- Small vessels join to form two (right and left) *endothelial heart tubes* that give rise to the endocardium.
- *Splanchnopleuric mesoderm* that lies between heart tube and pericardial cavity form a *myoepicardial mantle*.
- The myoepicardial mantle condense to form
  - Myocardium (cardiac muscles) [cardiac muscles develop from splanchnopleuric mesoderm.[Neet]]
  - Epicardium (visceral layer of pericardium)

Cardiovascular System I: Development of Heart

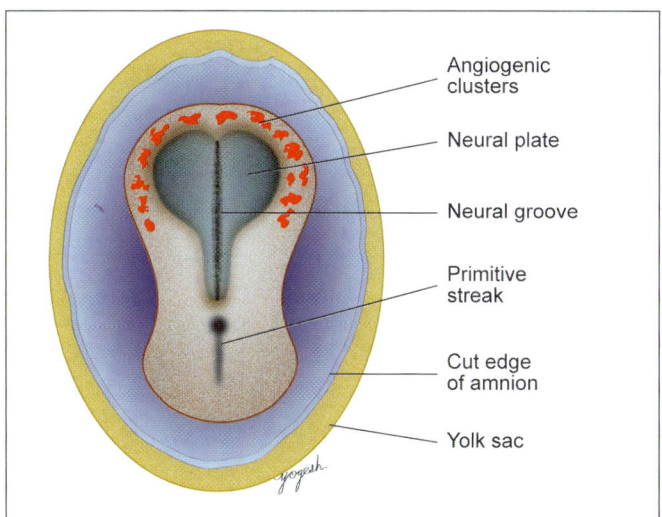

Fig. 18.1: Cardiogenic area is derived from intraembryonic mesoderm in the third week

- Somatopleuric mesoderm that surrounds pericardial cavity form parietal layer of pericardium.
- Primitive heart starts beating on the 22nd day.^{MCQ}
- Blood begins to circulate within the embryo by 24th day.^{MCQ}

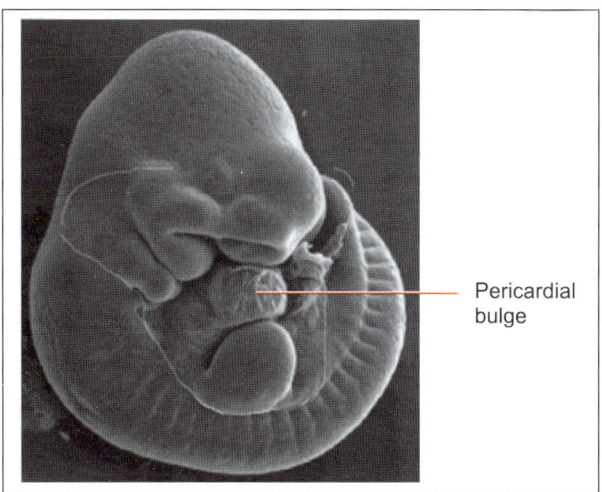

Scanning electron micrograph 18.1: SEM showing 6-week embryo showing pericardial bulge [Species: Mouse, approximate human age: 6 weeks, lateral view]

Heart Tubes

- In the third week, two heart tubes fuse and form a single heart tube. Ends of the heart tube remain bifurcated. Its cranial end is called *arterial end*, whereas caudal end is called *venous end* (Fig. 18.2).
- Heart tube soon forms five dilatations from cranial to caudal end as follows (Fig. 18.3, Practice Fig. 18.1):^{Viva}

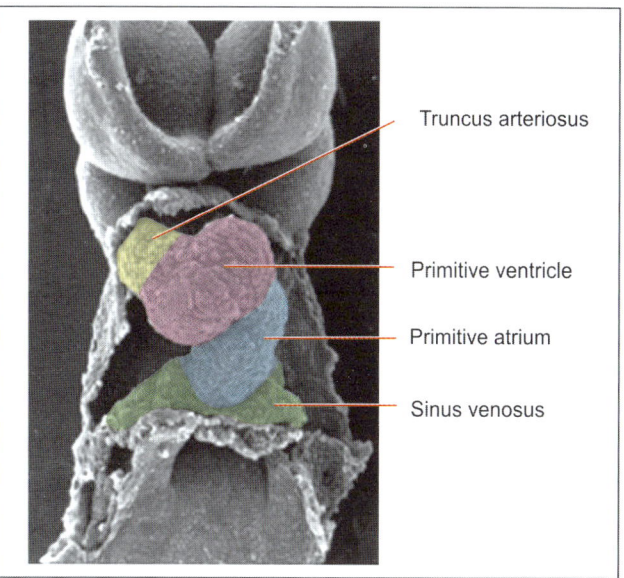

Scanning electron micrograph 18.2: Developing heart tube at week 4 development [Species: Mouse, approximate human age: 25 days, frontal view]

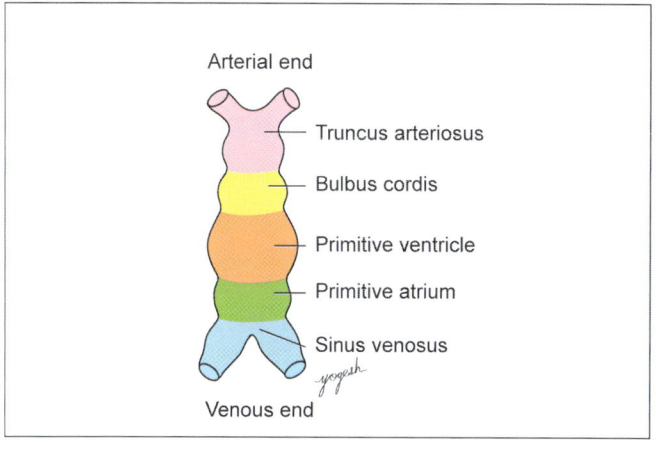

Practice Fig. 18.1: Parts of heart tube

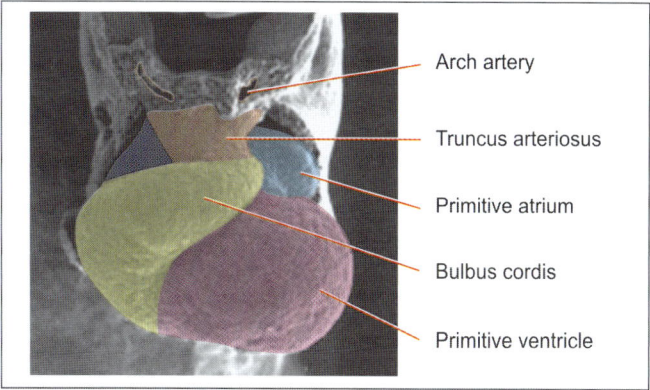

Scanning electron micrograph 18.3: Heart chambers and outflow tract. The truncus arteriosus carries blood out of heart into aortic sac and subsequently into aortic arch vessels. The conus cordis is a major contributor to the right ventricle [Species: Mouse, approx. human age: 27 days]

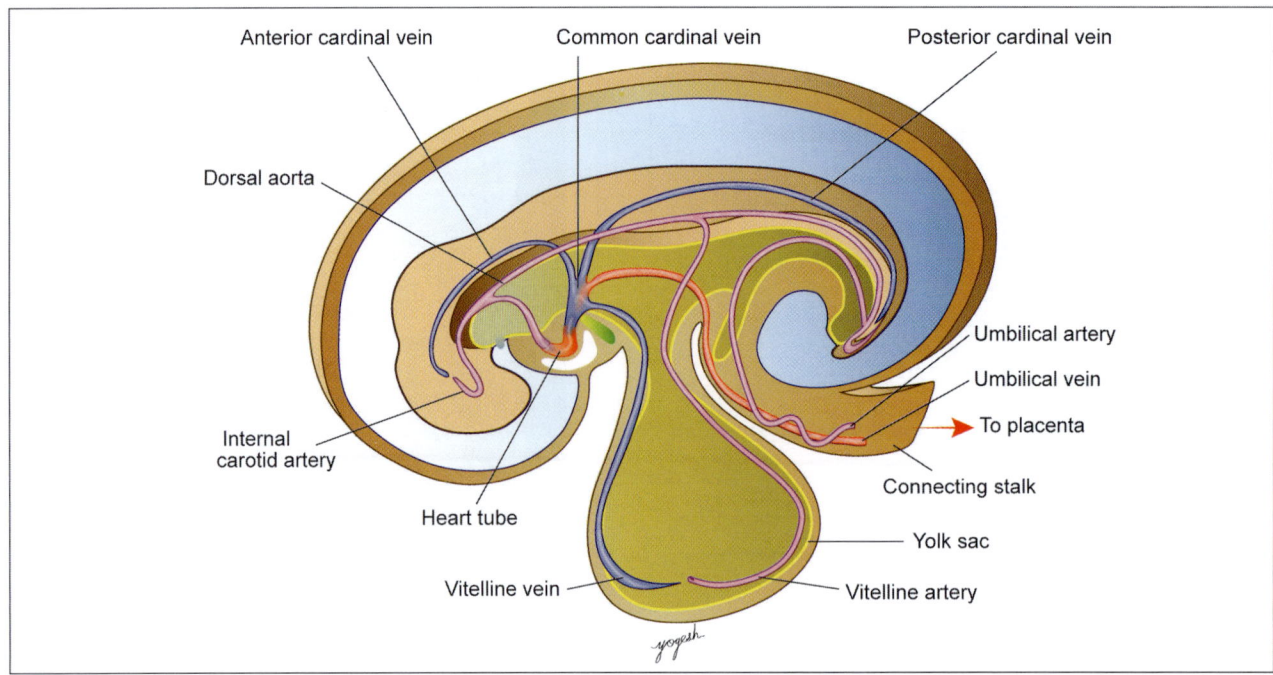

Fig. 18.2: Major vessels of embryo

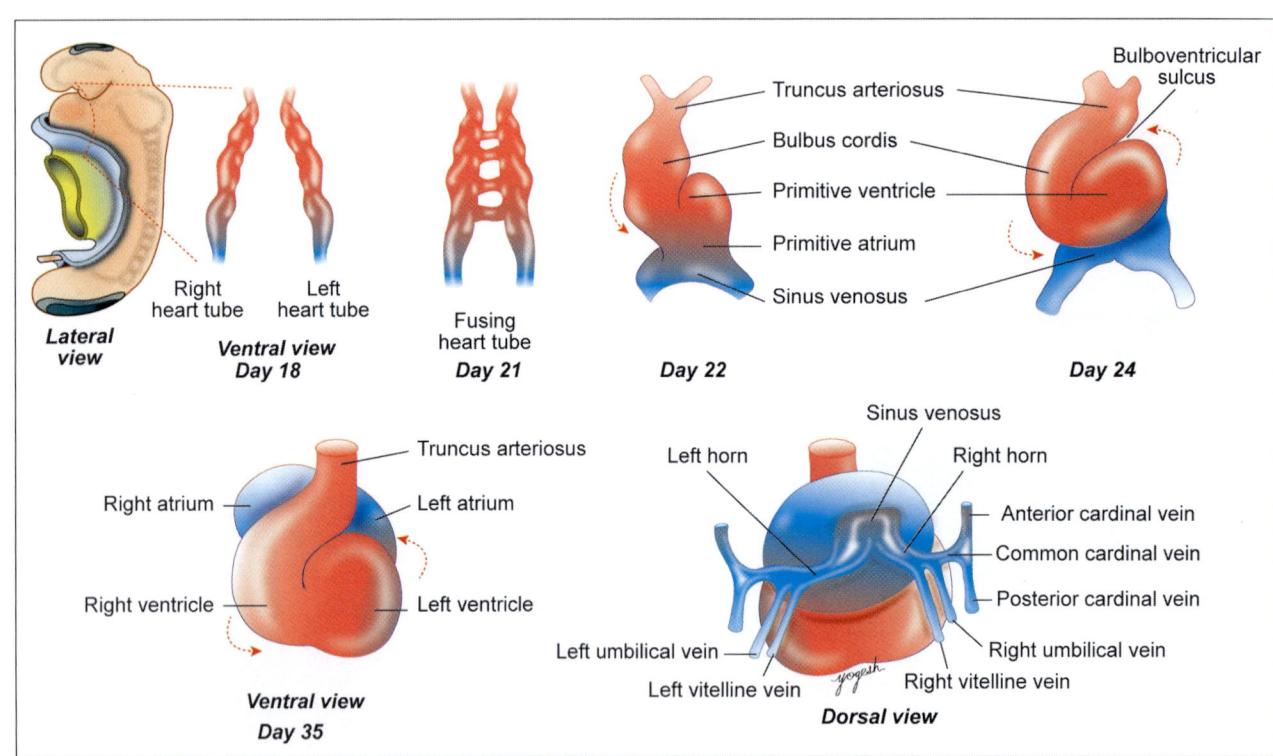

Fig. 18.3: Development of heart. External views

1. Truncus arteriosus
2. Bulbus cordis
3. Primitive ventricle
4. Primitive atrium
5. Sinus venosus

Ends of Heart Tube

- Arterial end or truncus arteriosus shows right and left limbs.
- These limbs (horns) are continuous with corresponding dorsal aorta through first pair of pharyngeal arteries (Fig. 18.2).

Cardiovascular System I: Development of Heart

- Soon six pairs of pharyngeal arch arteries connect truncus arteriosus with dorsal aorta. All pharyngeal arch arteries run on either side of foregut (primitive pharynx).

Venous End of Heart Tube

- Unfused part of sinus venosus (venous end of heart tube) forms two horns (right and left).
- Each horn receives three veins (from lateral to medial)[Neet] (Figs 18.2 and 18.3):
  1. Common cardinal vein from the body wall
  2. Umbilical vein from the placenta
  3. Vitelline vein from the yolk sac.[MCQ]

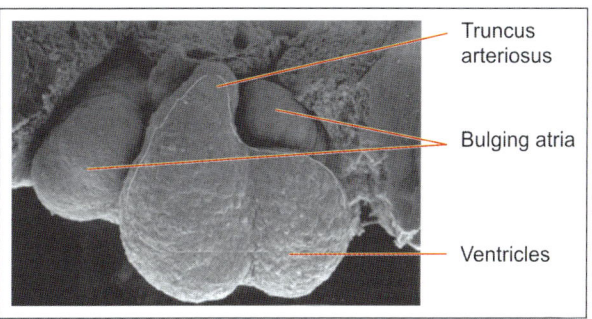

Scanning electron micrograph 18.4: External view of heart at 6 weeks [Species: Mouse, approximate human age: 6 weeks, ventral view]

FATE OF HEART TUBE[VIVA, MCQ]

The fate of the heart tube is summarised in Table 18.1.

Q. Enumerate derivative of different parts of heart tube.

Table 18.1	Fate of components of heart tube
Components of heart tube	Fate or derivative
Truncus arteriosus	• Ascending aorta • Pulmonary trunk
Bulbus cordis	• Conus arteriosus (smooth part of right ventricle) • Aortic vestibule (smooth part of left ventricle)
Primitive ventricle	• Trabeculated part of right and left ventricles
Primitive atrium	• Trabeculated part of right and left atrium
Sinus venosus[Neet]	• Right horn: Sinus venarum (smooth part of right atrium)[Neet] • Left horn: Coronary sinus and oblique vein of atrium[Neet]

ACQUISITION OF EXTERNAL FEATURES OF THE ADULT HEART

Heart tube undergoes growth and folding to acquire external features of the adult heart as follows (Figs 18.3 to 18.5):

- Initially, heart tube is placed longitudinally in pericardial cavity.
- Heart tube is suspended from dorsal wall of pericardial cavity by a fold of pericardium called *dorsal mesocardium* (Fig. 18.4).
- Formation of bulboventricular loop: Bulbus cordis and primitive ventricle grow ventrally and form bulboventricular loop (U-shaped).
- Formation of transverse sinus: The mesocardium connecting bulboventricular loop disappear to form a gap, that later called *transverse sinus* (Fig. 18.4).[Neet]
- Formation of S-loop: As primitive atrium and sinus venosus get freed from septum transversum, they come lie in the pericardial cavity dorso-cranial to the primitive ventricle and thus, S-shaped cardiac loop is formed.
- Bulbus cordis and primitive ventricle are separated by *bulboventricular sulcus* that later disappears and

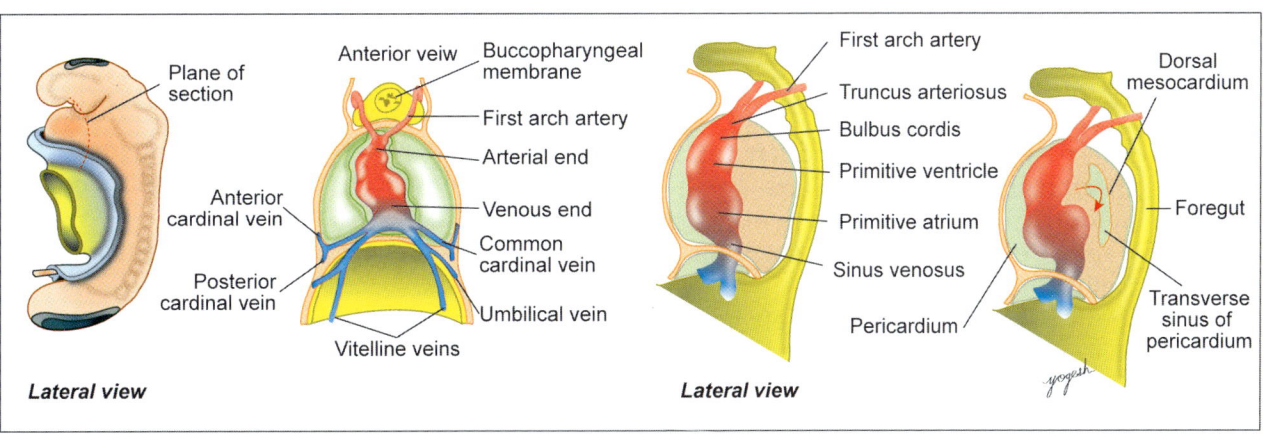

Fig. 18.4: Development of heart tube and mesocardium

bulbus cordis and ventricle fuse to form a single chamber (Fig. 18.5).

- **Formation of auricles:** Primitive atrium lies dorsal to (behind) the truncus arteriosus. On expansion, primitive atrium project forward on either side of truncus arteriosus as *auricles*.

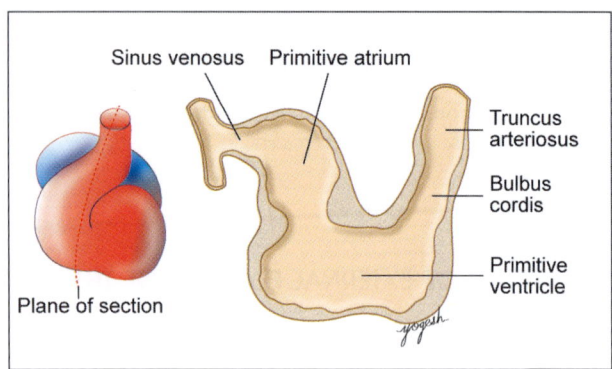

Fig. 18.5: Section of developing heart showing relationship of primitive atria and ventricles

DEVELOPMENT OF ATRIA

Atria of heart develop as follows.

Right Atrium^{MCQ}

Q. Write short note on development of right atrium.

Summary (Examination Guide)

1. Rough trabeculated part of right atrium and right auricle from right half of primitive atrium.
2. Smooth part of right atrium (sinus venarum) from sinus venosus.
3. Crista terminalis, valve of inferior vena cava and valve of coronary sinus develop from right venous valve.
4. A small area of most ventral smooth part develops from right half of atrioventricular canal.

Left Atrium^{MCQ, Viva}

Q. Write short note on development of left atrium.

Summary (Examination Guide)

1. Anterior rough part of left atrium and left auricle develop from left half of primitive atrium.
2. Posterior smooth part (between openings of pulmonary veins) develops from absorption of pulmonary veins.
3. Ventral smooth part develops from left half of atrioventricular canal.
   - Details of the development of atria are described in the following sections.

Sinus Venosus

Q. Write short note on sinus venosus.

Structure of sinus venosus (Figs 18.6 and 18.7)

- Sinus venosus is a caudal end of heart tube.
- It represents venosus end of developing heart.
- Its unfused part is called *right and left horns*.
- Each horn receives blood from various body parts as follows (Fig. 18.4):
  1. Vitelline vein from yolk sac
  2. Umbilical vein from placenta
  3. Common cardinal vein (duct of Cuvier) from body wall.
- Sinoatrial orifice: It is a communication between sinus venosus and primitive atrium.

Changes in left horn (Fig. 18.6)

- At the level of sinoatrial orifice, sickle-shaped sinoatrial fold develops. This fold separates left horn from primitive atrium, and thus left horn becomes just a tributary of the right horn.

Fate of sino-atrial orifice (Fig. 18.7)

- Initially, wide oval-shaped, transversely oriented sino-atrial orifice lies in the centre.
- On formation of sinoatrial fold, size of the orifice reduces and it becomes a narrow slit. Right margin of sinoatrial orifice is called *right venous valve*, whereas left margin is called *left venous valve*.
- Cranial fusion of these valves forms a fold called *septum spurium*, whereas caudal fusion form *sinus septum*.

Fate of tributaries of sinus venous^{MCQ}

- The tributaries of sinus venosus develop to form the following structures (Fig. 18.6):
  - Right common cardinal vein → part of superior vena cava
  - Right vitelline vein → terminal part of inferior vena cava
  - Left horn of sinus venosus and left common cardinal vein → coronary sinus
  - Left common cardinal vein → oblique vein of left atrium
  - Cephalic part of right posterior cardinal vein → arch of azygous vein
  - Right umbilical vein and left vitelline vein → obliterated by 5th week
  - Left common cardinal vein → obliterated by the 10th week.

For details, read Chapter 19. Right umbilical vein and left vitelline vein are obliterated in the fifth week. Left common cardinal vein is obliterated by 10th week.^{MCQ}

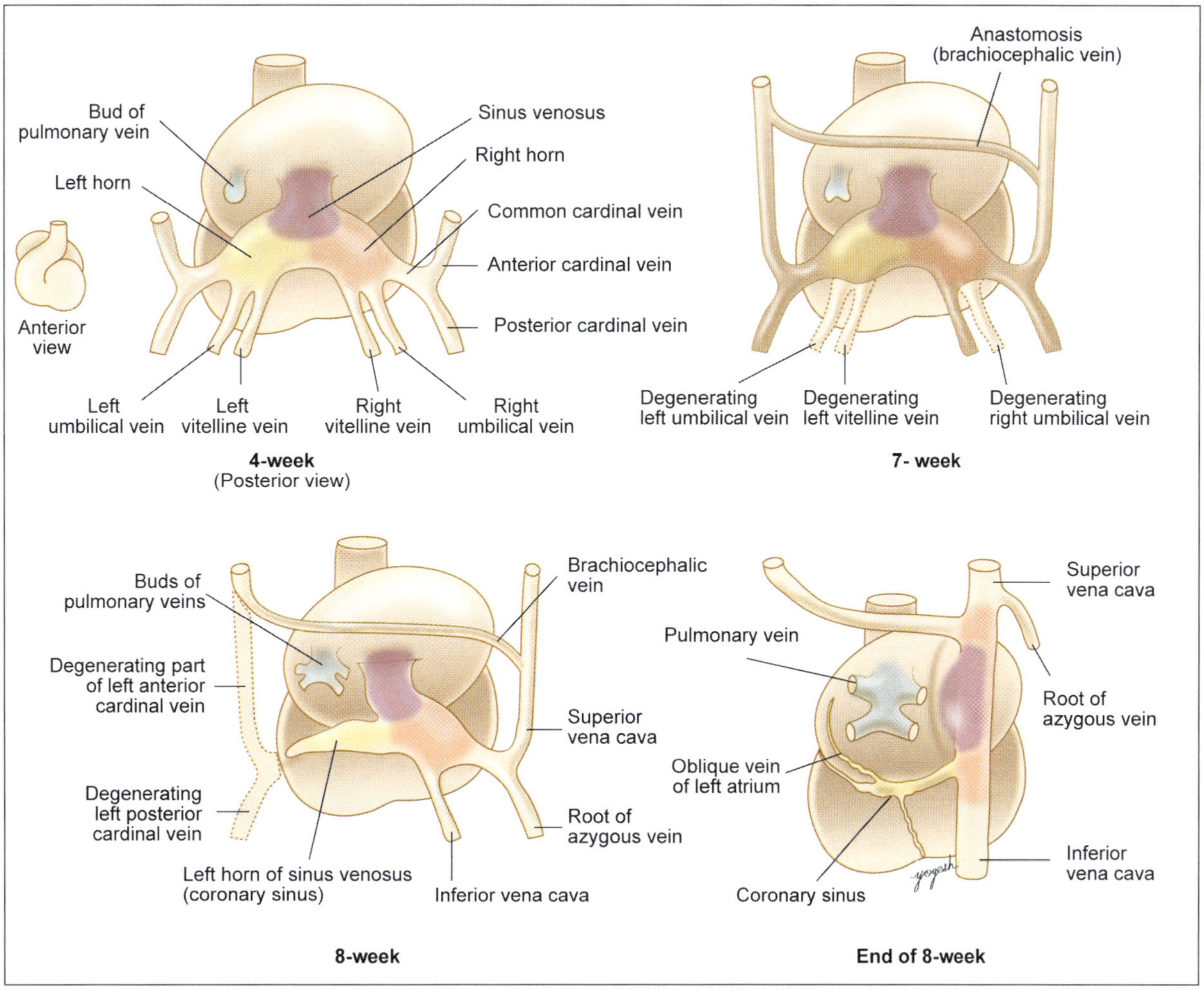

Cardiovascular System I: Development of Heart

Fig. 18.6: Development of sinus venosus and pulmonary veins

Changes in Atrioventricular Canal

- The communication between primitive atrium and primitive ventricle is an *atrioventricular canal*.
- AV cushions: Two atrioventricular (AV) cushions appear as thickening of subendocardial mesenchymal cells in ventral and dorsal wall of AV canal. Cardiac jelly forms around the heart tube during early development forms endocardial cushion and myocardium.^Neet
- Septum intermedium: AV cushions grow and fuse with each other to form *septum intermedium* and divide the AV canal into right and left halves.
- Major septa of heart are formed between 27th and 37th day of development.^MCQ

Development of Interatrial Septum

Q. Write short note on development of interatrial septum.

Interatrial septum develops in 5th week of intrauterine life from the following two sources (Practice Fig. 18.2):
1. septum primum and
2. septum secundum

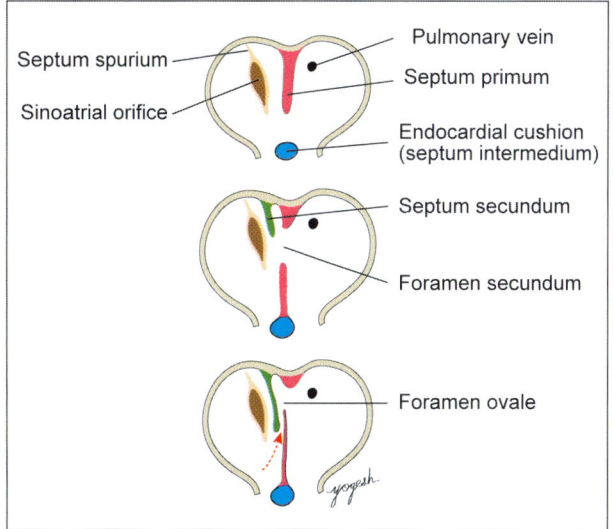

Practice Fig. 18.2: Development of interatrial septum

Stages of Development

1. *Septum primum*: At the end of fourth week, a *septum primum* starts developing from roof of primitive

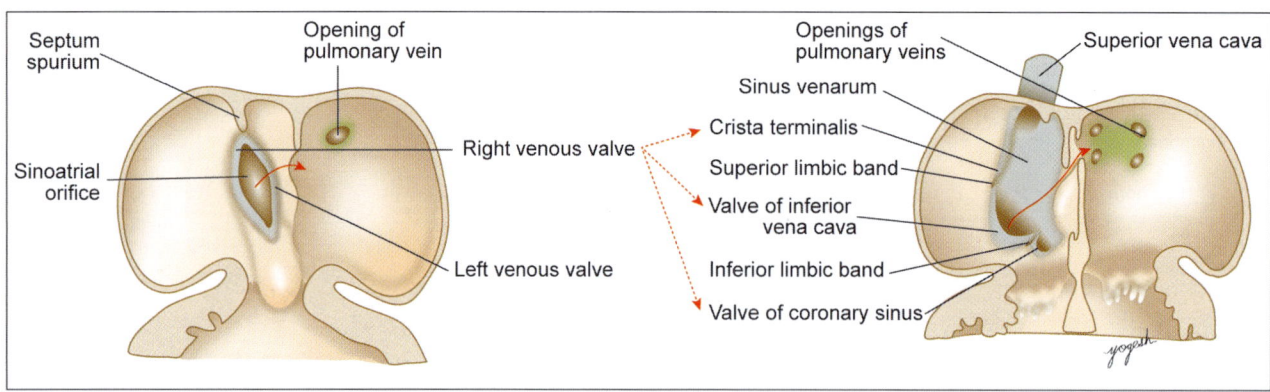

Fig. 18.7: Absorption of sinus venosus in the right atrium. Superior and inferior limbic bands divide right venous valve into three zones. Right venous valve forms crista terminalis, valve of inferior vena cava and valve of coronary sinus. Left venous valve fuse with the interatrial septum. Absorbed part of sinus venosus forms sinus venarum

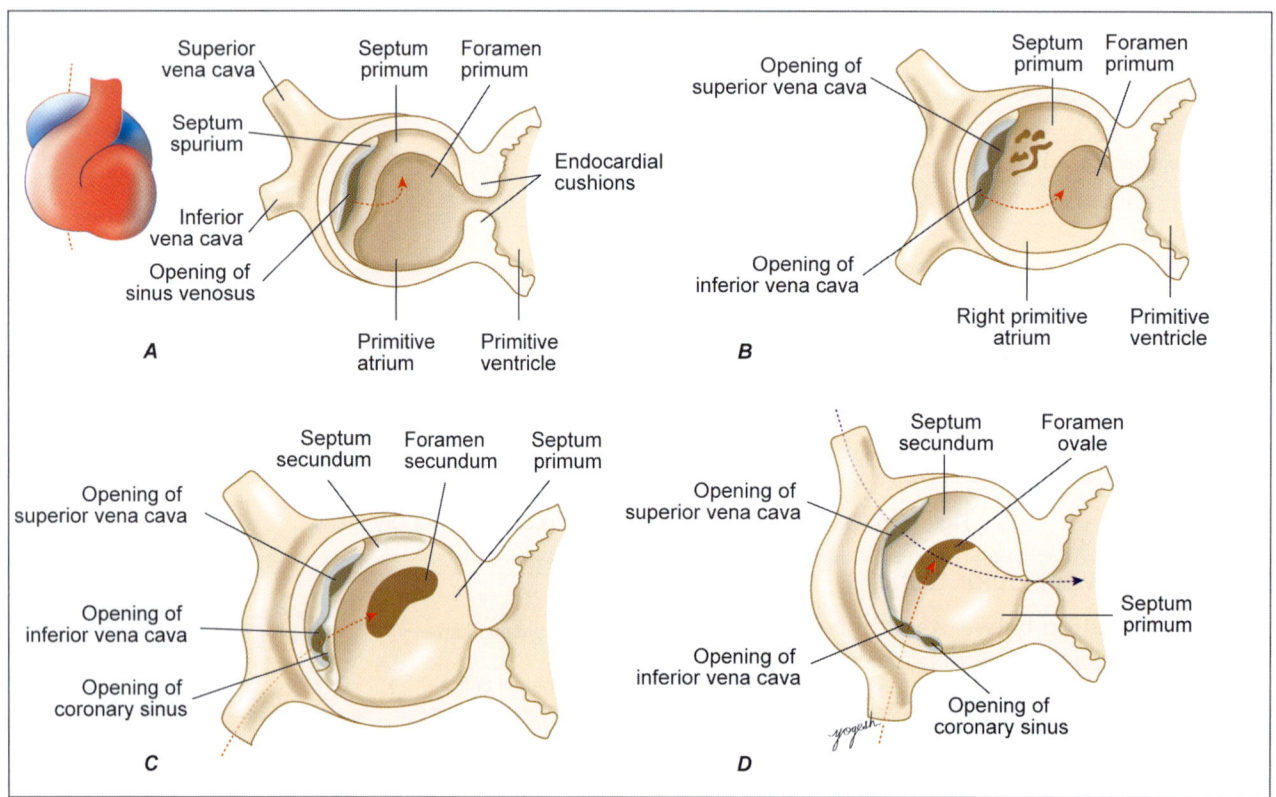

Fig. 18.8: Development of interatrial septum. Sagittal section of the developing heart seen from right side

atrium on left side of septum spurium and sinoatrial opening (Figs 18.8A, 18.9A).

2. *Foramen (ostium) primum*: Septum primum grows towards AV cushions (septum intermedium) and becomes sickle-shaped septum. A small gap between the growing septum primum and septum intermedium is called *foramen primum* (Fig. 18.8B).

3. *Foramen secundum*: Finally, septum primum fuses with AV cushions and that closes foramen primum. Simultaneously, a small gap as *foramen secundum* appears in the septum primum (Fig. 18.8C).

4. *Septum secundum*: A crescent-shaped *septum secundum* starts growing from roof of the primitive atrium between septum spurium and septum primum (Figs 18.8C, 18.9).

5. Foramen ovale: The septum secundum grows towards septum intermedium and overlaps foramen secundum. Overlapping septum secundum converts foramen secundum into an oblique passage called *foramen ovale* (Figs 18.8D, 18.9B).

6. After birth, foramen ovale obliterates and is represented as depression called *fossa ovalis*. The lower free margin of septum secundum forms the *annulus ovalis*.

Cardiovascular System I: Development of Heart

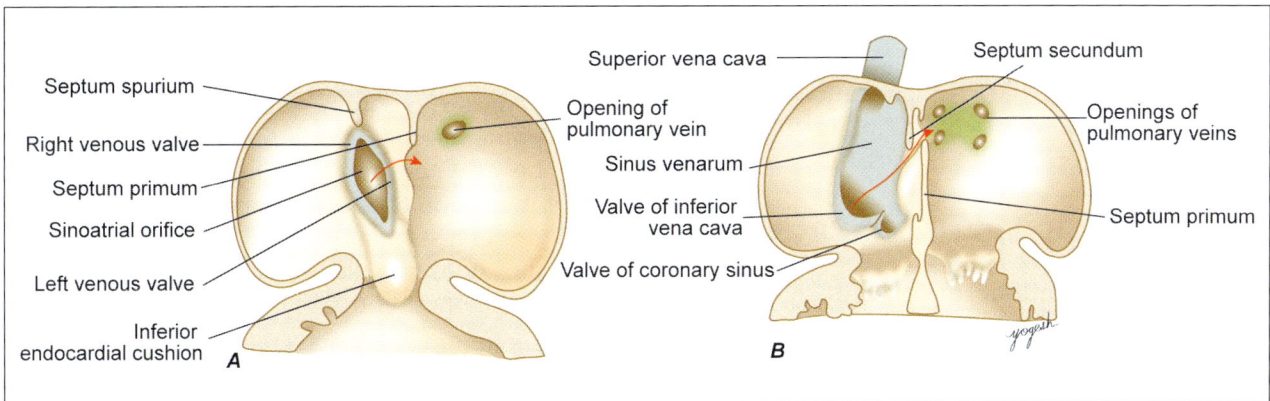

Fig. 18.9: Development of atria, interatrial septum and absorption of sinus venosus and pulmonary veins into the atria: (A) Coronal section passing through the atria at 5 weeks. Blue colour indicates the sinus venosus and green shading indicates pulmonary veins; (B) Coronary section of atria at the end of 8th week

Function of Foramen Ovale

- Foramen ovale is converted into a valve by opposition of thick-flap of septum secundum over thin mobile flap of septum primum.
- This valve allows transmission of blood from right atrium to left atrium, but blood cannot re-enter the right atrium.
- Thus, foramen ovale allows blood to bypass pulmonary circulation and shunts most of the blood from right atrium to left atrium instead of right ventricle.
- After birth:
  – Immediately after birth, pulmonary circulation begins and volume of blood returning to left atrium increases. It increases pressure in left atrium and produces physiological closure of foramen ovale (later it closes anatomically).

Formation of Sinus Venarum (absorption of sinus venosus in right atrium)

- The right and left horns of sinus venosus are absorbed into right atrium and results in segregation of openings of superior vena cava, inferior vena cava and coronary sinus from each other.
- Superior and inferior limbic bands (muscular bands) divide right venous valve into three zones.
- Right venous valve forms the following structures:
  1. Crista terminalis
  2. Valve of inferior vena cava
  3. Valve of coronary sinus
- Left venous valve fuse with interatrial septum.
- Absorbed part of sinus venosus forms sinus venarum.

Absorption of Pulmonary Veins into Left Atrium

- The dorsal wall of left atrium outpouches to form a primordial pulmonary vein.
- Single pulmonary vein divides into two and later into four pulmonary veins.
- Part of pulmonary veins get absorbed into dorsal wall of left atrium and openings of all four pulmonary veins get separated from each other.
- Absorbed portion of pulmonary veins forms smooth posterior part of left atrium.

Box 18.1: Dextrocardia

Definition

It is a congenital condition in that heart points to right side rather than the usual left side.
- Dexter in Latin means 'right' and Kardia in Greek means 'heart'.
- Dextrocardia is the most common positional anomaly of the heart.

Classification

It is classified as follows:
  A. Isolated dextrocardia: Only heart is placed on the right side of thorax.
  B. Dextrocardia invertus (situs invertus) refers to disposition (reversal) of all thoracic and abdominal viscera including heart.

Incidence: 1 in 7000 individuals.

Causes: Abnormal left-sided looping of heart tube instead of usual right-sided looping.

Ectopia Cordis

Q. Write short note on ectopia cordis.

- It is a rare congenital positional anomaly of heart.
- The heart lies exposed on anterior thoracic wall.
- Cause: Non-union of sternal halves.
- Treatment: Surgical repositioning of heart is not very successful due to high postpartum mortality (deaths).

Molecular Regulation

- Foregut endoderm secretes bone morphogenic proteins (BMP2 and BMP4) that induce expression of transcription factor NKX2.5 in splanchnic mesoderm and formation of heart tubes in cardiogenic area.
- NKX 2.5 is product of master gene for heart development. ^{MCQ}
- Simultaneously endoderm inhibits secretion of neural tube protein production as WNT proteins inhibit cardiogenic area.
- Laterality inducing genes (nodal and LEFTY-2 genes) are responsible for left sidedness of heart looping.

Box 18.2: Atrial septal defects (ASD)

- **Definition**
- Atrial septal defects are congenital anomalies that involve defective formation of interatrial septum resulting in an abnormal communication between right and left atria.
- **Incidence**
  6.4 in 10,000 births.
  More common in females (2:1) than in males.
- **Cause**: Mutation of NKX2.5.

- **Types**
  1. Ostium secundum defects (Fig. 18.10B)
     Failure of septum secundum to cover septum primum results in ostium secundum defect. It may be due to short septum secundum or more absorption of septum primum. Ostium secundum defect results information of large foramen ovale that does not close after birth. It is one of the commonest congenital heart diseases.
  2. Septum primum defect (Fig. 18.10C)
     Failure of septum primum to close foramen primum result in septum primum defect.
  3. Endocardial cushion defect ((Fig. 18.10D)
     Failure of fusion of septum primum with endocardial cushions (septum intermedium) results in persistent foramen primum.
  4. Sinus venosus ASD
     Incomplete absorption of sinus venosus in right atrium results in defective atrial septum near the opening of SVC.
  5. Common atrium/cortrioculare biventricularae (Fig. 18.10E) ^{MCQ}
     It is a rare condition with a failure of development of the interatrial septum.

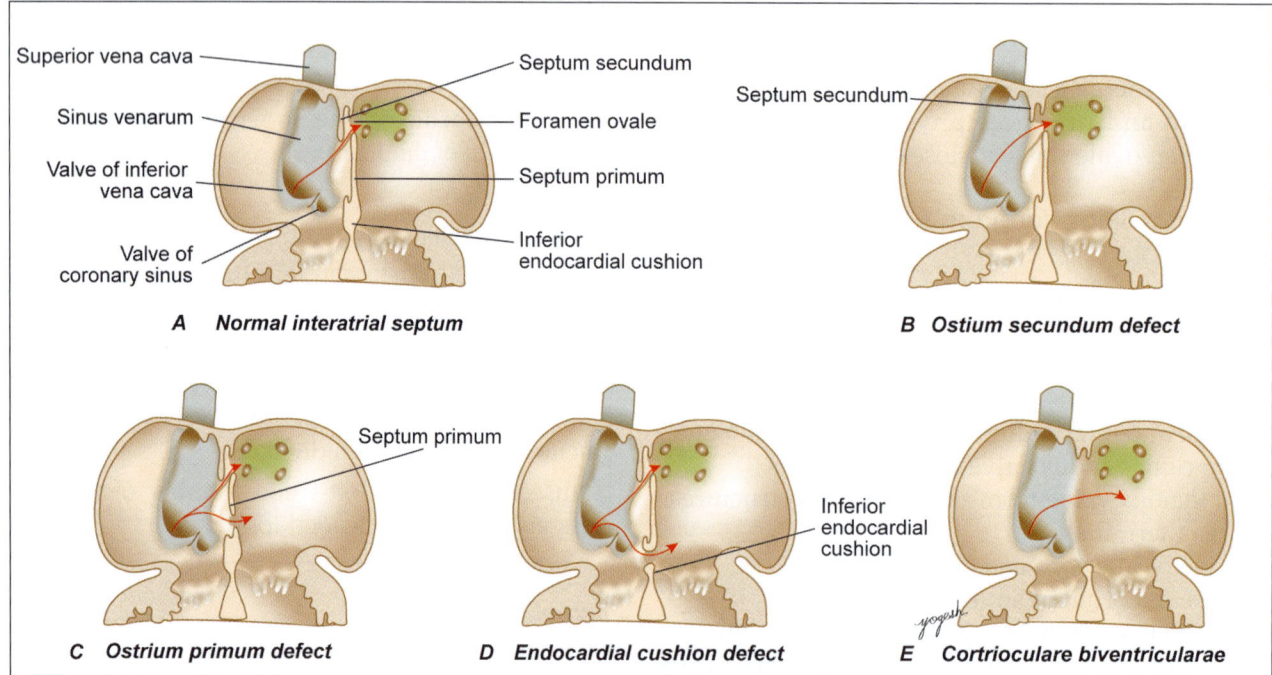

Fig. 18.10: Atrial septal defects involve the defective formation of interatrial septum resulting in an abnormal communication between the right and left atria. Ostium secundum defects are failure of septum secundum to cover septum primum. Ostium primum defect involves incomplete closure of foramen primum. Endocardial cushion defect is the result of failure of fusion of septum primum with endocardial cushions and persistent foramen primum. Common atrium or cortrioculare biventricularae is a failure of development of the interatrial septum

> **Box 18.3:** Probe patency of foramen ovale[Viva, MCQ]
> - Just after birth, foramen ovale closes physiologically by forced opposition of septum primum on septum secundum owing to:
>   1. Increased blood return to left atrium from lungs.
>   2. Increased pressure in left atrium.
> - Anatomical fusion also takes place soon.
> - In about 20% cases, anatomical fusion does not occur and a small probe can be passed through the foramen ovale.
> - Failure of fusion of septum primum with septum secundum results in patent foramen ovale.[Neet]

DEVELOPMENT OF VENTRICLES

Ventricles develop as follows:
  A. Rough (inflow) parts: From primitive ventricles.
  B. Smooth (outflow) parts (infundibulum of right ventricle and aortic vestibule of left ventricle): from conus or middle one-third of the bulbus cordis.

Bulbus Cordis

Q. Write short note on bulbus cordis.

- The arterial end of developing heart tube shows a dilatation called bulbus cordis.
- There are three parts of bulbus cordis as follows:
  1. Proximal one-third: It fuses with primitive ventricle to form *bulboventricular chamber*. Proximal one-third later form the trabeculated part of right ventricle.
  2. Middle one-third: It is called *conus cordis*. It forms outflow parts of both ventricles.
  3. Distal one-third: It is called *truncus arteriosus*. A spiral septum divides truncus arteriosus into pulmonary trunk and ascending aorta.

Formation of Interventricular Septum

Q. Write short note on development of interventricular septum.

- Interventricular septum separates right ventricle from left ventricle.

Summary (Examination Guide)

- It consists of three parts (Fig. 18.11, Practice Fig. 18.3):
  – Muscular part: Develops from muscular ridge arising on the floor of primitive ventricle.
  – Bulbar part: Develops from right and left bulbar ridges arising from conus cordis.
  – Membranous part: Develops from proliferation of AV cushion that fills the gap between muscular and bulbar parts.

Stages of Development

1. Muscular part
   - A muscular interventricular septum grows from the floor of bulboventricular cavity and divides ventricles into two halves.
   - It grows towards septum intermedium (AV cushion) and fuses partially with it.
   - Right and left ventricles communicate with each other through an interventricular foramen that lies cranial to the muscular interventricular foramen.

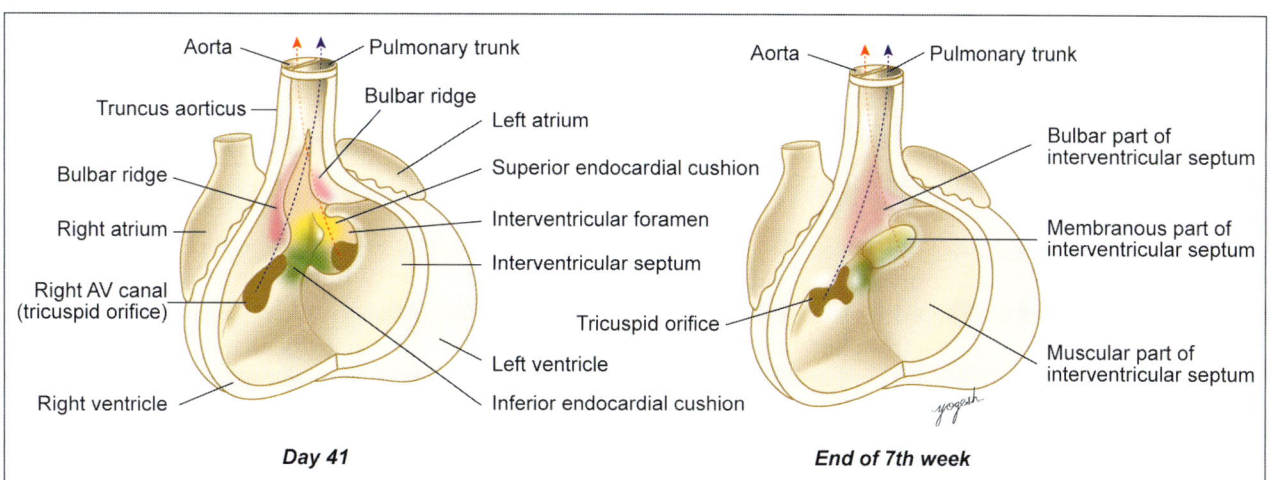

Fig. 18.11: Development of the interventricular septum. Muscular part of the interventricular septum develops from muscular ridge raising from the floor of primitive ventricle. Bulbar part develops from right and left bulbar ridges arising from conus cordis, whereas membranous part develops from the proliferation of AV cushion that fills the gap between muscular and bulbar parts

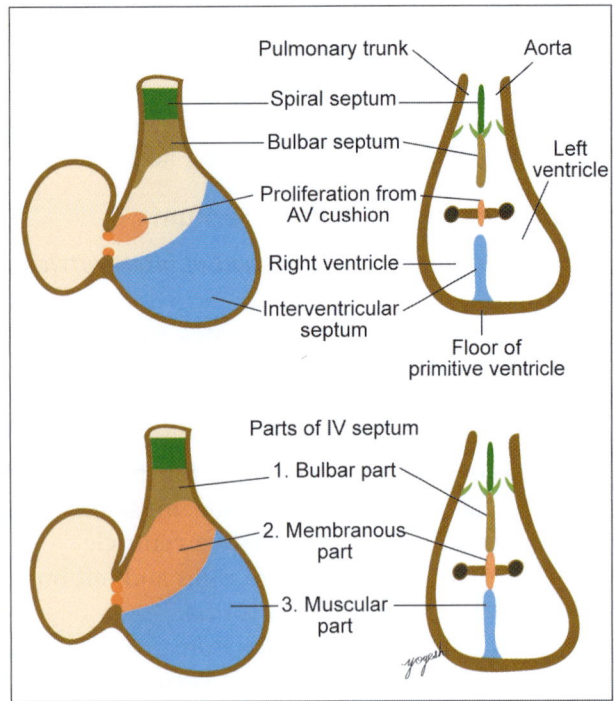

Practice Fig. 18.3: Development of interventricular septum

2. Bulbar part
   - From conical part of bulbar cordis, right and left bulbar ridges develop and later fuse to form a bulbar part of the septum.
   - Bulbar part grows caudally towards muscular part of interventricular septum.
   - The right and left ventricle communicate with each other through the interventricular foramen that lies between muscular and bulbar parts.
3. Membranous part
   - By 8th week, gap of interventricular foramen is filled by tissue that proliferates from right side of AV cushions and right and left bulbar ridges. It forms a membranous part.
   - Presence of interventricular foramen is essential until separation of bulbus cordis and truncus arteriosus.
   - Anterior portion of membranes part of interventricular septum is derived from AV cushions and it separates right and left ventricles.^{Neet}
   - Posterior atrioventricular portion of membranous part of IV septum is derived from AV cushions and it separates right atrium from left ventricle.^{Neet}

Formation of Aorticopulmonary Septum

- In the truncus arteriosus, a *spiral septum* called *aorticopulmonary septum* appears (Fig. 18.12).
- This septum divides truncus arteriosus (aorticus) into aorta and pulmonary trunk.

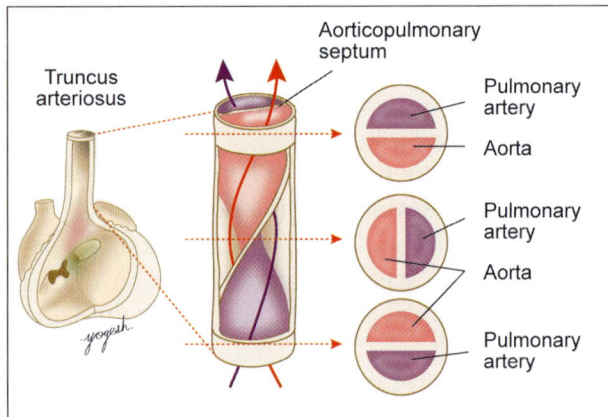

Fig. 18.12: Development of truncus arteriosus. Spiral aorticopulmonary septum divides the truncus arteriosus into aorta and pulmonary trunk. Note the changes in relationship of aorta and pulmonary trunk

Steps

1. Truncal ridges: Two truncal ridges appear in truncus arteriosus that grow and fuse to form the *spiral septum*.
2. Fusion with bulbar septum: Spiral septum lies in same plane as that of bulbar septum and grows to fuse with bulbar septum. Here, aorta lies behind the pulmonary trunk.
3. Spiralling of septum: Spiral septum separates aorta and pulmonary trunk in a spiral course. Aorta that lies behind the pulmonary trunk in the lower part, come to lie on the right side and finally anterior to the pulmonary trunk.

Transposition of great vessels

- Transposition of ascending aorta and pulmonary trunk may occur due to reverse spiral attachment of aortic-pulmonary septum. In this condition, aorta raises from the right ventricle, whereas pulmonary trunk from the left ventricle. Incidence of transposition of great vessels is 4.8 in 10,000 births.

DEVELOPMENT OF VALVES OF HEART

Atrioventricular Valves

- Tricuspid valve is present between right atrium and right ventricle, whereas mitral valve is present between left atrium and left ventricle (Fig. 18.13).
- Proliferation of subendocardial mesenchyme forms subendocardial cushions around atrioventricular canals.
- Excavation of these cushions forms cusps of AV valves.
- Free margins of these cusps get connected by thin chordae tendinae with papillary muscles of ventricular wall.

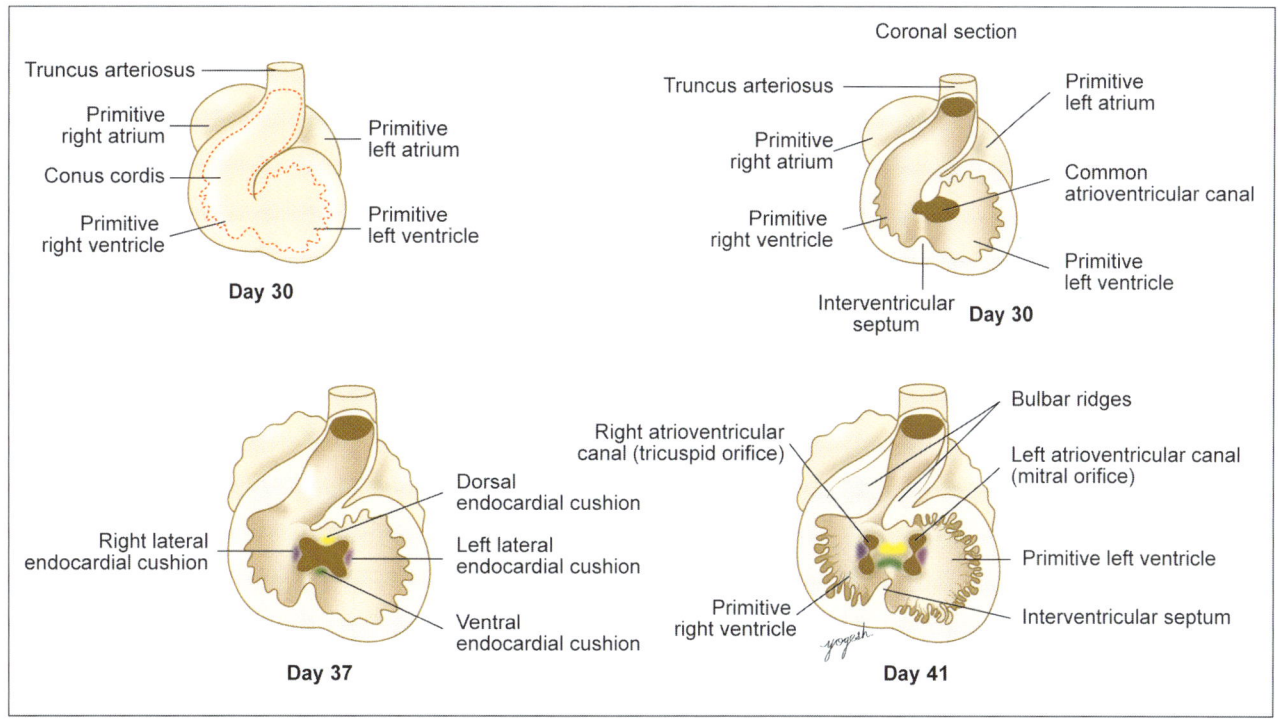

Fig. 18.13: Formation of septum in the atrioventricular canal

- On the right side, there are three cushions—anterior, posterior and septal, whereas on the left there are two cushions—anterior and posterior. Hence, on right, there is a tricuspid valve and on left, bicuspid (mitral) valve.

Pulmonary and Aortic Valves

- In trucus arteriosus, two endocardial cushions appear (right and left). Soon two more (anterior and posterior) cushions also appear (Fig. 18.14).
- On separation of the pulmonary trunk from aorta by a spiral septum, right and left cushions divide into two parts.
- Excavation of these cushions form cusps of aortic and pulmonary valves.
- Aorta and pulmonary trunk undergo spiral rotation and finally, valves show the following cusps:
  - Aortic valve: One anterior and two posterior
  - Pulmonary valve: One posterior and two anterior

DEVELOPMENT OF CONDUCTING SYSTEM OF HEART

Conducting system of heart is formed during 5th week. The components of conducting system of heart develop as follows:

1. SA node: SA node develops during the fifth week of IUL. After incorporation of sinus venosus into right atrium, SA node comes to lie near opening of SVC.
2. AV node and bundle of His: AV node and bundle of His are derived from interatrial septum near opening of the coronary sinus. It develops from dorsal endocardial cushion of AV canal in 6th week of IUL.
3. Purkinje fibres: Fibres from bundle of His form right and left bundle branches that get distributed as Purkinje fibres.

DEVELOPMENT OF PERICARDIUM

Q. Write short note on development of pericardium.

Summary (Examination Guide)

Pericardium is derived as follows:
- Serous pericardium
  - Visceral layer from splanchnopleuric mesoderm
  - Parietal layer from somatopleuric mesoderm
- Fibrous pericardium from somatopleuric mesoderm and septum transversum.
- Pericardial cavity from intraembryonic coelom.

Stages of Development

1. On head folding, pericardial cavity comes to lie on ventral aspect of foregut.
2. Heart tube with myoepicardial mantle invaginates pericardial cavity.
3. Layer of myoepicardial mantle that lines the pericardial cavity forms visceral layer of pericardium (epicardium).
4. Initially, heart tube is suspended in pericardial cavity by *dorsal mesocardium* (double-layer fold similar to mesentery).

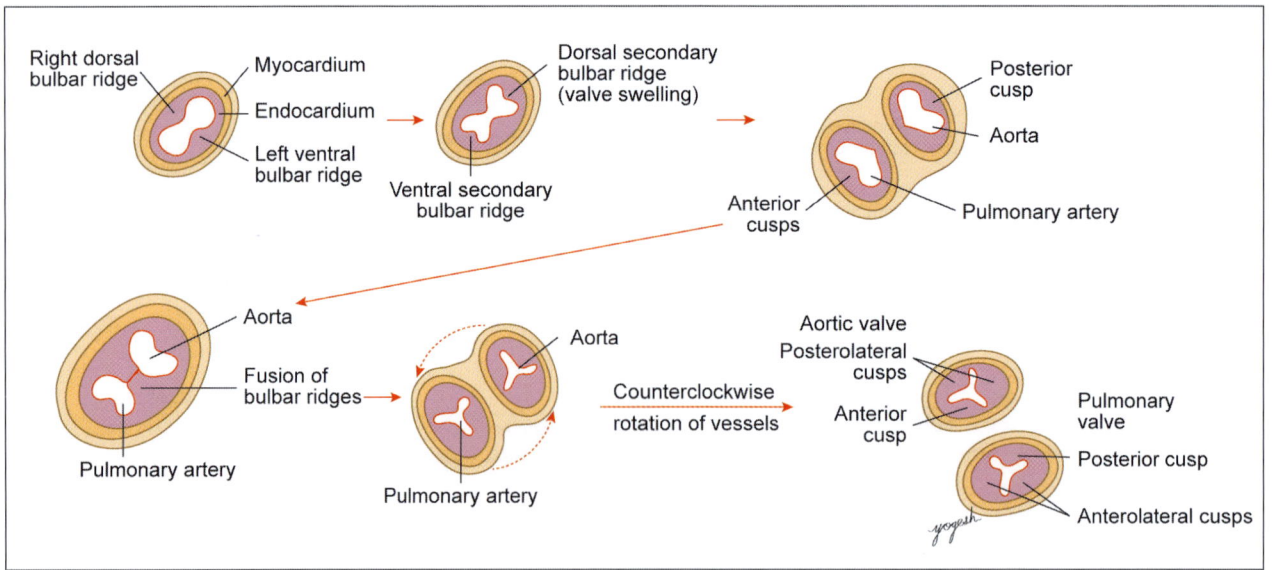

Fig. 18.14: Development of aortic and pulmonary valves (semilunar valves)

5. On formation of a cardiac loop, arterial and venous ends of heart tube come closer and dorsal mesocardium disappears to form *transverse sinus of pericardium*.
6. On formation of transverse sinus, fibrous and visceral pericardium become continuous with each other at arterial and venous ends of heart tube.
7. Somatopleuric layer of mesoderm lining pericardial cavity forms parietal pericardium and fibrous pericardium.
8. Reorientation of SVC, IVC and absorption of pulmonary veins in the left atrium results into formation of *oblique sinus of pericardium*.

Some Interesting Facts
- Appearance of paired angioblastic cords is first sign of development of heart.
- Heart is the first organ of the body to start functioning. Cardiovascular system is the earliest system that start functioning in foetus.^Neet
- Heart tubes are formed in the third week.
- Heart beats begin by 22nd day of IUL.^Neet
- Heart develops completely by 10th week (3rd month).^Neet
- Somatopleuric mesoderm forms myocardium, Purkinje fibres (conduction system of heart).^Neet
- Fallot tetralogy is the most common congenital cyanotic heart disease.
- Unequal division of conus cordis resulting for anterior displacement of conotruncal septum give rise to Fallot's tetralogy.^Neet

- Ventricular septal defect is almost common congenital anomaly of the heart.
- Between 18th and 22nd weeks of IUL, foetal heart echocardiography and Doppler ultrasonography is useful for detecting abnormal foetal heart anatomy.
- Real-time ultrasound can detect foetal heart anomalies even by 16th week.

Box 18.4: Tetralogy of Fallot (TOF)
Fallot's tetralogy

Q. Write short note on Fallot's tetralogy.
Q. Give embryological basis of Fallot's tetralogy.

- TOF is a congenital heart defect.
- Components (Fig. 18.15, Practice Fig. 18.4):
  1. Pulmonary stenosis
  2. Right ventricular or hypertrophy
  3. Ventricle septal defect (VSD)
  4. Overriding of aorta

Incidence
- It is the most common congenital cyanotic heart disease.
- Incidence of TOF is 9.6 in 10,000 births
- TOF is the most common cyanotic heart disease.
- TOF accounts for 6–10% of all CHDs.

Cause
- Mostly unknown.
- Associates with maternal phenylketonuria.
- Responsible genes: VAG1, NKX2.5.

Contd.

Cardiovascular System I: Development of Heart

Diagnosis
1. Echocardiography.
2. X-ray chest: *Coeur en sabot* (boot-like) appearance of a heart.^{MCQ}

Pathophysiology

Pulmonary stenosis causes concentric right ventricular hypertrophy without cardiac enlargement
↓
Increase in right ventricular pressure
↓
Blood shunts from right ventricle to left ventricle through VSD
↓
Ejection of mixed blood to aorta → cyanosis
↓
Overriding of aorta (disposition)

Clinical manifestation
- Blue-baby: Cyanotic lips and nail bed.
- Easy fatigability.
- Tell-spells: Acute hypoxic spells characterised by shortness of breath, cyanosis, agitation and loss of consciousness (syncope).

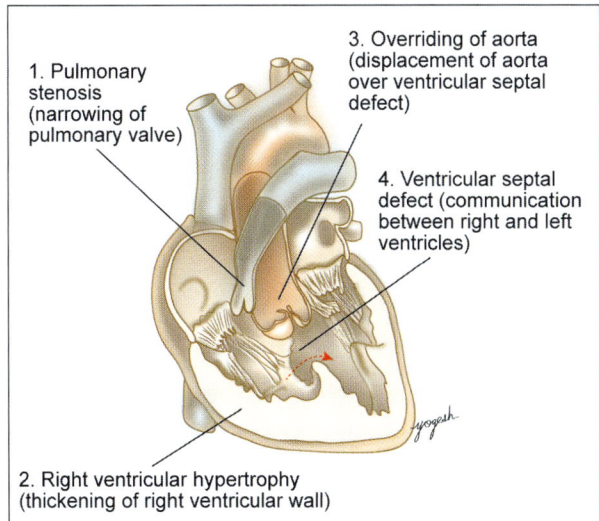

Fig. 18.15: Tetralogy of Fallot. It includes pulmonary stenosis, right ventricular hypertrophy, overriding of aorta and ventricular septal defect

Some Interesting Facts
- **Taussig-Bing syndrome:** It is a ventricular septal defect having a. Double outlet right ventricle, b. Subpulmonic ventricular septal defect (Fig. 18.16).

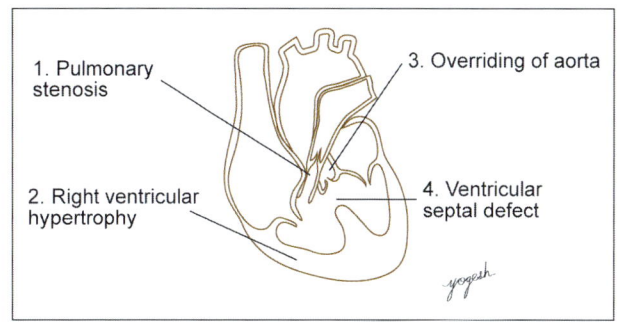

Practice Fig. 18.4: Tetralogy of Fallot

- **Holt-Oram syndrome**: Preaxial limb abnormalities with ASD. Cause: TBX5 gene mutation (autosomal dominant). *Note*: TBX5 gene is responsible for limb development and septation of heart.
- **Eisenmenger's complex**
  - It includes hypoplasia of pulmonary capillary plexus that causes
    1. Pulmonary hypertension
    2. Dilatation of pulmonary trunk
    3. Hypertrophy of right ventricle.
  - If Eisenmenger's complex is associated with ASD or VSD, then it is called Eisenmenger's syndrome.

Ventricular Septal Defects (VSD)
- VSD is the most common congenital anomaly of the heart.
- VSDs are more common in males than in females.
- VSD commonly involves the membranous part of interventricular septum.
- Incidence isolated VSD is 12 in 10,000 births.

Embryological basis

Failure of fusion of right and left bulbar ridges with AV cushions
↓
Communication between ventricles
↓
Shunting of blood from left ventricles to right ventricle

TIMING OF EMBRYOLOGIC HEART FORMATION

Days 21–22	Umbilical veins, vitelline veins, cardinal veins form
	Single heart tube forms
	Pericardial cavity forms
	Heart begins to beat
Day 23	Heart tube grows rapidly, heart folding begins
Days 25–28	Atrioventriculobulbar loop forms
	Septum primum appears

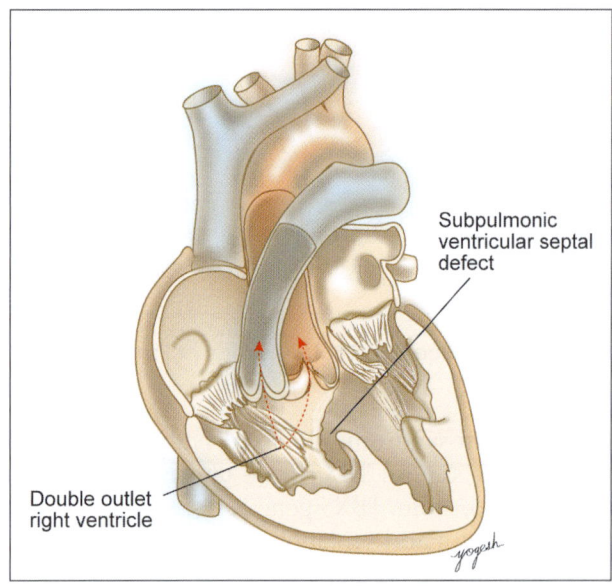

Fig. 18.16: Taussig-Bing syndrome. It is a ventricular septal defect having double outlet right ventricle and subpulmonic ventricular septal defect

Days 27–37	Endocardial cushions appear
Days 28	Ventricular septum appears as a small ridge in common ventricle
Days 28–35	Absorption of bulbous cordis and sinus venosus
	Four-chambered heart forms
Day 29	Pulmonary veins form
Days 31–35	Placental circulation begins
	Atrioventricular node develops
	Ostium secundum forms
	Sinoatrial node develops
Day 33	Tricuspid and mitral valves form
Days 35–42	Coronary arteries form
Days 36–42	Inferior vena cava forms
Days 43–49	Superior vena cava forms
	Coronary sinus forms
Day 49	Muscular interventricular septum forms
Day 56	Aorta and pulmonary arteries form
	Aortic and pulmonic valves form

CLINICAL EMBRYOLOGY

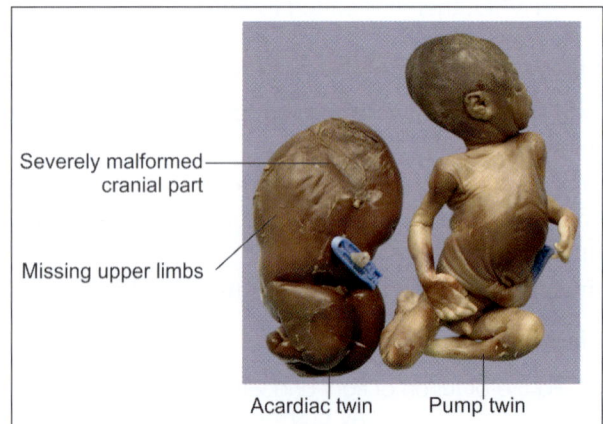

Clinical image 18.1: Acardiac twins [twin reversed-arterial perfusion (TRAP) sequence]: It is a rare and serious complication of monochorionic twins. The blood systems of twins are connected. One twin is acardiac and other one is pump twin. Acardiac twin is severely malformed. Its heart may be missing or deformed. The legs may be partially present or missing. Acardiac twin has reversed arterial perfusion because the blood flows in a reversed direction. The pump twin is usually normal and it drives blood through both foetuses (Image courtesy: *Dr Mamatha Gowda, Dr Haritha Sagili*)

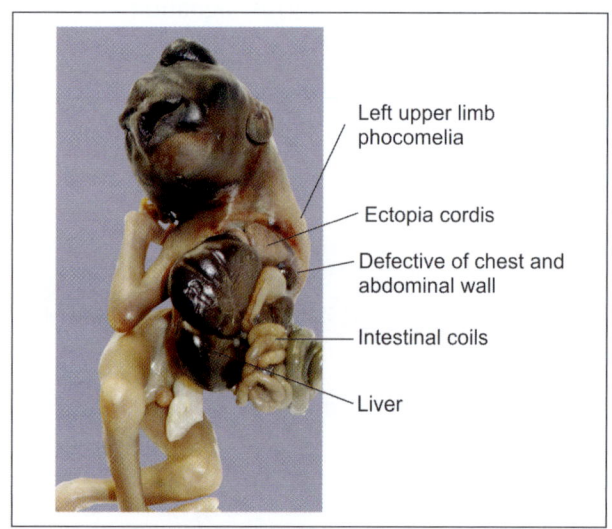

Clinical image 18.2: Ectopia cordis with left upper limb phocomelia. Congenital defect of chest wall associated with diaphragmatic hernia with ectopia cordis and omphalocele. Phocomelia is malformations of arms and legs. In the above case, left upper limb is completely absent. Thalidomide intake by mother may give rise to phocomelia (Image courtesy: *Dr Mamatha Gowda*)

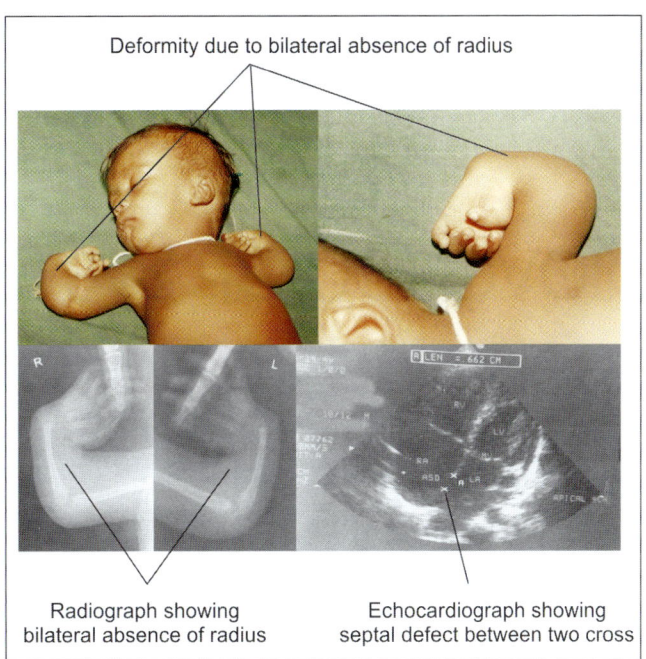

Clinical image 18.3: Holt-Oram syndrome (ventriculoradial syndrome): It is an autosomal dominant disorder caused due to TBX5 gene mutation. It includes absence of radius bone and atrial septal defect. Its incidence is 1 in 10,000 people. It may also show absence of carpal bones and heart block. Abbreviations: RA: Right atrium, RV: Right ventricle, LV: Left ventricle, LA: Left atrium, MV: Mitral valve, ASD: Atrial septal defect (Image courtesy: *Dr Kumaravel S*)

19

Cardiovascular System II
Blood Vessels and Foetal Circulation

Chapter Outline

- Erythropoiesis
- Development of arterial system
- Pharyngeal arch arteries
  - Changes in arch arteries and aortae
  - Patent ductus arteriosus
  - Unusual origin of aorta
  - Coarctation of aorta
  - Branches of dorsal aorta
- Umbilical arteries
- Development of vertebral artery
- Development of limb vessels
- Development of venous system
- Vitelline veins
- Umbilical veins
- Somatic veins
  - Primary head vein
  - Cervicothoracic vein
  - Anomalies of superior vena cava
  - Subcardinal veins
  - Supracardinal veins
  - Posterior cardinal veins
  - Azygous venous lines
- Renal collar
- Development of inferior vena cava
  - Anomalies of inferior vena cava
- Development of azygous venous system

Foetal circulation
- Special structures in foetal circulation
- Peculiarities of foetal circulation
- Circulatory changes at birth

Development of lymphatic system

INTRODUCTION

- Development of blood vessels begins in the third week of development.
- It involves vasculogenesis and angiogenesis.
- Vasculogenesis is formation of new vessels from mesenchymal tissue in the embryo (Fig. 19.1).
- Angiogenesis is the sprouting of vessels into adjacent area by endothelial budding (Fig. 19.1).
- Formation of vasculature begins in extraembryonic mesoderm of yolk sac, connecting stalk and chorion.
- Yolk sac is the first supplier of blood cells and it continues up to 60 days as a haematopoietic

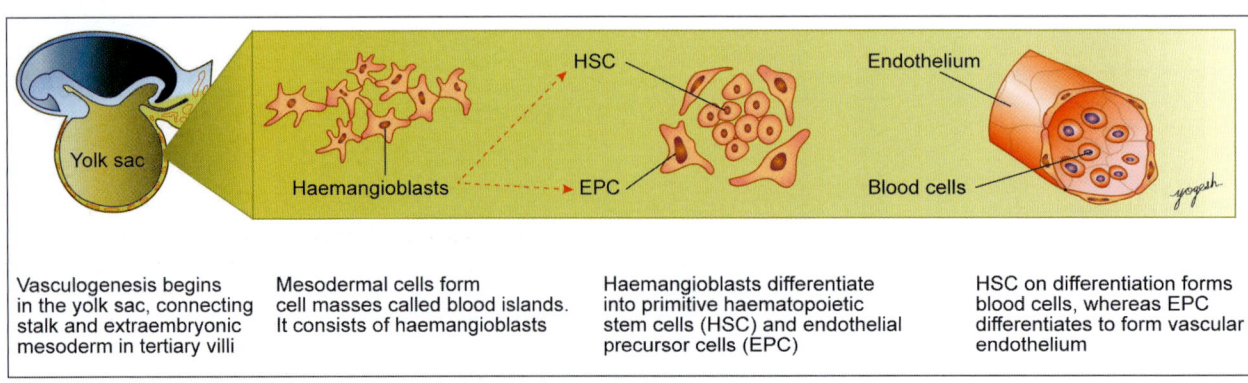

Fig. 19.1: Vasculogenesis

organ.^MCQ Later liver, spleen, thymus and bone marrow takes over the haematopoietic function.

> **Box 19.1:** Erythropoiesis
>
> - It is a process of formation of new red blood cells.
> - It begins in yolk sac wall and continue till death in the following phases.
>
> | Period/Phase ^Neet | Age | Organ |
> |---|---|---|
> | **Intravascular** | 3 weeks to 3rd month of intrauterine life | Wall of yolk sac |
> | **Hepatic and extramedullary** | 2–3 months^Neet to 5–7 months of IUL | Liver (major organ)^Neet Spleen, lymph nodes^Neet |
> | **Myeloid (medullary)** | 8–9 months of IUL and continue in post-natal life | Red bone marrow |

Note: After 20 years of age, erythropoiesis occurs mostly in flat bones such as sternum, ribs, ilium, vertebrae and in proximal ends of humerus, femur and tibia.

DEVELOPMENT OF ARTERIAL SYSTEM

In the fourth week, the following vessels are present in embryo (Fig. 19.2):
- A heart tube
- Arteries
  1. Aortic end of heart tube
  2. Aortic arch arteries connecting aortic end of heart to dorsal aortae (Fig. 19.3)
  3. Two dorsal aortae lie in front of notochord
  4. Vitelline arteries supply blood to yolk sac
  5. Umbilical arteries carry blood to placenta
- Veins
  1. Venous end of heart tube
  2. Common cardinal vein brings blood from embryo to heart tube through anterior and posterior cardinal veins
  3. Vitelline veins from the yolk sac
  4. Two umbilical veins from the placenta

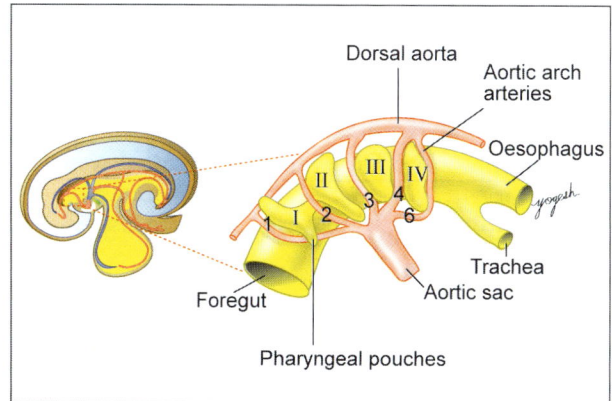

Fig. 19.3: Relation of the pharyngeal arch arteries with foregut

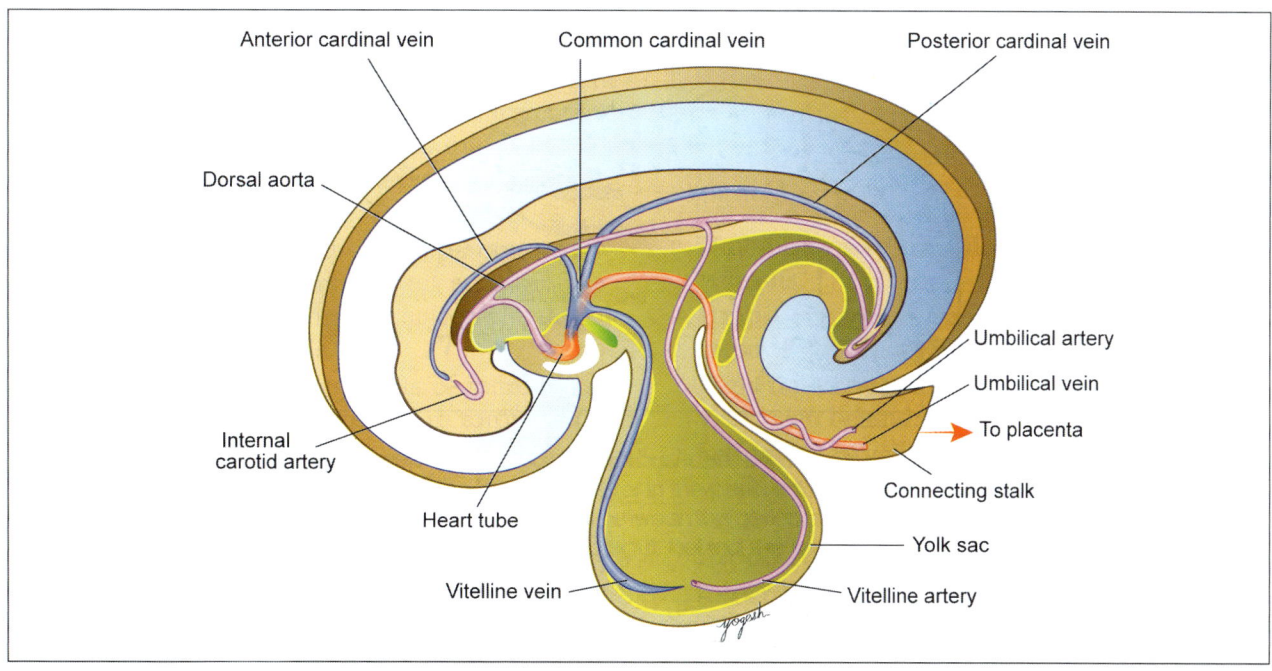

Fig. 19.2: Major vessels of embryo

Human Embryology

PHARYNGEAL ARCH ARTERIES

- Two primitive aortae arise from arterial end of heart tube (Fig. 19.4).
- These primitive aortae curve to reach near notochord and finally to reach caudal end of the foetus.
- Due to the course, primitive aortae are divided into three parts as follows:
  1. *Ventral aortae* that lies ventral to foregut.
  2. *Dorsal aortae* that lie dorsal to foregut.
  3. *First aortic arch artery* that connects ventral aortae with dorsal aortae and passes through first pharyngeal arch (Figs 19.3 and 19.4).
- Ventral aortae fuse in the midline to form heart tube.
- Near the fused heart tube, part of ventral aortae dilates to form *aortic sac*, whereas an unfused part of ventral aortae forms right and left horn of the sac (Figs 19.3 and 18.3 from Chapter 18).
- Also called *aortic arch arteries*.
- Pharyngeal arches appear during 4th and 5th weeks.
- Each arch is supplied by an artery called *pharyngeal arch artery*.
- Each pharyngeal arch artery connects aortic sac with dorsal aorta (Fig. 19.4).
- Initially, there are six pairs of aortic arch arteries. Later, fifth pair disappears along with fifth pharyngeal arch. In 50% of embryos, 5th aortic arch is never formed.^{Neet}
- Pharyngeal arch arteries are numbered craniocaudally as I, II, III, IV and IV.
- All 6 aortic arches are not present simultaneously.^{Neet}

Derivatives of Aortic Arch Arteries

Q. Write short note on development of: Arch of aorta, subclavian artery, pulmonary arteries, carotid arteries.

Derivatives of aortic arch arteries are as follows (Fig. 19.4, Table 19.1):

1, 2. First and second arch arteries mostly disappears leaving behind
   – Maxillary artery from first pharyngeal arch artery
   – Hyoid and stapedial arteries from second arch artery
3. Third arch artery forms common carotid artery, proximal part of internal carotid artery and external carotid artery
4. Fourth arch artery forms
   On left side: Part of arch of aorta
   On right side: Proximal part of right subclavian artery
5. Fifth arch artery disappears
6. Sixth arch artery:
   On left side: Left pulmonary artery and ductus arteriosus (ligamentous arteriosus after birth)
   On right side: Right pulmonary artery

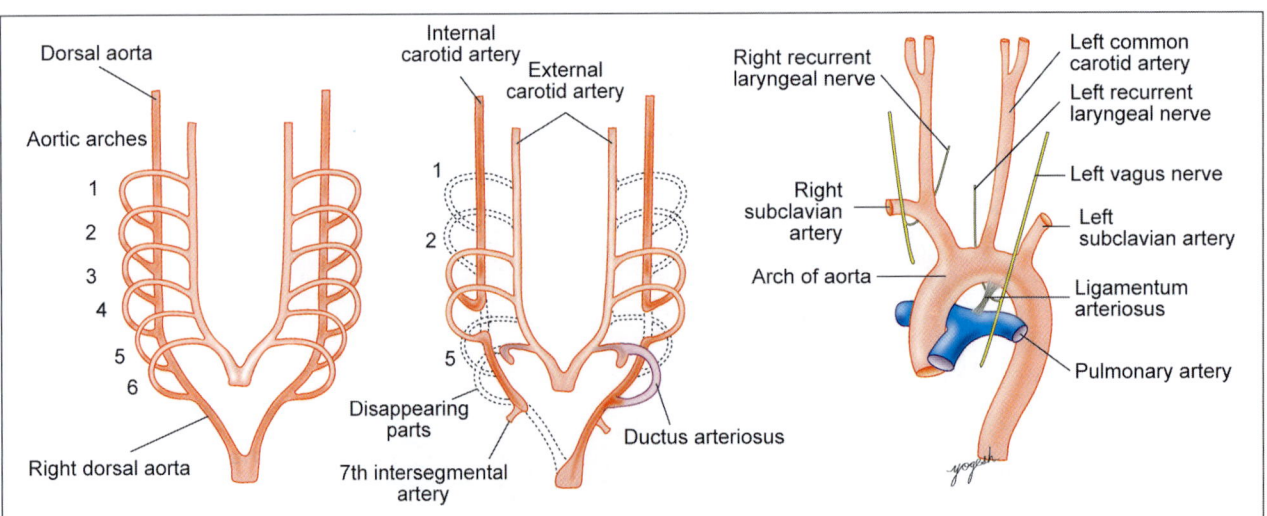

Fig. 19.4: Derivatives of pharyngeal arch arteries. First and second arch arteries mostly disappear leaving behind maxillary artery from first pharyngeal arch artery and hyoid and stapedial arteries from second arch artery (not shown in this Fig.). Third arch artery forms common carotid artery, proximal part of internal carotid artery and external carotid artery. Fourth arch artery forms part of arch of aorta on left side and proximal part of right subclavian artery on the right. Fifth arch artery disappears. Sixth arch artery forms left pulmonary artery and ductus arteriosus (ligamentous arteriosus after birth) on the left and right pulmonary artery on the right

Cardiovascular System II: Blood Vessels and Foetal Circulation

Table 19.1 Derivatives of pharyngeal arch arteries. In 50% of embryos, 5th aortic arch is never formed.*High yielding facts, Neet*

Arch artery	Fate
I	Maxillary artery
II	Stapedial artery; Hyoid artery
III	Common carotid artery Proximal part of internal carotid artery External carotid artery
IV	Left side: Part of arch of aorta Right side: Proximal part of right subclavian artery*Neet*
V	Disappears
VI	Left side: Left pulmonary artery ductus arteriosus (after birth: Ligamentum arteriosus) Right side: Right pulmonary artery

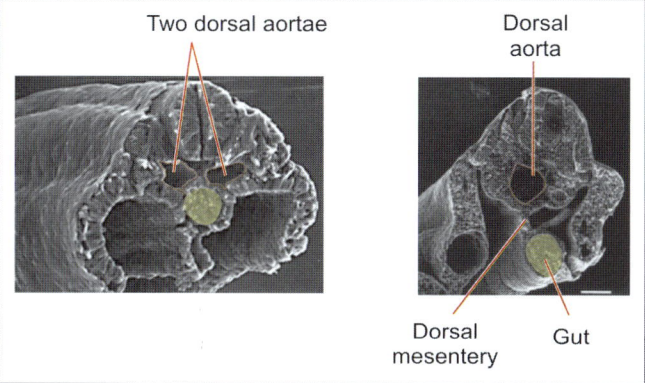

Scanning electron micrograph 19.1: Formation of single dorsal aorta. As development progresses, paired dorsal aortae form a single central vessel [Species: Mouse, approximate human age: 27–28 transverse section]

Changes in Arch Arteries and Aortae

- Dorsal aortae remain separated in the region of pharyngeal arch arteries. Caudal to sixth arch artery, dorsal aortae fuse to form a single dorsal aorta that later forms descending thoracic and abdominal aorta (Table 19.2).
- On development of spiral septum, ascending aorta blood enters third and fourth arch arteries, whereas pulmonary trunk blood is diverted to sixth arch arteries.
- Carotid duct (ductus caroticus): It is portion of dorsal aortae between third and fourth arch arteries. It disappears completely (Table 19.3).

Following Portions Disappear

1. Most of the part of first and second arch arteries
2. Ductus caroticus
3. Right dorsal aorta caudal to fourth aortic arch artery
4. Fifth aortic arch
5. Distal half of sixth arch artery on right artery

   – Ductus aorticus: It is distal portion of sixth aortic arch artery that connects left pulmonary artery with left dorsal aorta

Following Overgrowths Occur

1. Dorsal aortae grow cranially beyond the attachment of first aortic arch artery and form a part of internal carotid artery.
2. Bud form third artery gives rise to external carotid artery.*MCQ*
3. Communication of seventh intersegmental artery with dorsal aorta at the level of fourth arch artery and participate in formation of subclavian arteries.
4. Proximal part of right third and fourth arteries fuse to form brachiocephalic artery that arises from aortic sac.

Table 19.2 Development of major arteries*High yielding, Neet*

Artery	Embryonic source
Arch of aorta	Aortic sac (fused part of ventral aortae)
	Left horn aortic sac (unfused left ventral aortic arch)
	Left fourth arch artery
Brachiocephalic artery	Right horn of aortic sac (unfused right ventral aortic arch)
Right subclavian artery*Neet*	Proximal part: Right fourth arch artery, right dorsal aorta
	Distal part: Right seventh cervical intersegmental artery
Left subclavian artery	Left seventh cervical intersegmental artery
Pulmonary arteries	Proximal part of sixth arch artery
Descending aorta	Proximal part: Left dorsal aorta distal to attachment of fourth arch artery
	Distal part: Fused dorsal aorta

Note: Smooth muscles of dorsal aorta develop from splanchnopleuric layer of lateral plate mesoderm.*Neet*

Table 19.3 Development of carotid arteries

Artery	Embryonic source
Common carotid artery	Part of third arch artery proximal to the bud of external carotid artery
External carotid artery	Bud form third arch artery
Internal carotid artery	Part of third arch artery distal to the bud of external carotid artery Cranial extension of dorsal aortae distal to attachment of the third arch artery

Note: Left common carotid artery arising from brachiocephalic trunk is the commonest variation in arteries arising from arch of aorta.*Neet*

Patent Ductus Arteriosus (PDA)

Q. Write short note on patent ductus arteriosus.

Definition

Failure of closure of ductus arteriosus that connects left pulmonary artery with arch of aorta in the foetal life.

- Normal ductus arteriosus shunts blood between pulmonary trunk and descending aorta to bypass the lungs.^{Neet}
- Usual closure of ductus arteriosus occurs as follows:
  – Physiological (functional): Immediately after birth due to reflex contraction of muscles of arterial wall. Ductus arteriosus constricts at birth but shunting of blood from aorta to left pulmonary artery may continue up to 4 days after birth.^{Neet}
  – Anatomical: Within three months (12 weeks)^{Neet} after birth by proliferation of tunica intima into lumen, under the influence of transforming growth factor β (TGFβ).^{Neet}
- Patent ductus arteriosus occurs in 8 in 10,000 births.
- PDA leads to shunting of blood from aorta to pulmonary circulation.
- Prostaglandins keep ductus arteriosus open, whereas prostaglandin inhibitors (such as indomethacin) promotes closure of DA.
- Mechanism of closure: After birth, lungs release bradykinin during initial inflation. Bradykinin produces smooth muscle contraction in the wall of ductus arteriosus and closes it physiologically.
- Remnant of ductus arteriosus is called *ligamentum arteriosum*. Left recurrent laryngeal nerve loop around ligamentum arteriosum.

Coarctation of Aorta

Q. Write short note on coarctation of aorta.

Definition: Coarctation of aorta is congenital narrowing of the arch of aorta distal to origin of left subclavian artery (Fig. 19.5).

- Coarctation of aorta occurs in 3.2 in 10,000 births.

Types:
A. Preductal coarctation: It is narrowing of aorta proximal to ductus arteriosus.
B. Postductal coarctation: It is narrowing of aorta distal to ductus arteriosus

Unusual Origin of Aorta

1. Double aortic arches: It occurs due to *persistence of right dorsal aorta distal* to right seventh intersegmental artery (Fig. 19.6).^{Neet}
2. Right aortic arch: It occurs due to regression of left dorsal aorta distal to right seventh intersegmental artery instead of the same segment of right dorsal aorta (Fig. 19.7).
3. Abnormal (aberrant) origin of right subclavian artery: Right subclavian artery may arise from descending aorta. It occurs due to regression of right fourth arch artery (Fig. 19.8).^{Neet} It results in: (1) absence of brachiocephalic artery, (2) origin of right common carotid artery from arch of aorta and (3) absence of recurrent course of right recurrent laryngeal nerve.

Branches of Dorsal Aorta (Fig. 19.9)

Dorsal aorta gives three sets of arteries as follows:
1. Dorsolateral branches
   - These are also called *somatic intersegmental vessels*.
   - These arteries form
     – Arteries of limbs
     – Intercostal arteries
     – Lumbar arteries
     – Lateral sacral arteries
2. Lateral splanchnic branches
   - These branches develop
     – Phrenic arteries
     – Suprarenal arteries
     – Renal arteries
     – Gonadal vessels
3. Ventral splanchnic branches
   - These are of two groups:
     A. Vitelline arteries that form coeliac, superior and inferior mesenteric arteries.
     B. Umbilical arteries form superior vesical arteries and medial umbilical ligament.
4. Remnant of dorsal aorta below sacral segment form median sacral artery.

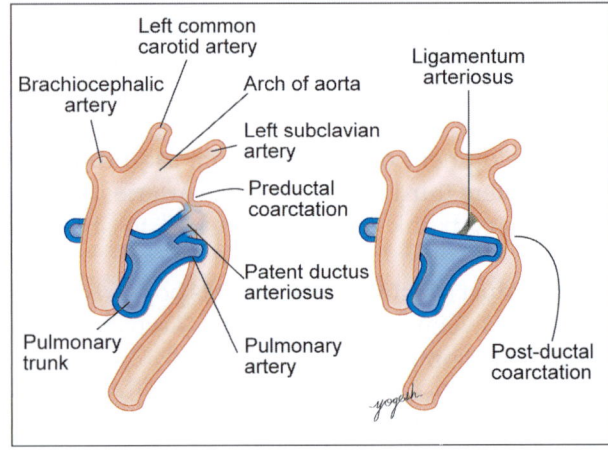

Fig. 19.5: Coarctation of aorta. Coarctation of aorta is a congenital narrowing of arch of aorta distal to the origin of left subclavian artery. Preductal coarctation is narrowing proximal to the ductus arteriosus, whereas post-ductal coarctation is a narrowing distal to the ductus arteriosus.

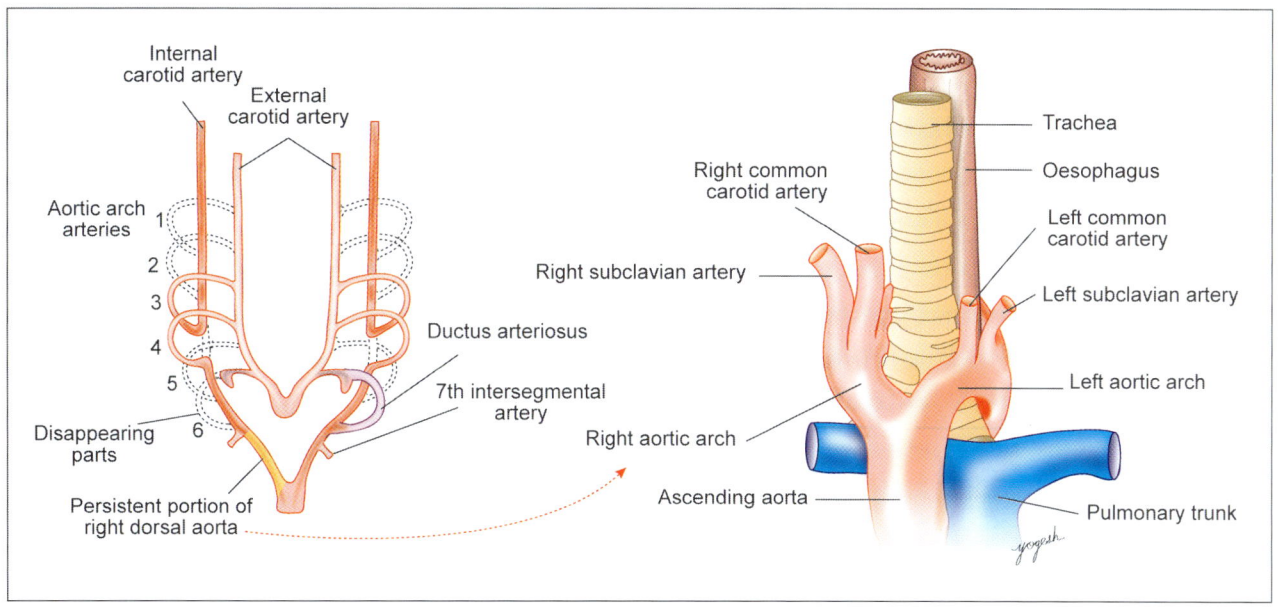

Fig. 19.6: Double aortic arches owing to persistence of right dorsal aorta distal to the right seventh intersegmental artery

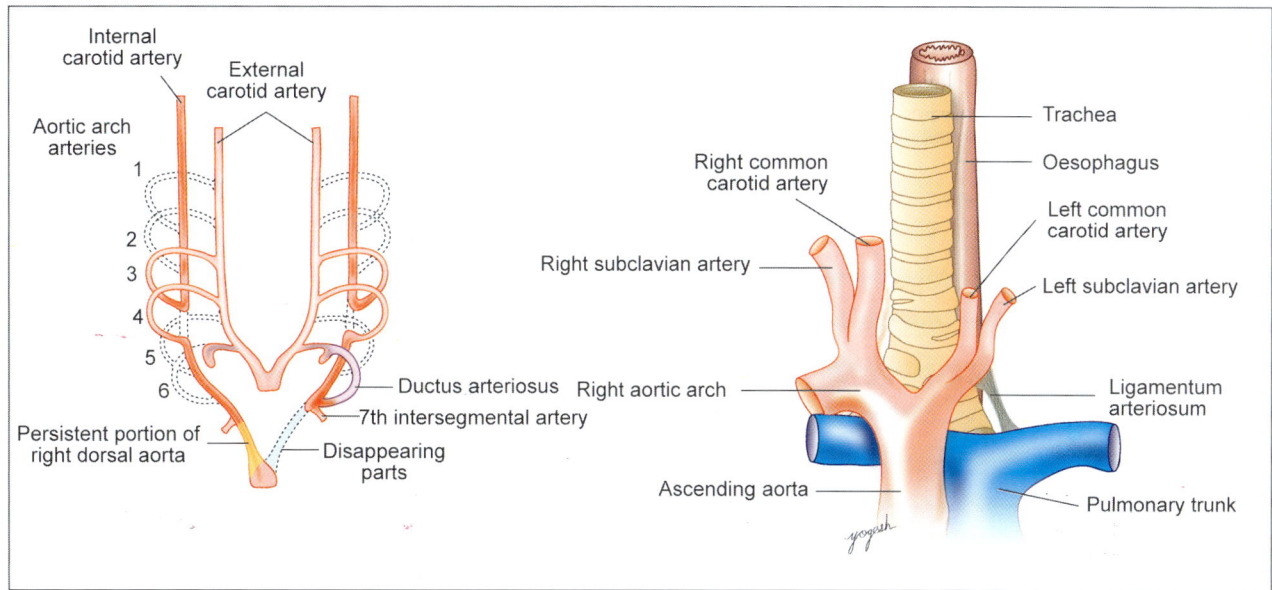

Fig. 19.7: Right aortic arch. Owing to regression of left dorsal aorta distal to the right seventh intersegmental artery instead of same segment of the right dorsal aorta results in right aortic arch

---

Box 19.2: Umbilical arteries

- Umbilical arteries are ventral splanchnic branches of dorsal aorta.
- Each umbilical artery supplies
  - Mesoderm of connecting stalk
  - Derivatives of allantois
  - Placenta
- Each umbilical artery gets communicated with part of fifth lumbar artery that forms the internal iliac artery.
- Portion of umbilical arteries between dorsal aorta and communication with internal iliac artery disappear. Thus, umbilical arteries become branches of internal iliac arteries.
- Single umbilical artery is present in 1% of cases and it is more common in twins and babies born to diabetic mothers.[Neet] Single umbilical artery is usually associated with renal abnormalities.[Neet]
- Post-natal change: After birth, umbilical arteries form
  - Superior umbilical artery from proximal part.
  - Medial umbilical ligament from distal obliterated part.

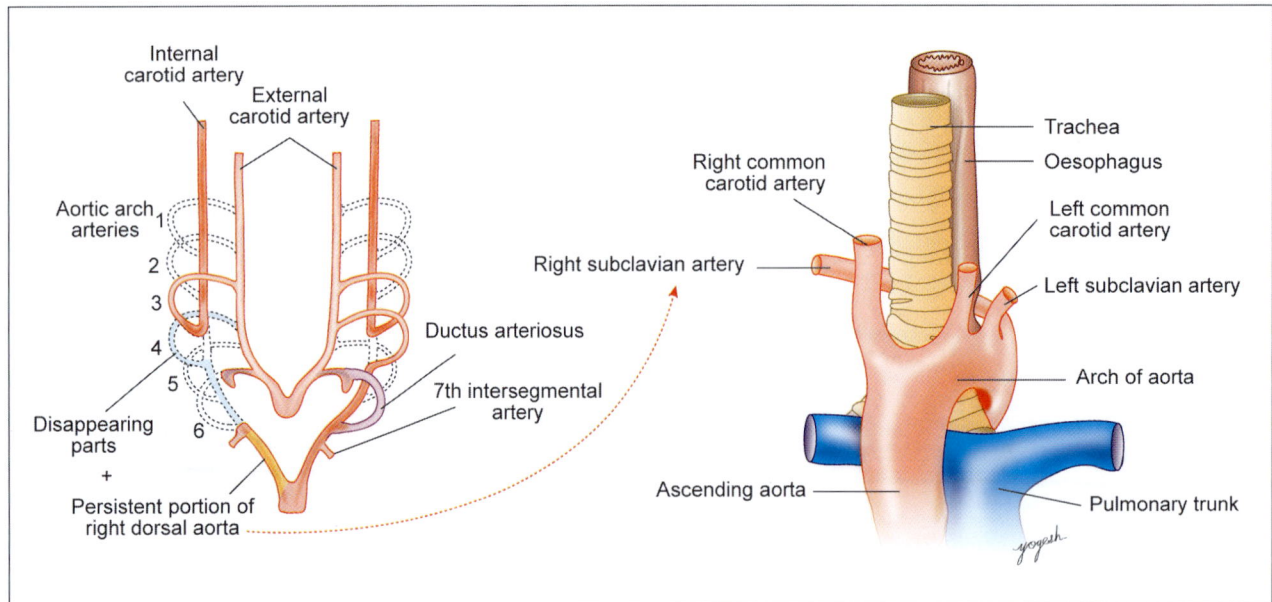

Fig. 19.8: Abnormal origin of right subclavian artery. Right subclavian artery may arise from the descending aorta. It occurs due to regression of right fourth arch artery. It results in absence of brachiocephalic artery, origin of right common carotid artery from arch of aorta and absence of recurrent course of right recurrent laryngeal nerve. This aberrant right subclavian artery may compress oesophagus

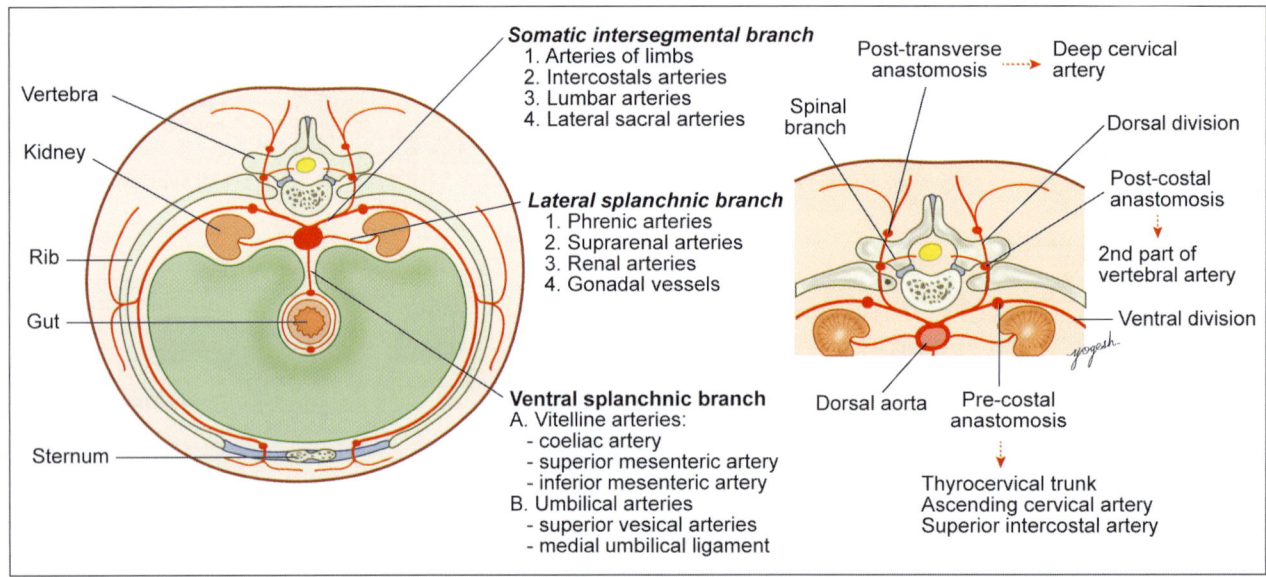

Fig.19.9: Branching pattern of dorsal aorta and its anastomoses

DEVELOPMENT OF VERTEBRAL ARTERY

Q. Write short note on development of vertebral artery.

- In cervical region, intersegmental arteries form longitudinal anastomotic channels as follows:
  A. *Pre-costal anastomosis*: Connects intersegmental arteries in front of the neck of the ribs.
  B. *Post-costal anastomosis*: Lies between costal elements (ribs) and transverse processes.
  C. *Post-transverse anastomosis*: Lies behind the transverse processes.
- Remnants or derivatives of cervical intersegmental arterial anastomosis are given in Table 19.4.

Summary (Examination Guide)

Vertebral artery consists of four parts (Fig. 19.9, Table 19.4):

1. **First part:** Extends from subclavian artery to foramen transversarium of sixth cervical vertebra—develops from dorsal division of seventh intersegmental artery.

2. **Second part:** Extends through foramina transversarium from sixth to first cervical segment—develops from postcostal anastomosis.
3. **Third part:** Extends from foramina transversarium and rest on posterior arch of the atlas—develops from spinal branch of first cervical intersegmental artery.
4. **Fourth part:** Intracranial part—develops from preneural division of spinal branch of basilar artery.

Table 19.4	Derivatives of cervical intersegmental arterial anastomosis
Anastomotic channel	Derivative
Precostal	Thyrocervical trunk, ascending cervical, superior intercostal arteries
Postcostal	Part of vertebral artery
Post-transverse	Deep cervical

DEVELOPMENT OF LIMB VESSELS

Q. Write short note on axis artery of upper and lower limbs.

- Each limb is supplied by an axis artery during development that runs along the central axis of limb.
- The axis artery is derived from intersegmental arteries.

Axis Artery of Upper Limb

- It is derivative of seventh cervical intersegmental artery (Fig. 19.10).

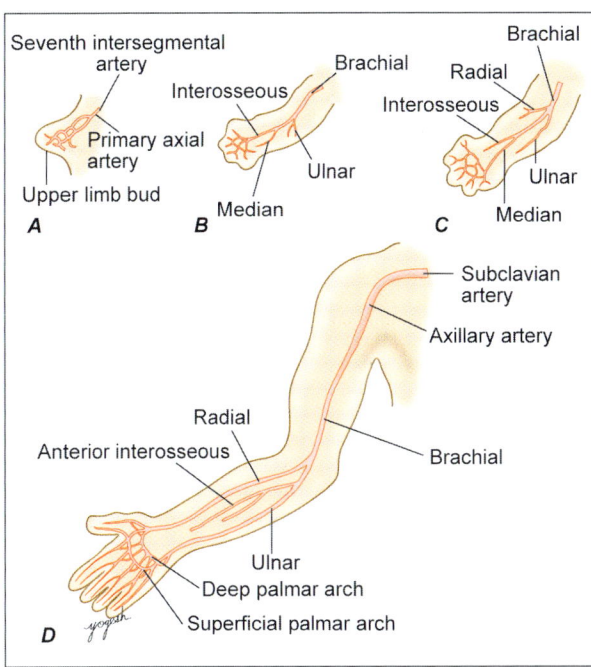

Fig. 19.10: Development of upper limb arteries. Axis artery of upper limb is a derivative of seventh cervical intersegmental artery. The axis artery later forms: Axillary artery, brachial artery, anterior interosseous artery and deep palmar arch. Radial and ulnar arteries arise as sprouts of the axis artery

- The axis artery of upper limb later forms:^{MCQ}
  - axillary artery
  - brachial artery
  - anterior interosseous artery^{Neet}
  - deep palmar arch

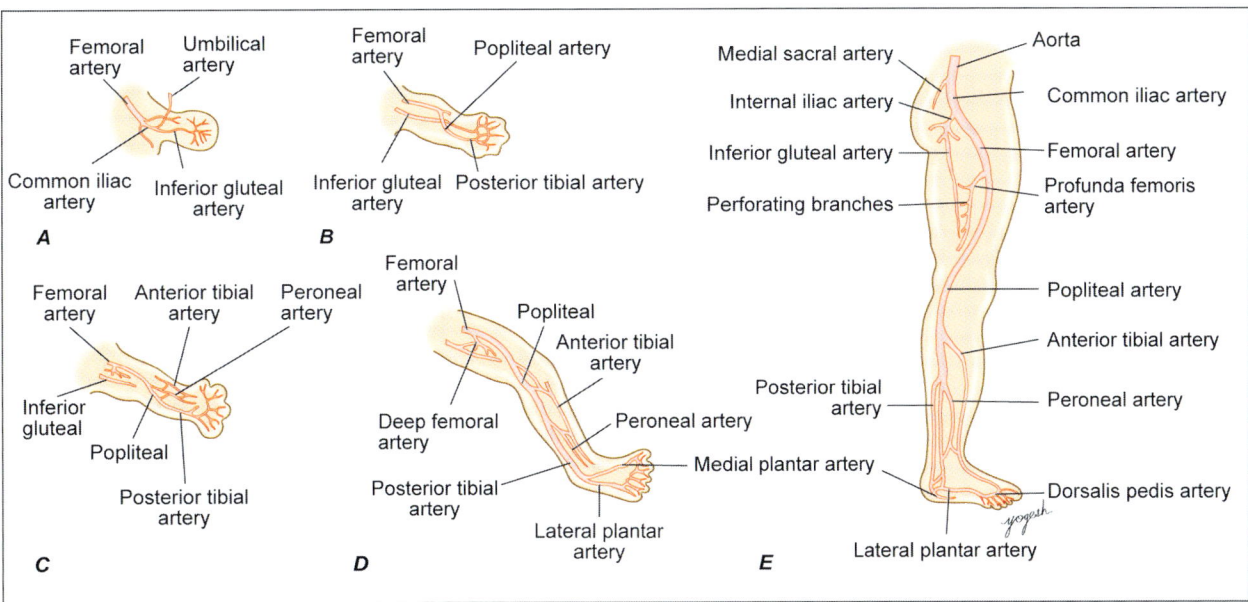

Fig. 19.11: Development of lower limb arteries. Axis artery of lower limb is derivative of fifth lumbar intersegmental artery. The axis artery of lower limb later forms arteria comitans nervi ischiadici, part of popliteal artery above the popliteus muscle, distal part of peroneal artery and part of plantar arch. Femoral artery develops from a capillary plexus present on ventral aspect of the thigh that later forms communication with external iliac artery and popliteal artery

- Radial and ulnar arteries arise as sprouts of the axis artery.

Axis Artery of Lower Limb

- It is derivative of *fifth lumbar intersegmental* artery.^Neet
- The axis artery of lower limb later forms:^MCQ
  - Arteria comitans nervi ischiadici (ischiadic artery that accompanies sciatic nerve)
  - Part of popliteal artery above the popliteus muscle
  - Distal part of peroneal artery
  - Part of plantar arch
- Femoral artery develops from a capillary plexus present on the ventral aspect of the thigh that later forms communication with external iliac artery and popliteal artery.

DEVELOPMENT OF VENOUS SYSTEM

INTRODUCTION

- Veins of developing embryo can be grouped as visceral and somatic veins (Flowchart 19.1, Fig. 19.12).
- **Visceral veins**
  These include
  1. Vitelline or omphalomesenteric veins—for draining yolk sac.
  2. Umbilical veins—for placenta.
- **Somatic veins**
  These are cardinal veins for draining body wall (cardinal = important).
  These are
  1. Anterior cardinal veins (right and left)
  2. Posterior cardinal veins (right and left)
  3. Common cardinal veins or *ducts of Cuvier* (right and left)
- Anterior and posterior cardinal veins join to form common cardinal veins.
- Anterior cardinal veins drain:
  - cranial half of embryo
  - upper limb buds
- Posterior cardinal veins drain
  - caudal half of embryo
  - lower limb buds
- Visceral and somatic veins finally drain into the sinus venosus.
- These visceral and somatic veins later in adult form
  - portal veins
  - caval veins
  - azygous veins

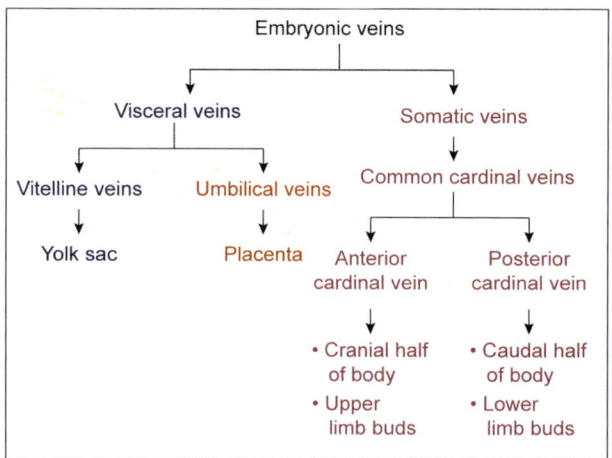

Flowchart 19.1: Embryonic veins

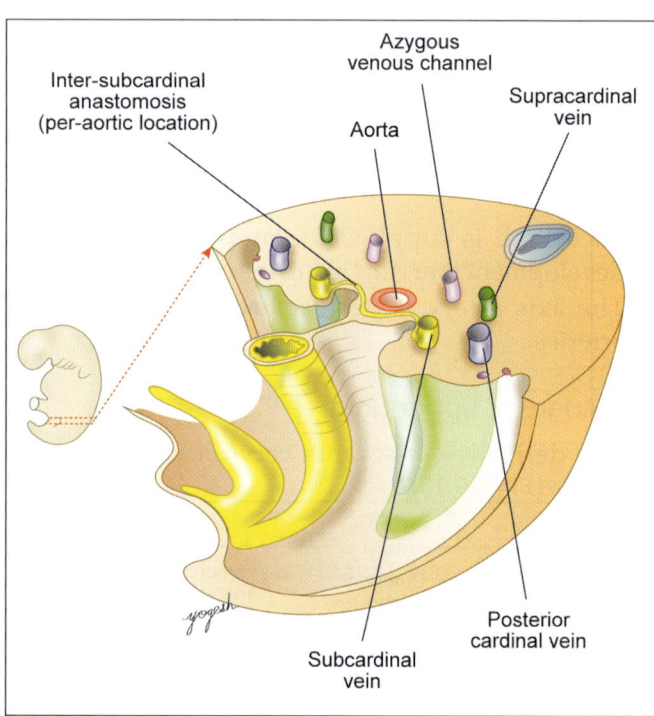

Fig. 19.12: Cross section of the embryo showing major embryonic veins

VITELLINE VEINS

Q. Write short note on development of portal vein.

- There are two vitelline (right and left) veins that drain yolk sac.
- On formation of head fold, part of the yolk sac participates in formation of gut.
- Both vitelline veins pass on either side of gut tube. They pass through septum transversum and finally open in sinus venosus.
- Developing liver in septum transversum divide vitelline veins into three parts: Infrahepatic, intrahepatic and suprahepatic parts (Fig. 19.13).

Cardiovascular System II: Blood Vessels and Foetal Circulation

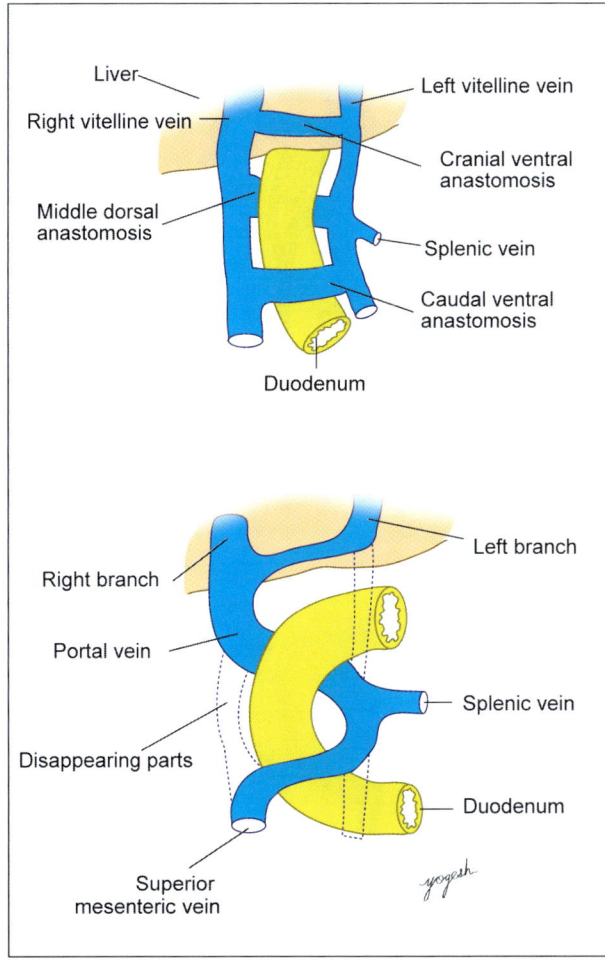

Fig. 19.13: Development of portal vein

A. Infrahepatic part
- Infra-hepatic parts lie caudal to septum transversum on either side of primitive gut.
- In zone of duodenum, right and left vitelline veins get communicated via three transverse anastomoses: Cephalic ventral, middle dorsal and caudal ventral to form a *Figure of 8*.^{MCQ}
- Communications:
  - Left umbilical vein develops communications with cranial ventral anastomosis, whereas splenic vein drain spleen into dorsal middle anastomosis.
  - Disappearance of segments of infrahepatic part of vitelline vein results in formation of (Table 19.5, Fig. 19.14):
    1. Superior mesenteric vein^{Neet}
    2. Trunk of portal vein^{Neet}
    3. Right branch of portal vein^{Neet}
    4. Left branch of portal vein^{Neet}

B. Intrahepatic part
- Intrahepatic plexus forms a capillary network that joins with developing hepatic sinusoids.
- This capillary network forms
  - afferent venae advehentes that develop branches of portal vein.
  - efferent venae revehentes that develop tributaries of hepatic vein.^{Neet}

C. Suprahepatic part
- Subdiaphragmatic anastomosis develops that connects right and left vitelline veins.
- Subdiaphragmatic anastomosis gets connected with cranial ventral intervitelline anastomosis.
- Left vitelline vein regresses (disappears).^{MCQ}
- Remaining portion of suprahepatic vitelline veins forms:
  1. Common hepatic vein that later forms terminal part of inferior vena cava^{Neet}
  2. Ductus venosus
  3. Left hepatic vein^{Neet}

Table 19.5	Development of portal venous system (Practice Fig. 19.1)
Derivative	*Embryonic source*
Superior mesenteric vein^{Neet}	– Infra-hepatic part of right vitelline vein distal to caudal ventral anastomosis – Caudal ventral anastomosis – Left vitelline vein between middle dorsal and caudal ventral anastomoses
Trunk of portal vein^{Neet}	– Middle dorsal anastomosis – Right vitelline vein between cranial ventral and middle dorsal anastomoses
Right branch of portal vein^{Neet}	– Infrahepatic part of right vitelline vein up to cranial ventral anastomosis
Left branch of portal vein^{Neet}	– Cranial ventral anastomosis – Infrahepatic left vitelline vein up to cranial ventral anastomosis

UMBILICAL VEINS
- Umbilical vein drains blood from placenta into sinus venosus.
- Umbilical veins pass through somatopleuric mesoderm and septum transversum.
- Right umbilical vein regresses, whereas left umbilical vein is left behind.^{MCQ, Viva}
- Left umbilical veins develop communication with left vitelline vein (that later form left branch of portal vein).
- A portion of left umbilical vein cranial to septum transversum disappears.
- Thus, blood from left umbilical vein pass through:
  1. Hepatic circulation via left branch of portal vein
  2. To inferior vena cava through ductus venosus.

Human Embryology

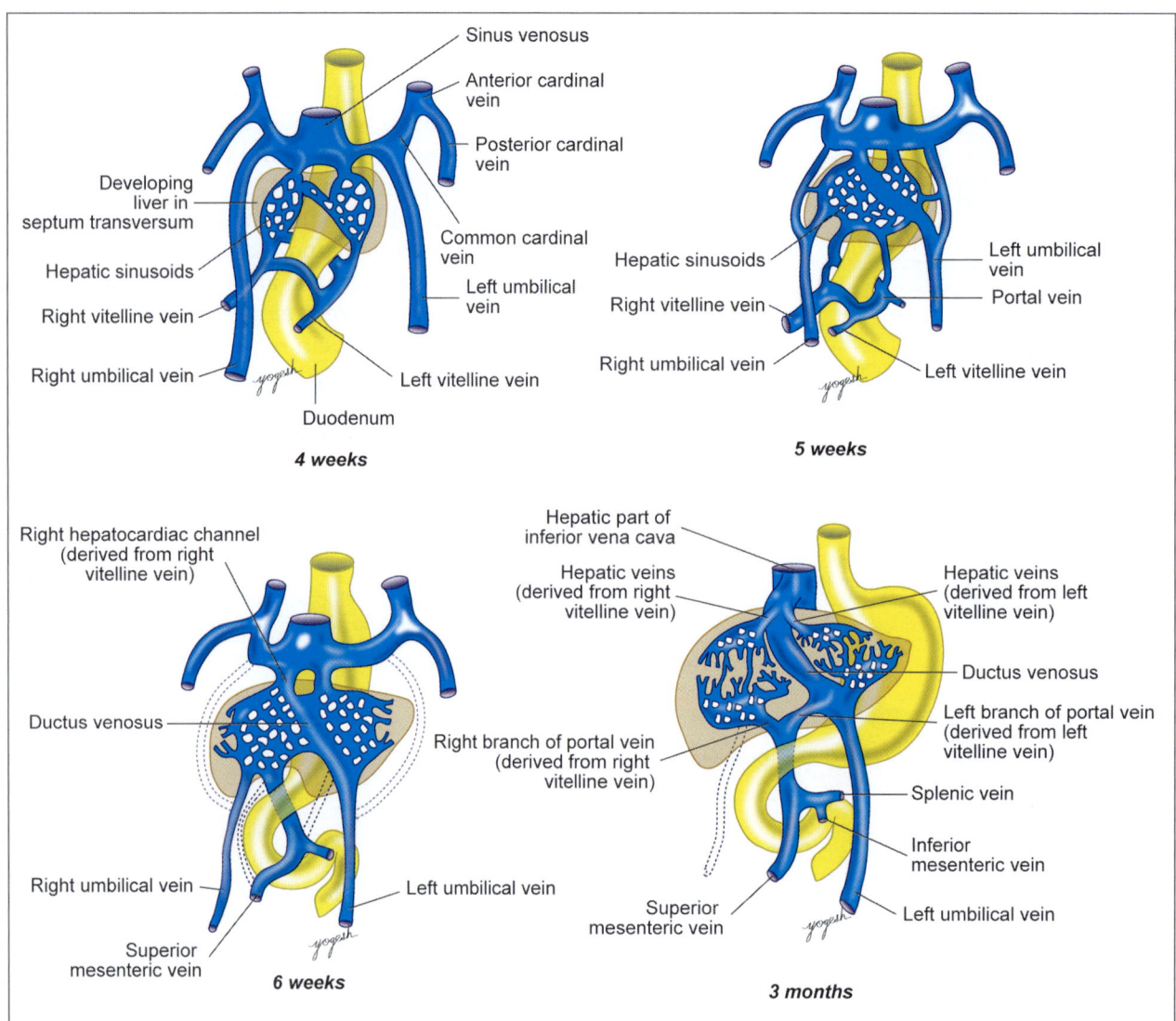

Fig. 19.14: Development of portal vein. Plexus around the duodenum develops hepatic sinusoid and ductus venosus. Terminal parts of the right and left vitelline veins form right and left hepatocardiac channels respectively. Note the formation of the portal vein, splenic vein, superior mesenteric vein and hepatic portion of the inferior vena cava

Note: Ductus venosus after birth forms ligamentum venosus, whereas left umbilical vein forms ligamentum teres hepatis.

SOMATIC VEINS

- There are two pairs of somatic veins:
  1. *Anterior cardinal veins* (right and left)
  2. *Posterior cardinal veins* (right and left)
- On each side, anterior and posterior cardinal veins join to form the *common cardinal vein* (duct of Cuvier).
- The common cardinal veins open into corresponding horns of sinus venosus.
- Anterior cardinal vein has two segments: Primary head vein and cervico thoracic vein.

Primary Head Vein

- It lies on side of cranial end of neural tube (or brain vesicles).
- It forms
  1. *Superficial venous plexus* that develops dural venous sinuses.
  2. *Deep venous plexus* that develops cerebral veins.
- Dural venous sinuses form three stems that terminate into primary head vein as follows:
  – cranial (ventral) dural stem for forebrain and midbrain
  – middle dural stem for metencephalon
  – caudal dural stem for myelencephalon
- Most of the part of primary head vein disappears and its small remnant develops *cavernous sinus*.

Cardiovascular System II: Blood Vessels and Foetal Circulation

- Communicating channels between dural stems form:
  - *Transverse sinus*: Channel between cranial and middle dural stem.
  - *Sigmoid sinus*: Channel between middle and caudal dural stem.
  - *Inferior petrosal sinus*: Channel between primary head vein and cavernous sinus.
  - *Superior petrosal sinus:* Middle dural stem
- *Primary maxillary vein* opens into primary head vein and later it forms superior ophthalmic vein.^{MCQ}
- *Sagittal plexus* develops on superolateral surface of the forebrain that forms:
  1. Superior sagittal sinus
  2. Straight sinuses
  3. Great cerebral vein

Cervicothoracic Vein

Q. Write short note on development of coronary sinus.

Cervicothoracic vein forms the following veins:
1. Internal jugular veins: From part of anterior cardinal veins cranial to opening of subclavian vein.
2. Subclavian vein: From seventh intersegmental vein.^{MCQ}
3. Right brachiocephalic vein: From part of right anterior cardinal vein between right subclavian vein and oblique intercardinal anastomosis.
4. Left brachiocephalic vein: From
   a. part of left anterior cardinal vein between left subclavian vein and oblique intercardinal anastomosis
   b. oblique intercardinal anastomosis
5. Superior vena cava:
   It has two parts:
   - Extra-pericardial part: Develops from part of right anterior cardinal vein caudal to oblique intercardinal channel. ^{MCQ}
   - Intrapericardial part: Develops from right common cardinal vein. ^{MCQ}
6. Left superior intercostals vein: A part of left anterior cardinal vein disappears. A small part of left common cardinal vein near oblique intercardinal channel form superior intercostal vein and ligament of left vena cava. ^{MCQ}
7. Oblique vein of left atrium (*oblique vein of Marshall*): From left common cardinal vein. ^{MCQ}
8. Coronary sinus: Develops from left horn of sinus venosus.

Note: Normal SVC and IVC develop from right embryonic veins. ^{Neet}

Anomalies of Superior Vena Cava

1. Double superior vena cava
   - It may occur due to failure of development of communicating channel between two anterior cardinal veins.
   - Usually, this channel forms left brachiocephalic vein.
   - In double superior vena cava cases, left superior vena cava develops from left anterior cardinal vein and left common cardinal vein. Left superior vena cava drains into coronary sinus (develops from left horn of sinus venosus).^{Neet}
2. Left superior vena cava
   - It occurs due to regression of caudal part of right anterior cardinal vein and right common cardinal vein.
   - Left superior vena cava develops from left anterior cardinal vein and left common cardinal vein.
   - Left superior vena cava drains into coronary sinus.^{Neet}

Subcardinal Veins

- These develop in relation to mesonephric ridge (future site of kidney formation) (Table 19.6).
- Pre-aortic anastomosis gets developed between two subcardinal veins.
- Subcardinal veins anastomose cranially and caudally with posterior cardinal vein on the same side.
- A communicating channel develops between right subcardinal vein and common hepatic vein. This channel is called *right hepatocardiac channel*.

Supracardinal Veins (Thoracolumbar Veins)

- These veins develop longitudinally and lie dorsolateral to posterior cardinal veins (Table 19.6).
- Supracardinal veins develop later than subcardinal veins.
- Cranially and caudally supracardinal veins develop communications with corresponding posterior cardinal veins.
- Supracardinal vein anastomoses with corresponding subcardinal vein through suprasubcardinal anastomosis.

Posterior Cardinal Veins

- Posterior cardinal vein joins with anterior cardinal vein to form common cardinal vein (Table 19.7).
- Posterior cardinal veins (right and left) join with each other by *iliac anastomosis* (transverse anastomosis).

Table 19.6	Subcardinal and supracardinal veins	
	Subcardinal vein	*Supracardinal vein*
Site	Ventrolateral to abdominal aorta	Dorsolateral to abdominal aorta
Communication (cranially and caudally)	Posterior cardinal veins	Posterior cardinal veins
Anastomosis	Intersubcardinal veins	Suprasubcardinal anastomosis
Right side derivatives	Right gonadal vein Right suprarenal vein Part of inferior vena cava	Postrenal segment of inferior vena cava
Left side derivatives	Left gonadal vein Left suprarenal vein	Disappears

Box 19.3: Renal collar

Definition: The ring of venous channels around aorta below origin of superior mesenteric artery is called *renal collar*.

Components: The renal collar is formed by the following communications:
1. Anastomosis between two subcardinal veins (preaortic)
2. Anastomosis between supracardinal and subcardinal veins.
3. Anastomosis between supracardinal and azygous veins
4. Anastomosis between azygous venous lines and subcentral veins.
5. Anastomosis between two subcentral veins (postaortic). *Note:* During embryonic period, right and left azygos lines are connected by subcentral vein that develops dorsal to the aorta.

Table 19.7	Right and left posterior cardinal veins	
Part	Derivatives of	
	Right posterior cardinal vein	*Left posterior cardinal vein*
Caudal to anastomosis	• Right common iliac vein • Right internal iliac vein	• Left internal iliac vein
Cranial to anastomosis	• Mostly degenerates • Cranial portion: Arch of azygous vein • Caudal portion: Most caudal part of IVC	• Mostly degenerates • Cranial portion: Part of left superior intercostal vein

- Tributaries of each posterior cardinal vein include:
  - 12 thoracic intersegmental veins
  - 5 lumbar intersegmental veins
  - Iliac veins—internal iliac vein from pelvic cavity and external iliac vein from lower limb bud
- Subset of veins in abdomen:
  - In the abdomen, pairs of subcardinal and supracardinal veins appear.

Azygous Venous Lines

- Longitudinal venous channels appear on medial side of sympathetic trunk.
- Cranially these channels communicate with corresponding posterior cardinal vein.
- Caudally, these channels communicate with corresponding subcardinal veins.
- *Intercommunicating channel* develops between azygous veins. This channel that runs dorsal to aorta.
- Azygous venous channel develops numerous venous channels with supracardinal vein. On disappearance of part of supracardinal vein, these communicating venous channels develop intersegmental veins and later intercostals and lumbar veins.

DEVELOPMENT OF INFERIOR VENA CAVA[High yielding]

Q. Write short note on development of inferior vena cava.

Inferior vena cava develops from the following components (Figs 19.15 and 19.16, Practice Fig. 19.1):[Neet]

1. Caudal segment of IVC: From caudal part of right posterior cardinal vein (between transverse interposterior cardinal veins and caudal to junction of right supracardinal vein with right posterior cardinal vein).
2. Postrenal segment of IVC: From right supracardinal vein
3. Renal segment: From right suprasubcardinal anastomosis
4. Prerenal segment: From right subcardinal vein
5. Hepatic segment: From anastomosis between right subcardinal vein and right vitelline veins (common hepatic veins)
6. Suprahepatic segment: From *right vitelline vein* or right hepatocardiac channel (left hepatocardiac channel disappears due to regression of left horn of sinus venosus).[Neet]

Anomalies of IVC

Owing to complex development of inferior vena cava, its anomalies may be present. These include:

1. Double IVC: It occurs due to failure of formation of ananastomosis between two posterior cardinal veins or persistence of left subcardianal and supracardinal veins. Left IVC develops from left posterior cardinal vein (below the level of renal veins).[Neet]
2. Absence of IVC: It occurs due to failure of development of communication between right subcardinal vein and right hepatocardiac channel.
3. Preuretic IVC: If infrarenal part of IVC develops from subcardinal vein (that lies anterior to ureter) instead

of supracardinal vein (that lies posterior to ureter), preureteric IVC develops (anterior to right ureter).
4. Azygous continuation of IVC: If a hepatic segment of IVC fails to develop, IVC opens in SVC via the route of azygous vein.

DEVELOPMENT OF AZYGOUS VENOUS SYSTEM

The azygous system of veins consists of three major veins: Azygous vein, hemizygous vein and accessory hemizygous vein (Fig. 19.17).

Azygous Vein

Azygous vein develops from the following sources:
1. Vein of right azygous line
2. Cranial most part of right posterior cardinal vein

Hemizygous Vein

It is derived from the following sources:
1. Lower part of vein of left azygous line
2. Caudal postaortic anastomosis between veins of right and left azygous lines

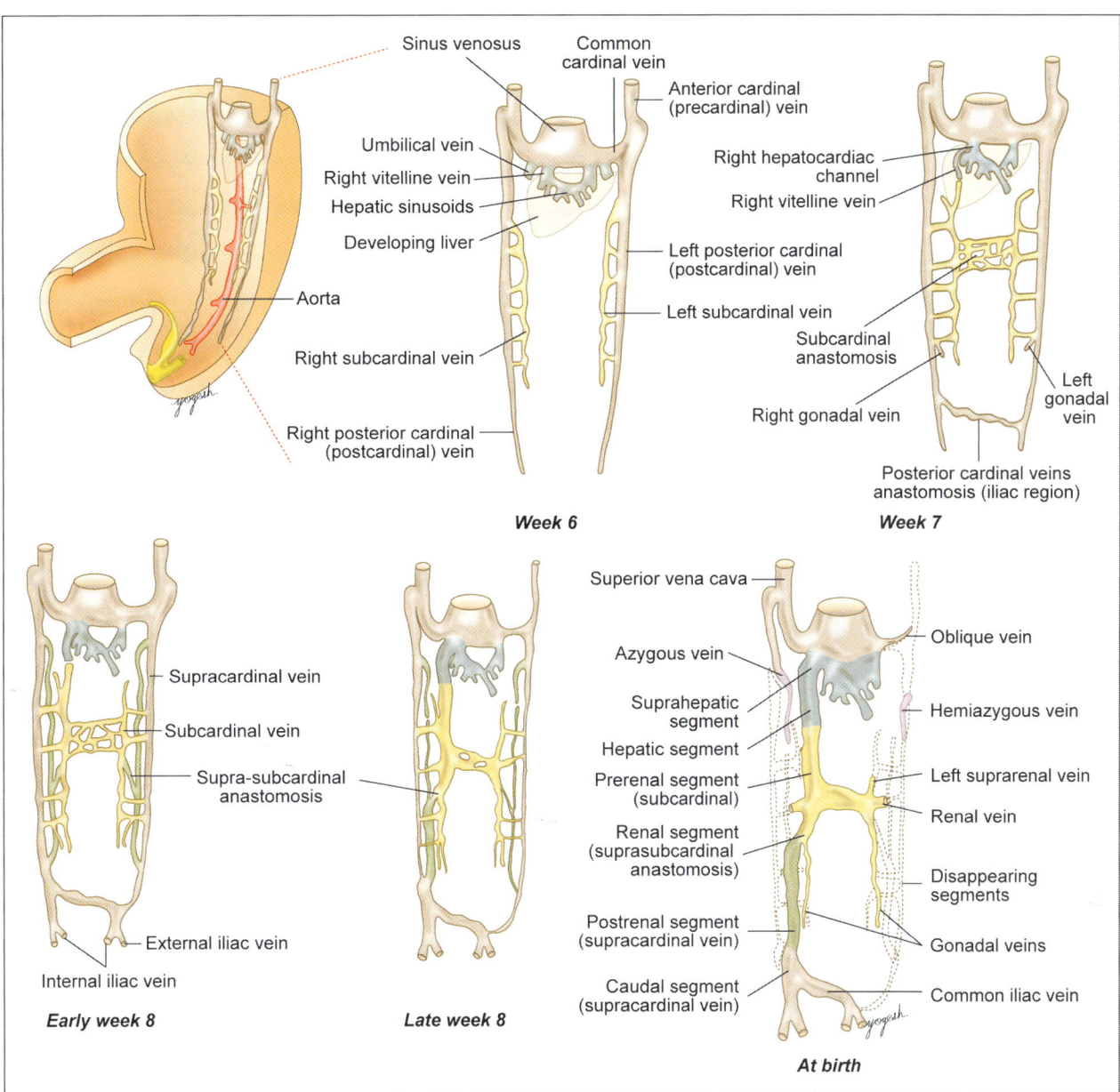

Fig. 19.15: Development of inferior vena cava. Segments of inferior vena cava develops by anastomosis channels of cardinal veins. Caudal segment of IVC develops from caudal part of the right posterior cardinal vein. Postrenal segment of IVC develops from right supracardinal vein. Renal segment develops from right supra-subcardinal anastomosis, prerenal segment from right subcardinal vein and hepatic segment from anastomosis between right subcardinal vein and right vitelline veins (common hepatic veins), suprahepatic segment from right hepatocardiac channel

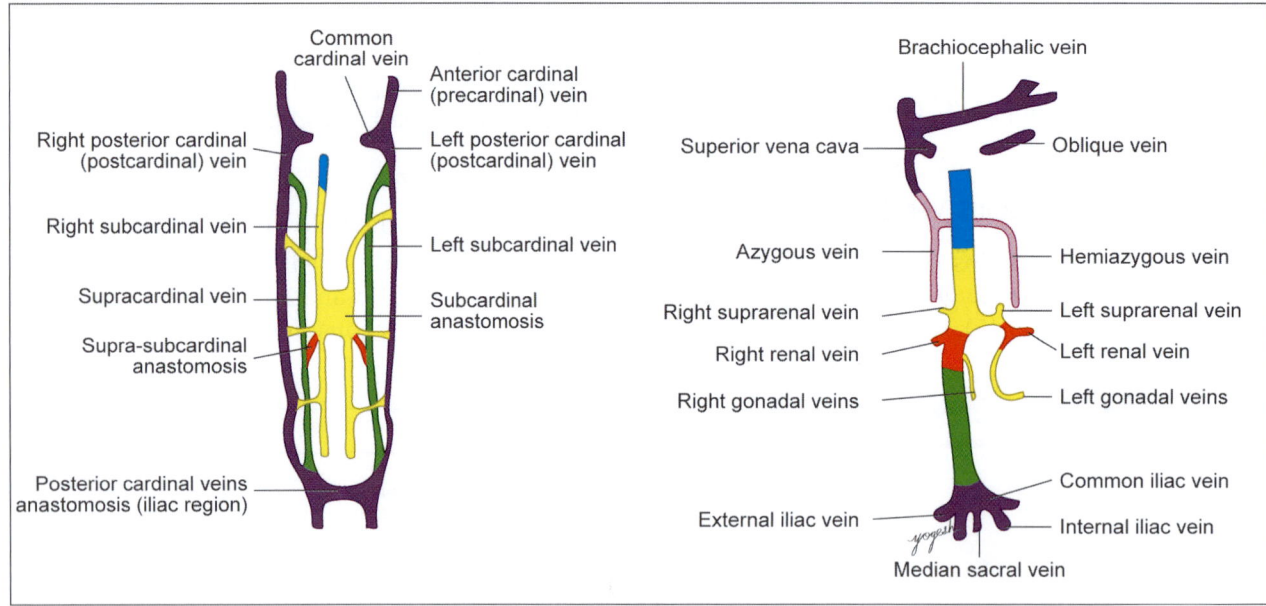

Practice Fig. 19.1: Development of inferior vena cava

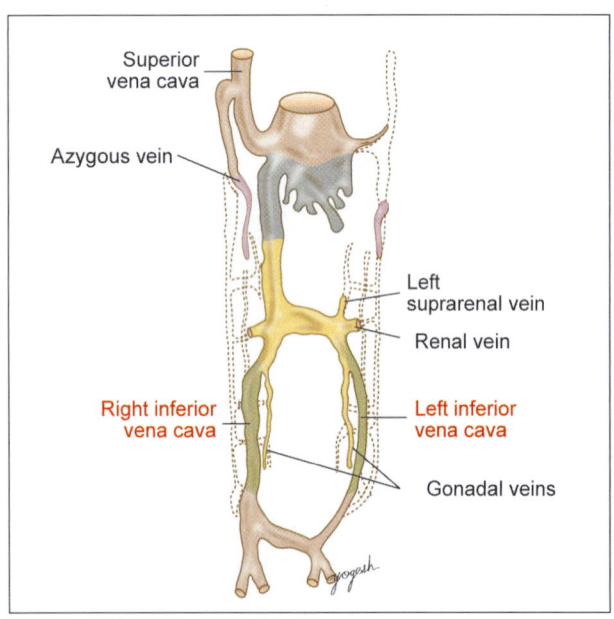

Fig. 19.16: Double inferior vena cava

Accessory Hemizygous Vein

It is derived from the following sources:
1. Upper part of vein of left azygous line
2. Cranial post-aortic anastomosis between veins of right and left azygous lines

FOETAL CIRCULATION

Q. Describe foetal circulation.

Developing foetus receives nutrition from placenta. The foetus is dependent on mother for:

1. Nutrients and oxygen intake
2. Carbon dioxide and waste product excretion

SPECIAL STRUCTURES IN FOETAL CIRCULATION
(Fig. 19.18 and Flowchart 19.2)

1. *Placenta*: It is a site of exchange of substances between mother and foetus.
2. *Umbilical vein*: Carries nutrients and oxygen to foetus.
3. *Umbilical arteries*: Carry waste products and carbon dioxide away from foetus. Oxygen saturation in umbilical arteries is approximately 58%.[MCQ]
4. *Foramen ovale*: Helps blood to bypass lungs. It transmits most of the blood from right atrium to left atrium.
5. *Ductus venosus*: Transmits oxygenated blood from umbilical vein and left branch of portal vein to inferior vena cava and thus blood bypass liver.[Neet]
6. *Ductus arteriosus*: Helps blood to bypass foetal lungs. It transmits the blood from left pulmonary artery to aorta.

PECULIARITIES OF FOETAL CIRCULATION

Q. Write short note on peculiarities of foetal circulation.

Following are the peculiarities of the foetal circulation:
1. **Blood shunts three times** in foetus at following places: Ductus arteriosus, foramen ovale and ductus venosus to bypass lungs and liver.[MCQ]
2. **Regulation** of oxygenated blood in foetal circulation: Sphincter at junction of left umbilical vein and ductus

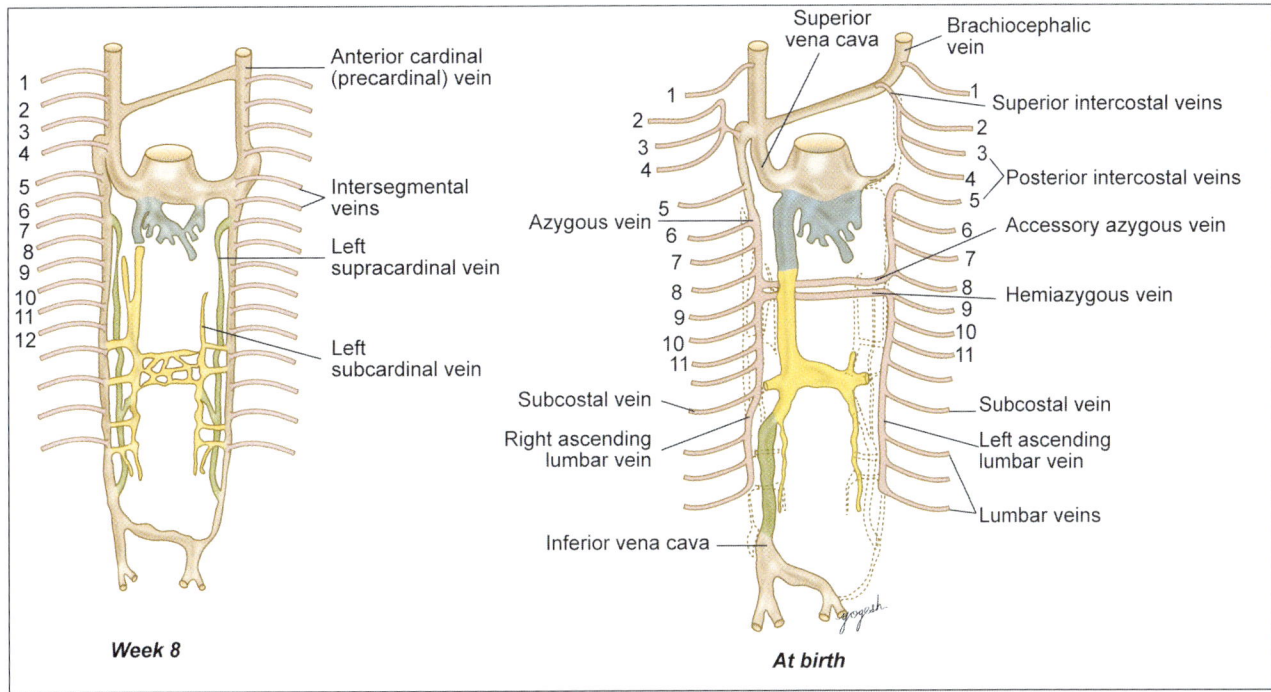

Fig. 19.17: Development of azygous vein and its tributaries

venosus regulates flow of oxygenated blood to the foetus.
3. **Mixing** of oxygenated and venous blood takes place at the following places: Liver, both atria, distal part of arch of aorta and terminal part of inferior vena cava.[MCQ]
4. **Trans septal blood circulation**: Through foramen ovale blood enters from right atria into left atria.
5. **Length** of the upper limb is more in foetus as upper limb bud receives more blood than lower limb bud.

CIRCULATORY CHANGES AT BIRTH

Q. Write short note on circulatory changes after the birth.

On birth, newborn starts respiration and lungs takeover functions of placenta. This produces the following changes (Table 19.8):
1. Muscle contraction in umbilical arteries occludes their lumen and prevents blood loss.
2. Umbilical vein contracts a few minutes after the umbilical arteries. This mechanism allows the newborn to receive more blood from placenta.[MCQ]
3. Occlusion of ductus arteriosus diverts right ventricular blood to lungs.
4. Closure of foramen ovale due to increased pressure in left atrium (owing to increased volume of blood that returns from lungs). *Note*: Premature closure of foramen ovale leads to right ventricular hypertrophy.[Neet]

Table 19.8 Remnants of embryonic vessels[High yielding, Neet]

Embryonic vessel	Remnant
Umbilical arteries	Superior vesical artery
	Median umbilical ligament
Left umbilical vein	Ligamentum teres hepatis
Ductus venosus	Ligamentum venosum
Ductus arteriosus	Ligamentum arteriosum
Foramen ovale	Fossa ovalis

- The embryonic communications close by vasoconstriction (physiologically) soon after the birth and later by proliferation of intima (anatomical closure).[MCQ] Completed obliteration of lumen of umbilical arteries and ductus arteriosus take place in 2–3 months after birth. Anatomical closure of foramen ovale takes in about 1 year.[MCQ]

Foetal heartbeat
- Foetal heart beat can be heard using a **stethoscope** and Doppler auscultation (**Doppler foetoscope**) (Table 19.9).[MCQ]

DEVELOPMENT OF LYMPHATIC SYSTEM

Q. Write short note on development of thoracic duct.
- At the end of sixth week, lymphatic system begins to develop.
- Lymphatic capillary plexuses join to form endothelium-lined lymph sacs.

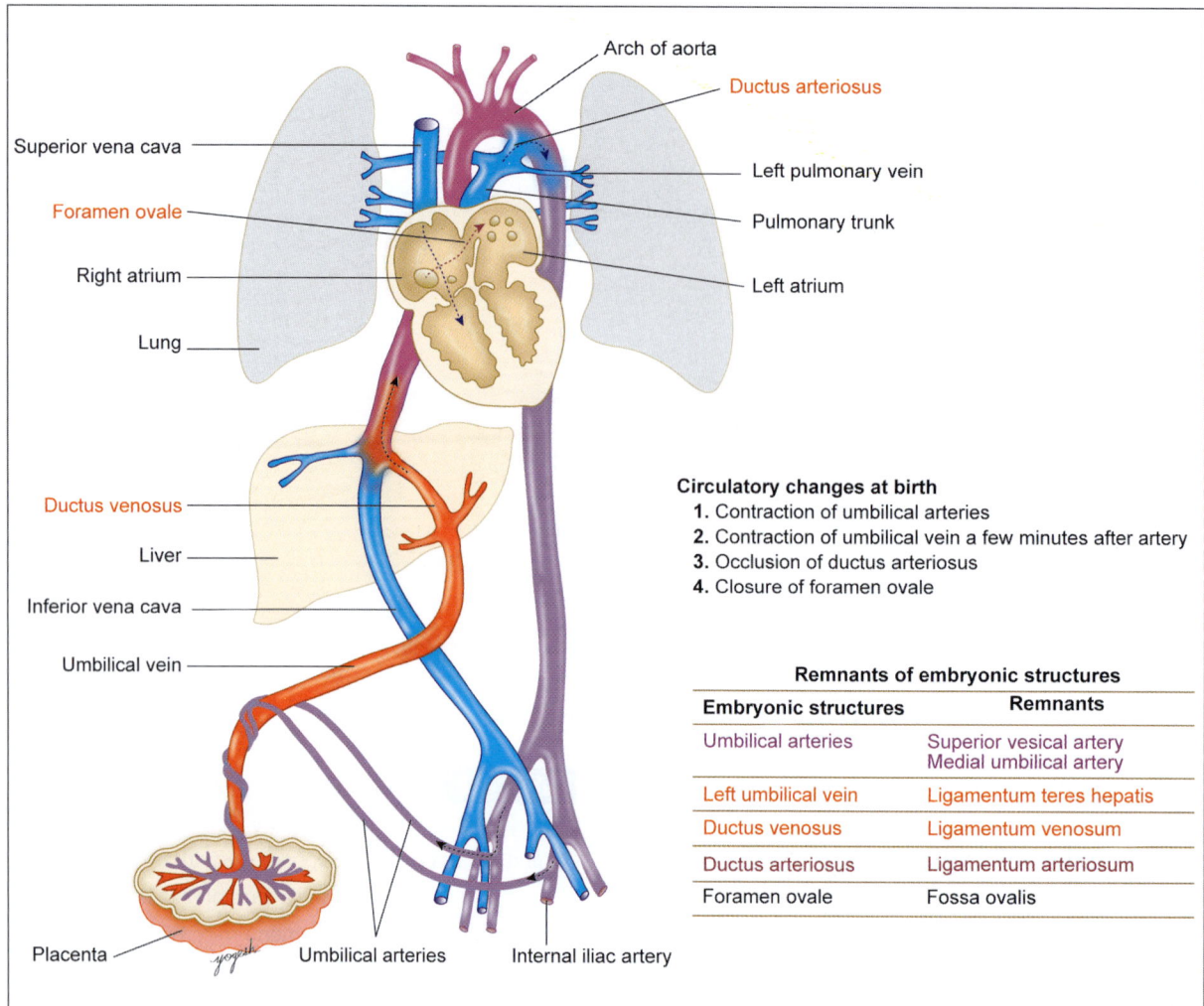

Fig.19.18: Foetal circulation. Blood shunts three times in foetus at following places: Ductus arteriosus from left pulmonary artery to aorta, foramen ovale from right atrium to left atrium and ductus venosus from left umbilical vein to inferior vena cava. The purpose of these shunts is to bypass lungs and liver

Table 19.9	Foetal heart rate
Gestational age	Heart rate (beats per minute)
5 weeks	80–103
6 weeks	103–126
7 weeks	126–149
8 weeks	149–172
9 weeks	155–195
12 weeks	120–160

- There are six primary lymph sacs as follows (Figs 19.19 and 19.20):
  - 1–2: Right and left jugular lymph sacs: Lie near junction of subclavian veins with anterior cardinal veins.
  - 3–4: Right and left posterior (iliac) sacs: Lie near junction of iliac veins with posterior cardinal veins.
  - 5: Single retroperitoneal sac: Lies in root of mesentery on posterior abdominal wall.
  - 6: Single cisterna chyli: Lies dorsal to retroperitoneal sac.
- Two large channels (right and left thoracic ducts) connects jugular sac with cisterna chyli.
- Thoracic ducts get communicated by a large anastomosing channel.
- Thoracic duct develops from
  - caudal part of primitive right thoracic duct
  - anastomosing channel
  - cranial part of primitive left thoracic duct
- Right lymphatic duct develops from cranial part of primitive right thoracic duct.
- Jugular lymphatic sac forms communication with venous junction of internal jugular and subclavian vein.

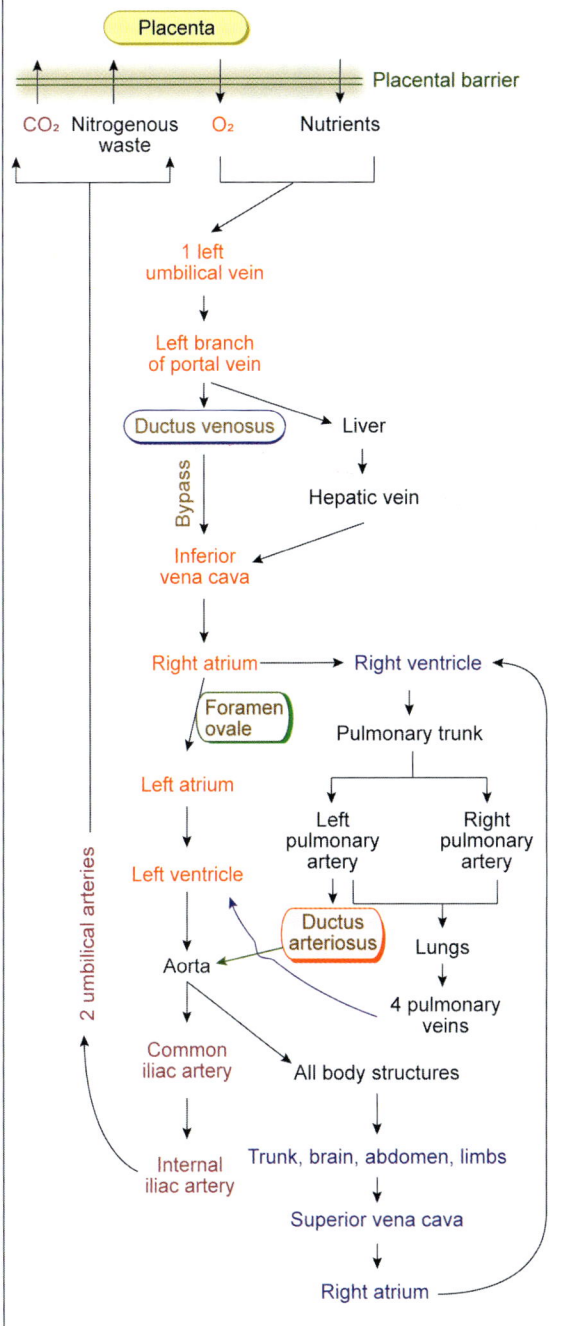

Flowchart 19.2: Foetal circulation

- Cystic hygromas (cystic lymphangioma/macrocystic lymphatic malformation): It is congenital multiloculated lymphatic lesion mostly present in left posterior triangle of neck and armpits. Hygromas arise from jugular lymph sac or from lymphatic spaces that fail to establish connections with primary lymphatic channels.

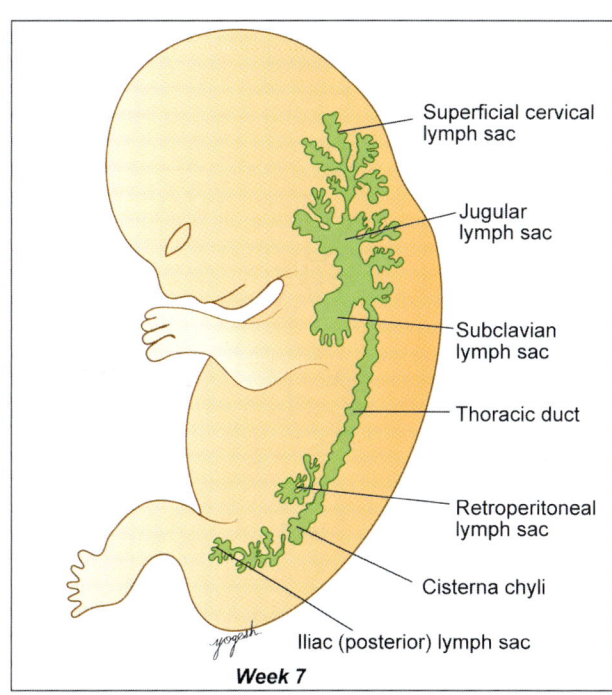

Fig. 19.19: Development of the lymphatic system

TIMING OF AORTIC ARCH FORMATION

Table 19.10	Timing of aortic arch formation
Timing	Event
Days 19–20	First pair of aortic arch forms
Days 20–23	Second pair of aortic arch forms
Days 24–25	Third pair of aortic arch forms Third pair of aortic arches becomes internal carotid arteries
Days 26–30	First and second pairs of aortic arches disappear Fourth pair of aortic arches forms Fourth left arch becomes definitive aorta Fourth right arch becomes right subclavian artery Fifth pair of aortic arches never fully develop
Day 30	Sixth pair of aortic arches forms Sixth right arch becomes right pulmonary artery Sixth left arch becomes left pulmonary artery (ductus arteriosus)

- Small lymphatic vessels drain body parts into lymph sac in the following manner:
  - head, neck, upper limb to jugular sacs
  - lower trunk and lower limb to iliac lymph sacs
  - primitive gut to retroperitoneal sac

Clinical Conditions

- Congenital lymph edema: It occurs due to dilation of primordial lymphatic channels.

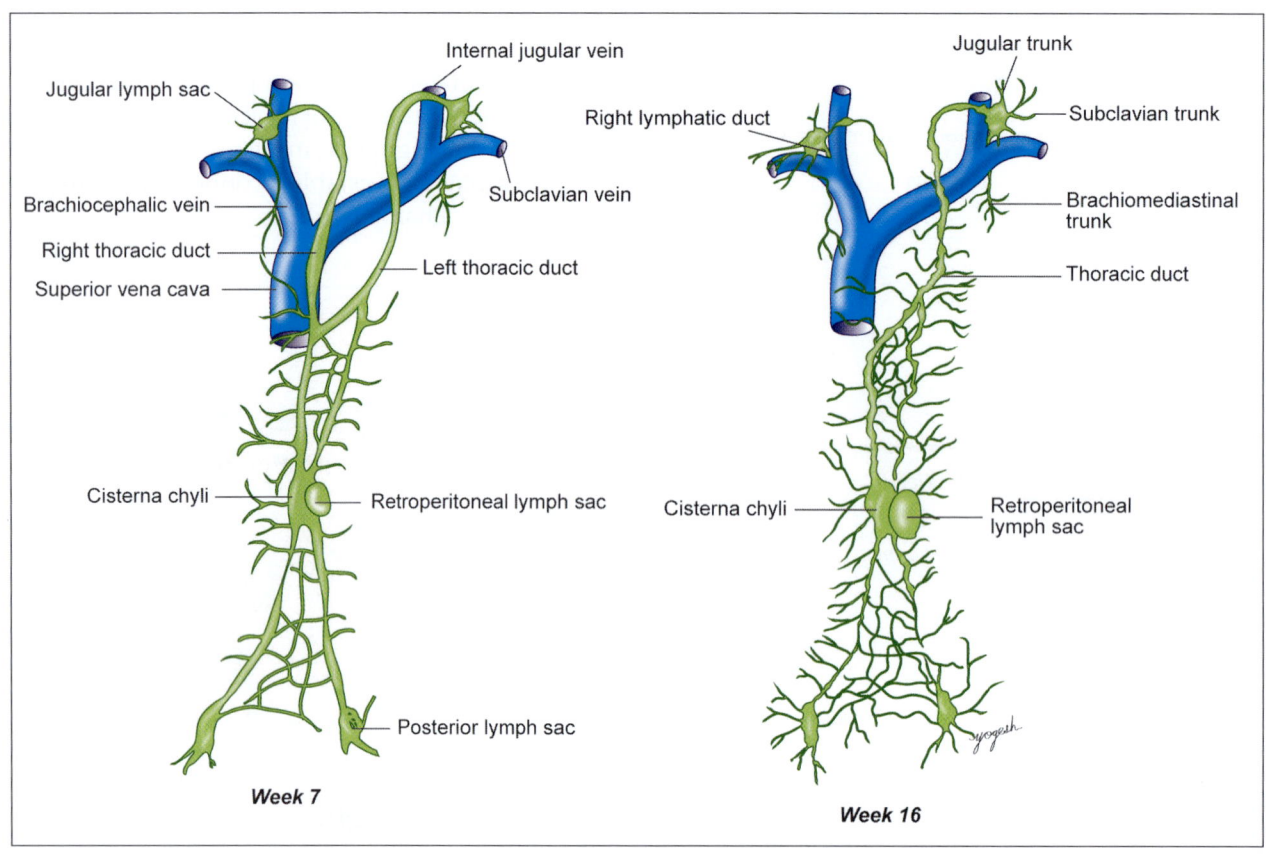

Fig. 19.20: Development of lymphatic system

20

Urinary System
Kidney, Ureter, Urinary Bladder, Urethra

Chapter Outline

- Introduction
  - Intermediate mesoderm
  - Cloaca
  - Mesonephric duct
  - Paramesonephric duct
- Development of kidneys
  - Evolutionary history of kidney
  - Stages of kidney development
  - Congenital anomalies of kidney
- Development of ureter
  - Anomalies of ureter
- Development of urinary bladder
  - Stages of development
- Ectopia vesicae
- Development of urethra
  - Development of female urethra
  - Development of male urethra

INTRODUCTION

- Urinary and genital systems develop from the common sources: Intermediate mesoderm and cloaca.

Intermediate Mesoderm

- On formation of the somites and intraembryonic coelom, the intraembryonic mesoderm is divided into three segments as follows (Fig. 20.1):
  - *paraxial mesoderm* that forms somties.
  - *intermediate mesoderm* that forms genitourinary system.
  - *lateral plate mesoderm* that forms somatopleuric and splanchnopleuric layers.
- Intermediate mesoderm forms bulging urogenital ridge on dorsal body wall just lateral to attachment of dorsal mesentery (Fig. 20.2).
- Urogenital ridge has two parts: Medial *genital ridge* and lateral *nephrogenic cord*.
- Nephrogenic cord extends from cervical to sacral segments of embryo.
- The nephrogenic cord passes through pronephric, mesonephric and metanephric phases that show formation of renal tubules and mesonephric ducts, paramesonephric duct and gonads (Fig. 20.3).

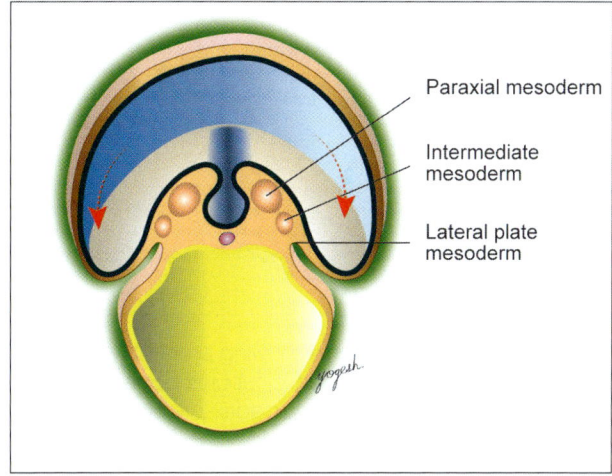

Fig. 20.1: Intraembryonic mesoderm. It is divided into three segments: Paraxial mesoderm, intermediate mesoderm (forms genitourinary system) and lateral plate mesoderm

Cloaca

- Cloaca is part of hindgut shared by genitourinary and digestive system (Fig. 20.4, Flowchart 20.1).
- The cloaca is divided into *primitive urogenital sinus* and dorsal *primitive rectum* by *urorectal septum*.
- Later, opening of mesonephric ducts divides primitive urogenital sinus into cranial *vesicourethral canal* and caudal *definitive urogenital sinus*.

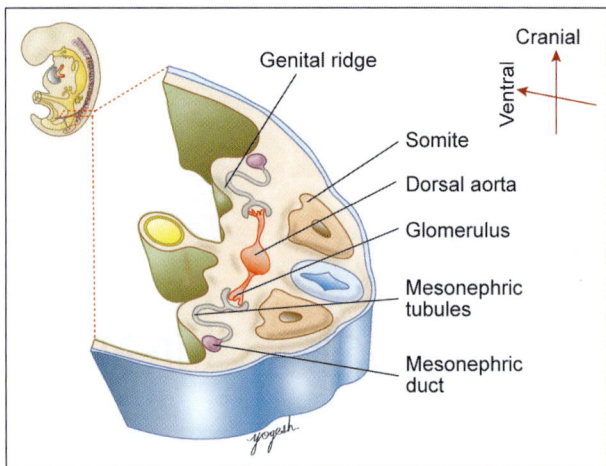

Fig. 20.2: Section of embryo with genital ridge and mesonephric duct and mesonephric tubules

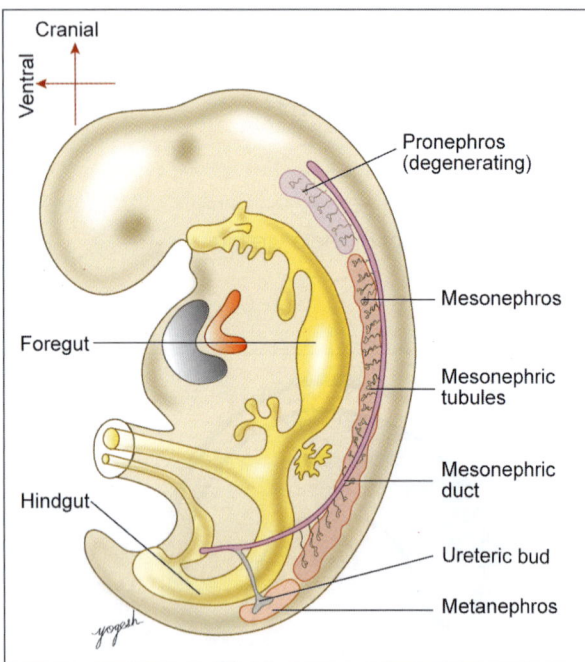

Fig. 20.3: A 28 days foetus showing pronephros, mesonephros and metanephros. Pronephric tubules appear in the cervical region and they soon disappears. Ureteric bud raises from mesonephric duct and grows towards metanephros

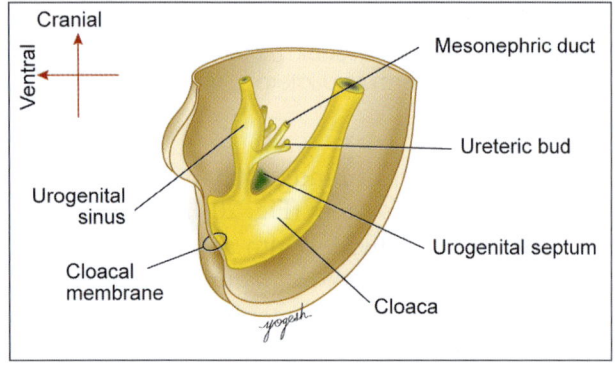

Fig. 20.4: Endodermal cloaca and allantois

Flowchart 20.1: Subdivisions of cloaca and development of urinary bladder

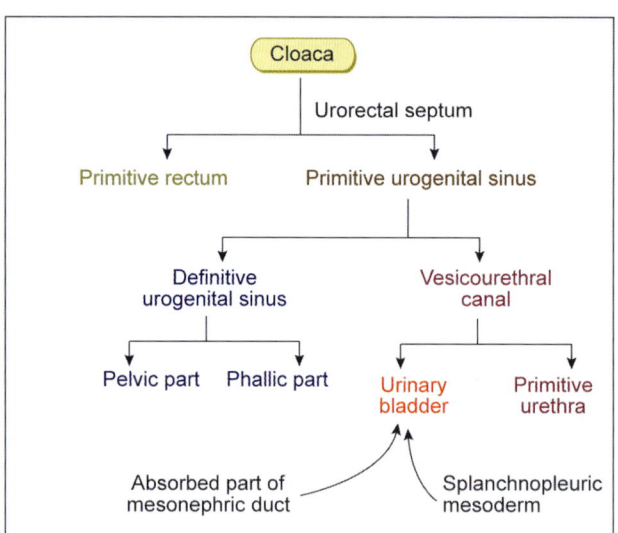

Mesonephric Duct (Wolffian Duct)^{High yielding}
(see Fig. 21.8)

Q. Write short note on mesonephric duct.
- A mesonephric duct is a paired duct that develops in the intermediate mesoderm that later communicates with primitive urogenital sinus.
- The mesonephric duct is also called Wolffian duct, Leydig's duct, archinephric or nephric duct.
- Casper Fredrich Wolf has first described the mesonephros (1759).
- Anti-müllerian hormone of Sertoli cells is absent in females. Hence, mesonephric duct regresses.

Derivatives[Viva, MCQ]
- Mesonephric duct forms the following structures:

In male
- Trigone of urinary bladder (in both sexes) [MCQ]
- Efferent ducts of testis, epididymis
- Vas deferens[Neet]
- Posterior wall of prostatic urethra, appendix of epididymis.[Neet] (*Note:* Hydatid of Morgagni is appendix of testis in male or paratubal cyst in female.)[Neet]
- Seminal vesicles, ejaculatory ducts[Neet]

In female
- Trigone of urinary bladder
- Epoöphoron
- Paraoöphoron
- Gartner's duct or cyst
- Skene's glands

Ureteric bud *arises from* Wolffian duct and it gives rise to ureter, renal pelvis, major and minor calyces, ampulla and 1–3 million collecting tubules.[Neet]

Paramesonephric Duct (Müllerian Ducts)^High yielding
(see Fig. 21.8)

Q. Write short note on paramesonephric ducts.

- Paramesonephric ducts are paired duct that develops in urogenital ridge of intermediate mesoderm lateral to the mesonephric ducts.
- In 6th week of IUL, lining epithelium of peritoneal cavity (*coelomic epithelium*) invaginates intermediate mesoderm and forms paramesonephric ducts.
- These ducts cross ventrally to mesonephric ducts (from lateral to the medial) and fuse with each other to form *uterovaginal canal* (uterine canal).
- Later, uterovaginal canal gets communicated with definitive urogenital sinus.
- Absence of anti-müllerian factor results in development of paramesonephric ducts in females, whereas in male, anti-müllerian factor secretion by Sertoli cells inhibits the development of paramesonephric ducts.

Derivatives^Viva, MCQ
In females
- Uterine tube
- Uterus
- Upper part of vagina

In males
- Appendix of testis
- Prostatic utricle (vagina musculina/vesicula-prostatica)

- *Note:* Prostatic utricle in male is homologous to uterus and vagina in female.

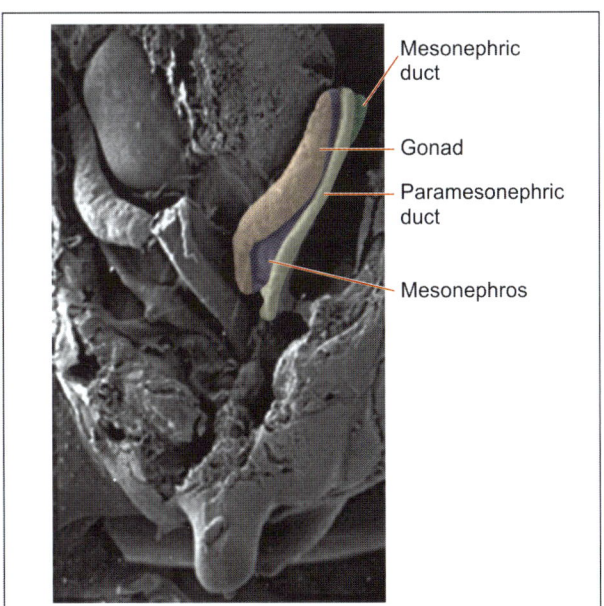

Scanning electron micrograph 20.1: Genital ducts and developing internal genitalia. The intact mesonephric and paramesonephric ducts, mesonephros and gonad of a 7-week human embryo are shown. [Species: Human, day gestation: 7 weeks]

DEVELOPMENT OF KIDNEYS

Q. Write short note on development of kidney.

Summary (Examination Guide) (Practice Fig. 20.1, Flowchart 20.2)

- Human kidney shows two developmental parts as
  A. Collecting part: It consists of collecting tubules, collecting ducts, minor and major calyces, renal pelvis and ureter.^Neet
  B. Secretory part: It consists glomeruli, Bowman's capsule, proximal and distal convoluted tubules and loop of Henle.
- Embryological sources:
  – Ureteric bud forms collecting part of kidney.
  – Metanephric blastema forms secretory part of kidney.
- Kidney ascends from sacral region to thoracolumbar region to get better blood supply.
- Primitive kidney initially gets supply from median sacral artery via renal atery. Later receives from common iliac artery.^Neet On ascent, kidney receives supply from lateral splanchnic branches of the aorta as renal artery.

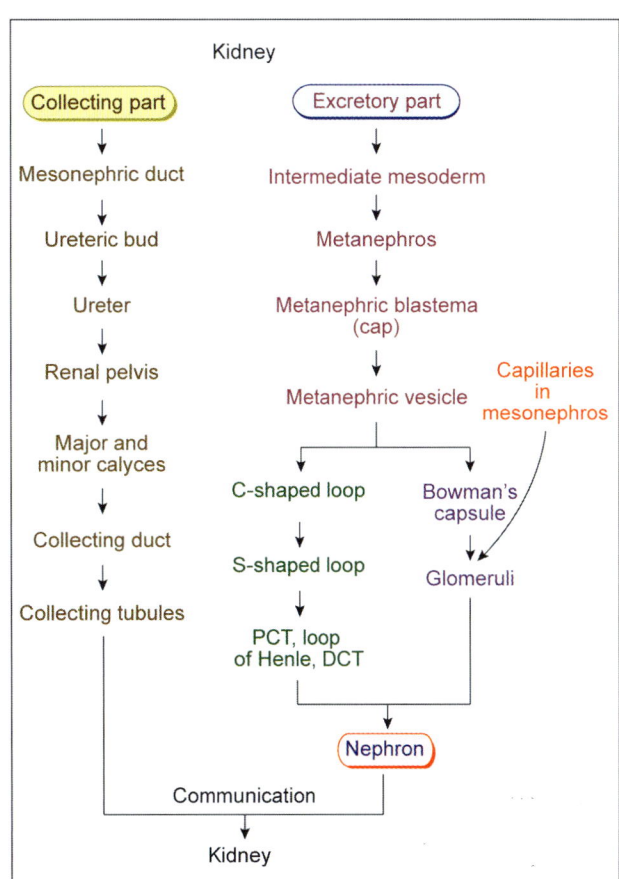

Flowchart 20.2: Development of kidney

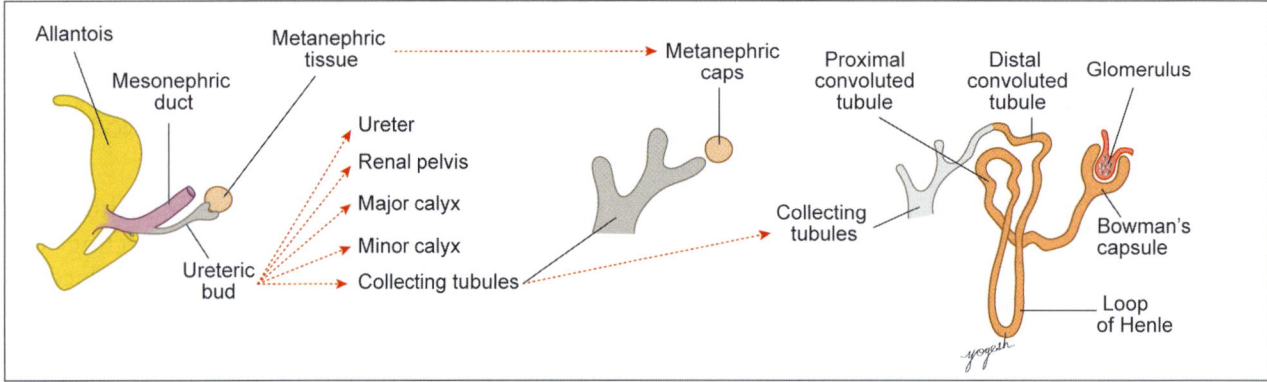

Practice Fig. 20.1: Development of kidney

- On rotation of kidney by 90° medially, hilus turns from ventral to medial side.
- Foetal kidney starts functioning by 12th week of IUL and excretes urine into amniotic cavity.^MCQ

Evolutionary History of Kidney

- Kidney develops from nephrogenic cord of intermediate mesoderm that extends from cervical to sacral region.
- Ontogeny repeats phylogeny in kidney development: Evolutionary history is repeated during the development of kidney.
- Pronephric kidney is present in some cyclostomes and some teleost fish.
- Mesonephric kidney is present in amphibians and most of fishes.
- Metanephric kidney is present in primates including human.
- Thus, evolutionary stages are pronephric kidney → mesonephric kidney → metanephric kidney^Viva
- During the development of human kidney, nephrogenic cord forms three sets of successive kidneys as follows:

1. Pronephros appears in cervical region at the beginning of 4th week and later it regresses and pronephric duct continues as mesonephric duct.
2. Mesonephros appears in thoracolumbar region at the end of 4th week. It also completely regresses. Mesonephric tubules mostly regress (some form vasa efferntia of testis). The mesonephric duct forms collecting part of the kidney and other parts in the male reproductive tract.
3. Metanephros appears in sacral region in the beginning of 3rd month. It forms secretory part of the human kidney.

Stages of Kidney Development

1. **Development of collecting system**
   - Ureteric buds arise from caudal region of mesonephric duct and grow towards metanephros (nephrogenic cord).
   - *Metanephric blastema* caps growing dilated end (ampulla) of ureteric bud.
   - Ampulla divides dichotomously for 12–14 generations to form renal pelvis, major calyces, minor calyces, collecting ducts and collecting tubules (Fig. 20.5).

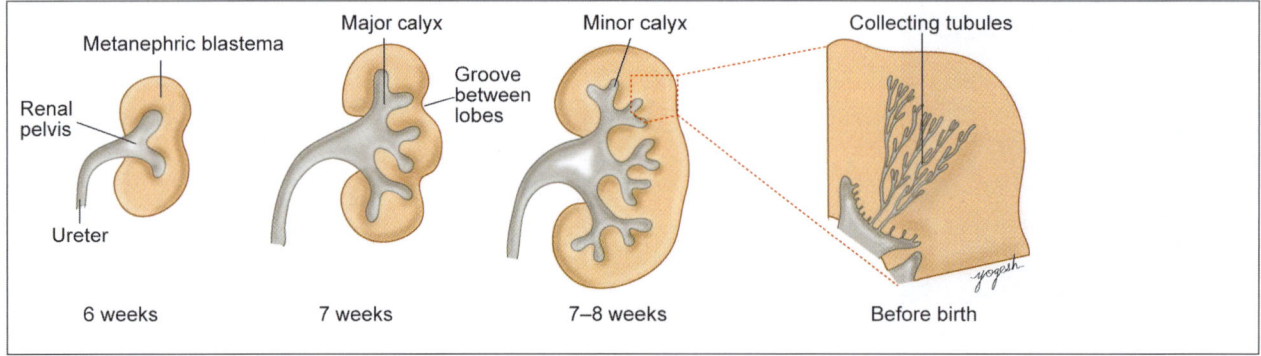

Fig. 20.5: Development of kidney. Ureteric bud divides dichotomously to form renal pelvis, major calyces, minor calyces and collecting tubules

2. Development of secretory (excretory) part
- Cells of the metanephros form metanephric blastema that caps dividing ureteric bud.
- Metanephric cap dilates to form a pear-shaped *metanephric vesicle* that later forms S-shaped *primitive renal tubule* (Fig. 20.6).
- One end of the primitive tubule dilates to form Bowman's capsule, whereas the other end communicates with collecting tubules (derived from ureteric bud).
- Primitive tubule finally forms Bowman's capsule proximal convoluted tubule, loop of Henle and distal convoluted tubule.
- Bowman's capsule is invaginated by a tuft of capillaries from adjacent mesoderm to form *renal corpuscles*.
- Thus, metanephros give rise to secretory unit or nephron up to collecting tubule that includes renal vesicle, glomeruli, Bowman's capsule, proximal convoluted tubule, loop of Henle and distal convoluted tubule.[Neet]

3. Ascent of kidney
Q. Write short note on ascent of kidney.
- Metanephric kidney develops in metanephros of nephrogenic cord that lies in pelvic cavity at sacral level (Fig. 20.7).
- Kidney ascends from its initial sacral position to thoracolumbar region (in 9th week).
- Cause for ascent of kidney[MCQ, Viva]
  - In search of better blood supply
  - Due to smaller pelvic cavity that fails to accommodate enlarging kidney
  - Differential growth of posterior abdominal wall
  - Reduction of foetal curvature
- Duration
  - Metanephros appears by 5th week of IUL
  - By 9th week, kidney ascends to their adult position within the abdomen.[MCQ]

4. Blood supply of kidney
- In initial phase, kidney is supplied by *median sacral artery* (continuation of the aorta).
- During ascent of kidney, lateral splanchnic branches of aorta supply it.
- Finally, one of the lateral splanchnic branches of aorta corresponding to L2 vertebra forms *definitive renal artery*.

5. Rotation of kidney
- On reaching thoracolumbar region, kidney rotates medially around the vertical axis. Hence, hilus changes its position from ventral to medial aspect of kidney.

Congenital Anomalies of Kidney
1. Renal agenesis (Fig. 20.8A)
   - Unilateral or bilateral, complete failure of kidney development is called renal agenesis.
   - Cause: Failure of ureteric bud formation.[Neet]
   - Genetic basis: Metanephros produces glial-derived neurotrophic factor (GDNF) that stimulates branching and growth of ureteric bud. Mutation in genes regulating GDNF production may cause renal agenesis (for example, SALL, PAX2, EYA1). SALL1 cause Townes-Brock syndrome. PAX2 causes coloboma syndrome. EYA1 cause branchio-otorenal syndrome.
2. Duplication: Early division of ureteric bud may produce extra kidney. There may be a separate or fused kidney. The ureters may be separate or partially fused with duplicate kidney (Fig. 20.8B).

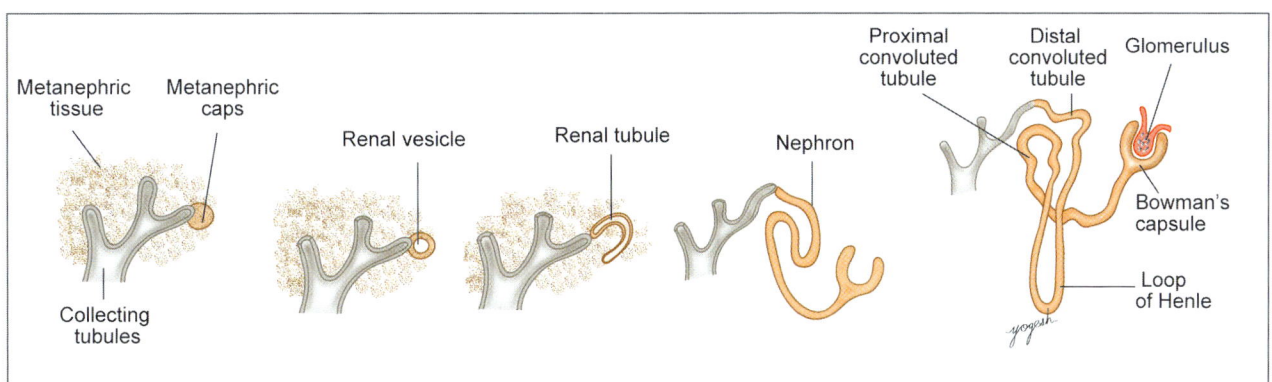

Fig. 20.6: Development of nephron from metanephric blastema. Excretory part of kidney develops from metanephric blastema (brown-coloured structure) and establishes communication with collecting tubules (ash-coloured structure) that develop from ureteric bud (mesonephric duct)

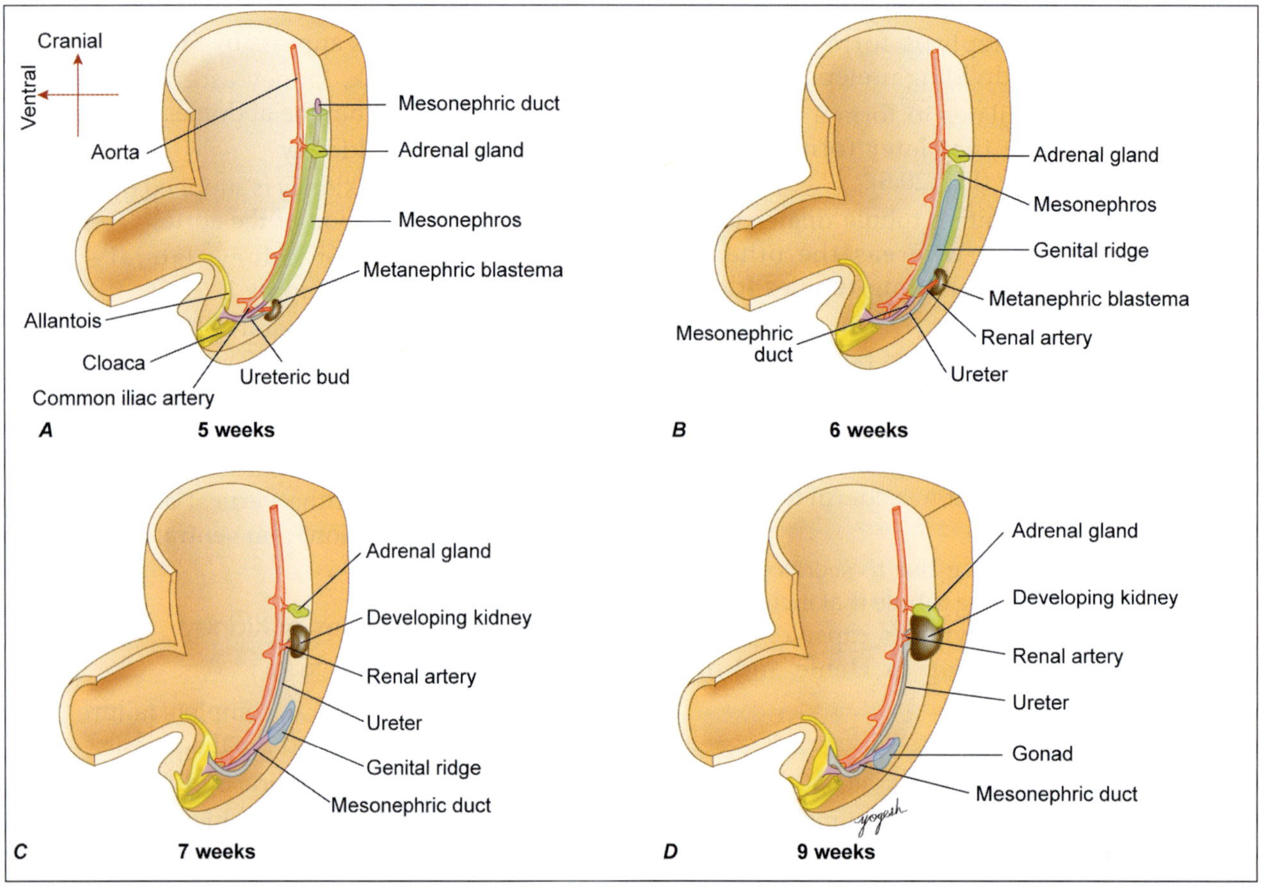

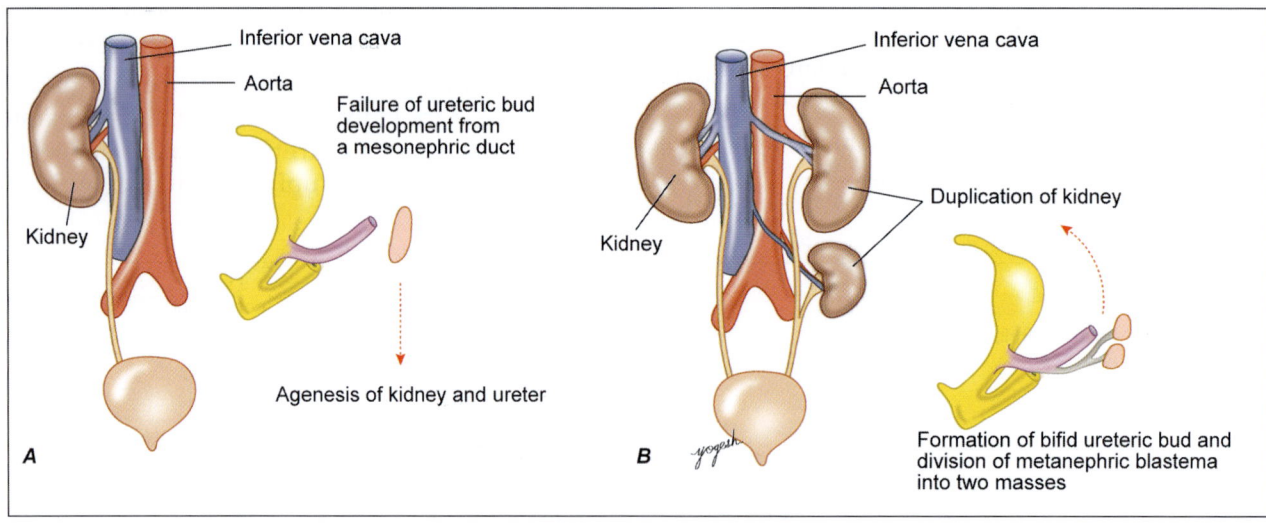

Fig. 20.7: Ascent of kidney. Kidney ascends from its sacral position to thoracolumbar region between 5th and 9th weeks of IUL. Simultaneously, size of mesonephros reduces

Fig. 20.8: Agenesis (A) and duplication (B) of kidney

3. **Horseshoe kidney:** Kidneys may be connected by an isthmus at lower poles. In this condition, kidney lies at the level of lower lumbar vertebrae as *inferior mesenteric artery* blocks the ascent of isthmus of horseshoe kidney (Fig. 20.9A).^{Neet} Horseshoe kidney is the most common congenital anomaly of kidney.^{Neet}

Urinary System: Kidney, Ureter, Urinary Bladder, Urethra

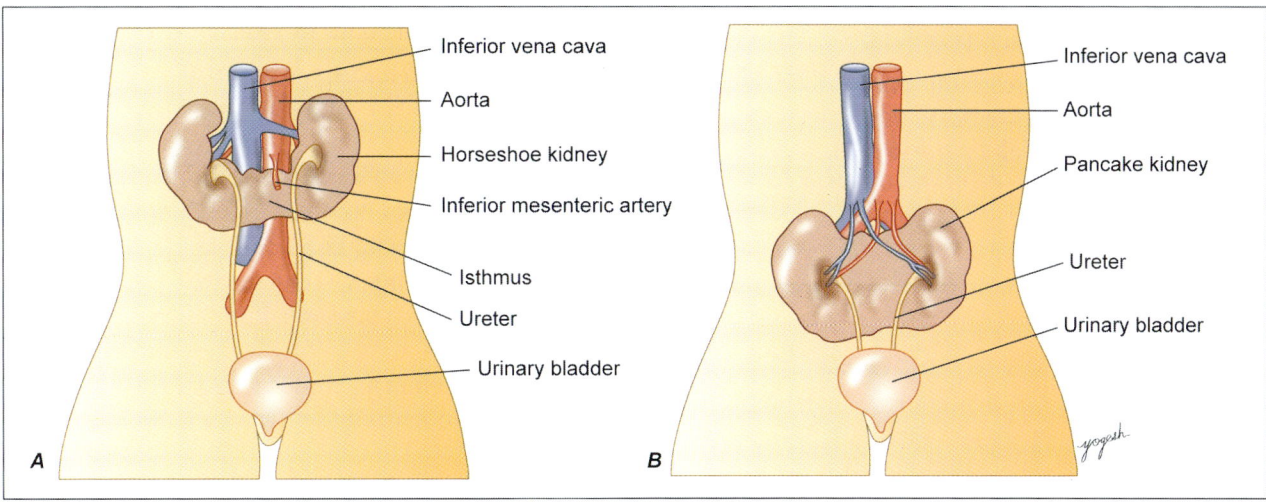

Fig. 20.9: Horseshoe kidney (A) and pancake kidney (B). Horseshoe kidney lies at the level of lower lumbar vertebrae as inferior mesenteric artery blocks ascent of isthmus of horseshoe kidney

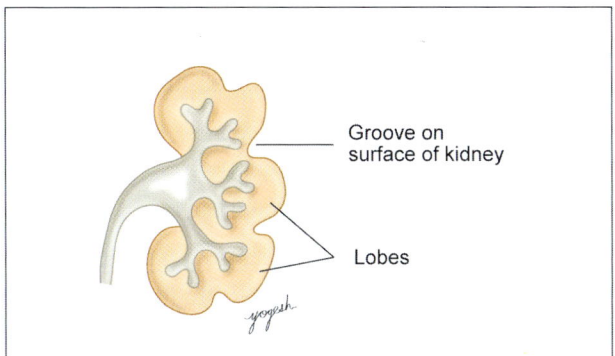

Fig. 20.10: Lobulated kidney. Usually, lobulation disappears in the first year of life. If it persists, it forms lobulated kidney

4. **Pancake kidney:** In this condition both the kidneys fuse to form a single mass (Fig. 20.9B).
5. **Lobulated kidney:** During development, kidney is lobulated. The lobulation disappears in the first year of life. If it persists, it forms lobulated kidney (Fig. 20.10).
6. **Anomalies of ascent of kidney** (Fig. 20.11)
   - Pelvic kidney: Kidney lies in pelvic cavity.
   - Lower lumbar kidneys: Kidney lies against lower lumbar vertebrae.
   - Thoracic kidneys: Abnormally high ascent of kidneys in thoracic cavity.
7. **Congenital polycystic kidney**
   - Polycystic kidney is the commonest congenital anomaly of kidney.^{MCQ}
   - Failure to establish communication between excretory and collecting part of kidney results in polycystic kidney.
   - These cysts are filled with urine.
   - The congenital polycystic kidney is usually bilateral.
   - Newer concept: This condition occurs due to abnormal dilation of uriniferous tubules.
   - It has two presentations:
     – Autosomal recessive polycystic kidney disease (ARPKD) (childhood): It is less common and symptoms appear shortly after birth.
     – Autosomal dominant polycystic kidney disease (ADPKD) (adult): It is more common and develops in adulthood (30–40 years).
   - Incidence of
     ARPKD: 1 in 5000 births
     ADPKD: 1 in 500–1000 births
   - Treatment: Kidney transplantation and dialysis.
   - ADPKD: Cause—mutation in short arm of chromosome 4 or chromosome 16.
8. **Accessory renal artery** (Fig. 20.12)
   - Persisting foetal renal arteries give rise to accessory or supernumerary renal arteries.^{MCQ}
   - Accessory renal artery is the most common renal vascular anomaly.^{Neet} It may cause ureter compression resulting in hydronephrosis.
9. Wilms' tumour is the most common primary renal tumour of the childhood that is produced due to mutation of WT1 gene (location—chromosome 11p13).

Development of Ureter

- Ureter develops from ureteric bud that raises from Wolffian duct (mesonephric duct).
- The part of ureteric bud that lies between renal pelvis and vesicourethral canal (a portion of cloaca) forms ureter.

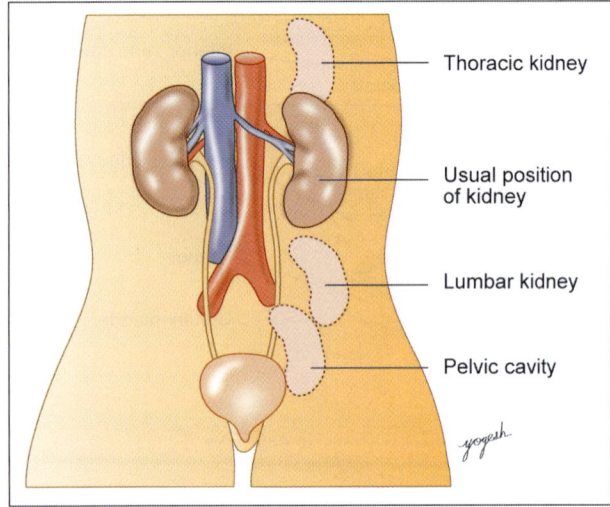

Fig. 20.11: Anomalies of ascent of kidney. Pelvic kidney lies in pelvic cavity, lumbar kidney lies against lower lumbar vertebrae and thoracic kidney lies in thoracic cavity

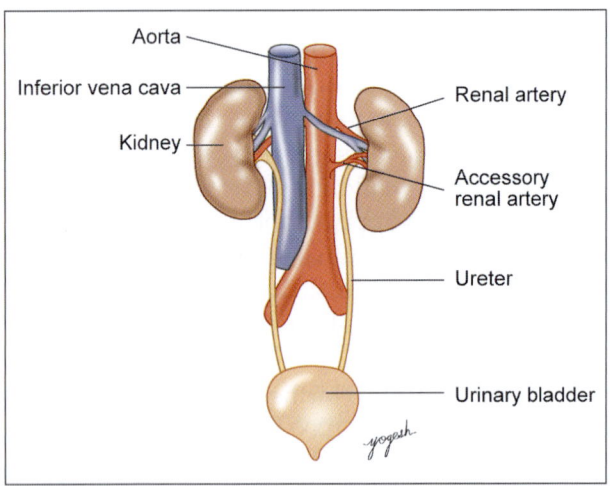

Fig. 20.12: Accessory renal artery represents persistent foetal renal artery

Anomalies of Ureter

1. Ectopic ureter
   - If ureter does not open into bladder at its usual site, it is called *ectopic ureter*.
   - Abnormal sites of ectopic ureteric openings are as follows:
     a. In male: Lower part of bladder, prostatic urethra, seminal vesicles, rectum (Fig. 20.13A).
     b. In female: Urethra, vagina, vestibule, rectum (Fig. 20.13B).
2. Ureteric obstruction (hydroureter): Congenital ureteric obstruction may result in dilation of ureter (hydroureter). Postcaval ureter (right ureter hooks around left side of inferior vena cava) may cause ureteric obstruction (Fig. 20.14).

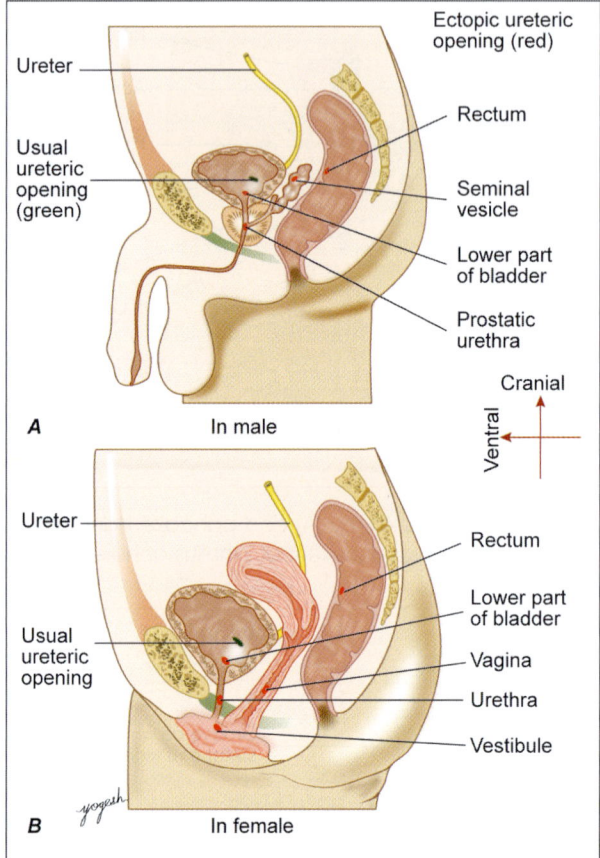

Fig. 20.13: Ectopic ureter. If ureter does not open into bladder at its usual site, it is called ectopic ureter. In male, ectopic ureter opens in lower part of urinary bladder, prostatic urethra, seminal vesicles or rectum, whereas in female in urethra, vagina, vestibule or rectum

3. Duplication: Ureter may be partially or completely duplicated. Duplication of ureter may or may not be associated with duplication of kidney. Duplicated ureter may open into bladder together or separately (Fig. 20.15A).
4. Blind ureter: It is a rare anomaly and can be diagnosed using intravenous urography. Blind ureter is not connected to kidney (Fig. 20.15B).

DEVELOPMENT OF URINARY BLADDER

Q. Write short note on development of urinary bladder.
Q. Write short note on primitive urogenital sinus.

- Urinary bladder shows three layers as inner lining (transitional) epithelium, middle connective tissue and smooth muscle layer and outer serous (connective tissue) layer.
- Interior of bladder shows a smooth triangular region called *trigone* of bladder. Ureters open at the superolateral angles of trigone, whereas its apex has a urethral orifice.

Urinary System: Kidney, Ureter, Urinary Bladder, Urethra

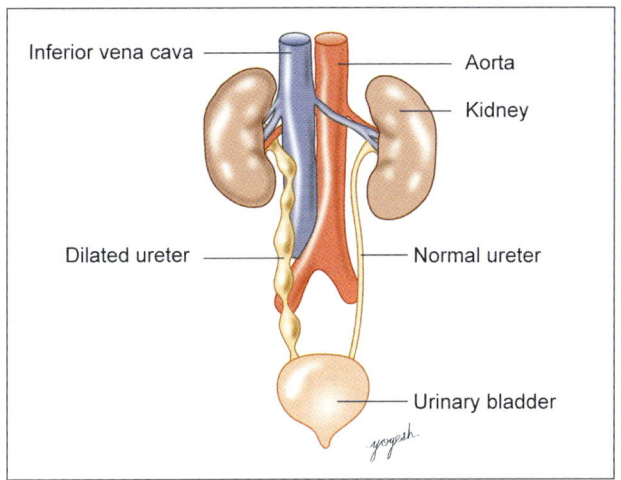

Fig. 20.14: Hydroureter (megaloureter). Congenital ureteric obstruction may result into dilation of ureter

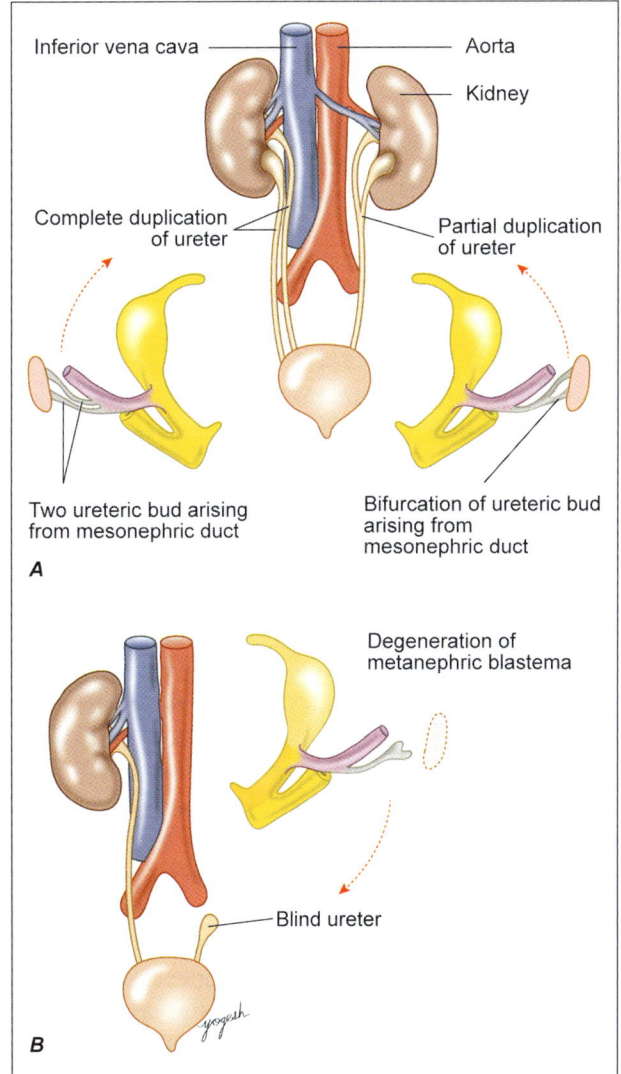

Fig. 20.15: Anomalies of ureter include partial or complete duplication of ureter (A) and blind ureter (B)

Summary (Examination Guide) (Table 20.1, Fig. 20.16, Practice Fig. 20.2)

Developmentally bladder shows following sources:

1. Lining epithelium of bladder except for trigone: It is derived from cranial dilated part of vesicourethral canal (endoderm).
2. Lining epithelium of trigone: It develops from mesoderm by absorption of mesonephric ducts in dorsal wall of vesicourethral canal.
3. Muscles and connective tissue coats: They develop from mesoderm—splanchnopleuric intraembryonic mesoderm surrounding vesicourethral canal.
4. Urachus (median umbilical ligament) is derived from allantois.^{Neet}

Stages of Urinary Bladder Development

1. Cloacal division:
   - Cloaca is divided by urorectal septum into ventral *urogenital sinus* and dorsal *primitive rectum*.
   - Urorectal septum establishes contact with cloacal membrane to divide it into ventral *urogenital membrane* and dorsal *anal membrane*.
   - Urorectal septum forms *perineal body*.^{MCQ}
   - Urorectal septum contains four ducts, a pair of mesonephric ducts and a pair of paramesonephric ducts.
   - In the 5th week, mesonephric ducts open into the urogenital sinus.
   - The opening of mesonephric duct divides the urogenital sinus in cranial *vesicourethral canal* and caudal *definitive urogenital sinus*.
   - Definitive urogenital sinus is subdivided into cranial *pelvic part* and caudal *phallic part*.

Table 20.1	Development of urinary bladder^{Neet}
Part of urinary bladder	*Embryological source*
Lining epithelium (transitional epithelium) of urinary bladder except for trigone	Endoderm: Cranial dilated part of vesicourethral canal^{Neet}
Lining epithelium of trigone	Mesoderm: Absorbed part of mesonephric ducts in vesicourethral canal
Connective tissue and muscles	Splanchnopleuric intraembryonic mesoderm surrounding vesicourethral canal
Urachus (median umbilical ligament), apex of urinary bladder	Allantois

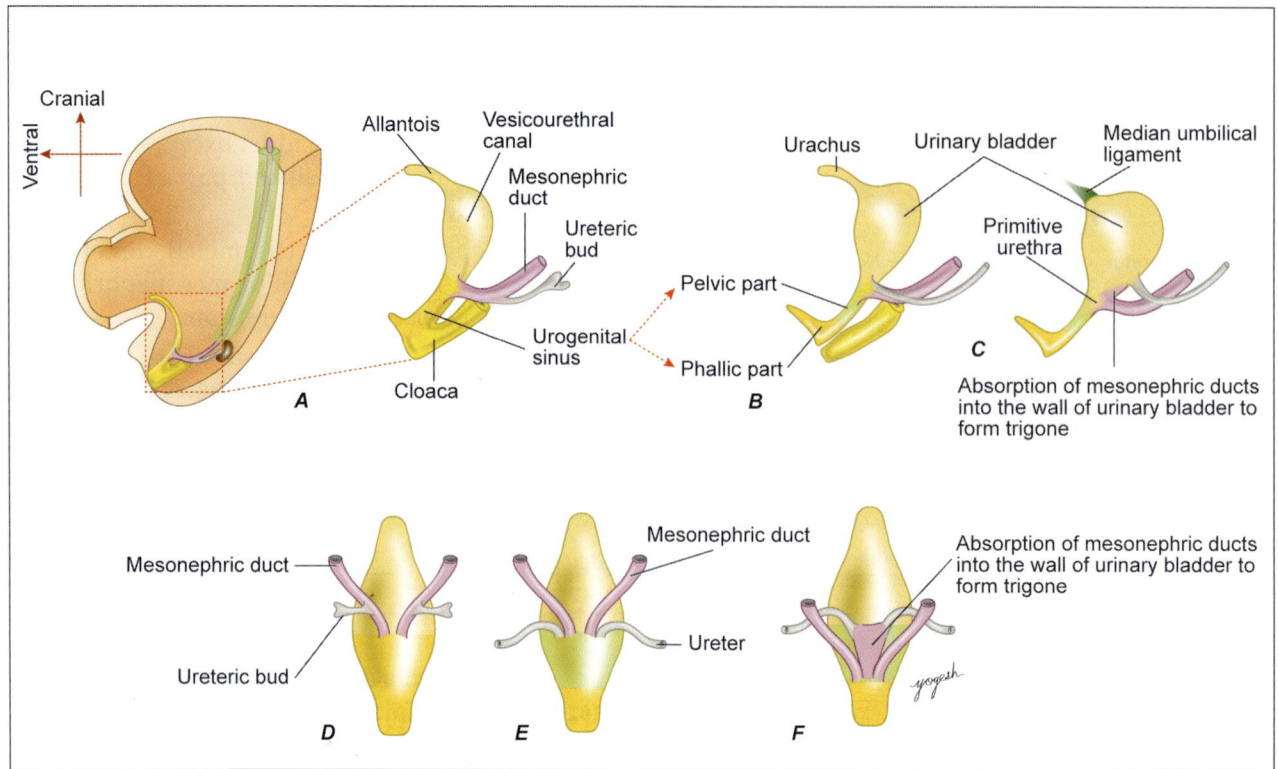

Fig. 20.16: Development of urinary bladder. A–C: Side view of developing urinary bladder; D–F: Dorsal view of the developing bladder showing changing relationship of ureter and mesonephric duct

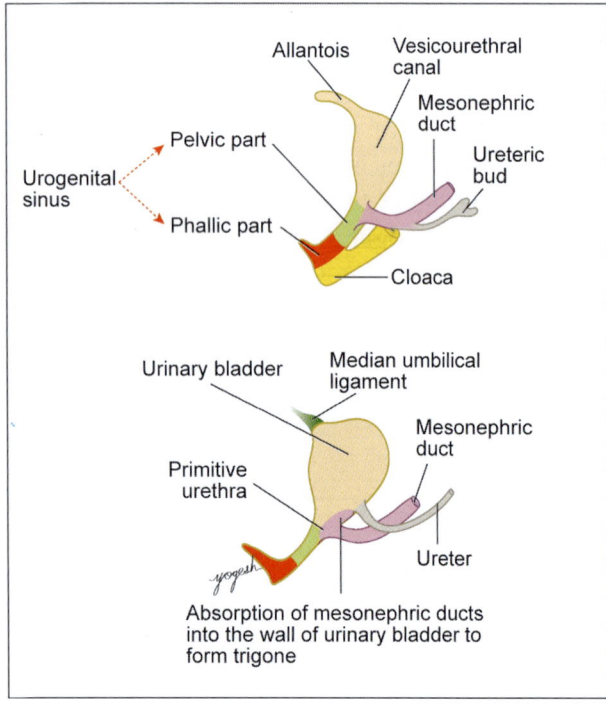

Practice Fig. 20.2: Development of urinary bladder

2. Absorption of mesonephric ducts into vesicourethral canal
   - Initially, ureteric bud (future ureters) and mesonephric ducts have a common opening in the vesicourethral canal.
   - Slow absorption (incorporation) of mesonephric duct in dorsal wall of vesicourethral canal separates openings of mesonephric ducts from ureteric buds.
   - Gradually absorption continues, and openings of ureteric buds move laterally and cranially.
   - Incorporated mesonephric ducts form a triangular zone on the dorsal wall of vesicourethral canal. This triangular part (trigone of urinary bladder) lies between the openings of ureters (ureteric bud) and mesonephric ducts.
   - *Note:* Terminal part of mesonephric ducts disappears in female and in male they formrs ejaculatory ducts (for details, read Chapter 21).
3. Development of muscular and connective tissue coats
   - Muscular and connective tissue coats (serous) of urinary bladder are derived from a

splanchnopleuric layer of intraembryonic mesoderm that surrounds vesicourethral canal.

Congenital Anomalies

1. Fistulas:
   a. Congenital rectovesical fistula: It develops due to incomplete urorectal septum.
   b. Congenital vesicovaginal fistula: Müllerian eminence is elevation in dorsal wall of the phallic part of the urogenital sinus formed by fused caudal ends of paramesopheric ducts. If müllerian eminence projects into the vesicourethral part of cloaca, it results in *vesicovaginal fistula*.
   c. *Urachal fistula*: It is persistent allantois.[Neet] In this condition, urinary bladder communicates with exterior at the umbilicus (Fig. 20.17A).
2. *Urachal cyst*: Urachal cyst develops from non-obliterated middle part of allantois.[Neet] It forms palpable midline cystic part of anterior abdominal wall (Fig. 20.17B).
3. *Urachal sinus*: It develops from nonobliterated distal part of allantois that shows opening at umbilicus (Fig. 20.17C).
4. Hourglass bladder: In this condition, urinary bladder is divided into upper and lower compartments by a constriction in middle zone (Fig. 20.18).

DEVELOPMENT OF URETHRA

Q. Write short note on development of urethra.

Development of Female Urethra

- Female urethra is short (4 cm).
- Female urethra is derived as follows:
  - Mostly from narrow caudal part of the vesicourethral canal.

Box 20.1: Ectopia vesicae

Q. Write short note on ectopia vesicae.

- It is also called *extrophy of urinary bladder*.
- Abnormality:
  - Deficient midline infraumbilical part of anterior abdominal wall
  - Deficient anterior wall of urinary bladder
  - Interior of bladder exposed
  - Urine dribbles from exposed bladder
- Embryological basis:
  - Failure of complete formation of lateral fold of embryo.
  - Failure of migration of mesoderm in lateral folds.
- Incidence: 1:10,000 births.
- Constant association: Ectopia vesicae is always associated with epispadias.

– Terminal part of urethra from pelvic part of definitive urogenital sinus (endodermal derivative).

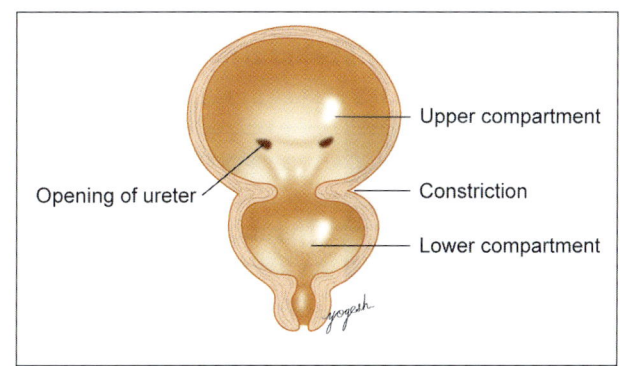

Fig. 20.18: Hourglass bladder is divided into upper and lower compartments by a constriction in middle zone

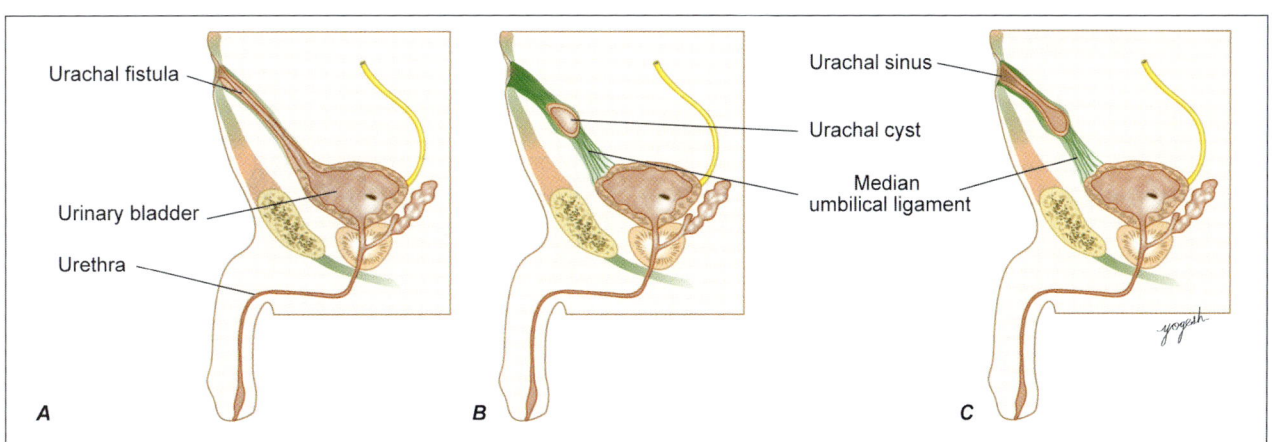

Fig. 20.17: Anomalies raising due to persistent urachus: (A) Urachal fistula; (B) Urachal cyst; (C) Urachal sinus

- A small part of dorsal wall from absorbed part of mesonephric ducts (mesodermal derivative) in vesicourethral canal.
- Female urethra corresponds to prostatic part of male urethra.^{MCQ}

Development of Male Urethra

Q. Write short note on development of male urethra.

- Male urethra has
  a. Prostatic part
  b. Membranous part
  c. Spongy part
  d. Glandular part

Summary (Examination Guide)

Male urethra develops as follows (Table 20.2):
1. Caudal part of vesicourethral canal forms prostatic part of urethra, above level of openings of ejaculatory ducts.
2. Pelvic part of definitive urogenital sinus forms:
   a. Prostatic part of urethra below level of openings of ejaculatory ducts
   b. Membranous part of urethra

Table 20.2	Development of urethra
Part	Embryonic source
Prostatic part	
– Above opening of ejaculatory ducts	Caudal part of vesicourethral canal
– Below openings of ejaculatory duct	Pelvic part of definitive urogenital sinus
Membranous part	Pelvic part of definitive urogenital sinus
Spongy (penile) part	Phallic part of definitive urogenital sinus
Glandular part (terminal part of glans penis)	Surface ectoderm

3. Phallic part of definitive urogenital sinus forms spongy part except near terminal opening that develops from surface ectoderm.

For further details, read the development of male external genitalia (Chapter 21).

CLINICAL EMBRYOLOGY

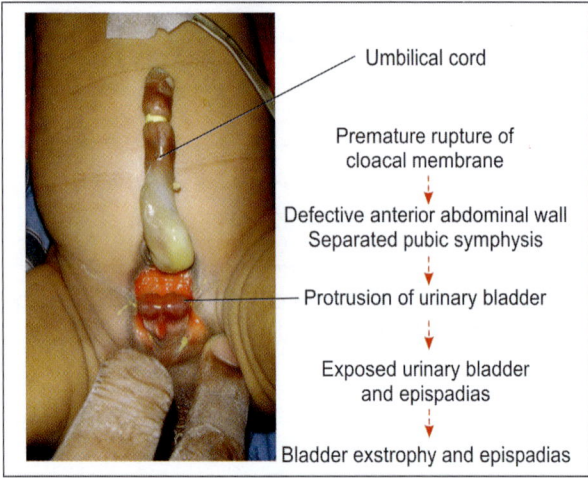

Clinical image 20.1: Bladder exstrophy (ectopia vesicae) is a congenital anomaly that includes exstrophy and epispadias with protrusion of the urinary bladder through a defect in the anterior abdominal wall. In this condition, posterior wall of the bladder is seen externally just below the umbilicus. Incidence is 1:10,000–50,000 live births with male preponderance (3:1) (Image courtesy: *Dr Kumaravel S*)

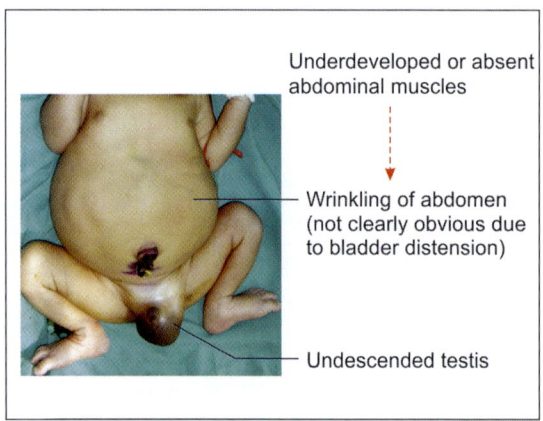

Clinical image 20.2: Prune-belly syndrome (Eagle-Barrett syndrome). It is a disorder of urinary tract that is characterised by the triad of anomalies: (1) Wrinkling of abdominal skin (due to underdeveloped or absent abdominal muscles, (2) cryptorchidism (undescended testis), (3) urinary tract malformations (megaloureter, hydronephrosis, vesicoureteral reflux of urine → renal failure). It has incidence of 1 in 40,000 births and affects male babies commonly (97%) (Image courtesy: *Dr Kumaravel S*)

21
Reproductive System
Male and Female Reproductive Organs

Chapter Outline

- Formation of primitive gonads
  - Genital ridge
  - Migration of primordial germ cells
  - Differentiation into definitive gonad
- Development of testis
  - Stages of development
  - Descent of testis
  - Anomalies of testis
- Cryptorchidism
- Development of ovary
  - Stages of development
- Descent of ovary
  - Anomalies of ovary
- Genital ducts
  - Mesonephric ducts
  - Paramesonephric ducts
- Development of uterus
  - Anomalies of uterus
- Development of vagina
  - Congenital anomalies of vagina
- Development of prostate
- Development of external genitalia
  - Male external genitalia
  - Female external genitalia
- Hypospadias
- Epispadias

INTRODUCTION

- The genital system consists of gonads and genital (sex) ducts.
- Gonads include testes in male and ovaries in females.
- Gonads develop from the genital ridge with incorporation of primordial germ cells.
- Genital ducts in male include efferent ductules of testis, epididymis, vas deferens, seminal vesicle and ejaculatory duct.
- Genital ducts in female include uterine tubes, uterus, and vagina.
- Accessory sex glands in male include prostate and bulbourethral glands, whereas in female include greater vestibular glands (Bartholin's glands).
- During early embryonic period, two paired ducts, namely mesonephric (wolffian) and paramesonephric (müllerian) are present. These ducts undergo further differentiation or regression depending on sex differentiation and finally form the genital duct system.

Primordial germ cells

- Primordial germ cells arise from epiblasts (primary ectoderm) in the second week.[Neet]
- These primordial germ cells remain within extraembryonic mesoderm of connecting stalk and wall of the yolk sac (Fig. 21.1).[Neet]
- On formation of the tail fold, primordial germ cells come to lie in splanchnopleuric mesoderm that surrounds hindgut.
- In **5th week**, coelomic epithelium covering mesonephric ridges proliferate to form genital ridges (Fig. 21.2). Formation of genital ridge is the first sign of gonad formation.[Neet]
- By 5th week, primordial germ cells migrate bilaterally through dorsal mesentery to the region of genital ridges (by amoeboid movements).

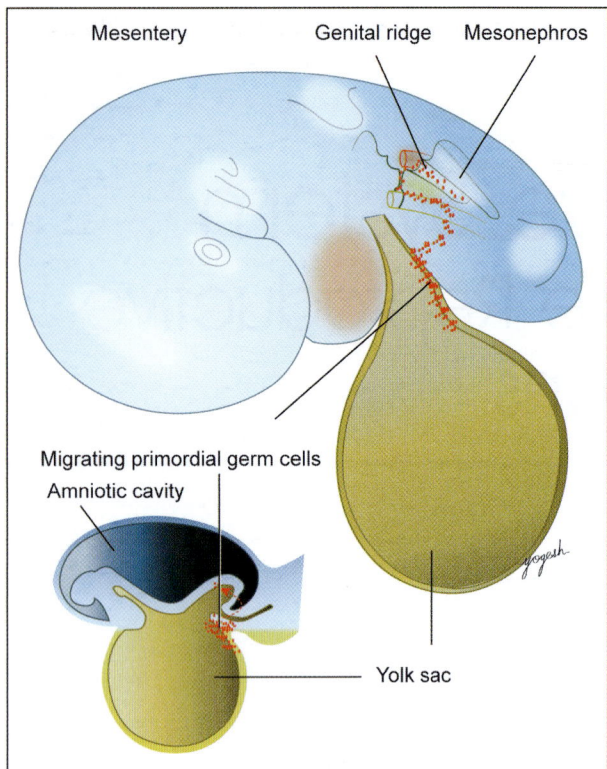

Fig. 21.1: Primordial germ cells (PGC). PGC resides in the yolk sac and migrates to wall of gut during fourth to sixth weeks. Later, these cells migrate through mesentery of gut to dorsal body wall and colonies to form gonadal ridge and subsequently gonads (testes or ovaries)

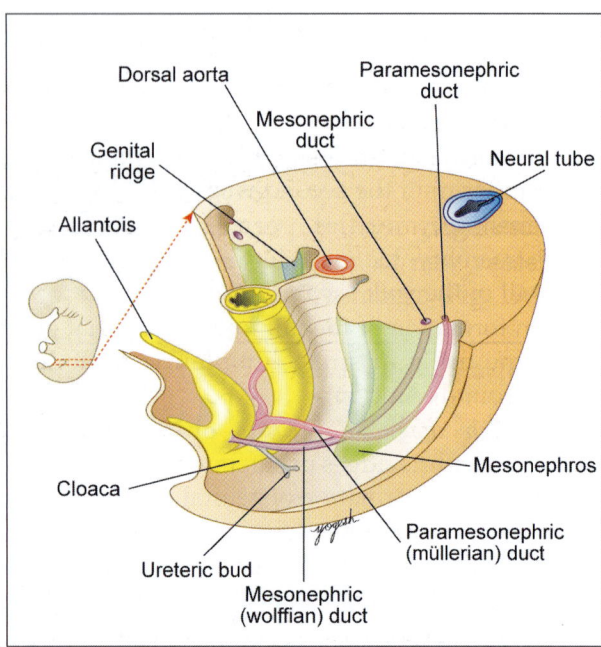

Fig. 21.2: Cross section of embryo showing mesonephric and paramesonephric ducts

FORMATION OF PRIMITIVE GONADS

Genital Ridge (Gonadal Ridge)

- In fifth week of intrauterine life, coelomic epithelium (lining epithelium of primitive peritoneal cavity) covering medial surface of mesonephros proliferates to form a *genital ridge*. Genitourinary system develops from genital ridge of intermediate mesoderm.[Neet]
- Genital ridge is an elevation of posterior abdominal wall, in between dorsal aorta and mesonephros (Fig. 21.2).
- Genital ridge consists of inner medulla and outer cortex.
- Testis or ovary arises from genital ridge (intermediate mesoderm) retroperitoneally, on the posterior abdominal wall in lumbar region (at T10 level).[Neet]

Migration of Primordial Germ Cells

- In fourth week, primordial germ cells migrate to genital ridge along dorsal mesentery (Fig. 21.1).
- Formation of primitive sex cords: From surface (coelomic) epithelium, numerous cord-like processes develop and enter the genital ridge to form finger-like cords called *primitive sex cords*.

Differentiation into Definitive Gonad

- *Up to 7th week* of IUL, gonad is ambisexual or indifferent.[Neet]
- Differentiation of genital ridge (undifferentiated gonad) into testis or ovary (definitive gonad) entirely depends on chromosomal constitution of the individual (Flowcharts 21.1 and 21.2).
- Y-chromosome determine testis formation as **testis-determining factor** (TDF) is located on short arm of chromosome Y. TDF is controlled by *SRY gene* (sex-determining region of Y chromosome).[MCQ]
- TDF induces differentiation of Sertoli cells.
- In the absence of TDF, cells of sex cords differentiate into follicular cells of ovary. Both X chromosomes should be genetically active to form primary ovarian follicles. After formation of definitive female gonad, only one X chromosome remains active, whereas the other X chromosome becames inactive to form the **Barr body**.[Neet] Barr body appears soon after the beginning of embryonic period, after 2nd–3rd week.[Neet]
- Genital ridge has an outer cortex and inner medulla.
- In female foetus, cortex differentiates to form ovary and medulla regresses.
- In male foetus, medulla differentiates to form testis and cortex regresses.
- TDF differentiate Sertoli cells that start producing **anti-müllerian substance** (AMS) or hormone. Anti-

müllerian substance inhibits development of the müllerian ducts.^MCQ

- Thus, absence of Y-chromosome (SRY gene) or TDF results in the formation of ovary.^Neet
- TDF also helps in differentiation of Leydig cells from mesoderm of gonadal ridge.^Neet Leydig cells start secreting testosterone and dihydrotestosterone 8 weeks onwards.^Neet Testosterone stimulates growth of mesonephric duct that forms male genital duct system. Dihydrotestosterone helps in formation of penis, penile urethra, prostate and scrotum.
- The absence of androgens (testosterone and dihydrotestosterone) allows differentiation of müllerian ducts into uterine tubes and uterus under influence of maternal and placental oestrogen. This oestrogen also differentiates genital swellings into female external genitalia.
- Differentiation of gonad starts after 7th week (2 months).^Neet

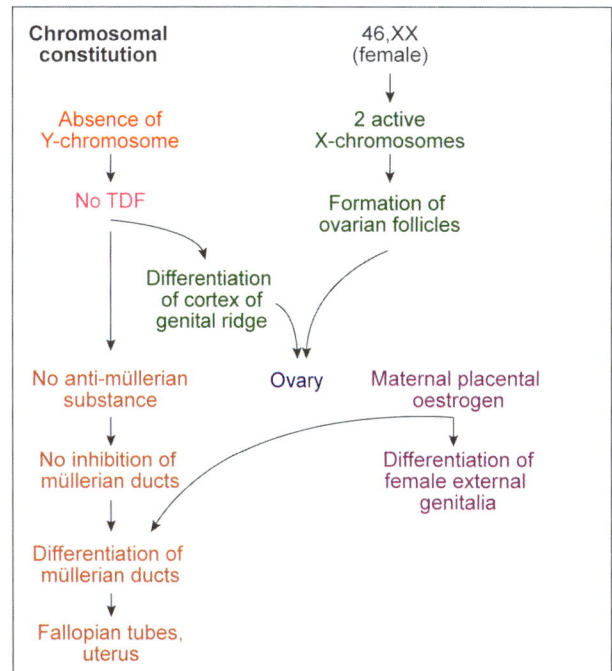

Flowchart 21.2: Sex differentiation in female

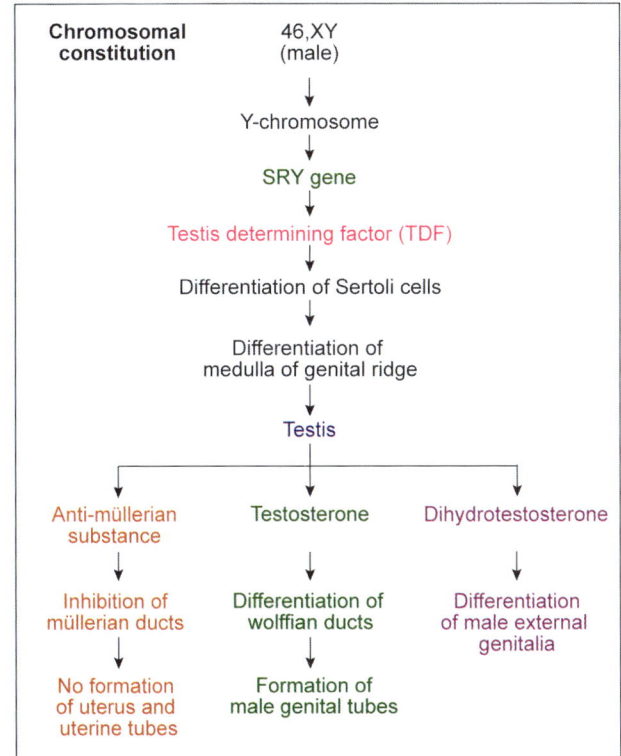

Flowchart 21.1: Sex differentiation in male

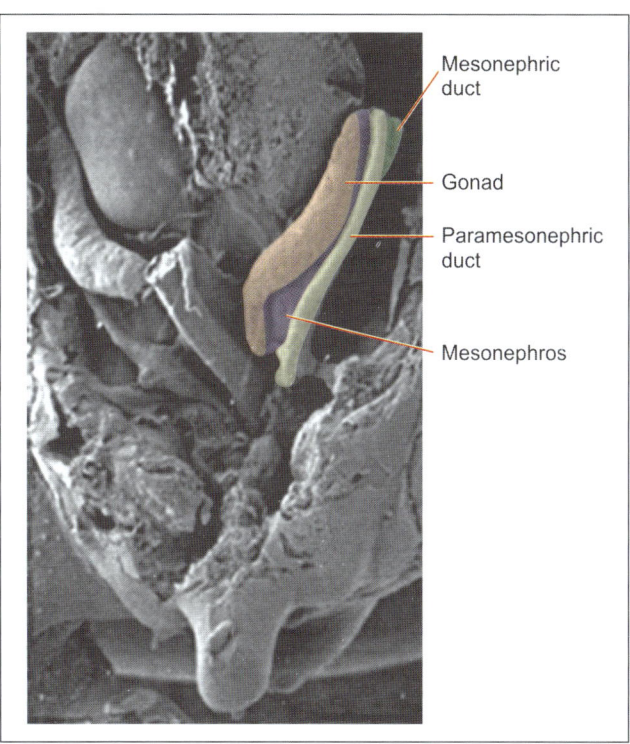

Scanning electron micrograph 21.1: Genital ducts and developing internal genitalia [Species: Human, gestational age: 7 weeks]

1. **Medulla of genital ridge:** It forms seminiferous tubules, rete testis, interstitial cells, fibrous septa and intrinsic coverings of testis.
2. **Mesonephric tubules:** 12–15 mesonephric tubules form efferent ductules.

DEVELOPMENT OF TESTIS

Q. Write a short note on development of testis.

Summary (Examination Guide)

- Testis is the male gonads. Various parts of the testis develop as follows (Table 21.1):

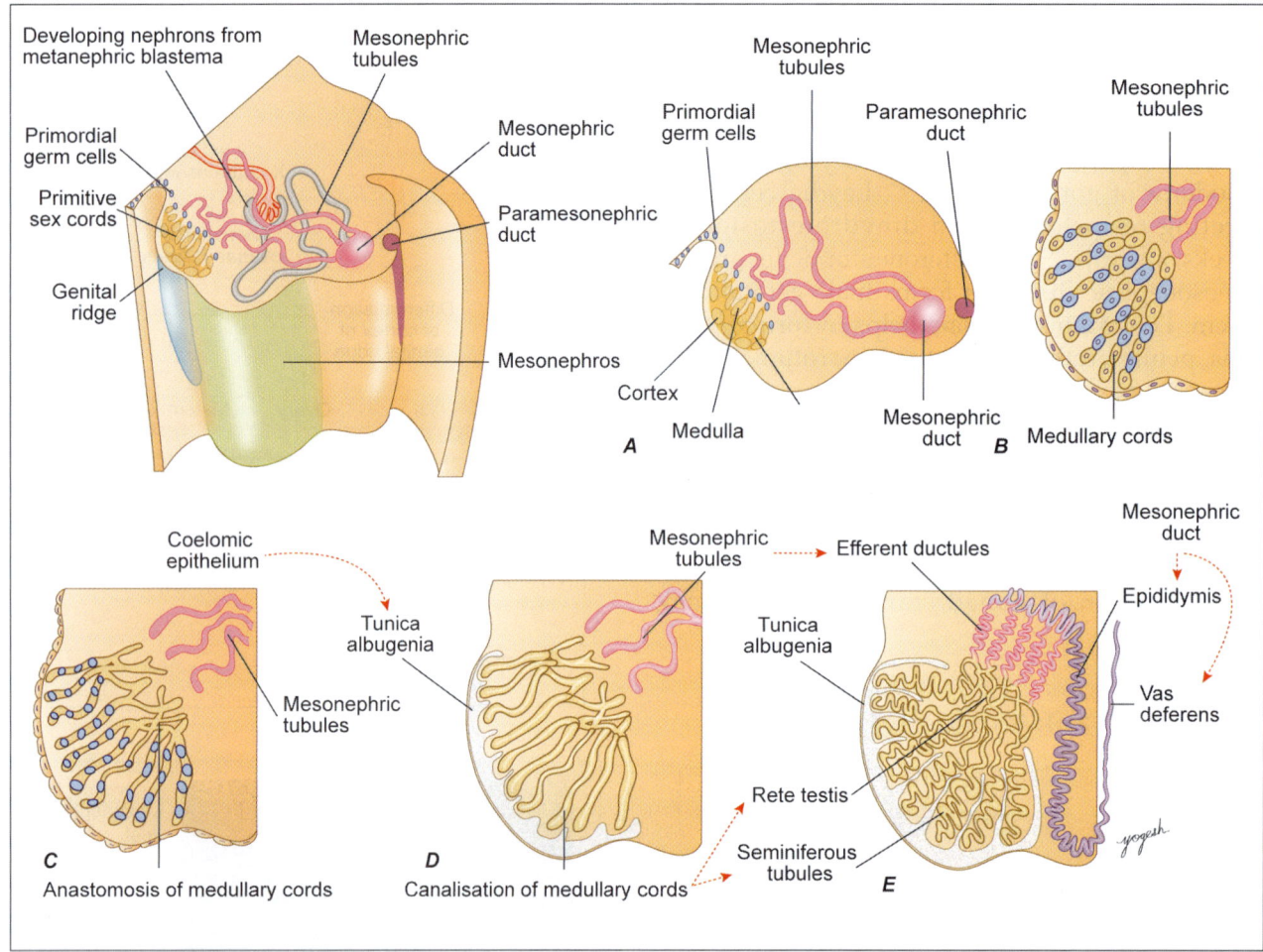

Fig. 21.3: Development of male gonad (testis). Medulla of genital ridge forms seminiferous tubules, rete testis and interstitial cells. Mesonephric tubules form efferent ductules. Mesonephric duct forms canal of epididymis and vas deferens. Paramesonephric (müllerian) duct gets degenerated except at appendix of testis. Mesonephros also degenerates, but its small remnant form appendix of epididymis

3. Mesonephric duct: It forms canal of epididymis and vas deferens.
4. Paramesonephric (müllerian) duct: It gets degenerated (remnants—appendix of testis).
5. Mesonephros: It degenerates (remnants—appendix of epididymis).

Table 21.1	Development of testis
Part of testis	Embryological source
1. Seminiferous tubules rete testis	Medulla of genital ridge (sex cords)
2. Interstitial cells of Leydig, fibrous septa and coverings of testis	Mesenchymal condensation of genital ridge
3. Efferent tubules	12–15 mesonephric tubules
4. Canal of epididymis and vas deferens	Mesonephric duct
5. Appendix of testis^{Neet}	Remnant of paramesonephric duct
6. Appendix of epididymis	Remnant of mesonephros

Stages of Development

- Testis-determining factor (TDF) produced by SRY gene located on short arm of chromosome Y influence development of testis.^{MCQ}
- Testis develops from medulla of genital ridge of primary gonads.
- In the genital ridge, primitive sex cords extend to form *medullary cords* that converge towards hilus of the developing testis (Fig. 21.3A).
- Near hilus, medullary cords anastomose with each other to form a network (Fig. 21.3B).
- Later, medullary cords get canalised to form *seminiferous tubules*, whereas anastomotic network forms the *rete testis* (Fig. 21.3B–E).
- Communication between rete testis and seminiferous tubules develop by fourth month of IUL.
- Sex cord cells derived from coelomic epithelium form *Sertoli cells*, whereas primordial germ cells form *spermatogonia*.

- In seventh week, mesenchymal tissue separates sex cords from coelomic epithelium and form a fibrous layer of *tunica albuginea; mediastinal septa* and *interstitial cells of Leydig* (Fig. 21.3D–E).
- The tubules of rete testis develop communication with adjacent 12–15 mesonephric tubules. These mesonephric tubules form *efferent ductules* of testis.
- Later, mesonephric duct form duct of *epididymis, vas deferens, seminal vesicles* and *ejaculatory duct*.

Descent of Testis

Q. Write short note on descent of testis.
Q. List the factors responsible for descent of testis.

- Testis develops in dorsal abdominal wall at the level of upper lumbar vertebrae.
- During development, testis descents slowly from lumbar region to the scrotum. After birth, testis lies outside the body (within the scrotal sac).

Summary (Examination Guide)^{High yielding, Neet}

Testis descent slowly with the following schedule (Fig. 21.4, Practice Fig. 21.1):
1. During 3rd month: Testis reaches to iliac fossa.
2. At the end of 6th month: It reaches to deep inguinal ring.^{Neet}
3. In 7th month: It travels through inguinal canal.^{Neet}
4. At the end of 8th month: It reaches to superficial inguinal ring.
5. By the end of 9th month: It reaches to scrotum.^{Neet}

Factors Responsible for Descent of Testis

The descent of the testis is influenced and assisted by the following factors (Table 21.2):
1. Differential growth of the posterior body wall.
2. Formation of inguinal bursa: Anterior abdominal wall forms an outpouching called *inguinal bursa*. Passage of inguinal bursa through anterior abdominal wall is given rise to the *inguinal canal*, whereas surface elevation forms the *scrotum*.
3. Gubernaculum testis: It is the mesenchymal band that connects *lower pole* of testis to bottom of scrotum (initially, to *anterior abdominal wall*).^{Neet} Body wall and embryo continue to grow rapidly but gubernaculum grows very slowly. Thus, testis progressively shifts to lower position. Gubernaculum also helps to dilate inguinal bursa and guide testis to scrotum.
4. Processus vaginalis: It is a diverticulum of the peritoneal cavity that extends into scrotum through inguinal canal. Processus vaginalis guide testis to the scrotum during descent and later it forms a covering

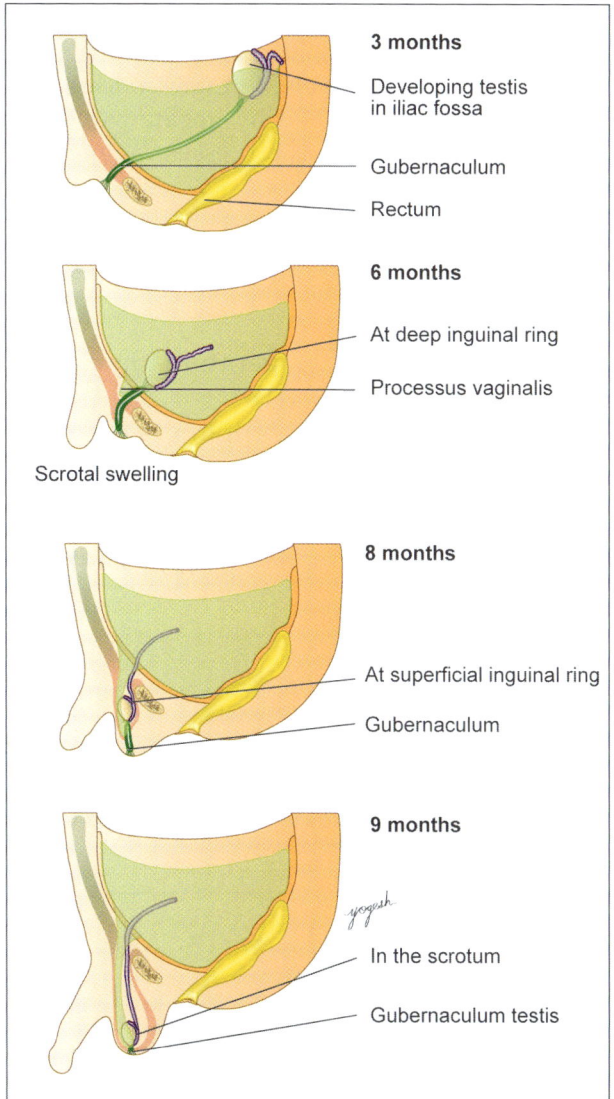

Fig. 21.4: Descent of testis

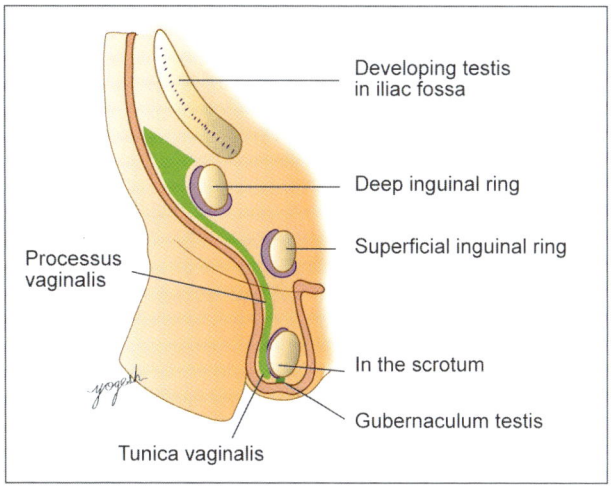

Practice Fig. 21.1: Descent of testis

of the testis called *tunica vaginalis*. Proximal part of processus vaginalis is obliterated by androgens (via calcitonin gene related peptide, CGRP, released from genitofemoral nerve) and by hepatocyte growth factor.^Neet Distal portion of processus vaginalis form tunica vaginalis.^Neet

5. Other factors:
   - Increased abdominal pressure due to growing abdominal viscera
   - Male sex hormones
   - High abdominal temperature than scrotal temperature (4°C higher)
   - Neurotransmitter (calcitonin gene-related peptide) secreted by the genitofemoral nerve cause contraction of the cremaster muscle.

Table 21.2	Factors assisting descent of testis
1. Differential body wall growth	
2. Formation of inguinal bursa	
3. Gubernaculum testis	
4. Processus vaginalis	
5. Other factors – Increased abdominal pressure – Male sex hormones – Higher abdominal temperature – Contraction of the cremaster muscle	

Anomalies of Testis

1. Cryptorchidism (Box 21.1)
2. Anorchism: Both the testis are absent or present as rudimentary gonads in abdomen.
3. Monorchism: Only one testis is descended, whereas another one remains intra-abdominal.
4. Ectopic testis: Testis deviated from its usual course of descent becomes ectopic testis (Fig. 21.5).

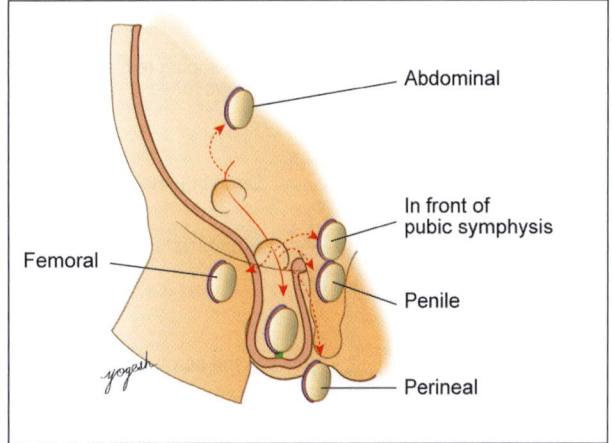

Fig. 21.5: Ectopic testis

The ectopic positions of testis are as follows:
- In superficial perineal pouch (perineal)
- In front of pubic symphysis
- In femoral canal (femoral)
- In skin of the penis (penile)
- Under skin in front of thigh

5. Congenital hydrocoele and congenital inguinal hernia (Fig. 21.6):
   - Processus vaginalis normally obliterates by one year.
   - Persistent processus vaginalis form a passage through which coils of intestine protrude and form *congenital inguinal hernia*.
   - Accumulation of fluid in part of processus vaginalis results in *congenital hydrocoele*.

Box 21.1: Cryptorchidism (undescended testis)

Q. Write short note on cryptorchidism.

Definition
- Cryptorchidism is a failure of descent of testis that results in absence of one or both the testes from scrotum.

Incidence
- 3% of full-term and about 30% of premature infant boys show undescended testis. Out of these in about 80% cases, testis descent during the first year of life.

Locations of testis in cryptorchidism
- In case of cryptorchidism, testis may be located at one of the following positions:
  1. High up in scrotum
  2. At superficial inguinal ring
  3. Within inguinal canal
  4. At deep inguinal ring
  5. In iliac fossa or lumbar region.

Signs and symptoms
1. Infertility: Exposure of undescended testis to higher temperature than scrotal temperature results in failure of spermatogenesis.
2. Undescended testis may result in malignancy or atrophy.

Treatment
1. Watchful waiting: Most of the times, testis descent within the first year of life.
2. Orchidopexy: Testis can be surgically moved to the scrotum.

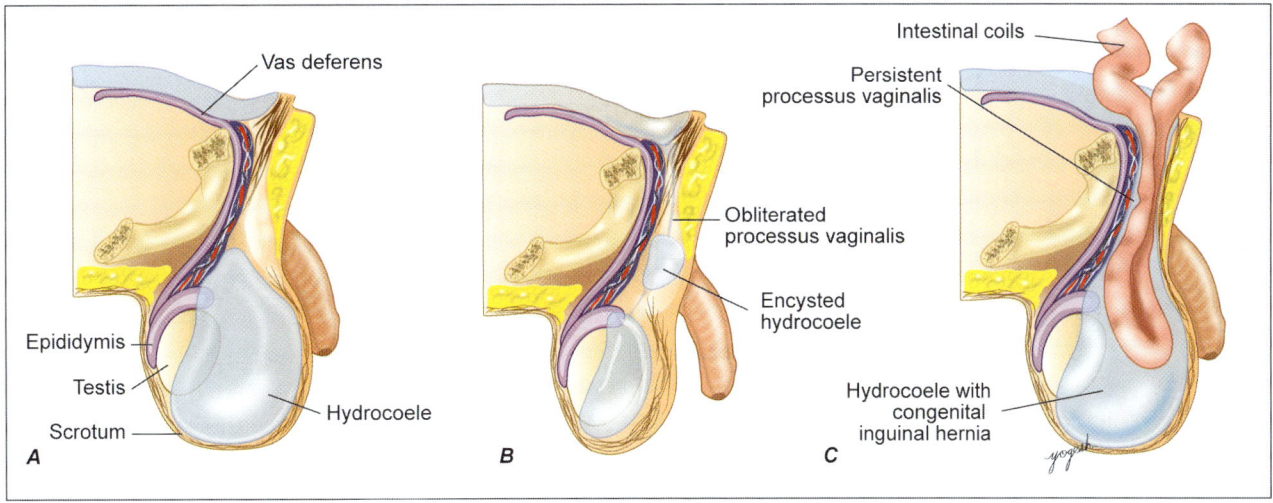

Fig. 21.6: Anomalies of processus vaginalis: (A) Hydrocoele; (B) Encysted hydrocoele; (C) Hydrocoele with congenital inguinal hernia

DEVELOPMENT OF OVARY

Q. Write short note on development of ovary.

Summary (Examination Guide)

- Ovaries are female gonads
- The components of ovary are derived as follows (Table 21.3):
  1. Oocyte develops from *primordial germ cells* that migrate from yolk sac.
  2. Follicular cells are derived from *cortical sex cords* that are raised from the coelomic epithelium.
  3. Germinal epithelium (cuboidal epithelium covering the ovaries) is derived from *coelomic epithelium* that covers genital ridge.
  4. Medulla of ovary is derived from degenerated *medullary sex cords*.

Table 21.3	Development of ovary
Part of ovary	Embryological source
Oocytes	Primordial germ cells
Follicular cells	Cortical sex cords
Germinal epithelium	Coelomic epithelium
Medulla	Degenerated medullary sex cords

Stages of Development

1. Primordial germ cells migrate from yolk sac in the genital ridge (Fig. 21.7).
2. Primitive medullary sex cords degenerate and form ovarian medulla.
3. In the seventh week, coelomic epithelium gives rise to second generation of sex cords called *cortical cords*. Cortical cords do not extend in the medulla.
4. In the third month, cortical cord form clusters of cells that surround each primordial cell.
5. Thus, primordial germ cell forms *oogonia* and surrounding cortical cell cluster form *follicular cells* to develop *primordial follicle*.
6. The coelomic epithelium forms a single-layered epithelial covering of the ovary called *germinal epithelium* (it is misnomer as it does not give rise to germ cells).
7. The ovary is suspended by a fold of peritoneum called *mesovarium*.

Descent of Ovary

- Ovaries develop in the posterior abdominal wall and descent to true pelvis.

Factors affecting descent of ovary

1. Gubernaculum ovarii: It is a fibromuscular band that extends from caudal end of ovary to genital swelling (future labium majus).
2. Developing uterus and broad ligament: They arrest the descent of ovary in true pelvis as the gubernaculum gets attached to the angle of uterus.
   Gubernaculum forms two derivatives:
   a. Ligament of ovary: It extends between ovary and uterus.
   b. Round ligament of uterus: It passes from uterus to labium majus through inguinal canal.

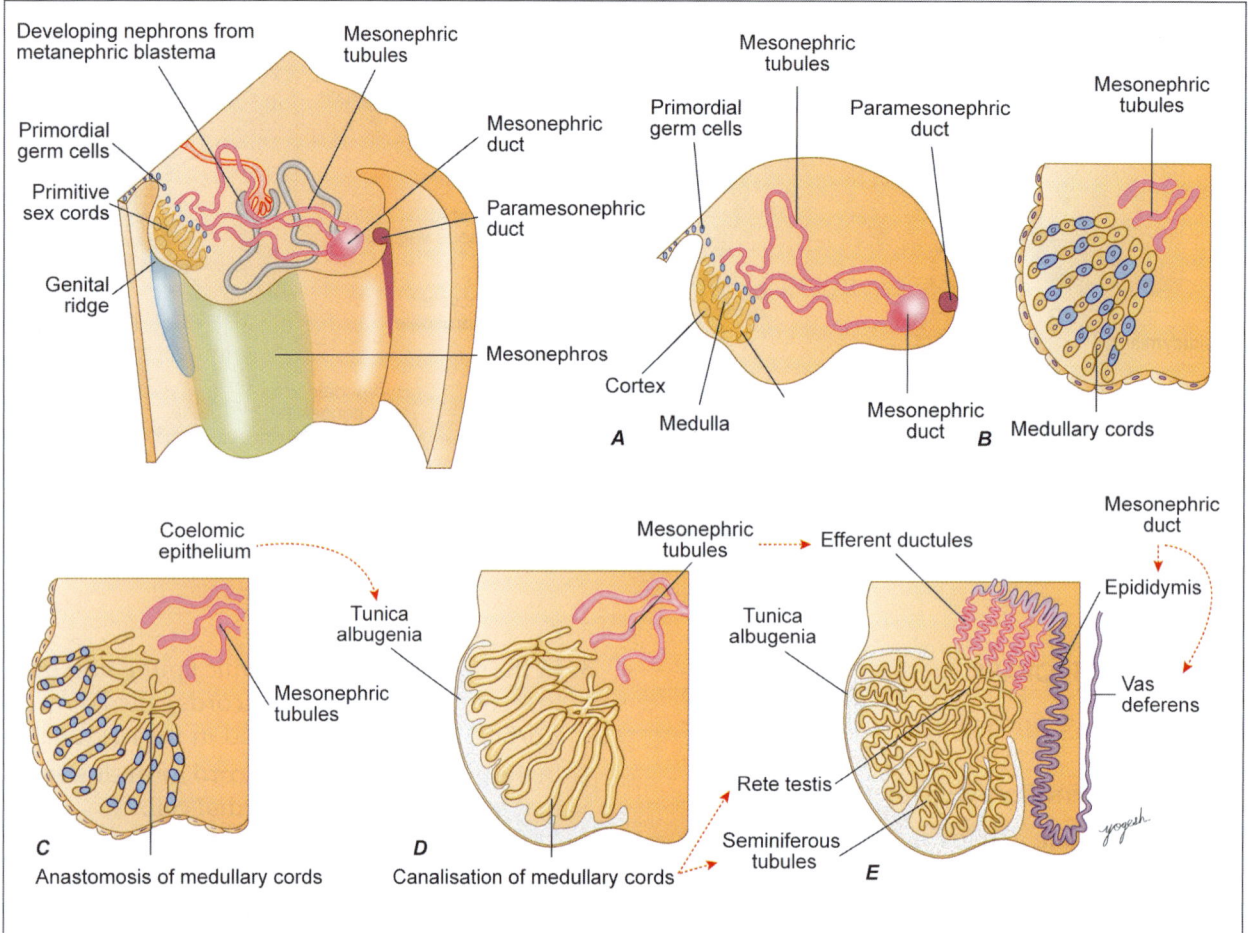

Fig. 21.7: Development of female gonad (ovary). Oocyte develops from primordial germ cells of cortical cords. Follicular cells are derived from cortical sex cords. Germinal epithelium is derived from coelomic epithelium that covers genital ridge. Medulla of ovary is derived from the degenerated medullary sex cords

Some Interesting Facts
1. Absence of Y chromosome (SRY gene, TDF proteins) and presence of two active X chromosomes are required for the formation of ovary.
2. Mesoderm does not form tunica albuginea (fibrous layer) during the development of ovary.
3. Processus vaginalis or canal of Nuck: It is a tubular prolongation of peritoneum that extends into inguinal canal is also present in females but get obliterated before birth.

Anomalies of Ovary
1. Ovary may be
   a. absent on one or both sides
   b. duplicated
   c. present in inguinal canal or labium majus.
2. Ovarian teratoma: It is a teratoma that may consist of derivatives of all germ layers such as adrenal or thyroid tissue, bone, cartilage, hair and so on.

GENITAL DUCTS
- In embryonic life, two pairs of ducts form primitive genital ducts. They are mesonephric (wolffian) and paramesonephric (müllerian) ducts.
- Mesonephric ducts form genital duct system in males, whereas paramesonephric ducts form genital duct system in females.

Mesonephric Ducts^{Highyielding, MCQ}
- Mesonephric duct develops in mesonephros and runs up to urogenital sinus through urorectal septum.
- Mesonephric duct gives rise to *ureteric bud* that later forms the collecting part of urinary system.
- Part of the mesonephric duct gets absorbed in *trigone* of urinary bladder.

Mesonephric Tubules and Ducts in Male^{Neet}

Q. Name the derivatives of mesonephric duct in male and female.

- Persistent mesonephric tubules form efferent ductules of the testis (Fig. 21.8).

Reproductive System: Male and Female Reproductive Organs

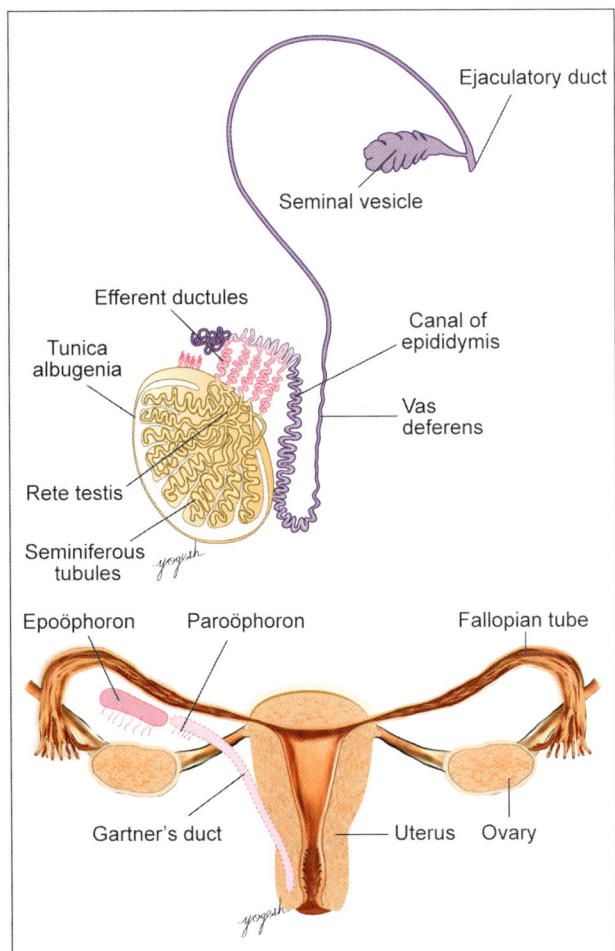

Fig. 21.8: Derivatives of mesonephric duct in genital system

- Remaining some mesonephric tubules form
  a. superior aberrant ductules
  b. inferior aberrant ductules and
  c. tubules of paradidymis
- Mesonephric duct forms
  a. canal of epididymis
  b. ductus deferens and
  c. ejaculatory duct
- Ductus deferens gives rise to seminal vesicles.

Mesonephric Tubules and Ducts in Female

- Mesonephric tubules form vestigial remnants such as tubules of epoöphoron and tubules of paroöphoron (Fig. 21.8).*MCQ*
- Mesonephric duct in female form the duct of epoöphoron (Gartner's duct) that joins with tubules of epoöphoron. *MCQ* Thus, organ of Rosenmüller (epoöphoron) is derivative of mesonephric tubules and duct.*Neet*
- All these structures (tubules of epoöphoron, paroöphoron, and Gartner's duct) are present in the broad ligament of uterus (fold of peritoneum attached to uterus).

Paramesonephric Ducts (Müllerian Ducts)*Highyielding, MCQ*

Q. *Name the derivatives of paramesonephric duct in male and female.*

- In 6th week, paramesonephric ducts develop from coelomic epithelial invagination into mesonephric ridge.
- Cranial ends of paramesonephric ducts open into peritoneal (coelomic) cavity.
- In the 8th week, caudal ends grow caudally and cross mesonephric ducts ventrally to enter urorectal septum.
- By the 3rd month, caudal ends of both (right and left) paramesonephric ducts meet and fuse to form *uterovaginal canal*.
- Fused uterovaginal canal bulge into dorsal wall of urogenital sinus to form bulging called *müllerian tubercle*.

Paramesonephric Ducts in Female

- Cephalic unfused part of each of paramesonephric duct forms the *uterine tube* (fallopian tube) (Fig. 21.9).
- Cranial opening of paramesonephric ducts in coelomic cavity forms the *pelvic ostium* of fallopian tubes.
- Degeneration of mesonephros develop *fimbriae* around pelvic ostium of fallopian tube.
- Fused caudal part of paramesonephric ducts forms *uterovaginal canal*.
- Cranial part of uterovaginal canal forms *uterus*.
- Blind caudal end of uterovaginal canal projects into dorsal wall of urogenital sinus as an elevation called *müllerian tubercle*.
- Part of the uterovaginal canal adjacent to the müllerian tubercle proliferates and form solid bar of tissue (*vaginal cord*).
- Endodermal urogenital sinus develops two cellular cord-like outgrows as *sinovaginal bulbs*.
- Sinovaginal bulbs later fuse and form a plate like structure called *vaginal plate*; that push vaginal cord (part of uterovaginal canal away from urogenital sinus).
- By the 5th month, vaginal cord and vaginal plate get canalised to form *vaginal canal*.
- Expansion of sinovaginal bulbs around the cervix of uterus form *fornix of vagina*.
- Central part of müllerian eminence degenerates to form **orifice of hymen** and remnant of peripheral part of müllerian eminence forms **hymenal membrane**.
- Thus, paramesonephric duct in female forms fallopian tube, upper part of vagina and vaginal fornices.*Neet*

Paramesonephric Ducts in Male

- Due to the presence of anti-müllerian hormone, paramesonephric ducts (müllerian ducts) in male degenerate.
- Remnant of paramesonephric ducts in male forms appendix of testis and prostatic utricle.^{MCQ}

DEVELOPMENT OF UTERUS

Uterus develops from the following sources (Fig. 21.9, Practice Fig. 21.2):

1. Epithelium from uterovaginal canal (fused part of paramesonephric ducts).
2. Myometrium from mesoderm surrounding paramesonephric ducts.
3. Fallopian tubes from unfused part of paramesonephric ducts.
4. At birth, cervix is twice in length than body of uterus. After puberty, the body of uterus elongates and becomes longer than the cervix.

Anomalies of Uterus

1. **Bicornuate uterus:** In this condition, body of uterus is duplicated and it forms horn or cornua of uterus. Each horn communicates with one fallopian tube. It occurs due to partial non-fusion of caudal part of paramesonephric ducts (Fig. 21.10A).
2. **Unicornuate uterus:** Due to failure of development of one paramesonephric duct, half of uterus and one fallopian tube are absent (Fig. 21.10B).
3. **Septate uterus:** In this condition, two paramesonephric ducts fuse but portion between them does not disintegrate (Fig. 21.10C).
4. **Absence of uterus:** Complete failure of uterus development is a rare condition.
5. **Double uterus:** In this condition, no fusion of paramesonephric ducts results in formation of two separate half of uteruses (**uterus didelphys**) (Fig. 21.10D).
6. **Double uterus with double vagina:** In this condition, failure of fusion of right and left sinovaginal bulbs and right and left paramesonephric ducts result in double uterus with double vagina.

DEVELOPMENT OF VAGINA

Summary (Examination Guide)

Various parts of vagina develops as follows:
- Above hymen (upper 3/4th):
  - Mucous membrane derives from sinovaginal bulbs (**endoderm**).^{Neet}
  - Muscles and connective tissue derive from **mesoderm** surrounding paramesonephric ducts.^{Neetj}
- Below hymen (lower 1/4th): Derives from urogenital sinus (endoderm).
- External vaginal orifice derives from genital folds after rupture of urogenital membrane.
- Hymenal membrane derives from müllerian eminence.

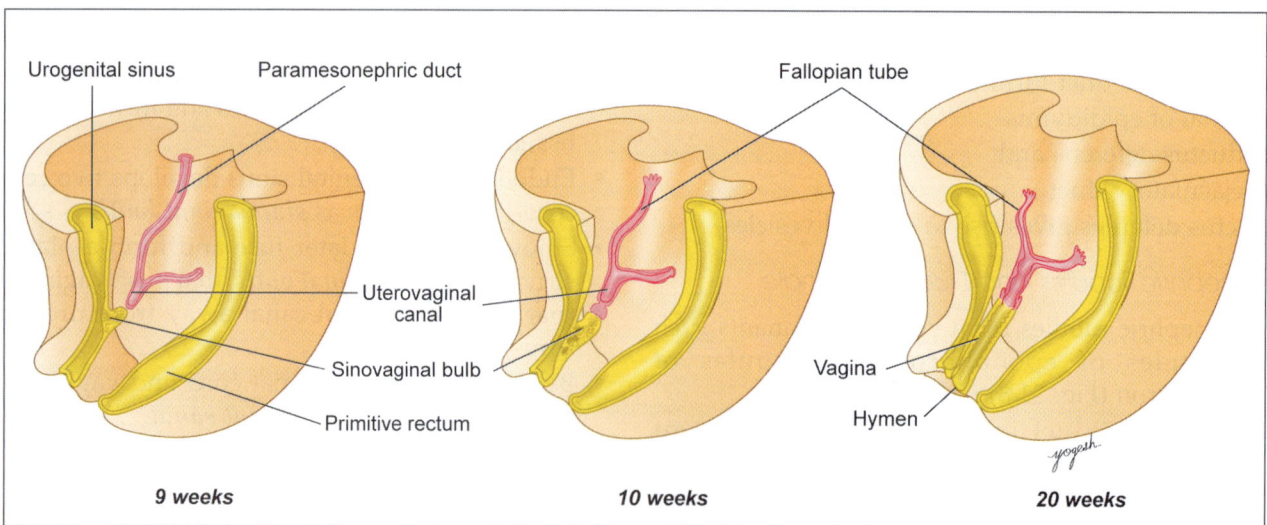

Fig. 21.9: Development of uterus and vagina. Paramesonephric ducts (müllerian ducts) grow caudally, fuse and form uterovaginal canal. The uterovaginal canal forms solid vaginal cord. Endodermal urogenital sinus develops two sinovaginal bulbs that later fuse and form vaginal plate. By the 5th month, vaginal cord and vaginal plate get canalised to form vaginal canal. Central part of müllerian eminence degenerates to form orifice of hymen and remnant of peripheral part of müllerian eminence forms hymenal membrane

Reproductive System: Male and Female Reproductive Organs

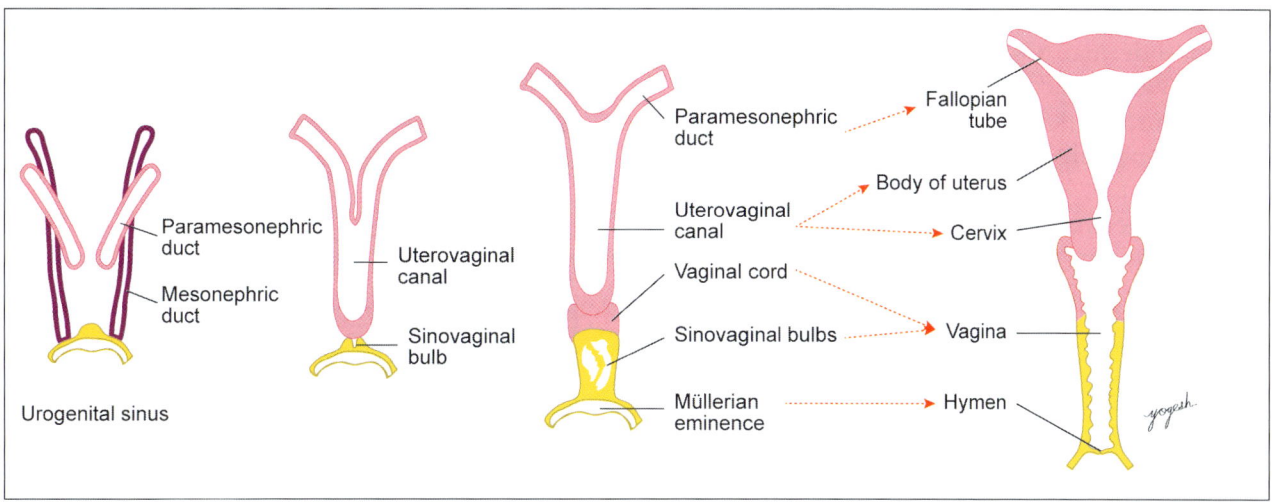

Practice Fig. 21.2: Development of uterus and vagina

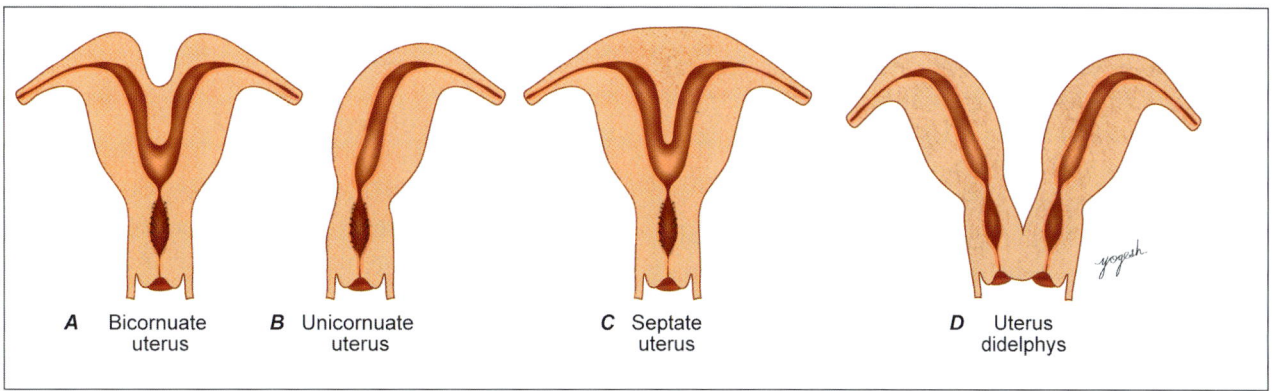

Fig. 21.10: Congenital anomalies of uterus

Congenital Anomalies of Vagina

1. Imperforate hymen: It occurs due to failure of canalisation of the central part of müllerian eminence.
2. Atresia of the vagina: It occurs due to failure of canalisation of vaginal plate.
3. Agenesis of vagina: It is absence of vagina due to failure of formation of vaginal plate by sinovaginal bulb.
4. Septate vagina: It occurs due to patchy disintegration of central part of sinovaginal bulb.
5. Rectovaginal or vesicovaginal fistula: It occurs if müllerian eminence projects into vesicourethral part of cloaca or primitive rectum.

DEVELOPMENT OF PROSTATE

Summary (Examination Guide)

Prostate develops from the following sources (Fig. 21.11):

A. Outer glandular zone: It develops from buds arising from prostatic urethra (endodermal in origin).

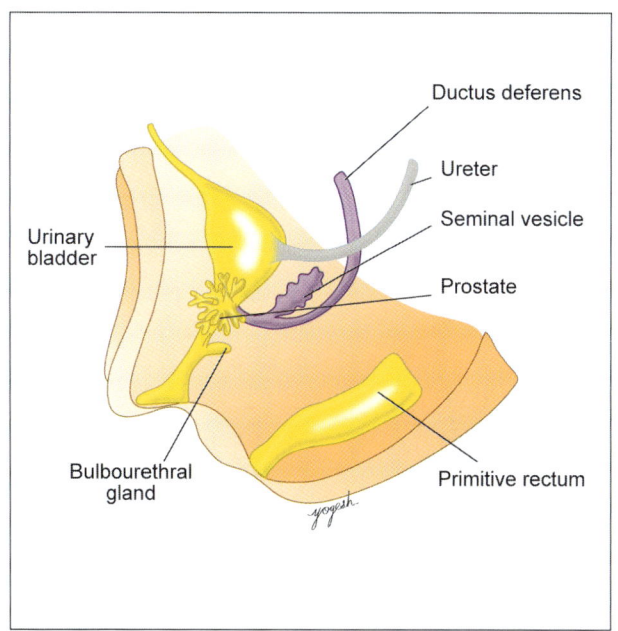

Fig. 21.11: Development of seminal vesicle, prostate and bulbourethral gland

B. **Inner glandular zone:** It develops from buds arising from mesodermal posterior wall of urethra above the openings of ejaculatory ducts.
- There are total five buds arising from the prostatic urethra, namely one anterior, two posterior and two lateral.

C. **Muscle, connective tissue and capsule:** They develop from surrounding mesoderm of urethra.

DEVELOPMENT OF EXTERNAL GENITALIA

- In initial stages, the development of male and female external genitalia is same.
- In 4th week, *somatopleuric lateral plate mesoderm* thickens on the side of cloacal membrane. This thickening produces surface elevation called *cloacal folds* (Fig. 21.12).[Neet]
- Urorectal septum divides the cloacal membrane into ventral *urogenital membrane* and dorsal *anal membrane*.
- Along with the division of cloacal membrane, cloacal fold is also divided into cranial larger *urethral folds* and caudal *anal folds* (Fig. 21.12).
- Lateral to urethral folds, another swelling called *genital swellings* appears (Fig. 21.12).
- Genital swelling forms scrotum in males and labia majora in females, whereas **genital tubercle** forms clitoris/glans penis.[Neet]

Development of Male External Genitalia

Stages of Development

- Development of male external genitalia can be divided into three stages as follows:
  1. Development of penile urethra
  2. Development of prepuce of the penis and
  3. Development of scrotum

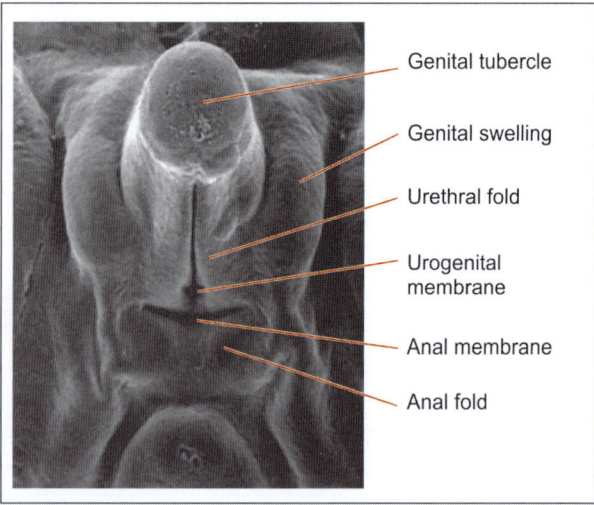

Scanning electron micrograph 21.2: Undifferentiated external genitalia. In 8th week of human development, male and female external genitalia appear the same. [Species: Human, gestational age: 52 days]

1. Development of penile urethra
   - Genital tubercle elongates to form *phallus* or *primitive penis* (Fig. 21.13).
   - Primitive urethral groove (ectoderm) appears on surface of urogenital membrane and it extends to tip of primitive penis.
   - Simultaneously, urethral folds and *primitive urethral groove* also elongate on the undersurface of primitive penis.
   - Endoderm of phallic part of urogenital sinus proliferates into phallus (primitive penis) and forms solid plate called *urethral plate*.
   - Soon solid urethral plate gets canalised and forms a tube (endodermal) that is closely attached to a urethral groove (ectoderm).

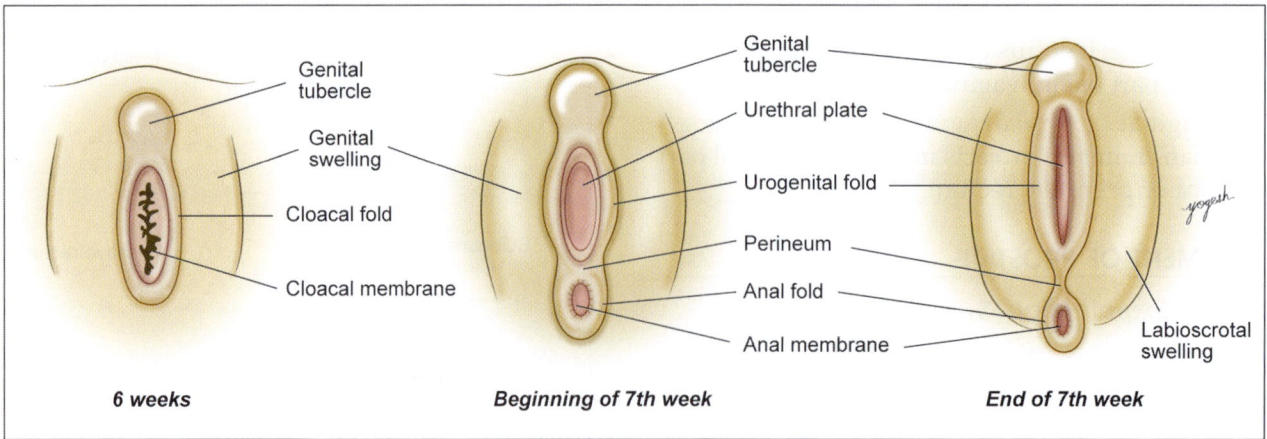

Fig. 21.12: Development of external genitalia: Indefinitive stage

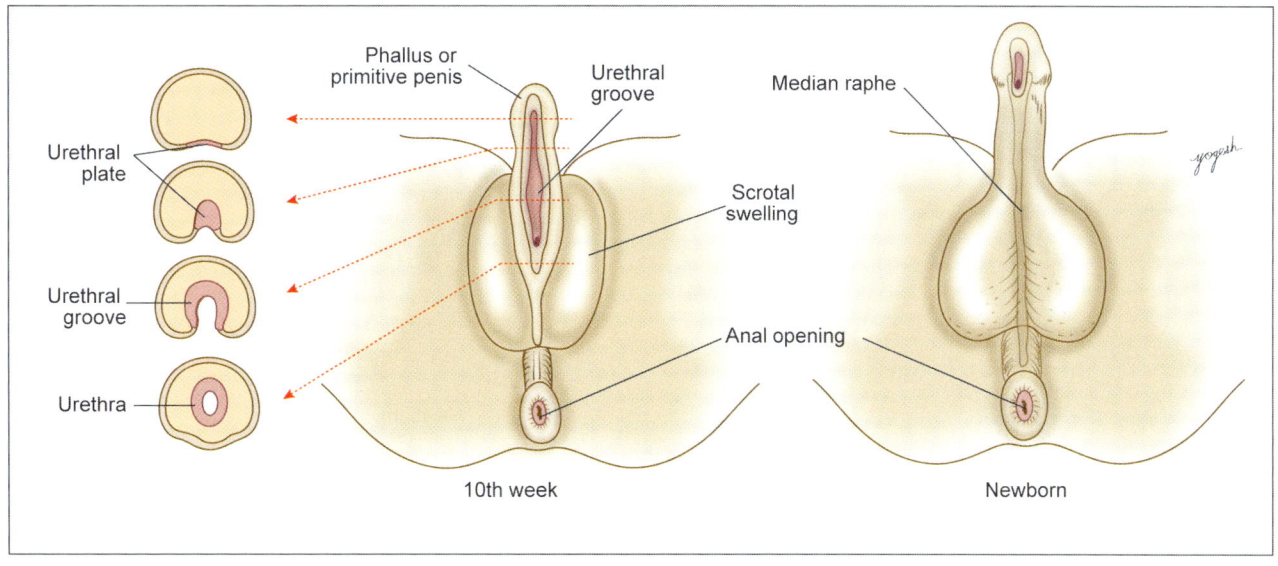

Fig. 21.13: Development of male external genitalia

- Urethral groove (urogenital membrane) ruptures and a deep groove called *definitive urethral groove* under the surface of phallus.
- Through definitive urethral groove, urogenital sinus communicate with the exterior. Margins of this groove are called *definitive urethral folds*.
- Definitive urethral folds fuse with each other in caudocranial direction (from base to the tip of primitive penis) to form *penile urethra*.
- Midline ectodermal fusion forms *penile raphe*.
- The terminal part of urethra develops from the solid ectodermal mass that later gets canalised (Fig. 21.14).
2. Development of prepuce of the penis (Fig. 21.14)
    - Near the tip of the primitive penis (phallus), a circular sulcus appears that separate glans penis from the rest of the penis.
    - Surface ectoderm proliferates and forms a fold called *prepuce* or foreskin.

3. Development of scrotum (Fig. 21.15)
    - On fusion of urethral folds, both the genital swellings enlarge to form scrotal swellings.
    - Scrotal swellings enlarge and fuse in the midline to form scrotum.

Development of Female External Genitalia
(Fig. 21.16)

Female external genitalia develops as follows:
1. Clitoris develops from genital tubercle (phallus).
2. Labia minora develops from primitive urethral folds.
3. Labia majora develops from genital swellings. Labia majora fuse posteriorly to form posterior labial commissure and anteriorly to form mons pubis and anterior labial commissure.
4. Vestibule of vagina develops by rupture of urogenital membrane.

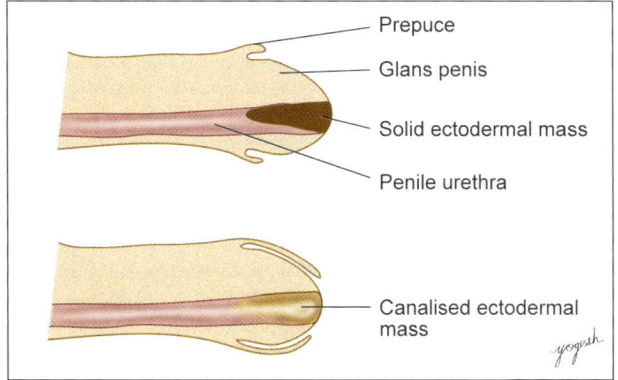

Fig. 21.14: Development of glandular portion of penile urethra

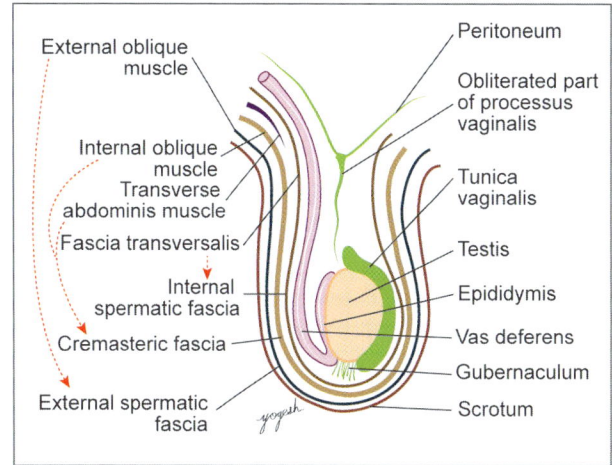

Fig. 21.15: Development of layers of scrotum from layers of anterior abdominal wall

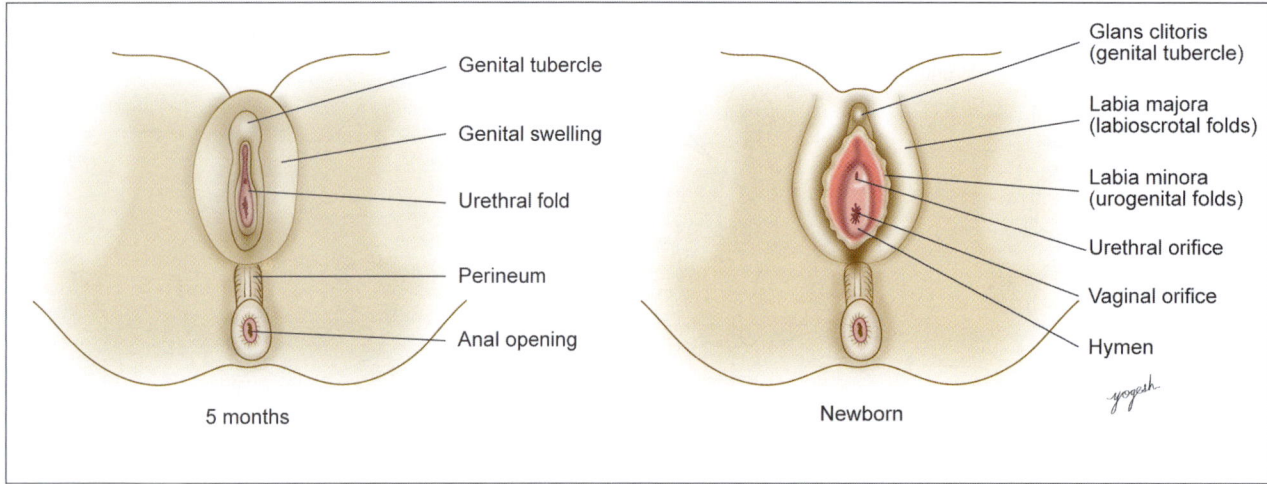

Fig. 21.16: Development of female external genitalia

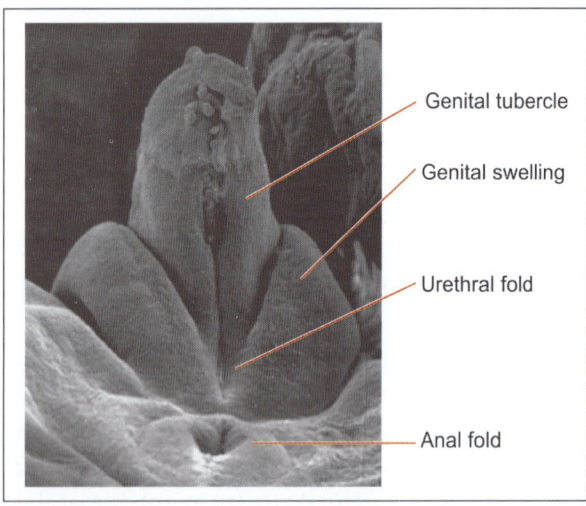

Scanning electron micrograph 21.3: Female external genitalia. In the female, urethral folds remain unfused and will form labia minora, while genital swellings become labia majora. [Species: Human, gestational age: 72 days]

1. **Glandular hypospadias:** Urethra opens on ventral surface of glans penis.
2. **Balanic hypospadias:** Urethra opens at the base of glans penis.
3. **Penile hypospadias:** Urethra opens on ventral surface of penis in between glans and scrotum.
4. **Penoscrotal hypospadias:** Urethra opens at the junction of penis and scrotum.
5. **Perineal hypospadias:** Urethra opens at unfused part of scrotum due to failure of fusion of labioscrotal folds.

Treatment
- Surgical correction is the treatment of choice.
- Hypospadias usually produces a condition called chordee. In this condition, head of penis curves downward that shows resistance during erection.

Box 21.2: Hypospadias

Q. Write note on hypospadias.

Definition
- It is a congenital anomaly of urethra; in that external urethral orifice is located on ventral aspect of penis, instead of at tip of penis.

Incidence: One in every 300 male births.

Embryological basis
- Hypospadias results due to
  1. Failure of canalisation of ectodermal cord that forms the terminal part of urethra in glans penis.
  2. Failure of fusion of urethral folds that completes formation of penile urethra.

Classification (Fig. 21.17)
- Hypospadias is classified according to location of external urethral opening into the following types:

Box 21.3: Epispadias

Definition
It is congenital anomaly of penis in that external urethral orifice is located on dorsal (upper) surface of penis.

Incidence: 1 in 30,000 births.

Embryological basis
- Embryological basis is not clear.
- Probably due to the formation of genital tubercle caudally.

Association
- Mostly epispadias is associated with bladder exstrophy (ectopia vesicae).

Treatment
- Comprehensive surgical correction is the treatment of choice.

Reproductive System: Male and Female Reproductive Organs

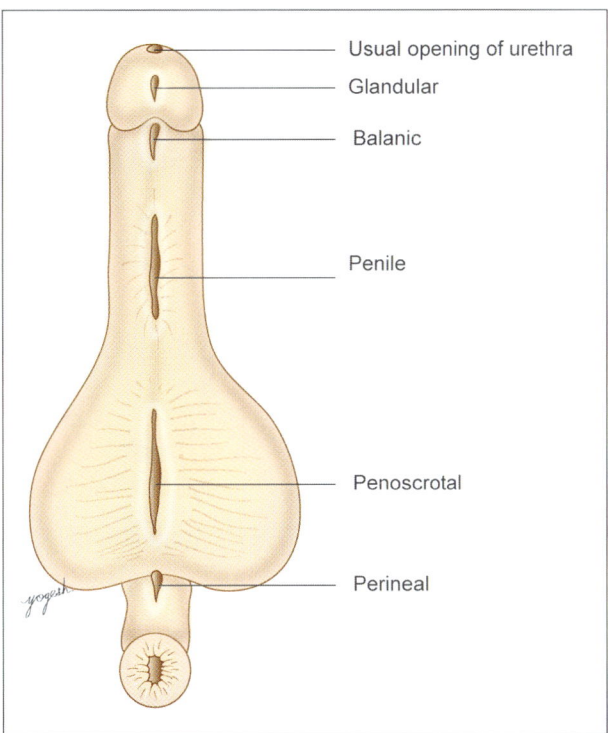

Fig. 21.17: Hypospadias. External urethral orifice is located on ventral aspect of the penis or scrotum, instead of at tip of the penis. It may be glandular (on ventral surface of glans), balanic (at base of glans), penile (on ventral surface of penis), penoscrotal (at junction of penis and scrotum), perineal (at unfused part of scrotum)

CLINICAL EMBRYOLOGY

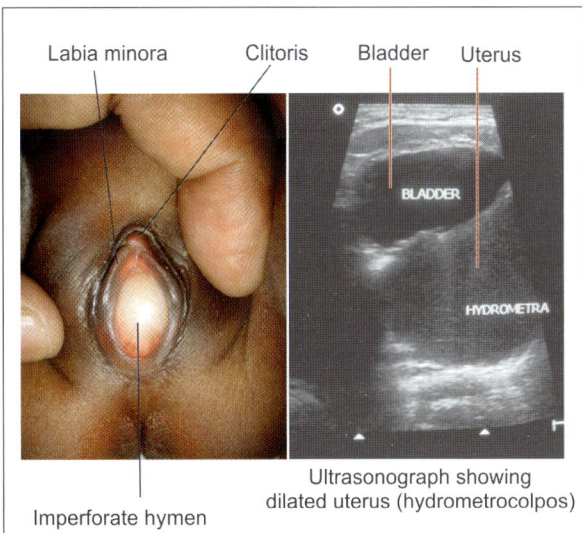

Clinical image 21.1: Imperforate hymen with hydrometrocolpos. During embryonic life, the remnant of peripheral part müllerian eminence forms the hymen and central degenerated part forms orifice of the hymen. Failure of the degeneration of müllerian eminence or failure of the sinovaginal bulb canalisation causes imperforate hymen. Its incidence is 1:1000–1:10000 females. In the infant babies, there may be hydrocolpos due to the accumulation of secretions in uterus and vagina or during puberty, there may be hematocolpos (Image courtesy: *Dr Kumaravel S*)

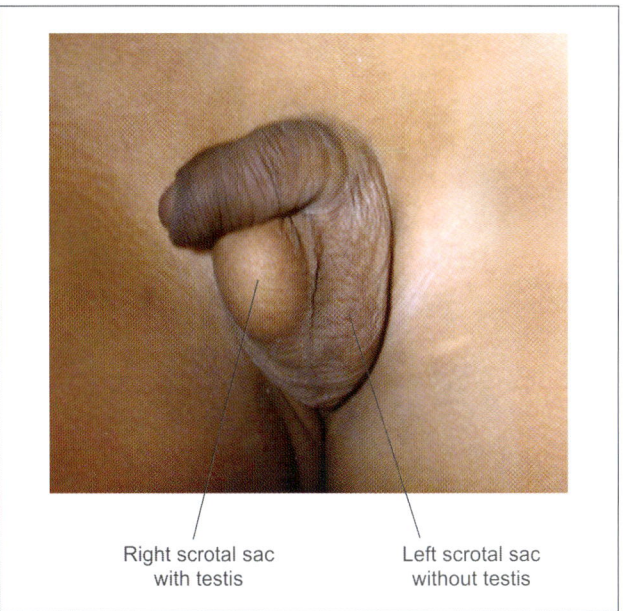

Clinical image 21.2: Undescended testis (left). Cryptorchidism is the failure of descent of testis. Undescended testis may descend on its own during the first year of life. If it does not descend, then it can be surgically placed in the scrotum (orchidopexy). Undescended testis cannot produce sperms (male infertility), but produces testosterone (normal secondary sexual characters) (Image courtesy: *Dr Kumaravel S*)

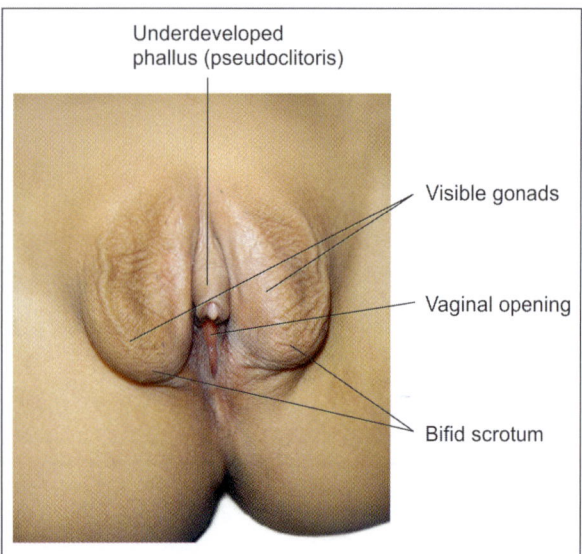

Clinical image 21.3: Male pseudohermaphrodite. Pseudohermaphrodite is the condition in which the individual has gonad of one sex and external genitalia of the other sex. Male pseudohermaphrodite shows testes with external genitalia that resembles female. These patients may have **androgen insensitivity** or they may not Leydig cells in testis (no secretion of testosterone). Hence, they do not have secondary sexual characters → feminine appearance. The above case shows underdeveloped phallus (pseudoclitoris), vaginal opening, bifid scrotum with testis. Unfused scrotal swellings give appearance of labia majora (Image courtesy: *Dr Kumaravel S*)

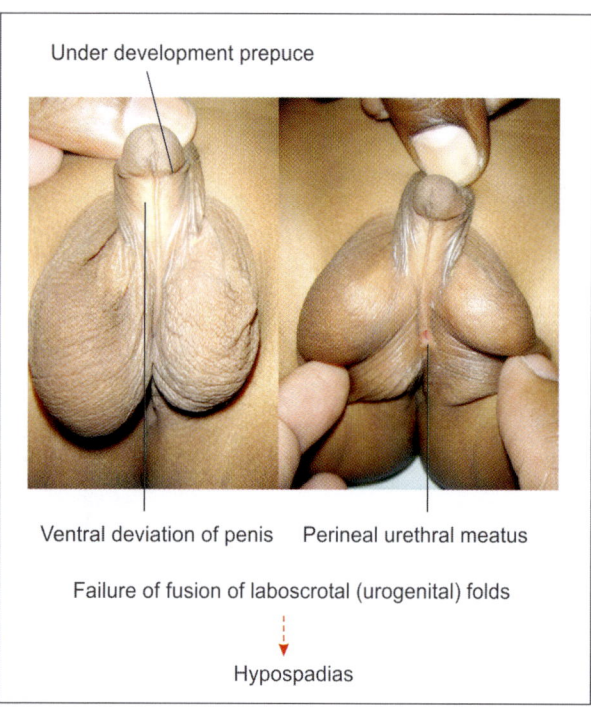

Clinical image 21.4: Perineal hypospadias: It is a congenital anomaly of the urethra in that external urethral orifice is located on the ventral aspect of penis instead of at the tip of penis. In perineal hypospadias, urethra opens at the unfused part of scrotum due to failure of fusion of laboscrotal folds. (Image courtesy: *Dr Kumaravel S*)

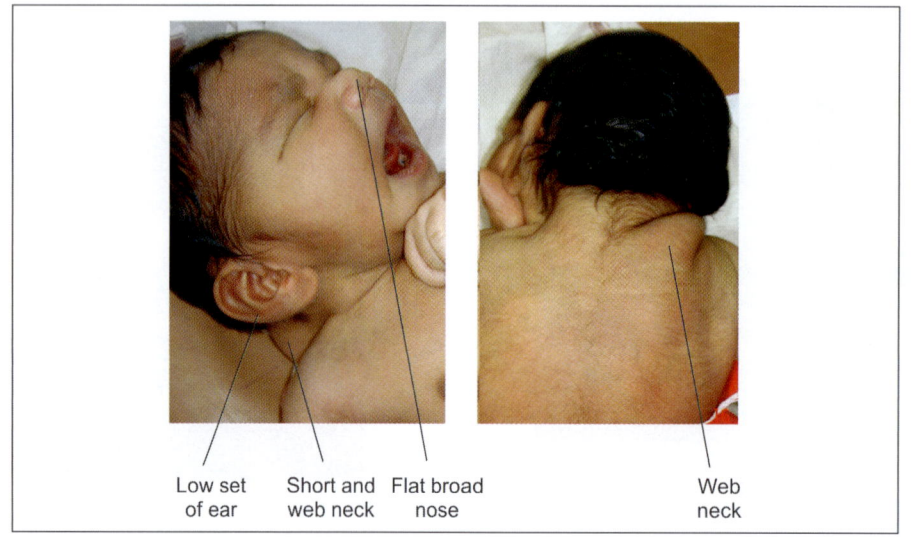

Clinical image 21.5: Webbed neck in Turner's syndrome or 45,X0 syndrome. Turner syndrome (karyotype: 45,X) occurs due to the absence of one X chromosome in female. The absence of second X chromosome result on ovarian dysgenesis. Incidence is 1 in 2500–3000 newborn girls. Female mainly has ovarian dysgenesis, infertility, webbing of neck, short stature, low set of ears and cubitus valgus (For details, refer *Principles of Clinical Genetics*, Chapter 4 by Dr Yogesh Sontakke). *Note:* Webbed neck is associated with Turner syndrome, Noonan Syndrome (mutations pathways) in RAS/mitogen activated protein kinase), Klippel-Feil syndrome (fused spinal vertebrae). (Image courtesy: *Dr Kumaravel S*)

22
Nervous System

Chapter Outline

- Neurulation
- Differentiation of neural tube
  - Flexures of neural tube
  - Cavity of neural tube
- Neural crest cells
- Spinal cord
  - Phases of development
  - Functional columns of spinal cord
- Myelination
- Neural tube defects
  - Spina bifida
- Hydrocephalus
- Functional columns of brainstem
- Development of medulla oblongata
- Development of pons
- Development of midbrain
- Development of cerebellum
- Evolutionary aspect of cerebellum
- Development of diencephalon
- Development of cerebrum

INTRODUCTION

- Nervous system includes brain, spinal cord, peripheral nerves and ganglia.
- Whole nervous system is derived from a part of surface ectoderm, called **neuroectoderm**.
- Neuroectoderm extends between primitive node to prechordal plate.
- Neural plate gets folded to form *neural tube* that later form central nervous system (Practice Fig. 22.1).

NEURULATION

Q. Write short note on neurulation.

Definition: The process of formation of neural tube from neural plate is called neurulation.

Stages of neurulation (Flowchart 22.1)

1. Neuroectoderm and neural plate stage
   - In presomitic period (16th–19th day): Surface ectoderm differentiates and thickens in the centre (between the prechordal plate and primitive node). This thickened zone is **neural plate** or **medullary plate**.
   - Notochord acts as a primary inducer for neural plate formation and differentiation (Practice Fig. 22.1).^{Neet}
   - Neural plate grows rapidly and elongates craniocaudally in the length.

2. Neural folding stage
   - Continuous growth of neural plate makes it depressed in the midline. This linear depression is called **neural groove**.
   - Elevated margins of neural groove form **neural folds**.
   - At the junctional zone of neural plate and surface ectoderm, the cells differentiate to form **neural crest**.
   - Neural crest forms peripheral and autonomic nerves.

3. Stage of neural tube formation
   - Due to rapid proliferation of neural plate, the neural folds come closer to each other and start fusion in the midline.
   - On fusion, it forms neural tube.
   - Fusion begins in cervical region and extends in cranio-caudal direction.^{Neet}
   - Neural tube forms central nervous system.

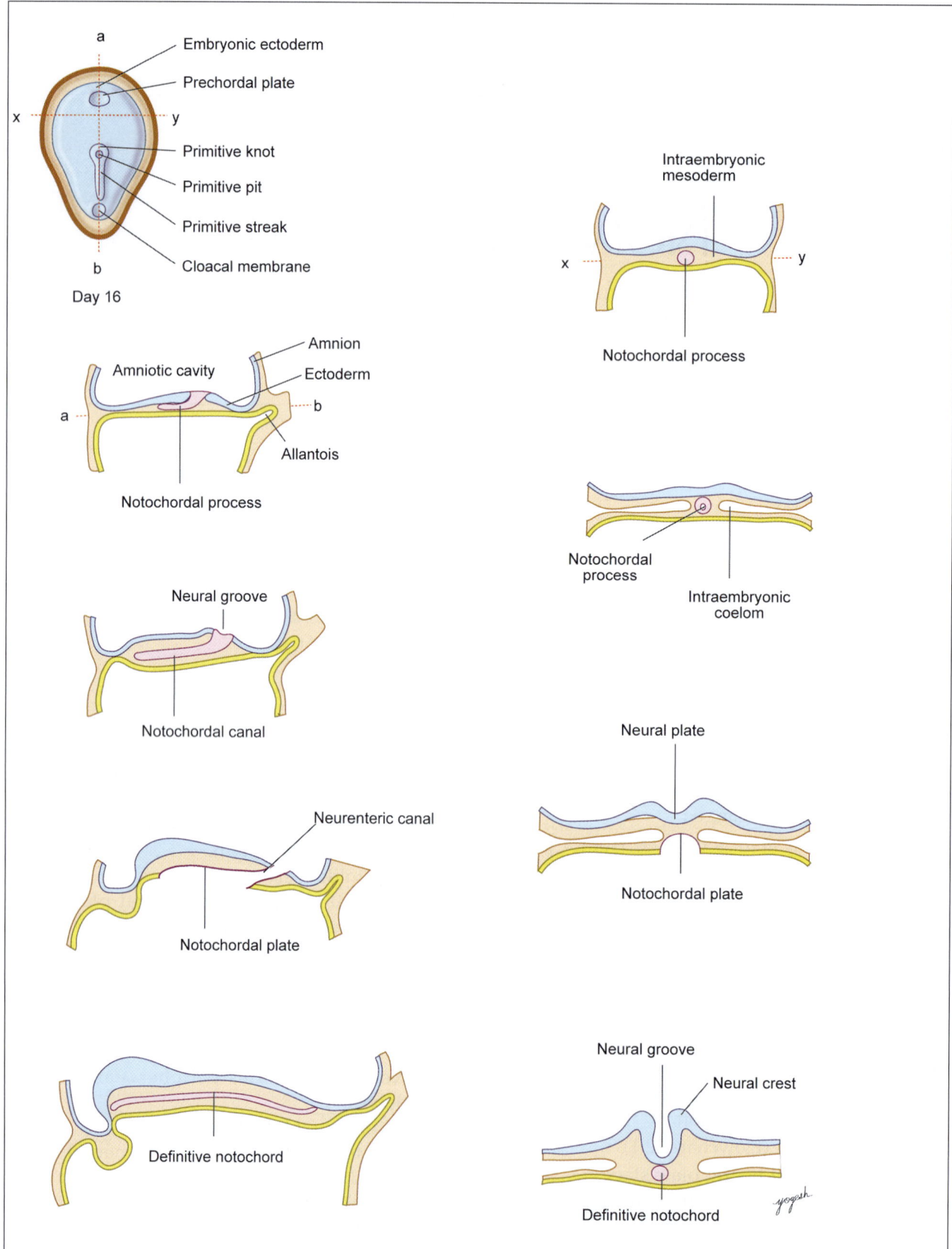

Practice Fig. 22.1: Formation of notochord and neural groove

Nervous System

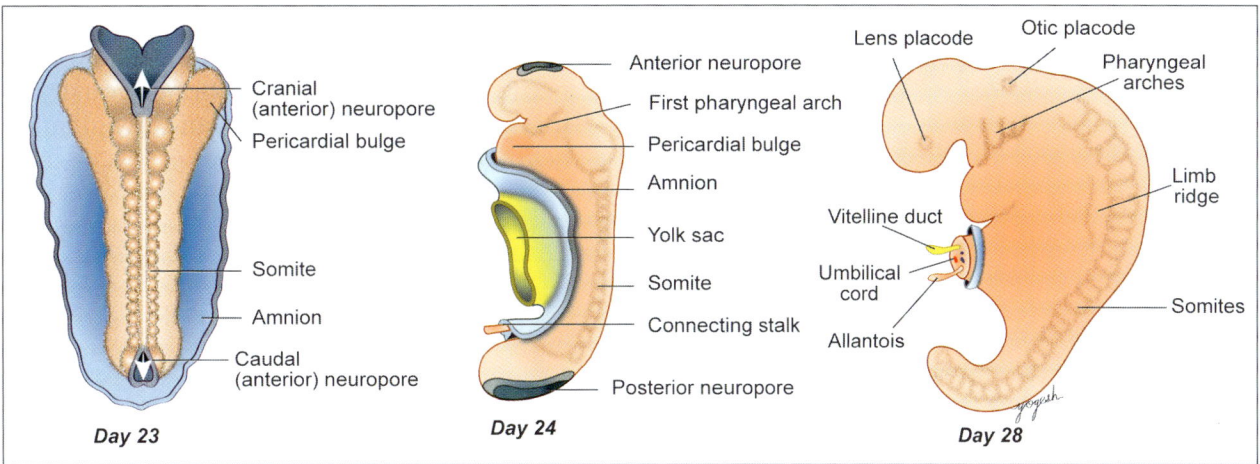

Fig. 22.1: Folding of neural plate and closure of anterior and posterior neuropores

4. Stage of neural tube closure
   - Neural tube remains open at cranial end as *cranial (anterior) neuropore* and at caudal end as *caudal (posterior) neuropore* (Fig. 22.1).
   - Open neural tube facilitates circulation of amniotic fluid through the lumen of neural tube. It provides nutrition to rapidly developing neuroectodermal cells before the establishment of sufficient uteroplacental circulation.
   - Cranial neuropore closes by 25th day of IUL, whereas caudal neuropore closes by 27th day of IUL.^{MCQ}
   - Closure of cranial neuropore occurs at the 20 somite stage, whereas closure of posterior neuropore occurs at 25 somite stage.
   - Non-closure of neuropore results in neural tube defects.
   - In later life, the location of anterior neuropore is represented by lamina terminalis, whereas posterior neuropore by terminal ventricle (lies in caudal end of spinal cord).^{MCQ}

DIFFERENTIATION OF NEURAL TUBE

- Neural tube has a central cavity (forms ventricles of brain and central canal of spinal cord) and a peripheral wall (forms tissue of nervous system).
- Neural tube elongates cranio-caudally.
- Cranial part of the cavity of neural tube dilates to form brain vesicles, whereas the caudal part of central cavity remains tubular.
- Dilated cranial part of neural tube forms 3 primary brain vesicles (Fig. 22.2, Practice Fig. 22.2, Scanning electron micrograph 22.1 and 22.2):
  1. prosencephalon (cranial most)
  2. mesencephalon (middle)
  3. rhombencephalon (caudal most)
- Prosencephalon, mesencephalon and rhombencephalon are also called forebrain, midbrain and hindbrain respectively.
- On further growth, 5 brain vesicles develop as follows:
  1. Prosencephalon divides into
     - Cranial telencephalon—gives rise to two cerebral hemispheres
     - Diencephalon—gives rise to optic vesicle, pineal gland, thalami and hypothalami, posterior hypophysis

Flowchart 22.1: Formation of neural tube

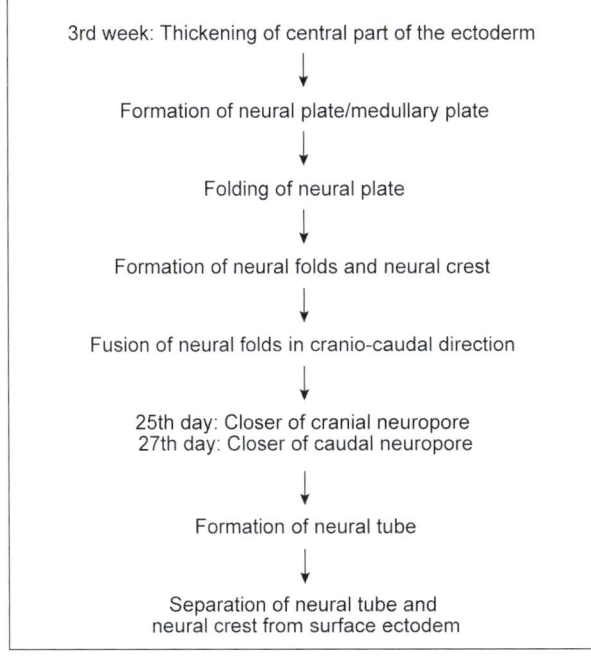

2. Mesencephalon—gives rise to midbrain
3. Rhombencephalon divides into
   - cranial metencephalon—gives rise to pons and cerebellum
   - caudal myelencephalon—give rise to medulla oblongata

Flexures of Neural Tube

- Unequal growth rates of various components of neural tube result in flexions, constrictions, thickenings, invaginations and evaginations of neural tube (Fig. 22.2).

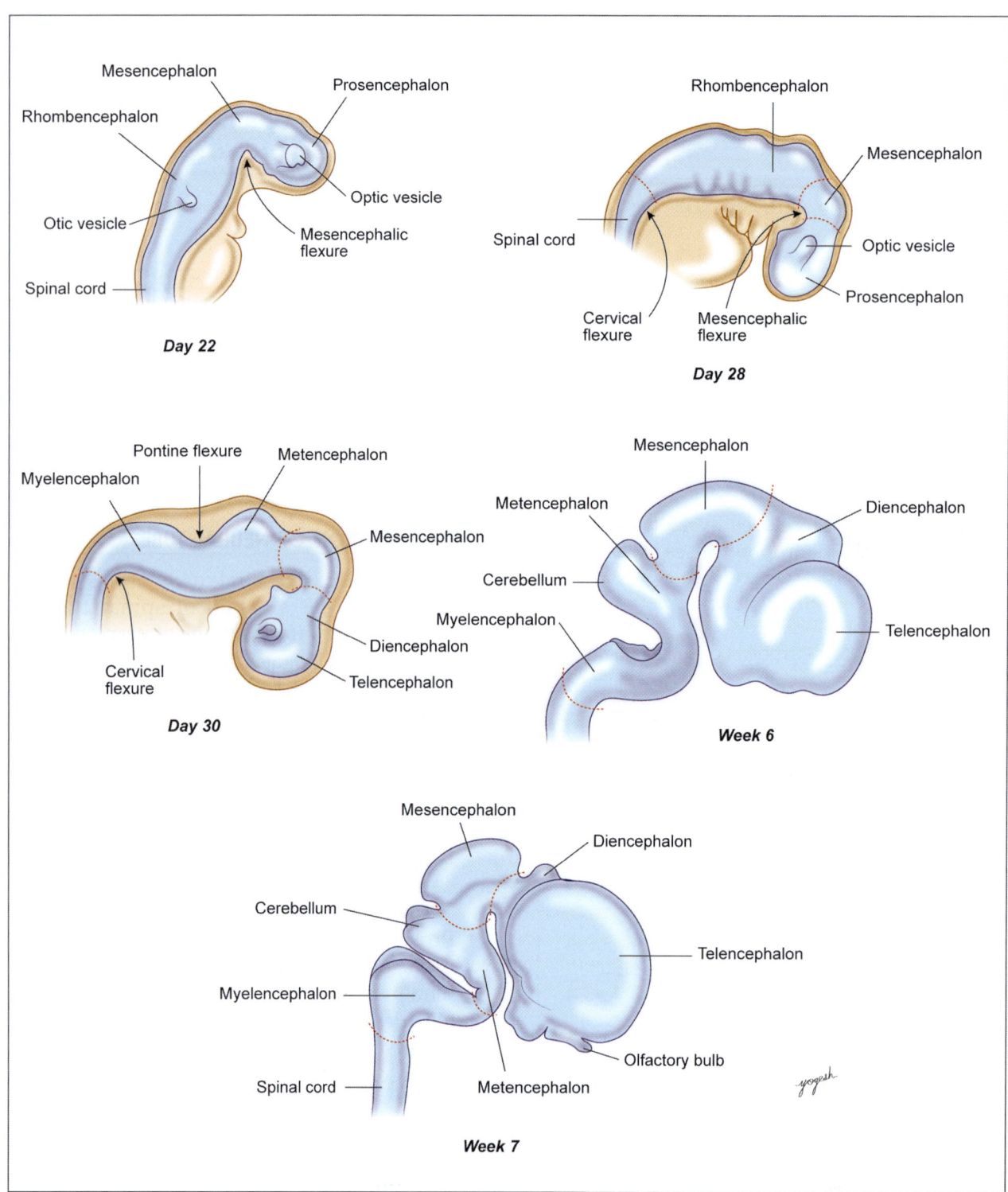

Fig. 22.2: Developing brain vesicles

Nervous System

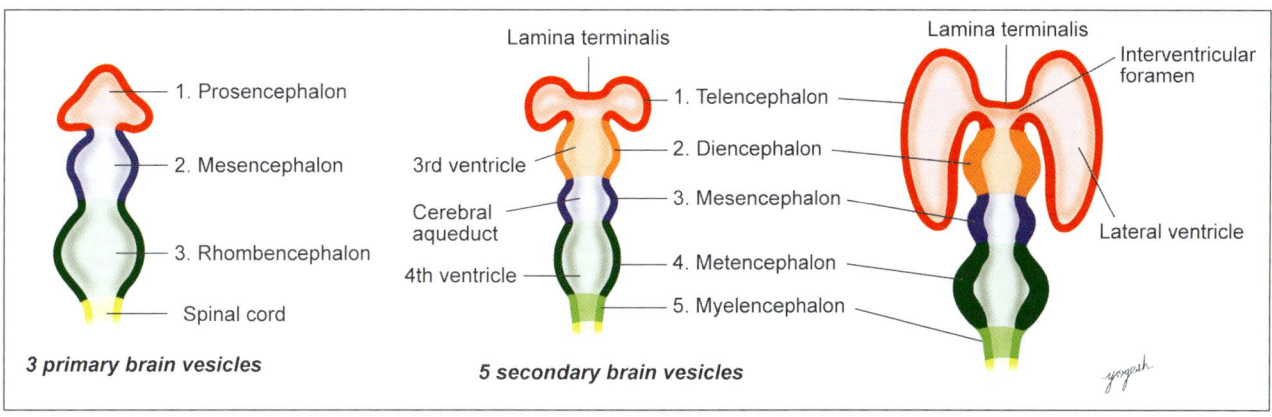

Practice Fig. 22.2: Developing brain vesicles

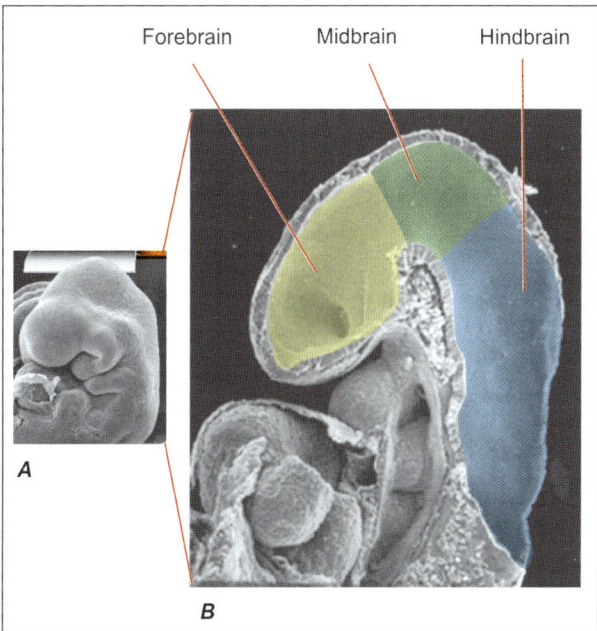

Scanning electron micrograph 22.1: A cut through the recently closed cranial neural tube illustrates the forebrain (prosencephalon), midbrain (mesencephalon), and hindbrain (rhombencephalon) [Species: Mouse, approximate human age: 5 weeks, lateral view in A and sagittal section in B]

Major Flexures of Neural Tube

- Flexion of embryo (folding) and differential growth of nervous tissue forms the following 4 basic flexures of neural tube:
  1. *Cervical flexure* at the junction of spinal cord and hindbrain. It makes 90° angle.
  2. *Cephalic flexure* (mesencephalic flexure): It occurs in the region of midbrain. It is concave ventrally.
  3. *Pontine flexure* at the junction of myelencephalon and metencephalon. It is convex ventrally.
  4. *Telencephalic flexure* at the junction of telencephalon and diencephalon.

Cavity of Neural Tube

- Cavity of neural tube gives passage to amniotic fluid till the closure of anterior and posterior neuropores. Flowing amniotic fluid nourishes rapidly growing brain and spinal cord.
- On the formation of brain vesicles, cavity of neural tube gets converted into ventricles and communications as follows:
  1. Cavity of telencephalon develops lateral ventricles.
  2. Communication between cavities of telencephalon and diencephalon develops interventricular foramina of Monro.
  3. Cavity of diencephalon forms 3rd ventricle.
  4. Cavity of mesencephalon forms cerebral aqueduct of Sylvius that connects the 3rd and 4th ventricle.^MCQ
  5. Cavity of rhombencephalon forms *4th ventricle*.
  6. Cavity of spinal cord forms central canal of spinal cord and its terminal ventricle (5th ventricle or ampulla caudalis). Terminal ventricle lies in conus medullaris (terminal part of spinal cord).
  7. Due to rupture of roof, the 4th ventricle communicates with subarachnoid space through (two lateral) foramina of Luschka and one central foramen Magendie.

NEURAL CREST CELLS

Q. List the derivatives of neural crest cells.

- During invagination of neural plate, a distinct group of ectodermal cells appears along the edges of neural groove. This group of cells is called *neural crest cells*.
- On the formation of neural tube, neural crest cells come to lie in zone between the neural tube and surface ectoderm.
- Neural crest cells get divided into *dorsal mass* and *ventral mass* that migrates freely and forms various derivatives.

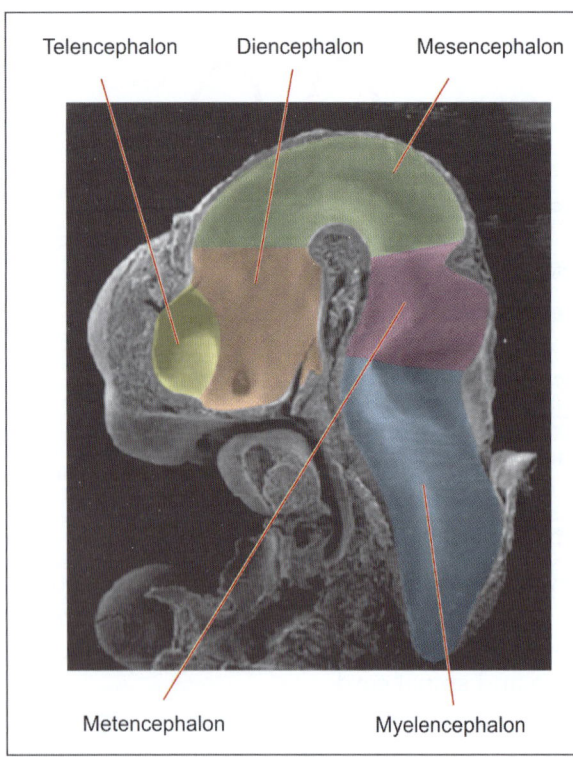

Scanning electron micrograph 22.2: Formation of brain vesicles [Species: Mouse, approximate human age: 6 weeks, sagittal section]

Derivatives of Neural Crest Cells (Fig. 22.3)

Dorsal Mass

A. Neuroblast cells
- Dorsal root ganglia
- Sensory ganglia of V, VII, IX and X cranial nerves
- Skeletal elements of pharyngeal arches
- Odontoblast of teeth
- Parafollicular cells of thyroid gland

B. Spongioblast cells
- Satellite cell in ganglion
- Schwann cells

C. Pluripotent cells
- Melanocytes

Ventral Mass

A. Sympatho-chromaffin organ
B. Sympathoblasts
- Sympathetic ganglionic neurons
- Parasympathetic ganglionic neurons (ciliary, pterygopalatine, submandibular and otic)

C. Chromaffin cells
- Chromaffin cells of medulla of adrenal gland
- Para-aortic body
- Argentaffin cells in respiratory system
- Enterochromaffin cells in gut

Other Derivatives

- Facial bones and vault of skull
- Dermis of face and neck
- Muscles of ciliary body
- Sclera and choroids of eyeball
- Substantia propria and posterior epithelium of cornea
- Pharyngeal arch cartilages
- Semilunar valves in heart
- Spiral and bulbar septum in heart

Some Interesting Facts

- Role of bone morphogenic proteins (BMPs)
  - Fibroblast growth factors (FGF) inhibit BMPs and transforming growth factor β (TGF-β).
  - Notochord produces noggin, chordin, follistatin that inactivate BMPs and causes neurulation.
  - Ectodermal cells
    1. that have high level of BMP get converted into surface ectoderm
    2. that have low level of BMP get converted into neural crest cells and
    3. that have absence of BMP form neural plate (neuroectoderm).
- Glomus (type I) cells are chemoreceptors that are located in carotid body and aortic body. They are derived from neural crest cells. Glomus (type II) cells are derived from neuroectoderm and they lie in arterial chemoreceptors.^{Neet}

Spinal Cord

- Parts of neural tube caudal to the hindbrain (rhombencephalon) form the spinal cord.
- Formation of spinal cord occurs in 4 phases as follows:
  1. Formation of mantle and marginal layers
  2. Formation of basal and alar plates
  3. Histogenesis of cells and
  4. Positional changes of spinal cord.

Phases of Development

Phase 1: Formation of mantle and marginal layers

- Neural tube is lined by a single layer called neuroepithelial cells.
- Neuroepithelial cells lining the lateral wall of central canal proliferate and get differentiates into three zones as follows:
  Innermost—primitive *ependymal cell layer*.
  Middle *mantle layer* that later forms neurons and neuroglial cells.

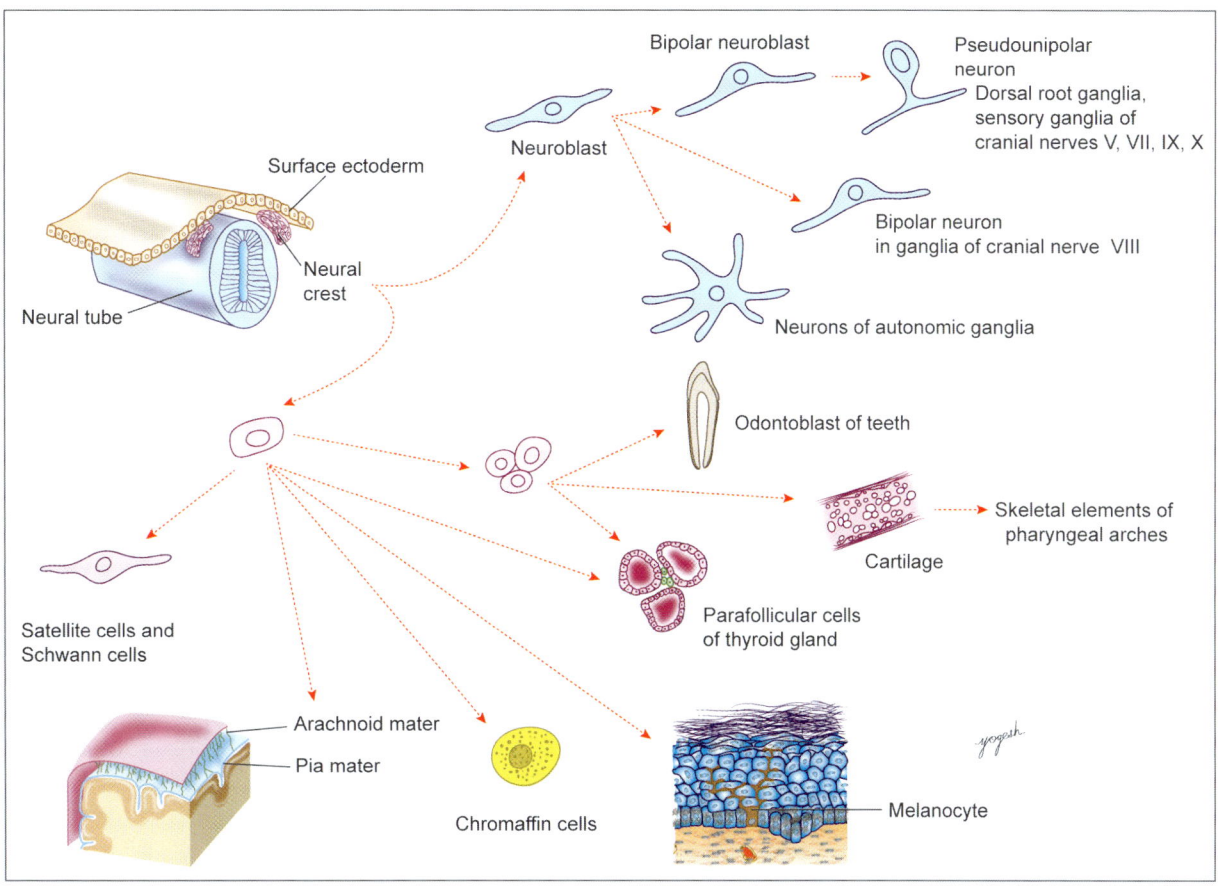

Fig. 22.3: Derivatives of neural crest cells

Outermost *marginal layer* that later forms supporting neuroglial cells and contain processes of neurons of mantle layer.

Phase 2: Formation of basal and alar laminae (Fig. 22.4, Scanning electron micrograph 22.3)

- The cells in mantle zone proliferate rapidly.
- Rapid growth in the mantle zone of ventral portion of the neural tube forms **basal plate** or lamina, whereas rapid growth in the dorsal portion forms **alar lamina** or plate.
- Dorsal and ventral portion of the neural tube are now called *roof* and *floor plates* respectively.
- A longitudinal groove called **sulcus limitans** appears in the canal of spinal cord. Sulcus limitans separates alar lamina from basal lamina.
- Continued growth of the alar lamina obliterates dorsal part of canal of neural tube that results in the formation of **dorsal median septum** of spinal cord.
- Continuous growth of the basal laminae produces bulging separated by *ventral median fissure*.
- A small remaining part of the central canal of neural tube form **central canal of spinal cord**.

Phase 3: Histogenesis of cells in neural tube
(Figs 22.5 and 22.6)

- The neuroepithelial cells of mantle and marginal laminae proliferate rapidly and get differentiated into two types of cells:

    A. Neuroblasts (form neurons) and

    B. Spongioblast (forms astrocytes, oligodendrocytes).

- *Histogenesis of neurons:*
    - *Neuroblast cells* in the mantle layer lose their cell processes to form *apolar neuroblasts*. From apolar neuroblasts, two processes develop at opposite pole and convert it into *bipolar neuroblast*.
    - Bipolar neuroblast loses one process to form *unipolar neuroblast*. Remaining single process of unipolar neuroblast elongates to develop *axon*.
    - Multiple small processes (primitive dendrites) appear on the surface of unipolar neuroblast to form *multipolar neuroblast*. These multipolar neuroblasts later form *mature neurons*.
    - Neuroblast loses mitotic activity. Motor neurons differentiate earlier than sensory neurons.^MCQ

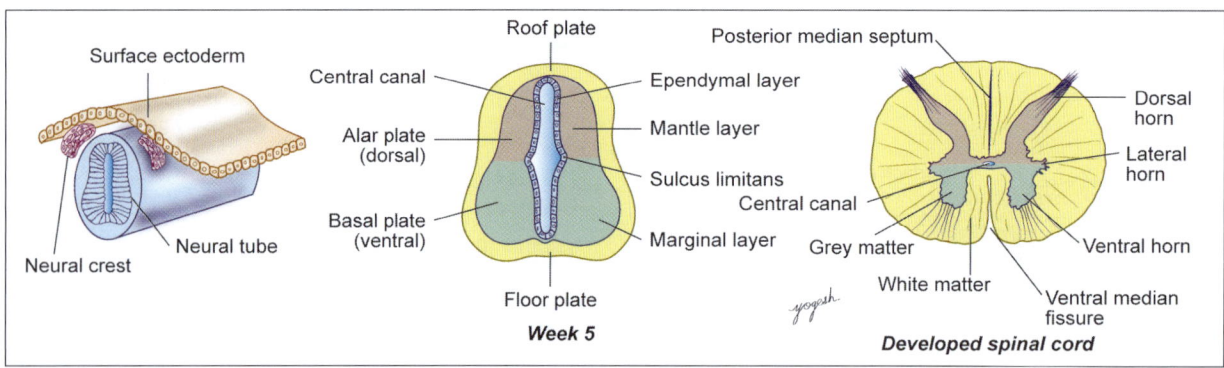

Fig. 22.4: Development of spinal cord

- Formation of grey and white columns
  - Neurons that develop in the mantle zone of basal lamina form neurons of anterior grey horn. Axons of these anterior grey horn neurons grow out at ventrolateral angle of spinal cord to form *ventral motor roots* of spinal nerves.
  - Nerve cells that develop in the mantle zone of alar lamina form neurons of *posterior grey horn*. Axons of these cells travel through marginal zone and form *ascending tracts*.
  - Many neurons of mantle zone form interneurons.
  - Neural crest cells form pseudounipolar neurons of *dorsal root ganglia* (spinal ganglia). Central processes of these pseudounipolar neurons enter the spinal cord at dorsolateral angle to form dorsal *sensory roots* of spinal nerve. Peripheral processes of these neurons run laterally as sensory fibres of spinal nerve.
  - Both sensory and motor roots join to form a typical spinal nerve.
  - Axons of neurons from various parts of the brain enter the marginal zone of spinal cord to form *descending tracts*.
  - Thus, mantle layer forms *grey matter*, whereas marginal layer forms *white matter* of spinal cord.
  - Cells at the junction of alar and basal laminae in the mantle zone proliferate to form *lateral horn* of spinal cord.
- Glial cells
  - Spongioblast (glioblasts) differentiate into astrocytoblast and oligodendroblast.
  - Astrocytoblast differentiates into *protoplasmic and fibrous astrocytes*, whereas oligodendroblast differentiates into *oligodendrocytes*.
  - *Microglial cells* (phagocytes) are derived from mesenchymal tissues.[Neet]
  - Lining epithelium of neural tube cavity differentiates to form *ependymal cells* and lining epithelium of choroid plexuses.

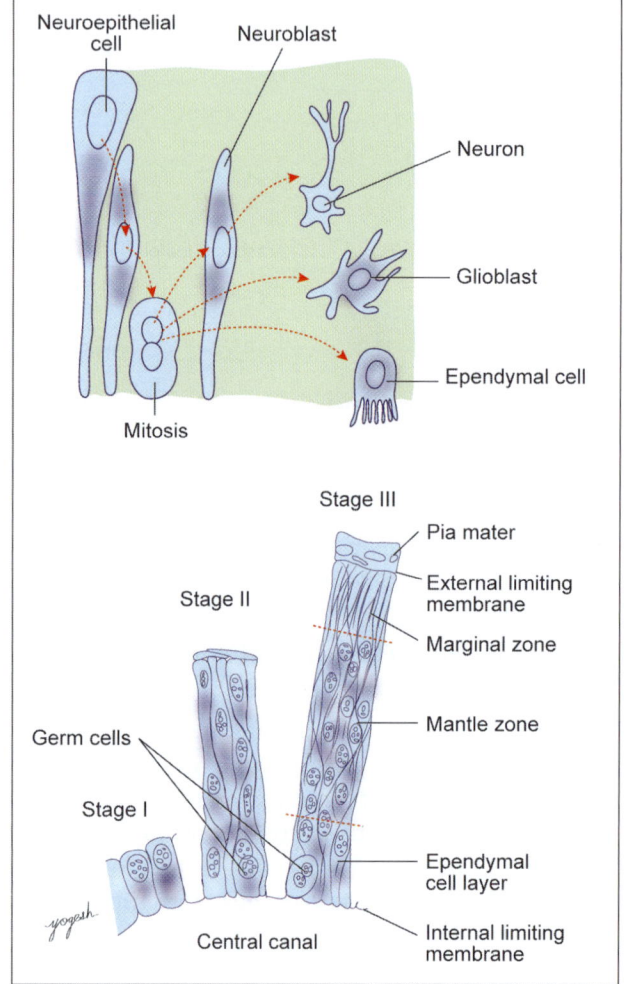

Fig. 22.5: Histogenesis of spinal cord

Phase 4. Positional changes in spinal cord (Fig. 22.7)

Q. *Write short note on positional changes of spinal cord.*

- Spinal cord extends through the entire length of vertebral canal up to 3rd month of IUL. Spinal nerves run horizontally and emerge from corresponding intervertebral foramina.[MCQ]

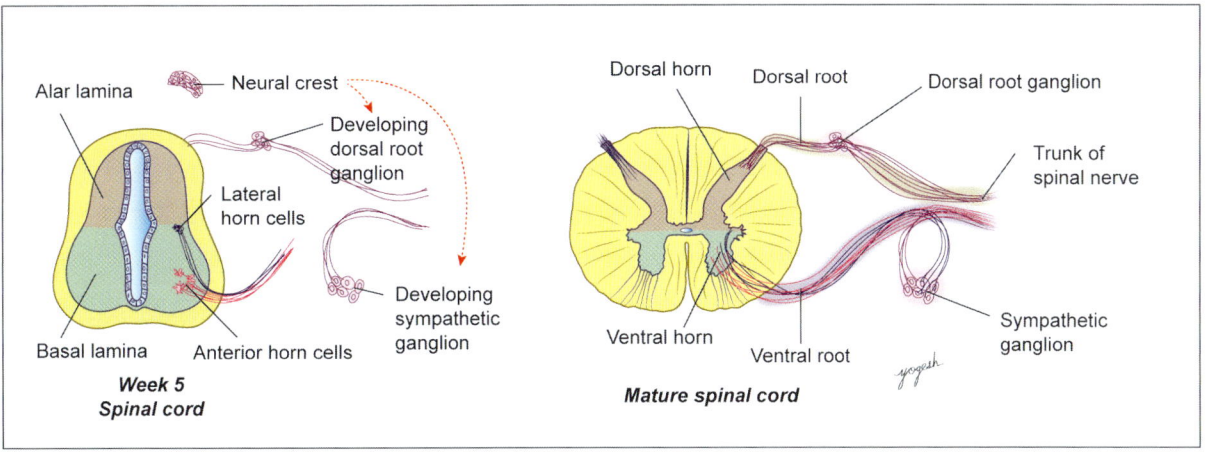

Fig. 22.6: Development of spinal nerve

- Due to differential growth, vertebral column elongates faster than spinal cord and terminal end of spinal cord shifts to a higher level.
- At birth, lower end of spinal cord is located at the level of 3rd lumbar vertebra.^{MCQ}
- The process of differential growth continues up to the adult life, hence, in adult, lower end of spinal cord is located at the level of lower border of first lumbar vertebra (or upper border of L2 vertebra).^{MCQ}
- Cauda equina is a derivative of neural tube.^{Neet}

Result of spinal cord recession

1. Spinal nerves do not arise at the level of corresponding intervertebral foramen.
2. Spinal nerves run obliquely downloads to reach corresponding intervertebral foramen.
3. Lower portion of pia mater form fibrous band called *filum terminale*, that extends from lower end of spinal cord up to the first coccygeal vertebra.^{MCQ}
4. Dura mater extends up to second sacral vertebra.^{MCQ}

Note: Pia mater is derived from neural crest cells, whereas arachnoid mater and dura mater are derived from condensation of mesenchyme that surrounds the neural tube.^{Neet}

Functional Columns of Spinal Cord

- The neurons of basal and alar lamina are arranged according to the designated function in the form of functional columns as follows:

Columns in basal lamina

1. *General somatic efferent*—provides innervations for skeletal muscles.
2. *General visceral efferent column*—present only in the thoracolumbar region and sacral region as lateral-horn of the spinal cord. It provides preganglionic sympathetic and parasympathetic fibres.

Columns in alar lamina

1. *General visceral afferent column*: It is present only in thoracolumbar and sacral regions of spinal cord and receives sensory inputs form viscera (organs).
2. *General somatic afferent column*: It receives exteroceptive and proprioceptive information.

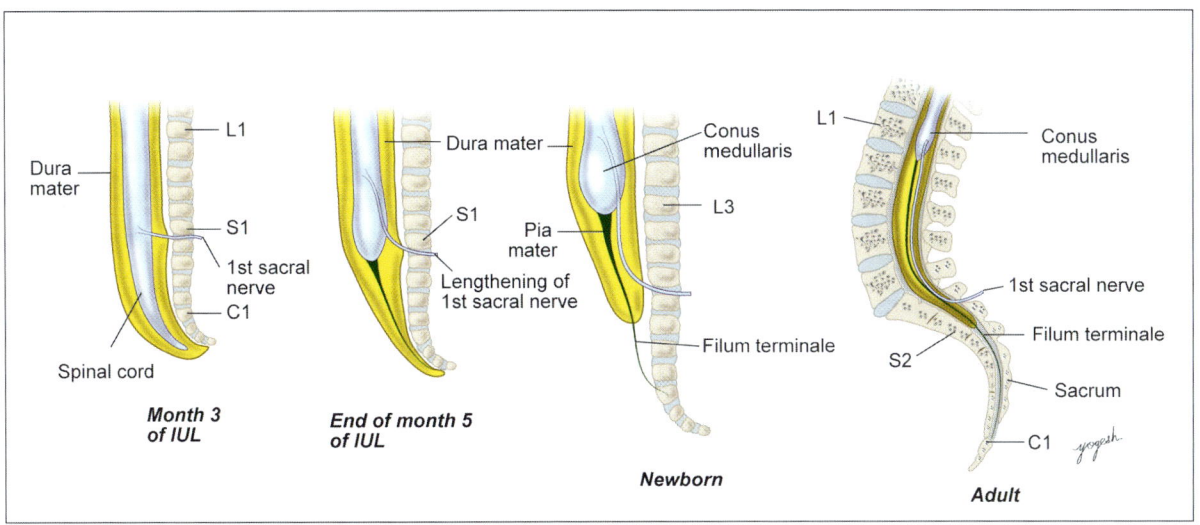

Fig. 22.7: Developing spinal cord—positional changes. Abbreviation: IUL, intrauterine life

Flowchart 22.2: Development of spinal cord

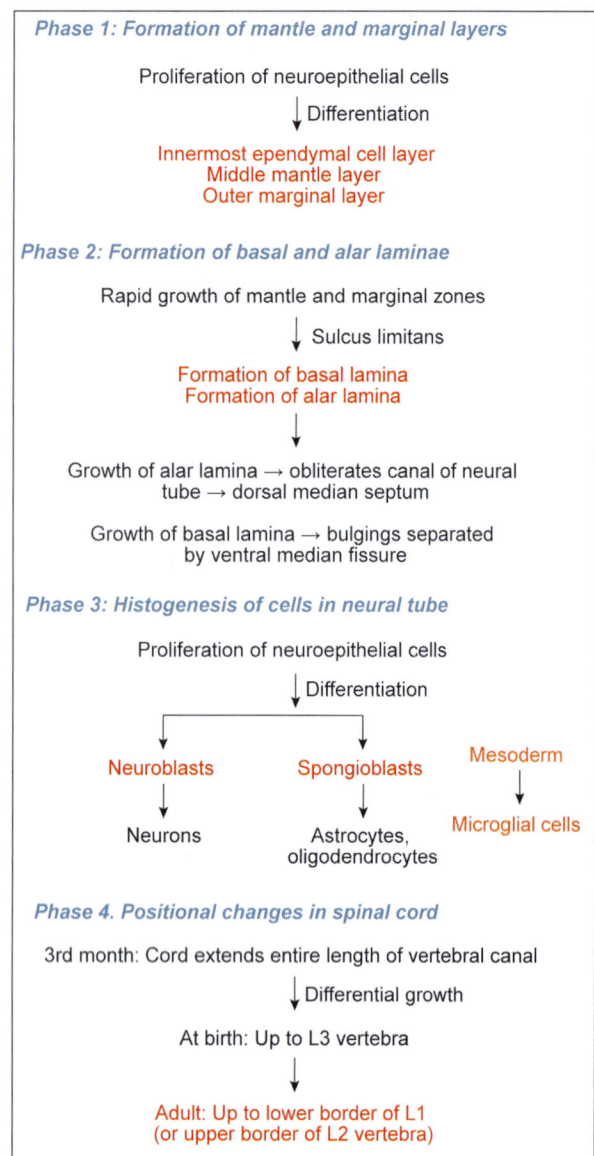

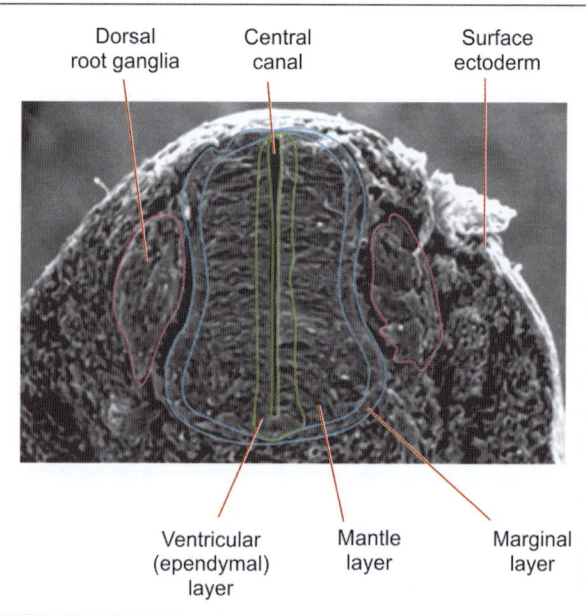

Scanning electron micrograph 22.3 Development of spinal cord. The cells of the neural tube form three layers, a ventricular ependymal layer of undifferentiated, proliferating cells, a mantle layer of differentiating neurons that will form the grey matter of the spinal cord, and a marginal layer that contains nerve fibres and will be the white matter [Species: Mouse, approximate human age: 6 weeks, transverse section]

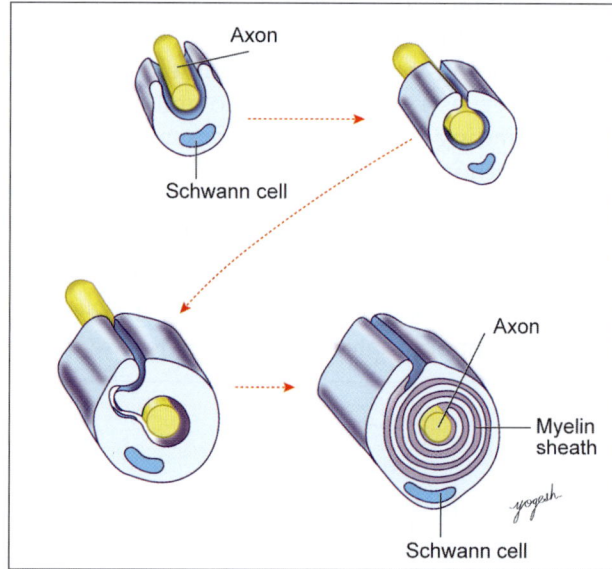

Fig. 22.8: Process of myelination of peripheral nerve fibres

Box 22.1: Myelination (Fig. 22.8)
- Myelination (myelinogenesis) is the process of formation of myelin around the axons.
- Myelination in the central nervous system is the function of oligodendrocytes, whereas in the peripheral nervous system, it is the function of Schwann cells. *Neet*
- Myelination begins when the nerve fibres start functioning.
- It begins during the 4th month of IUL and continues after the birth up to 2–3 years.
- Motor fibres myelinate earlier than sensory fibres. *MCQ*
- Myelination of corticospinal tract begins at 9 months of IUL and continues up to 2 years after birth. *Clinical fact*

NEURAL TUBE DEFECTS

Q. Write short note on spina bifida/ neural tube defects.

Definition: Neural tube defects (NTDs) are a group of conditions formed owing to non-closure of neural tube.
- Closure of the neural tube begins in the third week of IUL. Cranial neuropore closes by 25th day and caudal neuropore by 27th day of IUL.

- NTDs are the commonest birth defect.
- Most common cause for NTDs is folic acid (vitamin B9) deficiency.^{MCQ} Folate is essential for DNA/RNA synthesis, cell division and myelination.
- Folic acid supplements to the mother reduce chances of NTDs.
- Methylenetetrahydrofolate reductase (MTHFR) enzyme deficiency due to MTHFR gene mutation is also associated with neural tube defects.$^{Neet,\ Clinical\ fact}$
- NTDs are listed in Table 22.1.

Table 22.1 Neural tube defects

1. Spina bifida
   - Spina bifida occulta
   - Meningocele
   - Myelomeningocele
2. Anencephaly
3. Encephalocele
4. Iniencephaly
5. Rachischisis

Spina Bifida (Fig. 22.9, Practice Fig. 22.3)

Q. Write short note on spina bifida.

- Definition
  Spina bifida is a neural tube defect that occurs within the first four weeks of pregnancy due to the incomplete closure of neural tube.
- Pathology
  Folic acid deficiency or MTHFR gene defect !incomplete closure of neural tube → incomplete formation of vertebrae → bifid spines of vertebrae (spina bifida)

Types

A. *Spina bifida occulta*
   - In this condition, spine is bifid but not visible on the surface (occulta means hidden).
   - It commonly occurs in lumbosacral region.
   - Its location is marked by dimple on the skin and hairy skin.
   - Spinal cord and meninges are normal in position.
B. *Spina bifida cystica*
   It is of two types:
   1. Meningocele
      It is the protrusion of arachnoid and pia mater (only meninges) through the bifid spine.
      It produces cystic swelling covered with skin.
   2. Myelomeningocele (meningomyelocele)
      It is the protrusion of spinal cord through bifid spine.

It also produces cystic swelling covered with skin.

Prevention

- Supplementation of 0.4 mg/day folic acid from three months prior to conception up to the first 12 weeks of the pregnancy can prevent neural tube defects.

Screening

- Neural tube defects can be detected by
  1. Ultrasonography
  2. Increased maternal serum α-fetoprotein.^{Neet}

Treatment

- Spina bifida can be treated by surgery after delivery.

Other Defects

1. *Anterior spina bifida*: In this condition, two halves of vertebral body fail to fuse and results in a gap. Through this gap, spinal meninges protrude ventrally.
2. *Anencephaly*: It occurs due to the failure of closure of anterior neuropore. It shows irregular degenerated brain mass.
3. *Encephalocele*: Due to failure of formation of skull vault bones, brain tissue and meninges protrude outside the skull cavity and form encephalocele.
4. *Iniencephaly* (inion = nape of neck in Greek): It involves defective occipital bone, spina bifida of cervical vertebrae and retroflexion of head (backward bending).
5. *Rachischisis* (myeloschisis): It is the failure of closure of neural folds to form neural tube. It results in the exposure of flattened neural tissue onto the surface.

Box 22.2: Hydrocephalus

Q. Write short note on hydrocephalus.

- Hydrocephalus is the excess of CSF in the ventricular system.
- **Causes**
  - Obstruction of CSF passage
  - Excess production of CSF
  - Impaired communication between ventricles and subarachnoid space
- **Pathology**
  Dilatation of ventricular system results in separation of cranial bones. It produces large head size and degeneration of nervous tissue.
- Enlargement of central canal of spinal cord is called **syringomyelia**.^{Neet}

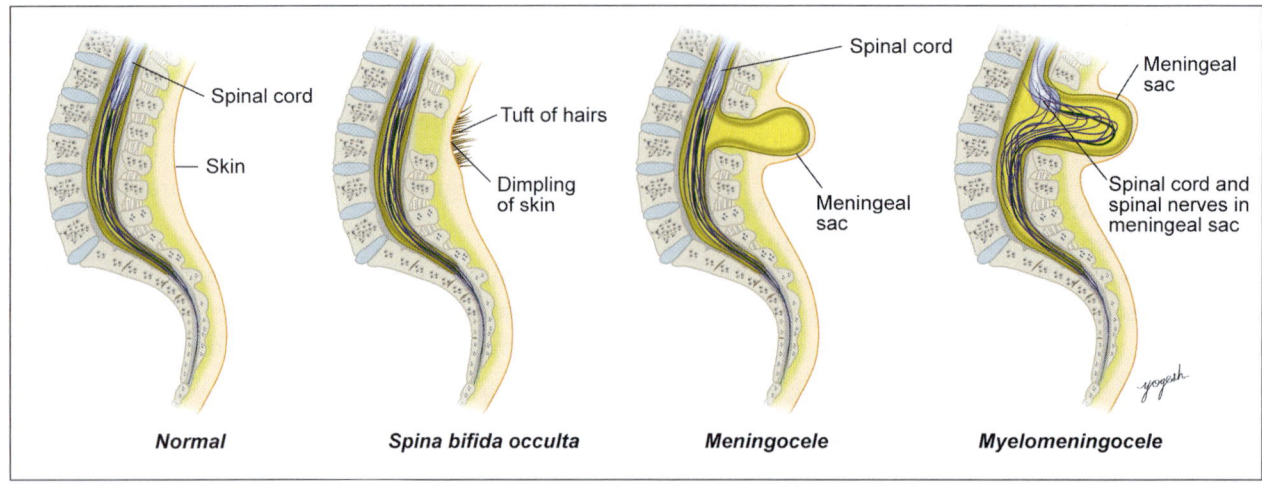

Fig. 22.9: Spina bifida

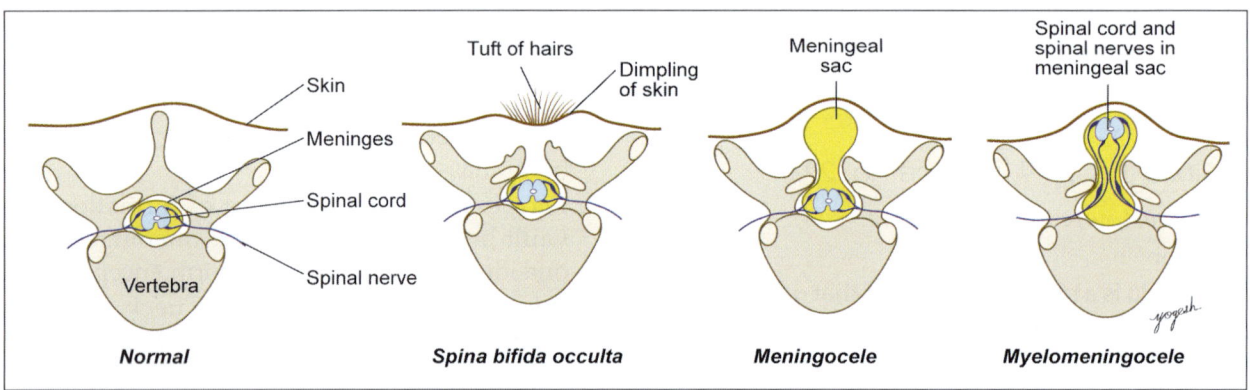

Practice Fig. 22.3: Spina bifida

FUNCTIONAL COLUMNS OF BRAINSTEM

- Medulla oblongata, pons and midbrain together constitute the brainstem.
- Sulcus limitans divide lateral part of the brainstem into dorsal *alar lamina* and ventral *basal lamina*.
- Cells of basal lamina form the efferent group of neurons (*efferent columns*), whereas cells of alar lamina form afferent group of neurons (*afferent columns*).
- These columns show group of neurons that perform specific function via cranial nerves. Such group of neurons in the brainstem form *cranial nerve nuclei*.

Division of Functional Columns (Fig. 22.10)

- According to functions, nuclear columns are divided as follows:
  1. *General somatic efferent* (GSE): For striated muscles of head that are not originated from the pharyngeal arches.
  2. *Special visceral efferent* (SVE) or branchial efferent: For striated muscles of pharyngeal arches, trapezius and sternocleidomastoid muscles.
  3. *General visceral efferent* (GVE) as preganglionic parasympathetic fibres.
  4. *General visceral afferent* (GVA) for visceral sensation via vagus nerve.
  5. *Special visceral afferent* (SVA) for taste sensation.
  6. *General somatic afferent* (GSA) for proprioception, tactile sensation from face and oral, nasal and pharyngeal mucosa via trigeminal nerve.
  7. *Special somatic afferent* (SSA) for auditory and vestibular impulses.

For further details, refer Tables 22.2 and 22.3 and read cranial nerves from Gross Anatomy book.

DEVELOPMENT OF MEDULLA OBLONGATA

Q. Write short note of development of medulla oblongata.

- Rhombencephalon (hindbrain) is divided into two parts:
  - *Myelencephalon* (caudal part) that forms medulla oblongata.

Nervous System

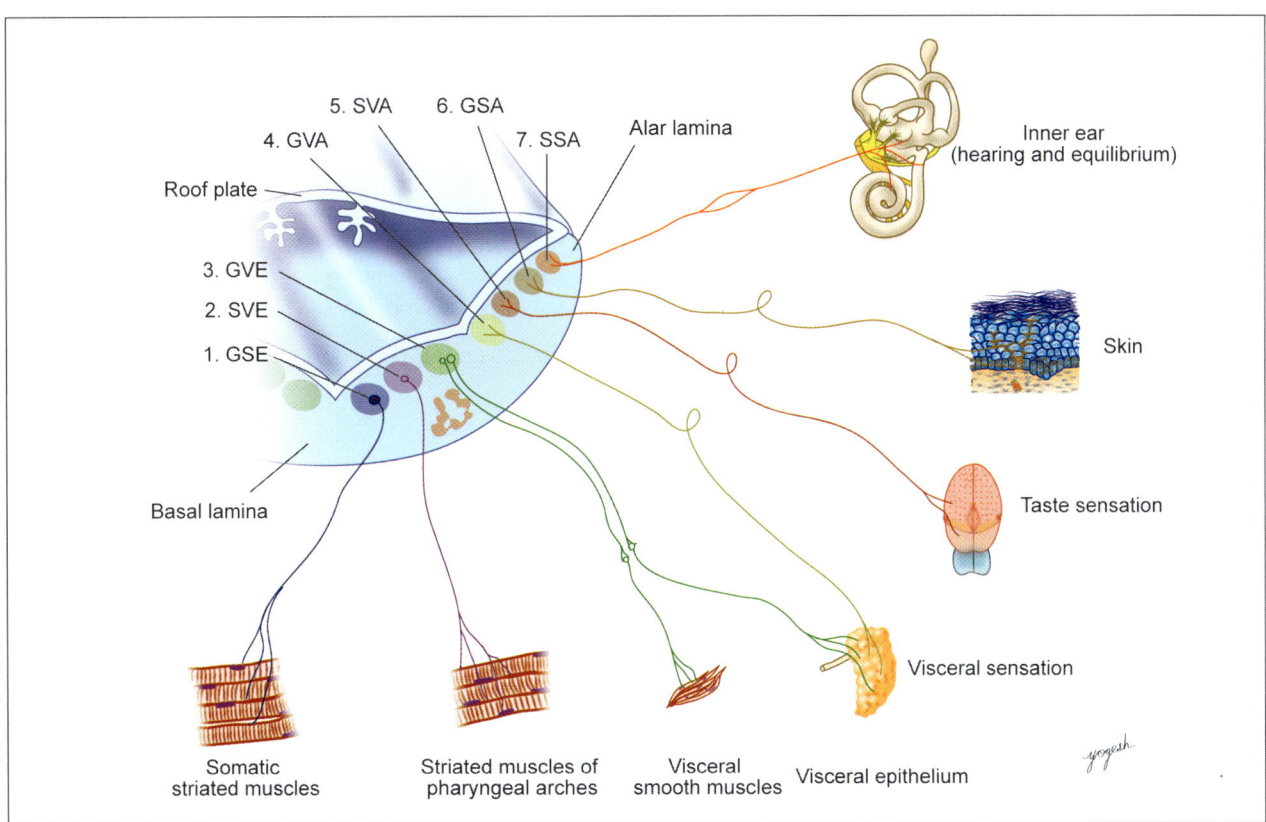

Fig. 22.10: Organisation of functional columns of cranial nerve nuclei in brainstem. GSE: General somatic efferent, SVE: Special visceral efferent, GVE: General visceral efferent, GVA: General visceral afferent, SVA: Special visceral afferent, GSA: General somatic afferent, SSA: Special somatic afferent

Q. List the functional columns of basal lamina of brainstem.

Table 22.2	Functional columns of brainstem—part I: Efferent columns				
Component	Function	Nucleus	Location	Cranial nerve	Remark
General somatic efferent (GSE)	Striated muscles of head not of pharyngeal arch origin	Third cranial nerve nucleus	Midbrain	3rd nerve	Extraocular muscles except lateral rectus and superior oblique muscles
		Fourth cranial nerve nucleus	Midbrain	4th nerve	Superior oblique muscle
		Sixth cranial nerve nucleus	Pons	6th nerve	Lateral rectus muscle
		Twelfth cranial nerve nucleus	Medulla	12th nerve	Muscles of tongue except palatoglossus
Special visceral efferent (SVE) (branchial efferent)	Striated muscles of pharyngeal arch origin as well as trapezius and sternocleidomastoid	Motor nucleus of trigeminal nerve	Pons	5th nerve	Muscles of the first arch via mandibular nerve
		Motor nucleus of facial nerve	Pons	7th nerve	Muscles of the second arch
		Nucleus ambiguus	Medulla	9th nerve	Muscle of the third arch—stylopharyngeus
		Nucleus ambiguus	Medulla	10th nerve	Muscles of 4th arch via superior laryngeal nerve
		Nucleus ambiguus	Medulla	11th nerve	Muscles of sixth arch (fibres of 11th nerve via recurrent laryngeal branch of vagus)

Contd.

Table 22.2	Functional columns of brainstem—part I: Efferent columns (Contd.)				
Component	Function	Nucleus	Location	Cranial nerve	Remark
General visceral efferent (GVE)	Preganglionic autonomic fibres	Edinger-Westphal nucleus	Midbrain	3rd nerve	Sphincter pupillae, ciliaris
		Superior salivatory nuclei	Pons	7th nerve	Submandibular and sublingual gland
		Lacrimatory nucleus	Pons	7th nerve	Lacrimal gland
		Inferior salivatory nucleus	Medulla	9th nerve	Parotid gland
		Dorsal nucleus of vagus	Medulla	10th nerve	

Q. List the functional columns of alar lamina of brainstem.

Table 22.3	Functional columns of brainstem- part II: Afferent columns				
Component	Function	Nucleus	Location	Cranial nerve	Remark
General visceral afferent (GVA)	Visceral sensation	Dorsal nucleus of vagus	Medulla	10th nerve	
Special visceral afferent (SVA)	Taste	Nucleus tractus solitarious	Pons and medulla	7th, 9th, 10th nerve	Taste sensation
General somatic afferent (GSA)	Proprioception, tactile sensation from face, and oral, nasal and pharyngeal mucosa	Mesencephalic nucleus of trigeminal nerve	Midbrain	5th nerve	
	General sensation from face, and oral, nasal and pharyngeal mucosa	Spinal nucleus of trigeminal nerve	Pons and medulla	5th nerve	
Special somatic afferent (SSA)	Auditory (hearing) and vestibular (equilibrium) impulses from inner ear (Sight is also SSA)	Cochlear and vestibular nuclei	Pons and medulla	8th nerve	Hearing and equilibrium

- *Metencephalon* (cranial part) that forms pons and cerebellum.
- Cavity of rhombencephalon forms the 4th ventricle.^{Neet}
- Fusion between mesencephalon and rhombencephalon is marked by a construction called *rhombencephalic isthmus*.
- On appearance of the fifth vesicle of brain, external appearance of myelencephalon changes markedly.
- Cavity of myelencephalon forms upper part of the 4th ventricle.

Developmental Stages

- *Sulcus limitans* divide alar and basal lamina.
- Roof plate of cranial part of medulla widens to form *roof* of the 4th ventricle.
- Widening of the roof plate brings alar lamina dorsolateral to the basal lamina and thus, both the laminae form *floor* of 4th ventricle.

Differentiation of Basal Lamina (Fig. 22.11)

- Basal lamina of myelencephalon differentiates into the following columns:
  1. General somatic efferent (GSE): It includes hypoglossal nuclei (XII) for the muscles of tongue.
  2. Special visceral efferent (SVE): It includes nucleus amibuguus for the muscles of third arch (glossopharyngeal nerve), muscles of fourth arch (superior laryngeal branch of vagus) and sixth arch (recurrent laryngeal branch) of vagus via spinal accessory nerve.
  3. General visceral efferent (GVE): It includes dorsal nucleus of vagus and inferior salivatory nucleus for parotid gland (glossopharyngeal nerve).

Differentiation of Alar Lamina (Fig. 22.11)

- Cells from each alar lamina migrate ventrally in the marginal layer to form **bulbo-pontine extension** and finally develop into olivary group of nuclei.^{MCQ}

- Due to growth and appearance of white matter, the nuclei shift from their initial positions to the definitive positions.
- Remaining cells of the alar lamina differentiate to form the following columns:
  1. General visceral efferent (GVE): It includes dorsal nucleus of vagus.
  2. Special visceral efferent (SVE): It includes nucleus tractus solitarious to receive taste sensation via 9th and 10th nerves.
  3. General somatic efferent (GSE): It includes spinal nucleus of trigeminal (for V nerve), nucleus gracilis and cuneatus (for tract of Goll and Burdach).
  4. Special somatic afferent (SSA): It includes cochlear and vestibular nuclei (for VIII nerve).
- White matter of medulla oblongata is mostly derived from ascending and descending tracts.

Formation of Tela Choroidea and Choroid Plexus

- Widening of roof plate of the myelencephalon results into formation of single cell layered ependymal roof plate of the 4th ventricle. This roof plate is surrounded by vascular pia mater called *tela choroidea*.
- The vascular proliferation of pia mater invaginates underlying ependyma. Thus, formed vascular tuft covered with ependyma called *choroid plexus*.
- Choroid plexus produces cerebrospinal fluid (CSF).
- Tela choroidea ruptures to form *foramina of Luschka* that communicates the 4th ventricle with subarachnoid space.

DEVELOPMENT OF PONS (FIG. 22.12)

Q. Write short note of development of pons.

- Rhombencephalon (hindbrain) is divided into cranial *metencephalon* and caudal *myelencephalon*.
- Metencephalon is divided into ventromedial part that forms *pons* and dorsolateral part called *rhombic lip* that forms cerebellum.^MCQ
- Roof plate of metencephalon also becomes thin and broad (similar to myelencephalon) to form roof of the 4th ventricle. The alar lamina becomes dorsolateral to the basal lamina.

External Features

- *Pontine flexure* separates pons from the medulla oblongata at pontomedullary junction.
- Bulging basilar part of pons shows midline groove (basilar sulcus).
- Pontocerebellar fibres form *middle cerebellar peduncles*.
- Dorsal surface shows elevation in the floor of 4th ventricle as *facial colliculus*.

Formation of Pontine Nuclei

- Cells of alar lamina of medulla oblongata (myelencephalon) migrate ventrally to form **bulbopontine extension**.
- This bulbopontine extension forms *olivary group of nuclei* and cranial migration of bulbopontine extension forms *pontine nuclei* in the ventral basilar part of pons.^Neet
- Axons of pontine nuclei form *middle cerebellar peduncle*.

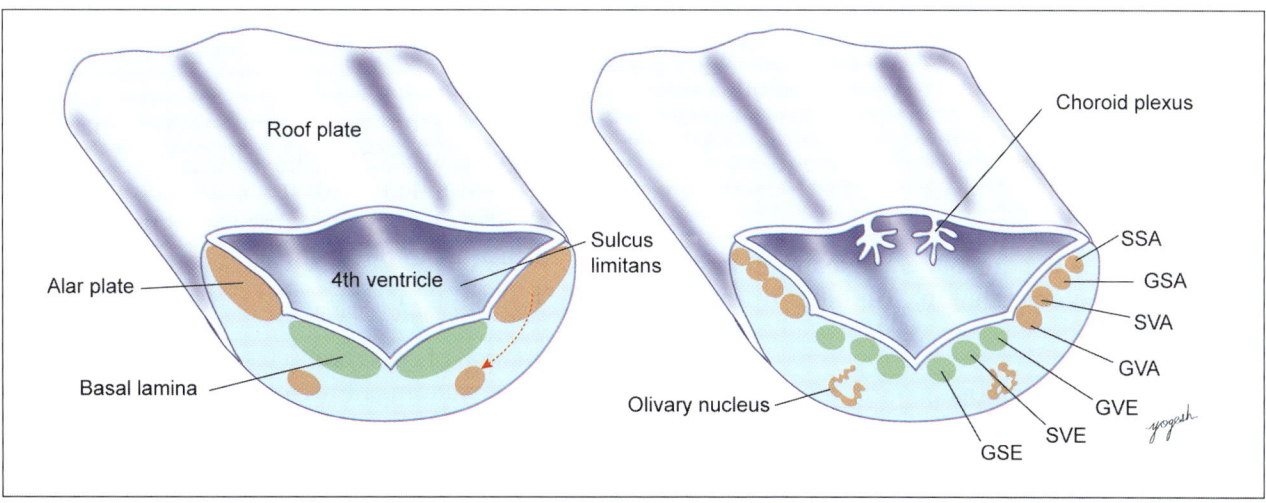

Fig. 22.11: Section of myelencephalon (medulla). Basal and alar lamina of myelencephalon. Roof plate connects alar laminae and forms the roof of the 4th ventricle. Cells of the alar laminae migrate in marginal zone that later forms olivary group of nuclei. GSE: General somatic efferent, SVE: Special visceral efferent, GVE: General visceral efferent, GVA: General visceral afferent, SVE: Special visceral efferent, GSA: General somatic afferent, SSA: Special somatic afferent.

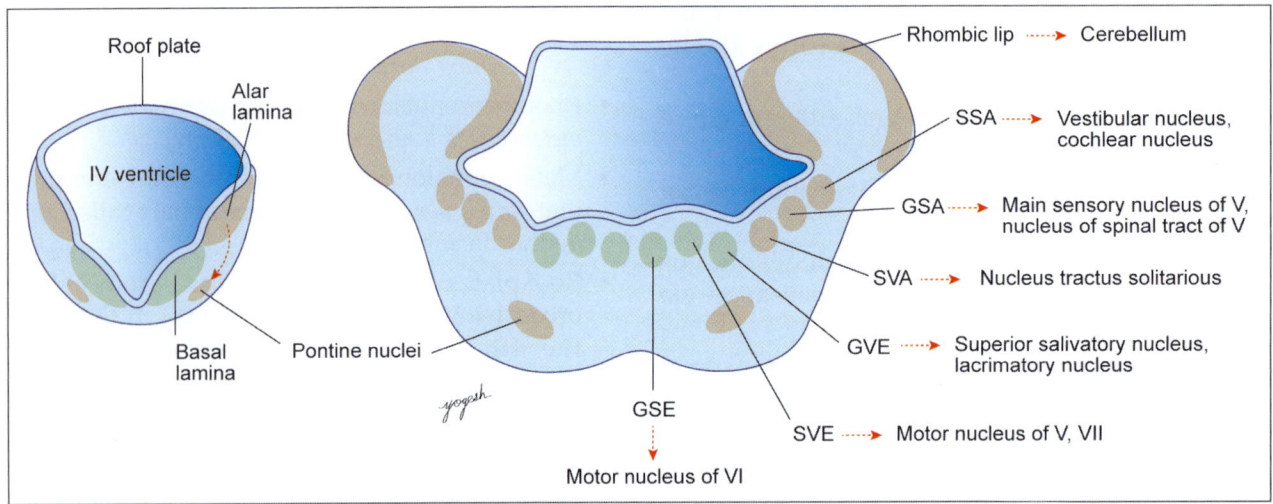

Fig. 22.12: Development of pons

Differentiation of Basal Lamina

- Basal lamina of pons differentiates into the following columns:
  1. General somatic efferent (GSE): It includes motor nucleus of VI nerve for the lateral rectus muscle.
  2. Special visceral efferent (SVE): It includes motor nucleus of V nerve for muscles of 1st pharyngeal arch and facial nucleus for muscles of 2nd arch.
  3. General visceral efferent (GVE): It includes superior salivatory nucleus for submandibular and sublingual gland (via VII nerve) and lacrimatory nucleus for lacrimal gland (via VII nerve).

Differentiation of Alar Lamina

- Alar lamina of pons differentiates to form the following columns:
  1. Special visceral afferent (SVA): It includes nucleus tractus solitarious for taste sensation via VII nerve.
  2. General somatic afferent (GSA): It includes the main sensory nucleus of V nerve and nucleus of spinal tract of trigeminal nerve.
  3. Special somatic afferent (SSA): It includes vestibular and cochlear nuclei.
  4. Rhombic lip is the dorsolateral expansion of alar lamina of metencephalon. Rhombic lip forms cerebellum.

DEVELOPMENT OF MIDBRAIN (Fig. 22.13)

Q. Write short note of development of midbrain.

- Midbrain develops from mesencephalon.

Stages of Development

- Sulcus limitans divide the mantle layer into dorsal alar lamina and ventral basal lamina.

Differentiation of Basal Lamina

- Basal lamina along with floor plate of mesencephalon forms tegmentum of midbrain.
- Basal lamina of midbrain differentiates into the following columns:
  1. General somatic efferent (GSE) column: It includes oculomotor nucleus (III nerve) and trochlear nucleus (IV nerve) for extraocular muscles.
  2. General visceral efferent (GVE): It includes Edinger-Westphal nucleus (III nerve).

Differentiation of Alar Lamina

- Alar lamina gives rise to stratified zones of colliculi (superior and inferior) and pretectal nuclei.
- Cells of the alar lamina migrate ventrally to form *red nucleus* and *substantia nigra*.
- Remaining cells of alar lamina along with basal lamina forms periaqueductal grey matter.
- Alar lamina of midbrain differentiates to form the following columns:
  1. General somatic afferent: It includes mesencephalic nucleus of trigeminal nerve.
  2. Special somatic afferent: It includes superior colliculus (reflex centre for light) and inferior colliculus (reflex centre for hearing).

White Matter of Midbrain

- Formation of crus cerebri (cerebral peduncles): Most of the descending fibres (corticospinal, corticobulbar, corticopontine) pass through the marginal zone of ventral part of midbrain that forms the crus cerebri.

Cerebral Aqueduct

- The cavity of mesencephalon forms *cerebral aqueduct of Sylvius* that connects the 3rd ventricle with 4th ventricle.[MCQ]

Nervous System

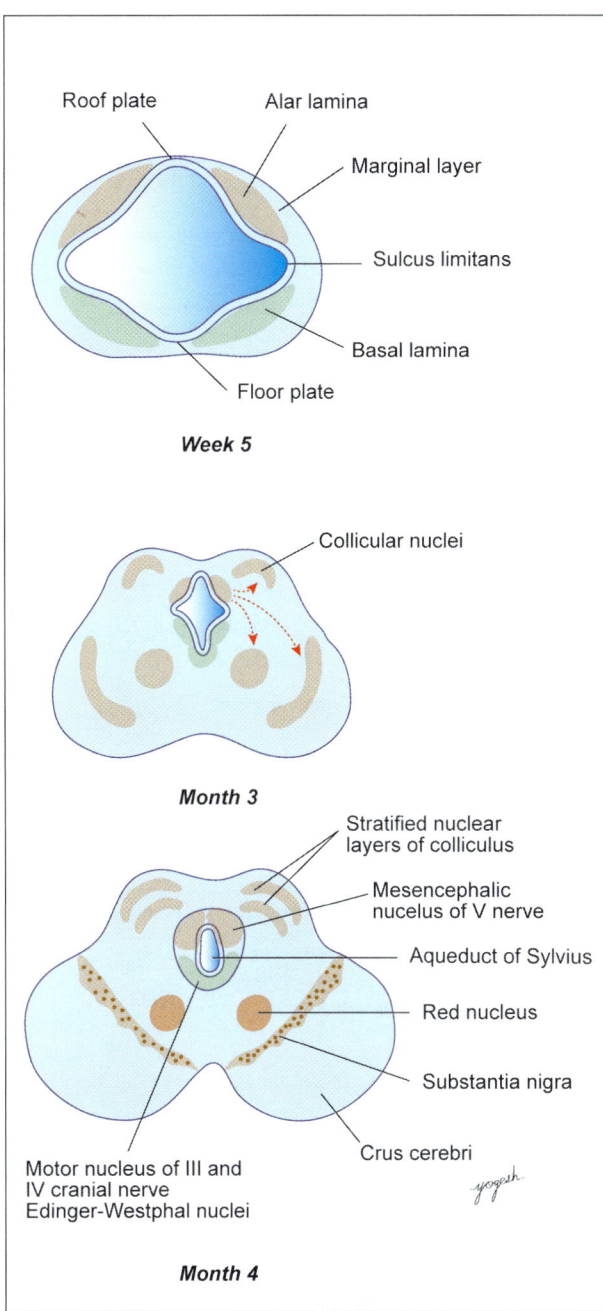

Fig. 22.13: Development of mesencephalon

- Some cells of mantle layer migrate outwards to form *external granular layer*, whereas remaining cells of mantle layer form *cerebellar nuclei*.
- External granular layer differentiates to form *cerebellar cortex*.
- Axons of dentate nucleus form superior cerebellar peduncles, axons of pontine nuclei form middle and axons of olivary nuclei form inferior cerebellar peduncles.

Stages of Development (Fig. 22.14)

- Development of cerebellum begins on 40–45 days of IUL.
- Two rhombic lips (right and left) appear in the caudal part of metencephalon.
- Initially, rhombic lips are separated by roof plate of metencephalon.
- Later, both the rhombic lips fuse across the midline to form *cerebellar plate*.
- In 12 weeks, cerebellar plate shows a small midline swelling called *vermis* and two lateral swellings called lateral *cerebellar lobes*.
- A transverse sulcus separates flocculus from lateral lobes and nodule from vermis and thus, *flocculonodular lobe* arises.
- Many transverse fissures appear and give cerebellum its characteristic adult appearance.
- Primary fissure separates anterior lobe from middle lobe (Table 22.4).

Table 22.4	Parts of cerebellum
Lobe	*Components*
Anterior lobe	Lingula
	Central lobule
	Culmen
	Ala of central lobule
	Quadrangular lobule
Middle lobe	Declive
	Folium
	Tuber
	Pyramid
	Uvula
	Lobulus simplex
	Biventral lobule
	Semilunar lobule
	Tonsil
Flocculonodular lobe	Nodule
	Flocculus

DEVELOPMENT OF CEREBELLUM

Q. *Write short note of development of cerebellum.*

Summary (Examination Guide)

- Bilateral rhombic lips arising from alar lamina of metencephalon form cerebellum.
- Rhombic lips produce bulging that fuse in midline to form *cerebellar plate*.
- Cerebellar plate differentiates to form *vermis* and *cerebellar hemispheres*.

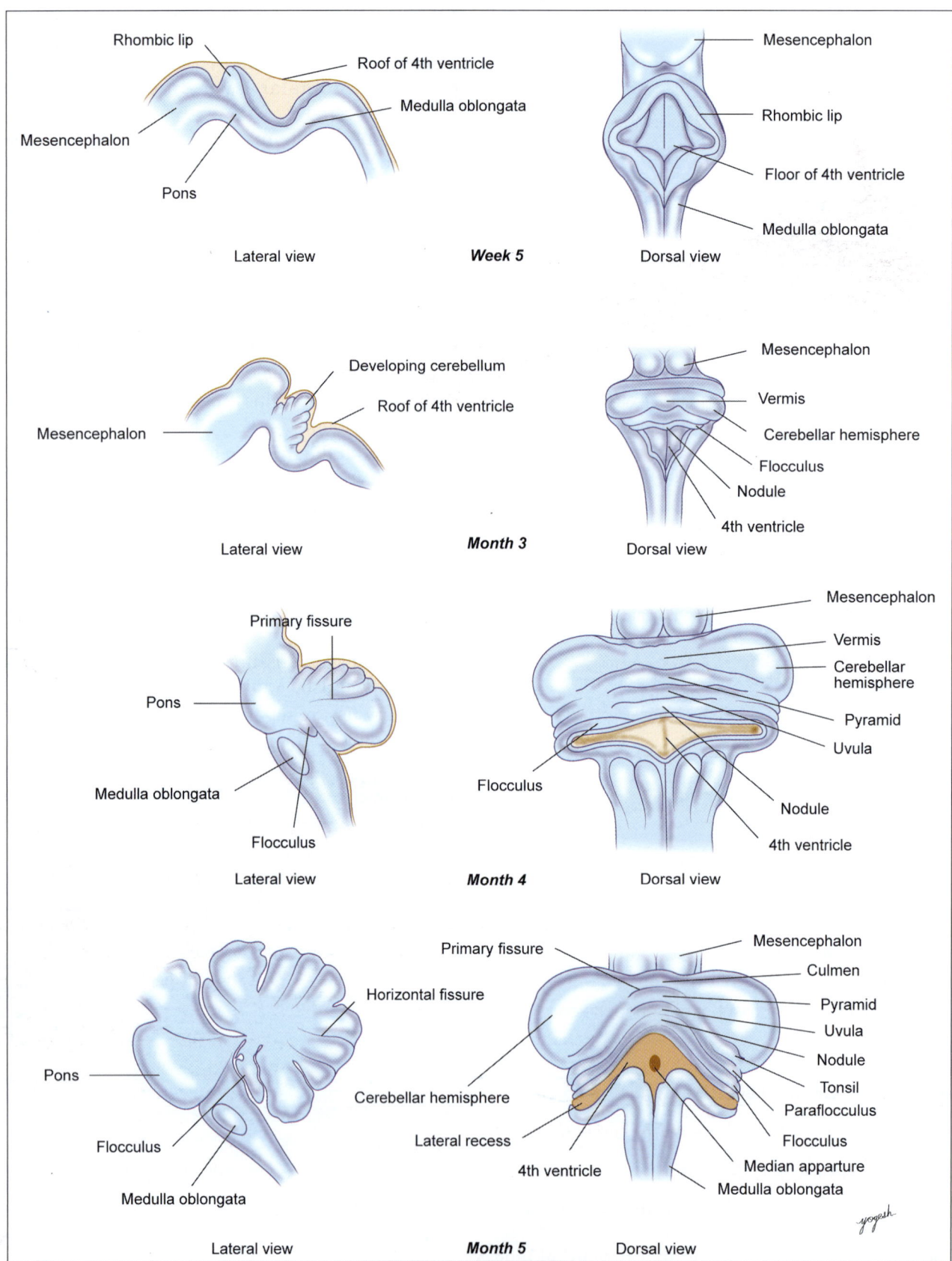

Fig. 22.14: Development of cerebellum

Flowchart 22.3: Development of cerebellum

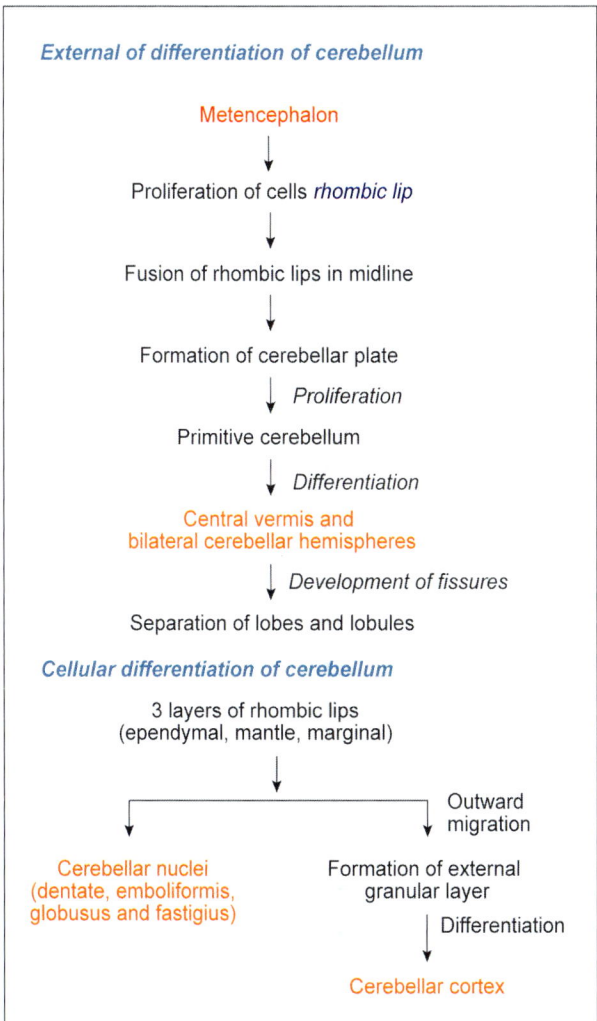

Histogenesis of Cerebellum (Fig. 22.15)

- Initially, *cerebellar primordium* consists of outer marginal and inner mantle zone of neuroepithelial cells.
- Cells from mantle zone migrate through the marginal zone to form *external granular layer*.
- Cells of external granular layer proliferate and migrate inward to form *cerebellar cortex*.
- It consists of outer molecular layer (stellate cells and basket cells), middle single cells layer (Purkinje cell layer) and inner granular layer (granule cells and Golgi cells).
- Formation of cerebellar cortex continues from 6th month of IUL till 1 ½ years after birth.^{MCQ} Note: DNA synthesis inhibitors (antiviral drugs) given up to the age of 2 years may cause cerebellar damage.
- Remaining cells of mantle layer (non-migrated cells) form dentate, emboliform, globose and fastigial nuclei.
- The part of the roof plate of 4th ventricle (with pia mater) that do not participate in the formation of cerebellum forms *superior* and *inferior medullary velum*.

Cerebellar Peduncles

The fibres passing through the marginal layer (white matter) of cerebellum form 3 cerebellar peduncles as follows:

- Superior cerebellar peduncle mainly consists of outgoing axons from dentate nucleus.^{MCQ}
- Middle cerebellar peduncle mainly consists of ingrowing axons of pontine nuclei.^{MCQ}
- Inferior cerebellar peduncle mainly consists of ingrowing axons of inferior olivary nuclei.^{MCQ}

DEVELOPMENT OF DIENCEPHALON (Fig. 22.16)

- Prosencephalon is divided into cranial *telencephalon* (cerebral hemispheres) and caudal *diencephalon*.
- Diencephalon has a cavity that forms 3rd ventricle.^{MCQ}

Box 22.3: Evolutionary aspect of cerebellum

- Phylogenetically cerebellum is divided into archicerebellum (older part), paleocerebellum and neocerebellum (newest part).
- Their functions and components are given in Table 22.5.

Table 22.5	Phylogenetic parts of cerebellum		
Phylogenetic part of cerebellum	*Example*	*Components*	*Function*
Archicerebellum	Aquatic vertebrates	Flocculonodular lobe, lingula	Maintenance of equilibrium
Paleocerebellum	Terrestrial vertebrates	Anterior lobe except lingula, pyramid and uvula	Controls tone, posture and crude movements of limbs
Neocerebellum	Higher animals	Middle lobe except pyramid and uvula	Regulation of fine movements of body

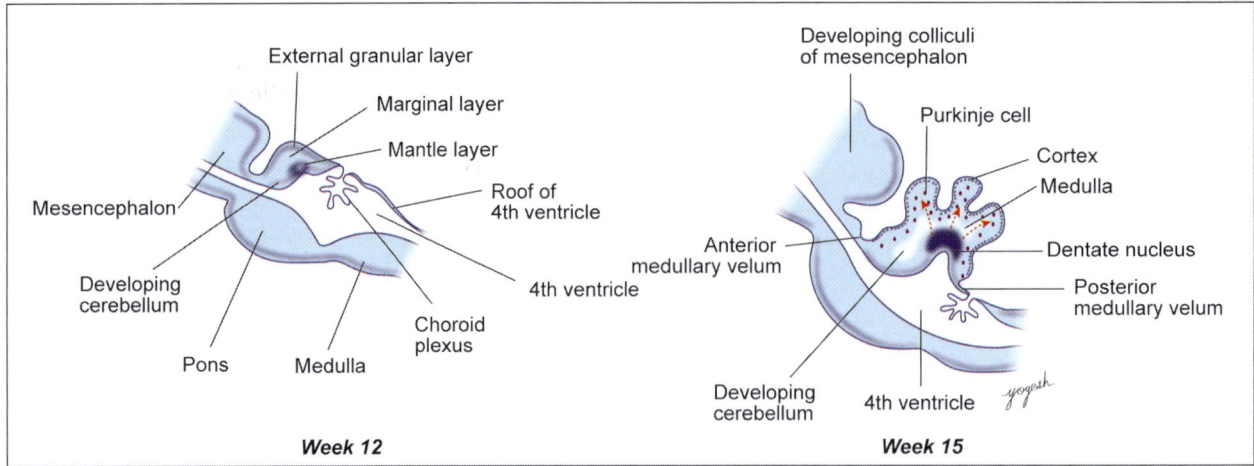

Fig. 22.15: Histogenesis of cerebellum. Cross-sectional view. Mantle layer gives rise to external granular layer that further produces cerebellar cortex and Purkinje cells. Mantle layer cells that left behind form deep cerebellar nuclei (dentate, emboliform, fastigus, globosus)

- The 3rd ventricle communicates with lateral ventricles through interventricular foramen of Monro and caudally with 4th ventricle through cerebral aqueduct.^{MCQ}
- Diencephalon has a roof plate and alar plates.

Differentiation of Roof Plate

- Roof plate is made up of ependymal cell layer covered by vascular pia mater.
- A portion of ependymal layer with tuft of capillaries from pia mater invaginates 3rd ventricle and forms *choroid plexus of 3rd ventricle*.
- Caudal part of roof plate forms *pineal body*.

Development of epithalamus

- Roof plate of diencephalon gives rise to epithalamus.
- It lies in the form of group of nuclei around the pineal gland.
- It includes habenular nuclei and habenular commissure.
- It is concerned with olfactory pathway.
- A small posterior commissure connecting epithalimi also develops caudal to pineal gland.
- Some authors consider pineal gland in the entity of epithalamus.

Differentiation of Alar Plates

- Alar plates form lateral wall and floor of diencephalon.
- Alar plates are divided into three zones by two sulci (hypothalamic sulcus and epithalamic sulcus) into three zones: Hypothalamus (lower part), thalamus (middle part) and epithalamus (upper part).
- *Thalamus* gradually bulges into the cavity of 3rd ventricle and differentiates to thalamic nuclei.

- *Hypothalamus* get pushed caudoventrally (antero-inferiorly in adult) due to enlarging thalamus.
- In the floor of cavity of diencephalon, a group of neurons assembles to form *mamillary body*.
- *Note:* On the 22nd day, in the region of hypothalamus, the lateral wall of diencephalon forms *optic sulcus* and later it becomes *optic vesicle* (optic cup). Optic cup forms retina and muscles of iris.
- From the floor of diencephalon, a downward growth develops that forms *infundibular process*. Later, the infundibular process develops posterior pituitary gland (neurohypophysis).

DEVELOPMENT OF CEREBRUM

- Telencephalon is divided into *prosencephalon* and *diencephalon*.
- Prosencephalon consists of two lateral outpouchings as *cerebral hemisphere* and a median *lamina terminalis*.
- Cavity of prosencephalon forms *lateral ventricles* (right and left) that communicates with 3rd ventricle through interventricular foramen.^{MCQ}
- The development of cerebral hemisphere can be studied as development during first two months and development after 2nd month.

Development During First 2 Months

- Each cerebral hemisphere consists of two parts:
  A. Thin *superior pallium*
  B. Thick *basal part*
- Cells from basal part migrate into the pallium that forms *cerebral cortex*.
- Remaining cells of basal part forms *corpus striatum*.

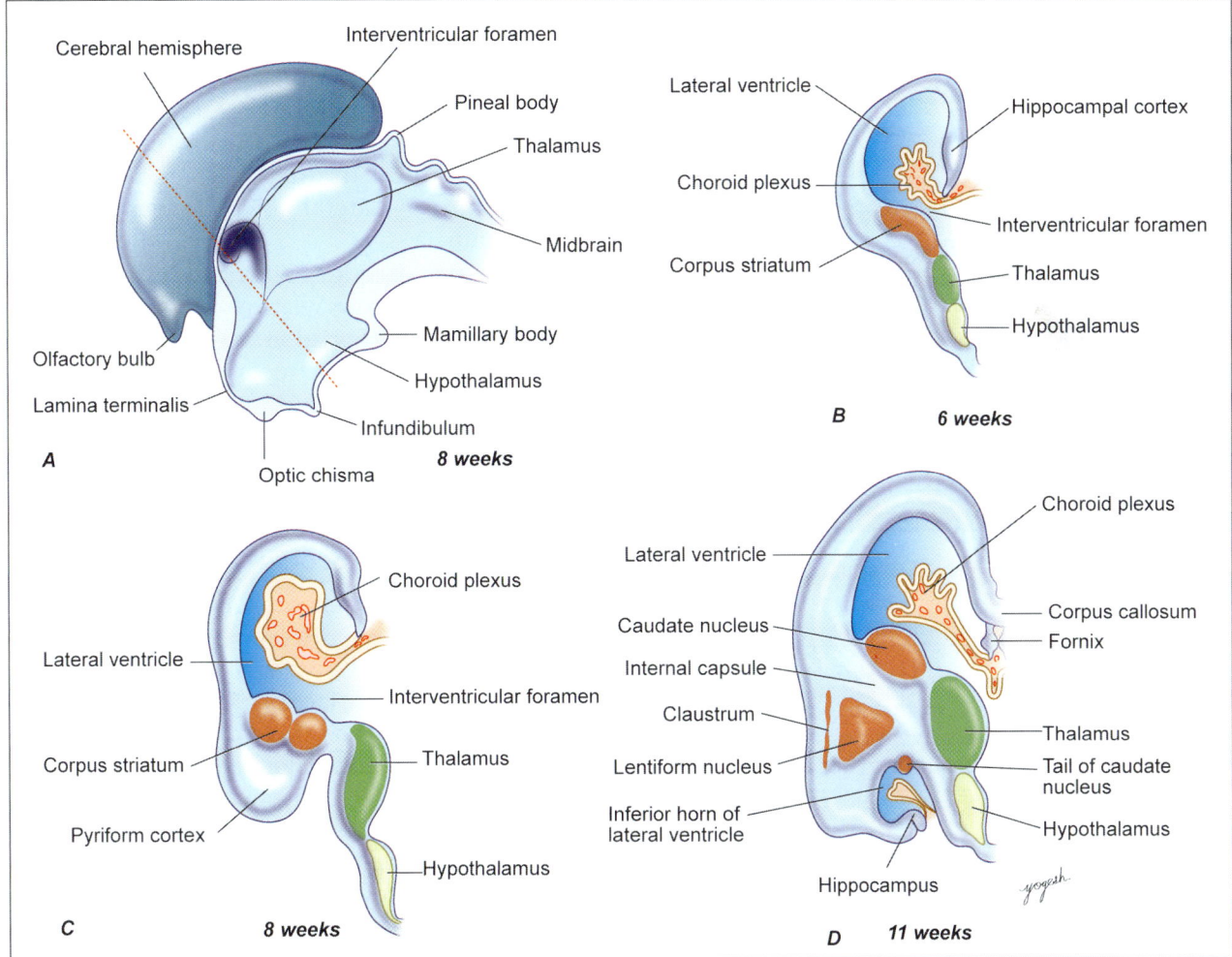

Fig. 22.16: A: In 8-week embryo, section showing medial surface of the right half of the telencephalon and diencephalon (red broken line indicates the plane of the section for B, C and D). B, C and D: Transverse sections through the right half of the telencephalon and diencephalon at the level of the broken lines in A

- The junctional zone of two pallium (cerebral cortex) is very thin and gets invaginated by choroid plexus.
- Pallium grows and gets differentiated into allocortex and neopallium. Human brain consists of 90% of neopallium.
- Allocortex = archipallium + paleopallium.
- Efferent and afferent fibres from the cerebral cortex form *internal capsule*.

Development after 2nd month

- Neopallium overgrows and compresses the allocortex.
- Increase in the cortical mass reduces ventricular cavity.
- In the floor of cerebral hemisphere, group of neurons condenses to form *striated nuclei*.
- These striated nuclei get transversed by fibres (axons) of *internal and external capsule*.

- Striated nuclei differentiate into three groups
  1. Lateral neostriatal nuclei: They form caudate nucleus, putamen and claustrum.
  2. Medial paleostriatal nuclei: They form globus pallidum.
  3. Archeostriatal nuclei: They form amygdaloid nucleus below the lenticular nucleus.
     Soon, the putamen and globus pallidum fuse to form lentiform nucleus.

Development of Lobes of Cerebral Hemispheres
(Fig. 22.17, Scanning electron micrograph 22.4)

- Cerebral cortex grows in various directions to form various lobes in the following manner:
  - Ventral growth forms *frontal lobe*.
  - Dorsal growth forms *occipital lobe*.
  - Parietal (lateral) growth forms *parietal lobe*.
  - Occipital pole expands ventrally to form *temporal lobe*.

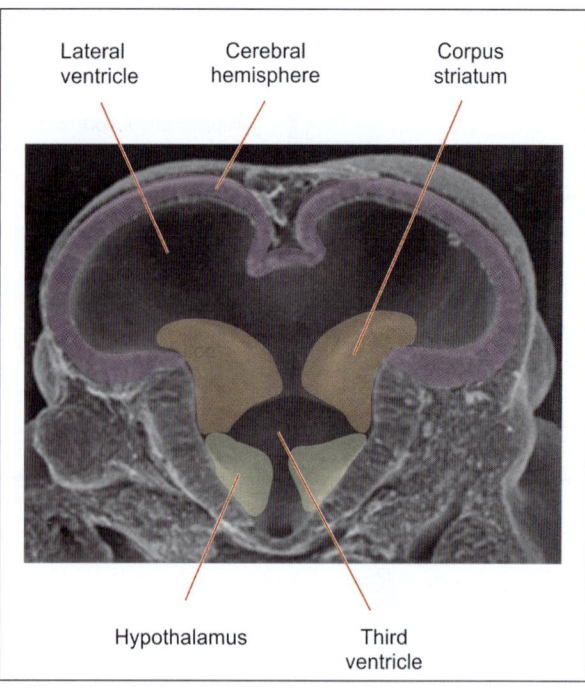

Scanning electron micrograph 22.4: A cut through the forebrain at the level of the line illustrates the expanding cerebral hemispheres surrounding the lateral ventricles, the third ventricle, hypothalamus and corpus striatum [Species: Mouse, approximate human age: 6 weeks, sagittal section]

Effects of development of cerebral hemispheres

1. Effect on lateral ventricle: Growth of occipital lobe and temporal lobe result in expansion of lateral ventricle to form *inferior horn* and *posterior horn* of lateral ventricle.

2. Effect on caudate nucleus: Expanding caudate nucleus turns around the developing ventricle and becomes 'C' shaped.

3. Formation of sulci and gyri: Continued growth of cerebral cortex starts formation of fissures. Parietooccipital fissure of Rolando appears by 7th month.[Neet] Lateral sulcus appears during the 4th month.[Neet]

4. Insula: A part of cortex covering the external surface of corpus striatum grows relatively slower. This part forms *insula*. Insula gets buried in the depth of lateral sulcus by overgrown cortex of frontal and temporal lobes.

5. Formation of olfactory bulb and tracts: From the frontal lobe, elongated evagination develops to form *olfactory bulb*. A stem that connects to the frontal lobe forms the *olfactory tract*.

Differentiation of Allocortex (Fig. 22.16)

- Allocortex differentiates to form limbic structures as follows:
  1. Allocortex has two parts: *Archipallium* that initially lies on medial surface of cerebral hemisphere and *paleopallium* that lies on ventral surface of hemisphere (ventrolateral to the corpus striatum).
  2. Allocortex differentiate to form *limbic lobe*. Limbic lobe differentiates into the following structures:
     a. Hippocampal cortex: Its *dorsal part* forms a thin band of grey matter called *induism griseum* on the dorsal surface of corpus callosum.
        Its *ventral part* forms *hippocampus* and *dentate gyrus* that projects into the cavity of inferior horn of lateral ventricle.

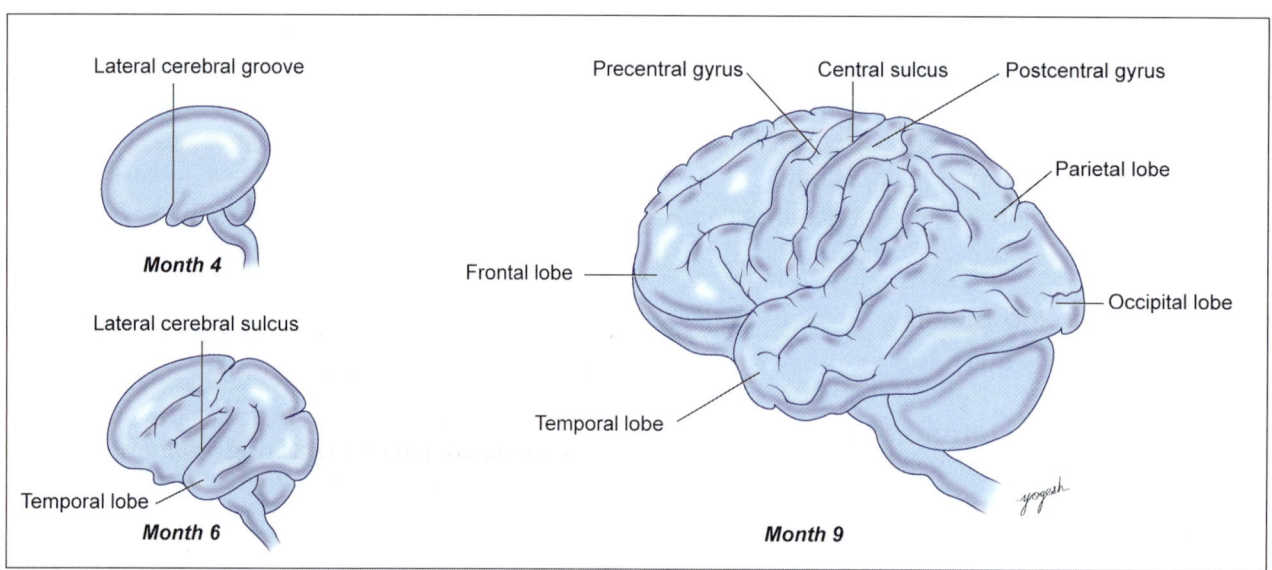

Fig. 22.17: Development of cerebral hemisphere during foetal life

b. *Projection fibres of hippocampal cortex*: The axons from hippocampal cortex forms *fimbria*, *fornix* and its *commissure*.
3. Allocortex also forms *olfactory bulb and tract*.

Some Interesting Facts
- Brain of mature infant has 9–14 billion neurons.
- Only neuroglial cells continue to multiply after birth.
- Total surface of adult cerebral cortex is about 285,000 mm^2.

Commissures of Telencephalon (Fig. 22.18)

- Lamina terminalis is the cranial most part of telencephalon and it connects two cerebral hemispheres. Hence, commissural fibres that connect two cerebral hemispheres pass through lamina terminalis.^{MCQ}
- Thickened band of fibres develops in lamina terminalis as follows:
  1. *Anterior commissure* connects two temporal lobes.
  2. *Corpus callosum* connects right and left cerebral hemispheres. With the growth of cerebral hemispheres, the size of corpus callosum also increases and it gets separated from fornix by *septum pellucidum*.
  3. *Hippocampal (fornix) commissure*: Connects right and left hippocampus.
  4. *Posterior commissure* is essential for light reflex (connections not yet discovered fully).
  5. *Habenular commissure* connects habenular nuclei of both sides. Habenular nuclei are part of epithalamus.
  6. Optic chiasma.

Some Interesting Facts
- Neural tube is covered by loose mesenchymal tissue that forms arachnoid and dura mater.
- Neural crest cells form pia mater.
- Pia mater and arachnoid mater together form leptomeninges (soft meninges).
- Leptomeninges coalesce to form subarachnoid space.

Developmental Anomalies

- *Anencephaly* is 4 times more frequent in females and 4 times more frequent in whites.
- Anencephaly in last trimester of pregnancy is associated with hydramnios due to lack of swallowing mechanism in the foetus.
- *Encephalocele* is defective closure of neural groove. It results in the herniation of parts of brain under the skin through a hole in the skull.
- *Dandy-Walker malformation*: Atresia of foramina of Magendie and Luschka (that communicate 4th ventricle with subarachnoid space) results in dilation of 4th ventricle and agenesis of cerebellum.
- *Microcephaly*: It is underdeveloped brain causing gross mental retardation. It is autosomal recessive disorder or may be produced due to antenatal cytomegalovirus infection or exposure to radiation.
- *Arnold-Chiari malformation*: It is downward displacement of cerebellar tonsil through foramen magnum.

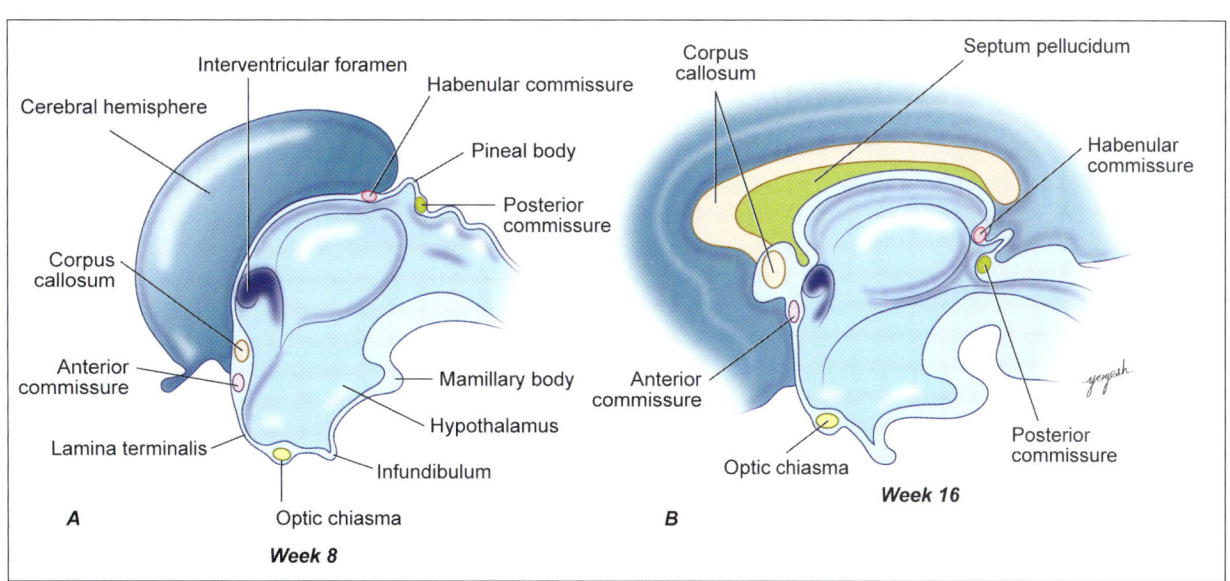

Fig. 22.18: Formation of commissures of telencephalon at 8 weeks: (A) and 16 weeks (B) For integration of the activity of right and left cerebral hemispheres, commissures play a key role

CLINICAL EMBRYOLOGY

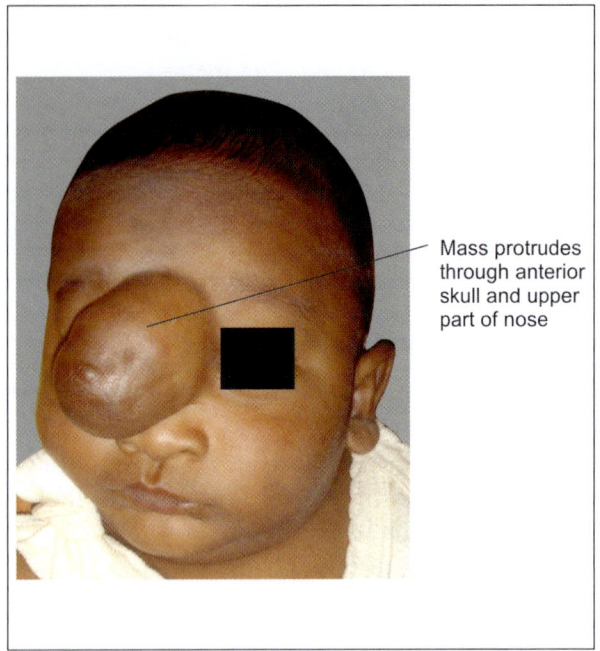

Clinical image 22.1: Frontonasal (anterior) encephalocele is a sac-like protrusion of the brain and meninges through a gap in the skull due to the failure of the neural tube closure (Image courtesy: *Dr Kumaravel S*)

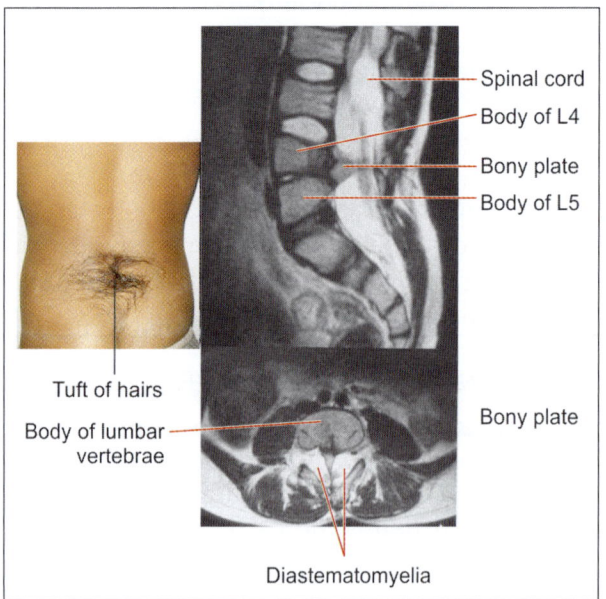

Clinical image 22.3: Spina bifida occulta with diastematomyelia. It occurs due to the failure of fusion of vertebral arches (neural arches) dorsally in the midline. Due to non-fusion, the spine becomes bifid and the defect is filled with connective tissue. Site of the defect usually shows a dimple and tuft of hairs. In this case, spina bifida occulta is present in the association of a bony plate arising from posterior surface of the body lumbar vertebrae. This bony plate splits the spinal cord into two halves hence called diastematomyelia or ***split cord malformation*** (Image courtesy: *Dr Kumaravel S*)

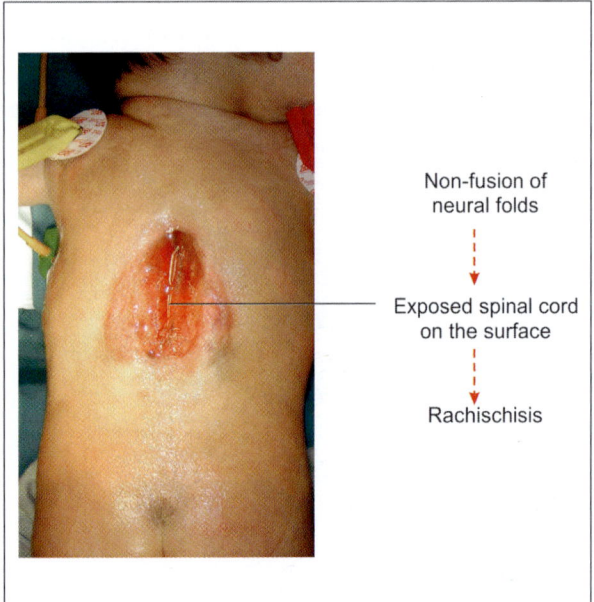

Clinical image 22.2: Rachischisis. Rachischisis is the severe neural tube defect that occurs due to failure of neural tube folding. In this defect, a portion of spinal cord is exposed on the surface and there is always failure of fusion of vertebral arches (spina bifida) due to non-fusion of neural folds. If rachischisis involves brain, it is called craniorachischisis or cranioschisis (Image courtesy: *Dr Kumaravel S*)

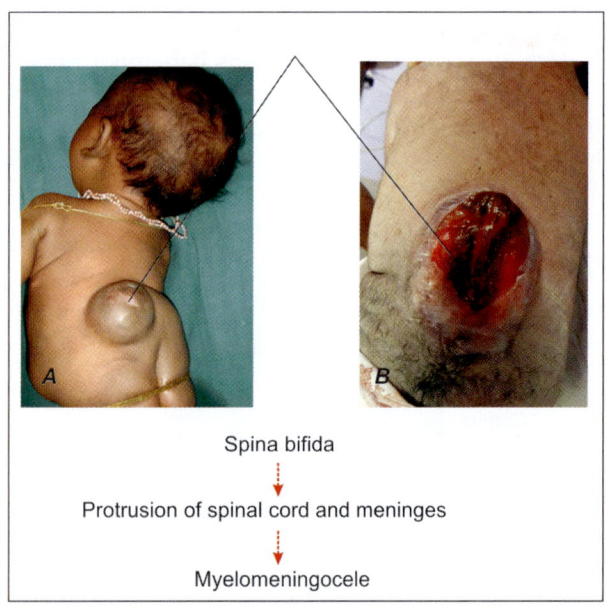

Clinical image 22.4: Myelomeningocele. It is a type of spina bifida (form of neural tube defect) in that spinal canal and backbone do not close. The spinal cord and the meninges along with tissue that covers spinal cord protrude through the skin on the back of newborn. Folic acid deficiency before and during early pregnancy may result in neural tube defects (Image courtesy: A: *Dr Adhisivam B*, B: *Dr Prakhar Mohniya*)

Nervous System

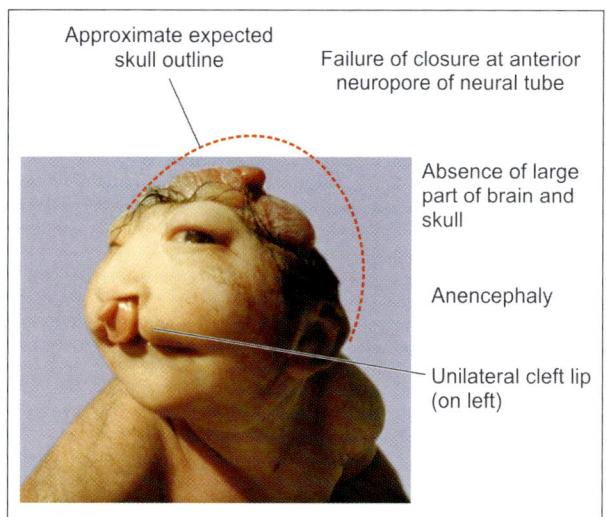

Clinical image 22.5: Anencephaly with unilateral cleft lip and cleft palate. A newborn with absence of a large part of brain and skull. Anencephaly occurs due to failure of closure at anterior neuropore of the neural tube. Cleft lip is a congenital split in the upper lip that occurs due to failure of fusion of the maxillary processes with the medial nasal process (part of frontonasal process). Cleft palate is a congenital split defect of the palate that causes communication between oral and nasal cavities. Cleft palate occurs due to the non-fusion of the median and lateral palatine processes (Image courtesy: *Dr Adhisivam B*)

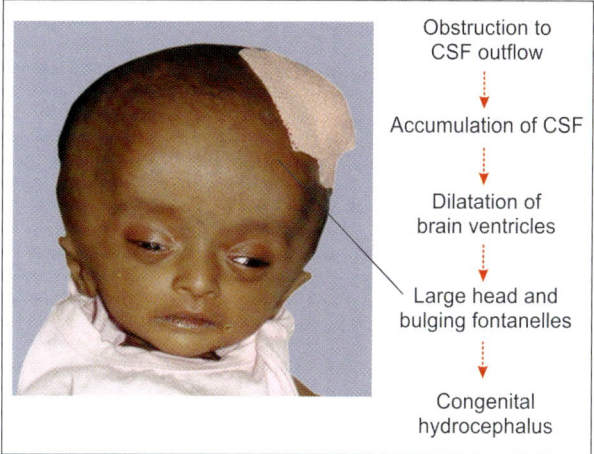

Clinical image 22.7: Congenital hydrocephalus. It is caused by excessive cerebrospinal fluid (CSF) accumulation in brain ventricles and subarachnoid space. This causes increased intracranial pressure and increases size of the ventricles. Infants with hydrocephalus show an unusually large head and a bulging fontanelle (Image courtesy: *Dr Adhisivam B*)

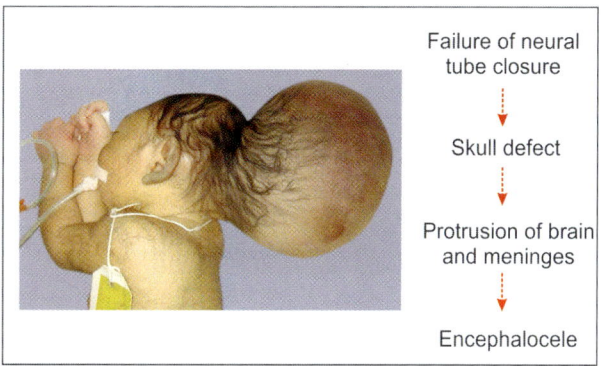

Clinical image 22.6: Encephalocele (cranium bifidum). It is neural tube defect having sac-like protrusions of brain with meninges through a defect in skull. It is caused by failure of neural tube to close completely during foetal development (Image courtesy: *Dr Adhisivam B*)

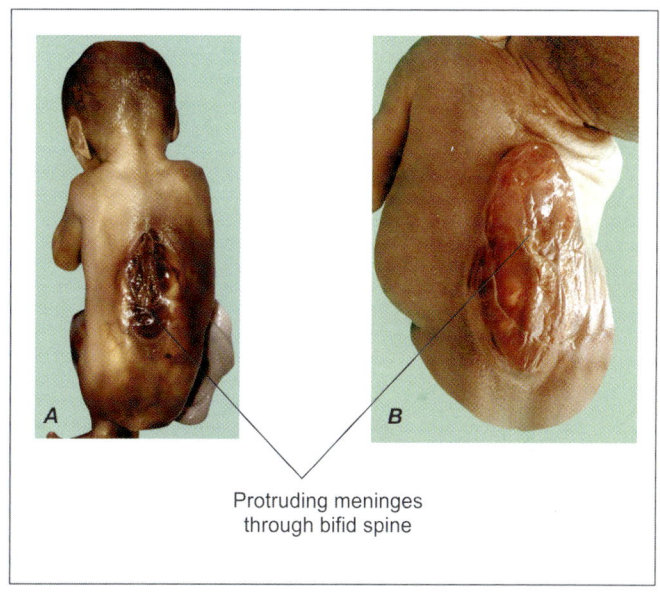

Clinical image 22.8: Meningocele (A and B are two separate cases). It is protruding arachnoid and pia mater (only meninges) through bifid spine that causes cystic swelling partially covered with skin (Image courtesy: *Dr Mamatha Gowda*)

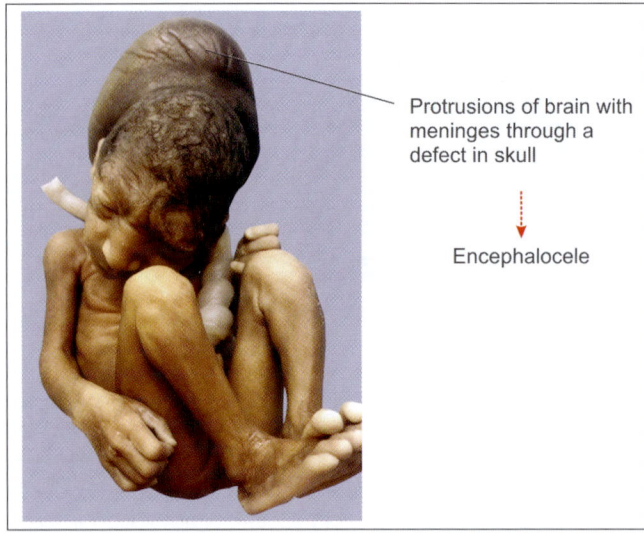

Clinical image 22.9: Encephalocele (cranium bifidum). It is a neural tube defect having sac like protrusions of brain with meninges through a defect in skull. It is caused by failure of neural tube to close completely during foetal development. (Image courtesy: *Dr Mamatha Gowda*)

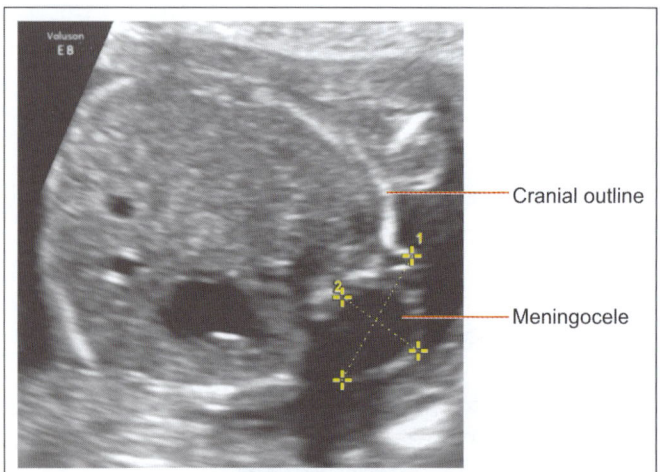

Clinical image 22.10: Ultrasound image of invitro foetus showing encephalocele (cranium bifidum) (marked by yellow dotted line). Skull outline shows defect through that sac of meninges is protruding. Encephalocele/meningocele is protrusion of arachnoid and pia mater (only meninges) through bifid spine or skull defect that cause cystic swelling partially covered with skin. (Image courtesy: *Dr Mamatha Gowda*)

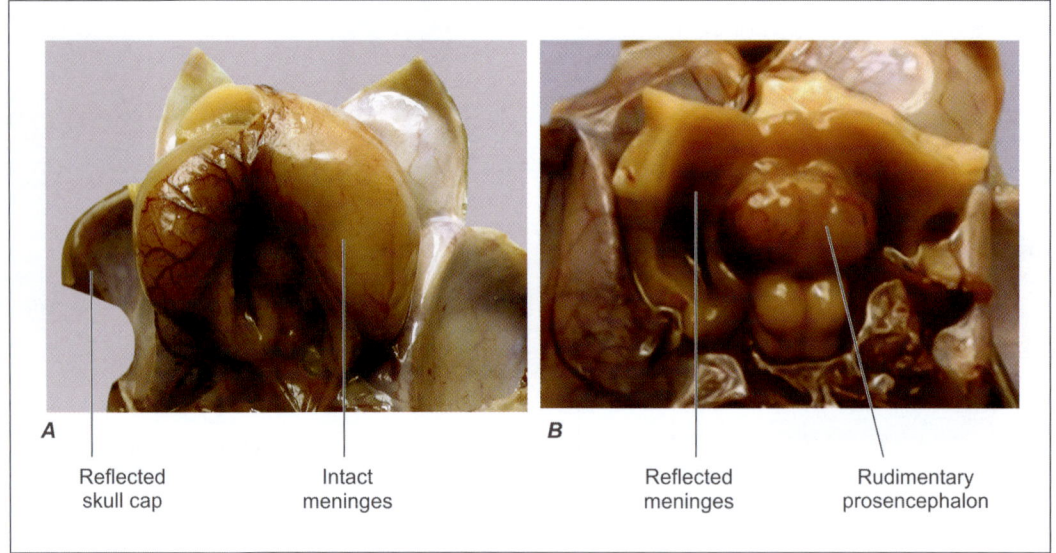

Clinical image 22.11: Holoprosencephaly (HPE) is a cephalic disorder with failure of prosencephalon (the forebrain of the embryo) development. Normally, the forebrain is formed and face begins to develop in 5th–6th weeks of intrauterine life; (A) Skull coverings are dissected to show the intact meninges; (B) Meninges are dissected to expose brain—holoprosencephaly (Image courtesy: *Dr Mamatha Gowda*)

23

Development of Eye

Chapter Outline

Development of various parts of eyeball
- Cornea
- Lens
- Retina
- Optic nerve
- Sclera and choroid
- Ciliary body
- Iris
- Vitreous
- Accessory structures of eyeball
  - Extraocular muscles
  - Eyelids and conjunctival sac
  - Lacrimal apparatus

Congenital anomalies of eye

INTRODUCTION

- The eyeball development begins early in the 4th week of intrauterine life with formation of optic vesicle (a diverticulum) from diencephalon.
- Various components of eyeball are derived from the following sources:
  1. Retina, iris and optic nerves are derived from optic vesicle that arises from neuroectoderm of diencephalon.
  2. Lens and corneal epithelium are derived from lens placode that arises from surface ectoderm.
  3. Fibrous and vascular coats of eyeball are derived from mesodermal condensation surrounding the optic vesicle.
  4. Choroid and sclera are derived from migrating neural crest cells.

Optic Vesicle and Lens Vesicle

- On 22nd day, wall of the diencephalon shows thickening and depression to form *optic sulcus*.^{MCQ} Formation of the optic sulcus or groove is the first indication for development of the eye.^{Neet}
- Optic sulcus further invaginates laterally in the surrounding mesoderm and form a bulging called *optic vesicle*.
- Optic vesicles grow laterally but remain connected to forebrain by a stalk-like structure called *optic stalk*.
- Optic vesicle meets surface ectoderm. In region of contact, the surface ectoderm forms localised thickening called *lens placode*.
- Lens placode depresses to form *lens pit* and later, *lens vesicle*.
- Lens vesicle loses contact with surface ectoderm by 33rd day.
- Lens vesicle invaginates the optic vesicle and converts it to a double layered *optic cup*.
- By 6th week, margins of the optic cup overgrow and cover lens vesicle except on caudal side of the lens and partly on caudal surface of optic stalk. This gap is called *choroidal fissure* or foetal fissure.^{MCQ}
- In a mesodermal encroachment along the choroidal fissure, *hyaloid vessels* develop that supply optic and lens vesicles. The distal part of hyaloid vesicles degenerates, whereas the proximal parts from *central artery of retina* and *central vein of retina*.

DEVELOPMENT OF VARIOUS PARTS OF EYEBALL

Cornea

- Cornea consists of outer stratified squamous epithelium resting on basement membrane, lamina propria, Descemet's membrane and inner corneal epithelium.

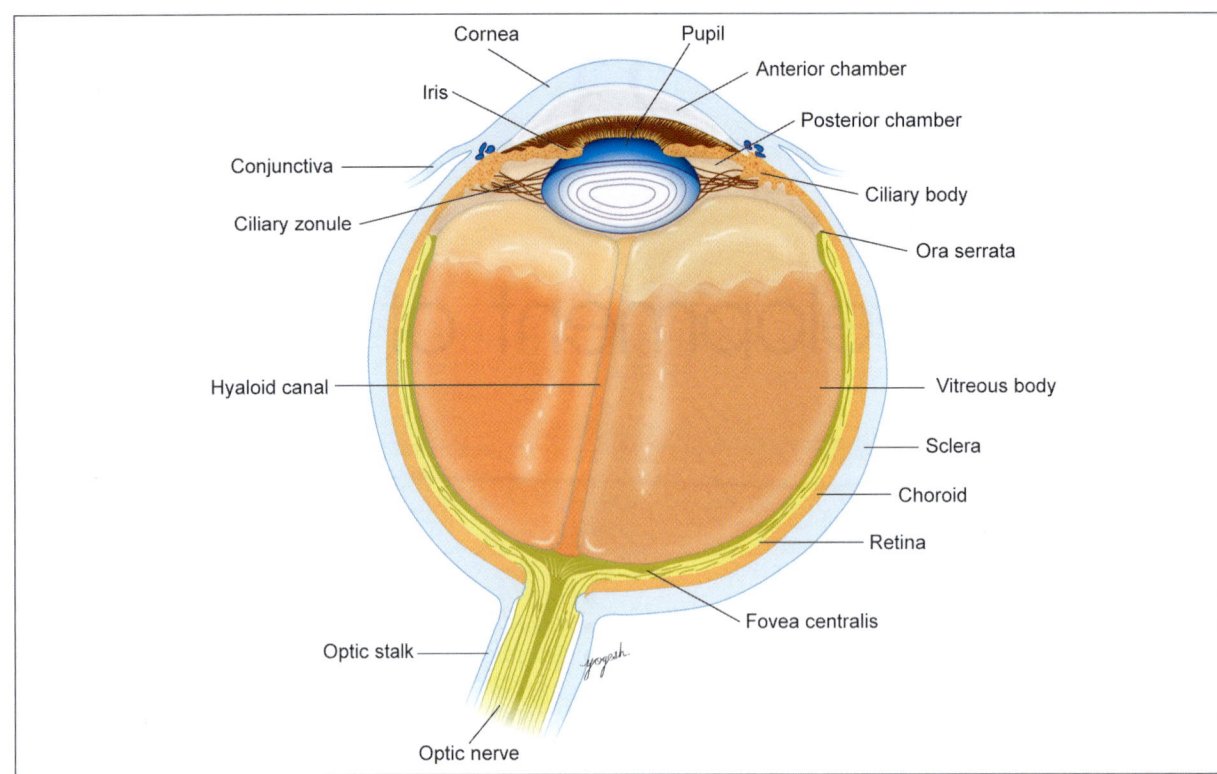

Fig. 23.1: Fully developed eyeball

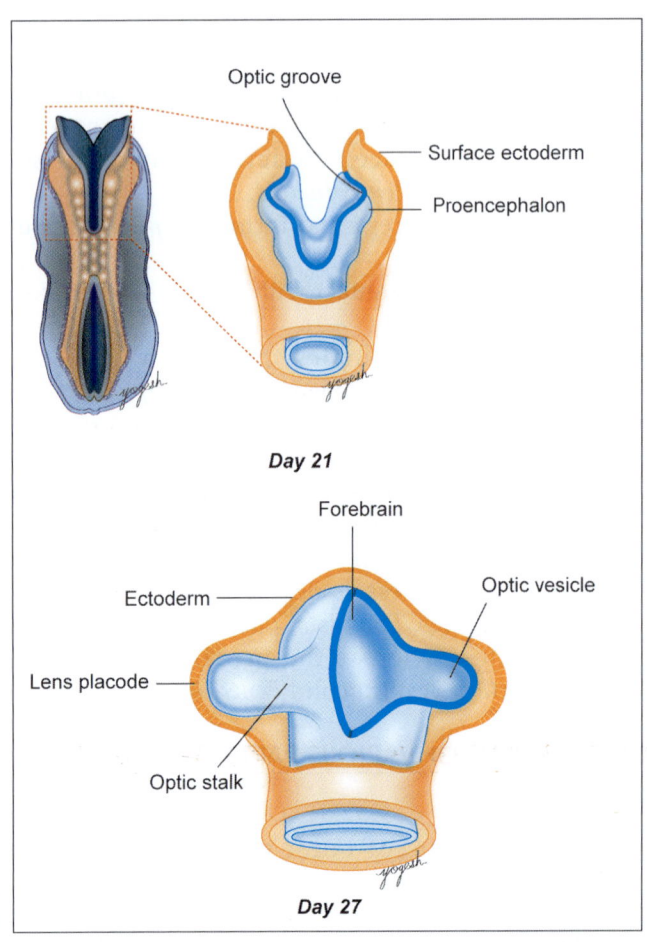

Fig. 23.2: Development of eyeball on day 21 and 27

- All these layers are derived from the following sources:
  1. Surface ectoderm forms outer stratified squamous epithelium and its basement membrane (Bowman's layer). *Neet*
  2. Lamina propria or stroma is derived from mesoderm.
  3. Neural crest cells form Descemet's membrane and inner corneal epithelium. *Neet*

Lens

Q. Write short note on development of lens.

- Lens is a transparent, biconvex structure that lies between aqueous and vitreous of the eyeball.
- Lens has three main parts:
  1. Lens capsule
  2. Lens epithelium (simple cuboidal epithelium)
  3. Lens fibres

Stages of Development

- By 33rd day of IUL, lens vesicle gets separated from surface ectoderm.
- Initially lens vesicle is lined by a single layer of cuboidal epithelium.
- Cells of ventral wall of lens vesicle remain cuboidal. Cells of deep wall of lens vesicle elongate, become columnar and occupy cavity of the lens vesicle.
- These elongated cells of posterior wall lose their nuclei and form transparent ***primary lens fibres***.

Development of Eye

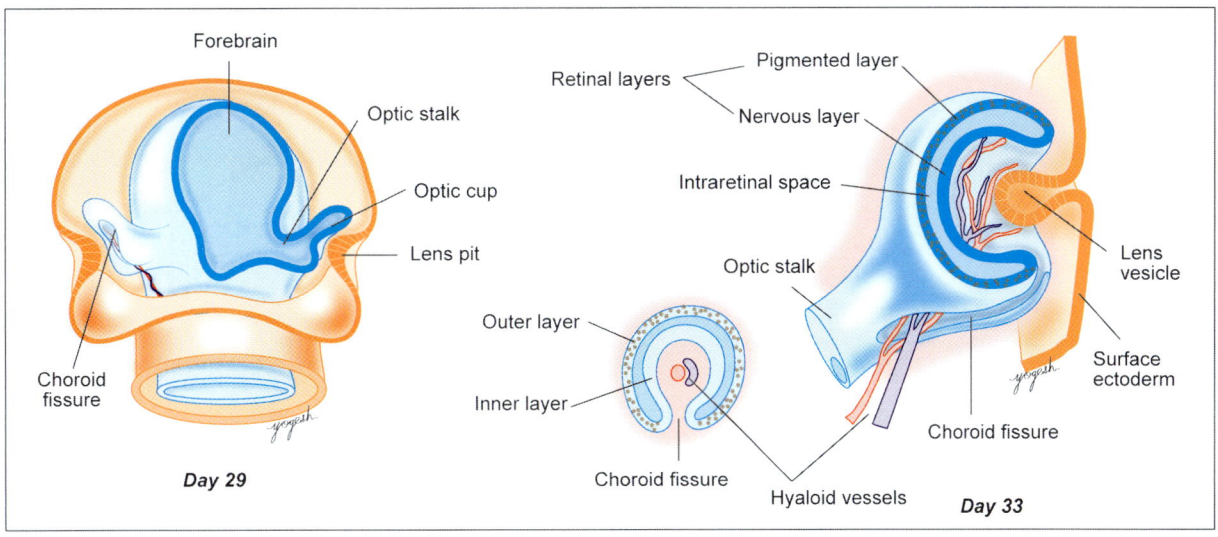

Fig. 23.3: Further development of eyeball (day 29 and day 33)

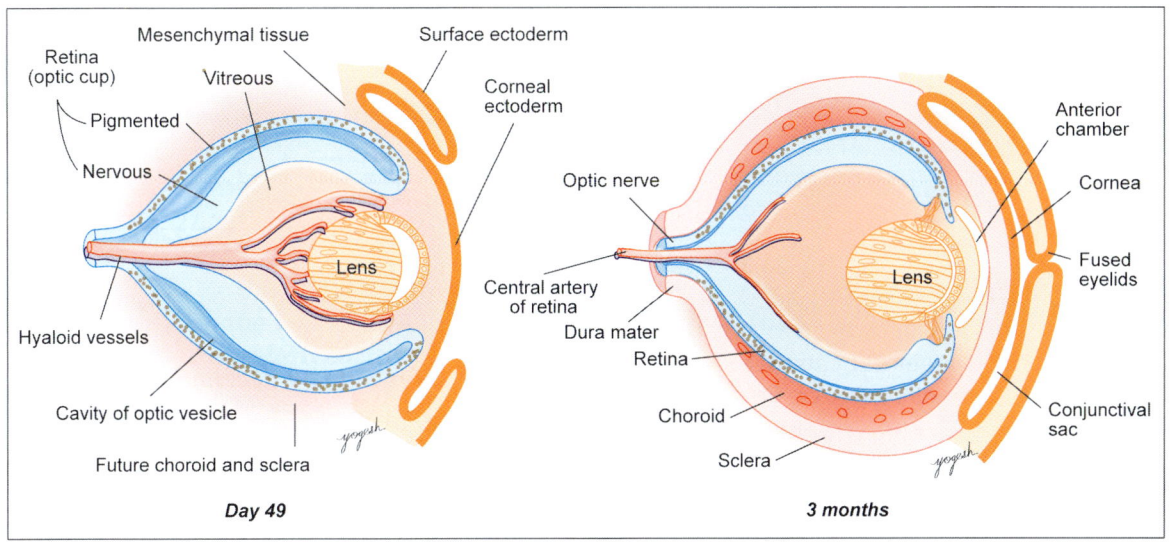

Fig. 23.4: Further development of eyeball (day 49 and 3 months)

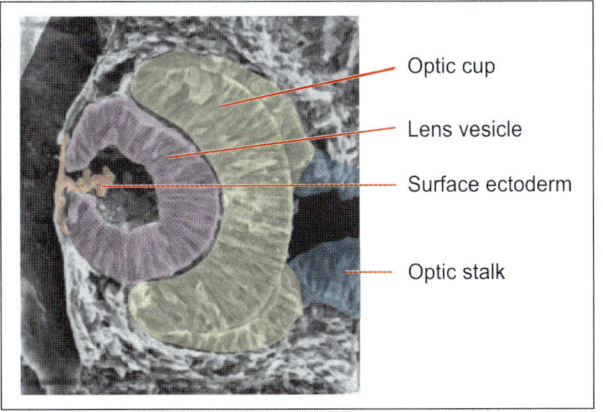

Scanning electron micrograph 23.1: SEM showing developing eye. The invaginating lens placode forms lens vesicle that pinches off surface ectoderm. Invagination of optic vesicle forms bilayer optic cup that remains connected to forebrain via optic stalk [Species: Mouse, approximate human age: 36 days, coronal section]

- The equatorial cells continue to contribute new lens fibres and lens grow. These fibres later become hard and form *secondary lens fibres*.
- Cells of anterior wall persist and form *epithelium of lens*.
- On degeneration of hyaloid artery (that supplies lens), lens becomes avascular structure.
- In 7th week, solid lens is formed.^{MCQ}

Congenital Cataract

- Congenital cataract is an opacity of lens that is present at birth.
- Congenital cataract may be unilateral or bilateral
- Causes: It may be due to rubella virus, toxoplasmosis infection, Down's syndrome or inborn error of metabolism such as galactosemia.

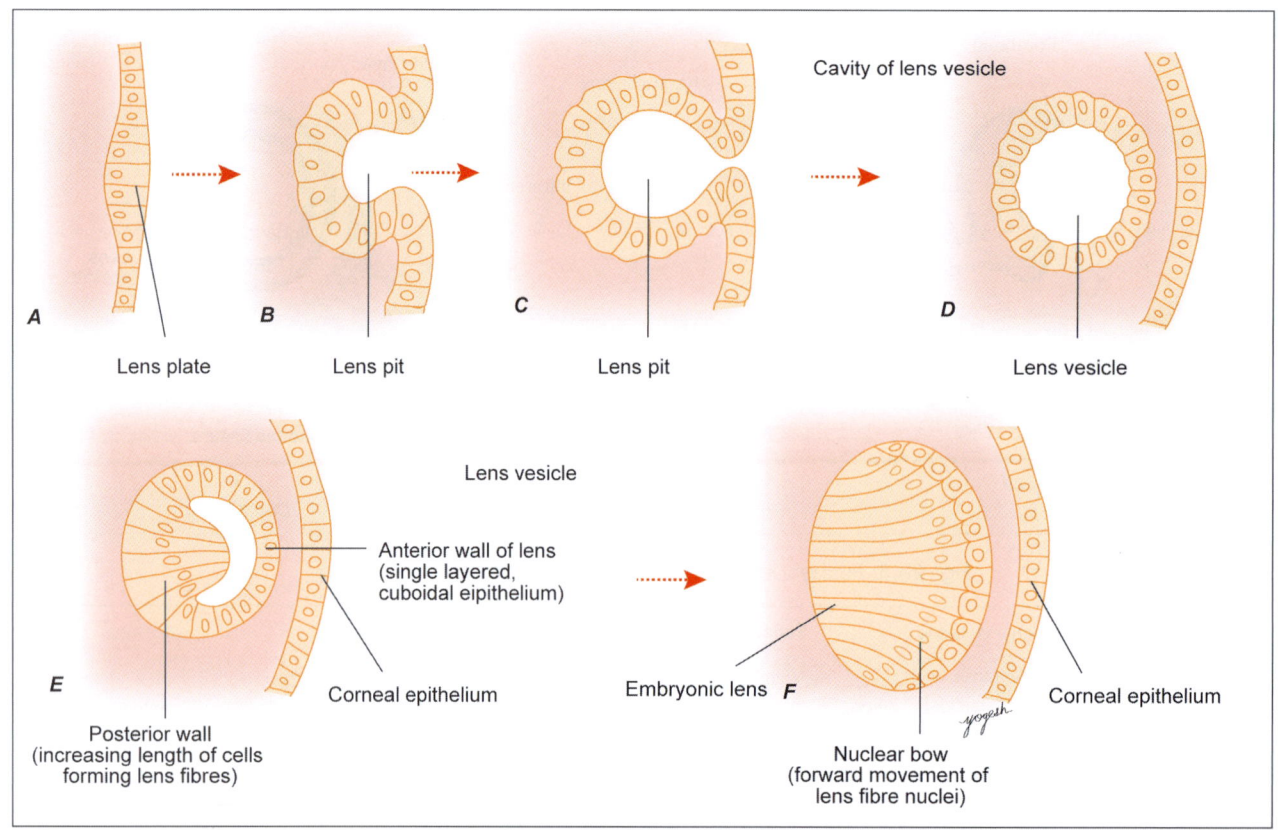

Fig. 23.5: Development of the embryonic lens

- Treatment: Congenital cataract can be treated surgically. Bilateral congenital cataract should be removed before the age of 10 weeks.

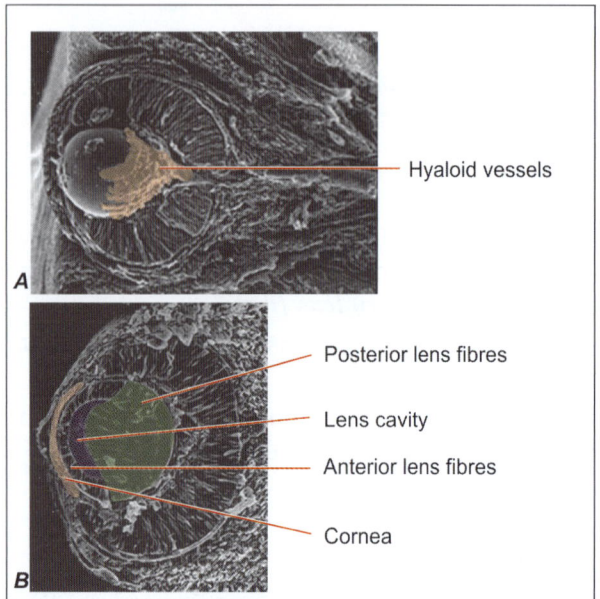

Scanning electron micrograph 23.2: Developing eye: (A) The hyaloid vasculature surrounds the back of the lens; (B) Following separation of the lens from the surface, the posterior lens fibres elongate to obliterate the lens cavity and the cornea begins to differentiate. [Species: Mouse, approximate human age: 7 weeks, coronal section]

Retina

Q. Write short note on development of retina.

- Cellular layers of retina from outside inwards include:
  1. Pigmented cell layer
  2. Layer of rods and cones
  3. Bipolar neuron layer
  4. Ganglionic cell layer
- All these layers are derived from the optic cup.

Stages of Development

- From wall of diencephalon, optic vesicle arises that grows laterally but remains connected by optic stalk with the diencephalon.
- Optic vesicle comes in contact with lens vesicle and gets converted to optic cup.
- Optic cup has two parts, anterior and posterior.
- Anterior part of optic cup forms an epithelial covering of ciliary body and iris.
- Posterior part of optic cup forms various layers of retina as follows:
  – Outer wall: Forms pigmented layer of retina.
  – Inner wall: Gets differentiated into three layers as

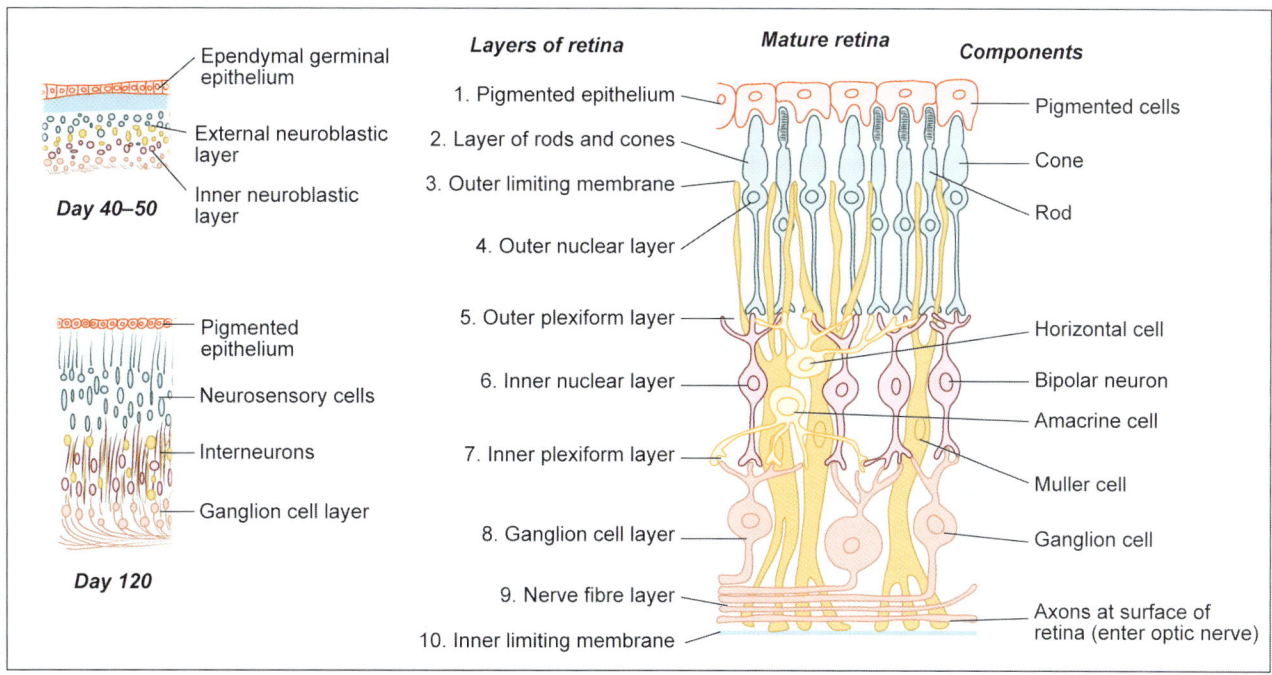

Fig. 23.6: Histogenesis of retina

1. Matrix layer—forms rods and cones.
2. Mantle layer—forms bipolar cells and ganglionic cells as well as other neurons of retina.
3. Marginal layer—forms optic nerve. Axons of ganglion cells form marginal layer that converges towards optic stalk and finally, forms optic nerve.
- Space between outer and inner wall of the optic cup is called *intraretinal space*. This space gets obliterated by increasing number of retinal neurons.

Optic Nerve

- Optic stalk contains
  1. Hyaloid artery and vein
  2. Axons of ganglionic cell layer
- On inferior (caudal) surface of optic stalk, choroid fissure is present, that closes by 7th week.
- Later, optic stalk forms optic nerve, whereas hyaloid vessels form central artery and vein of retina.

Congenital Retinal Detachment

- It involves separation of pigmented epithelium from neuronal layers of the retina.
- Congenital retinal detachment mostly occurs as an autosomal recessive disorder.
- It results in permanent blindness from birth.

Sclera and Choroid

- Sclera (white of eye) is opaque, fibrous protective outermost layer of eyeball.
- Choroid is a vascular coat of eyeball that lies between outer sclera and inner retina.
- During the 6th and 7th weeks, mesenchyme that surrounds external surface of optic cup condenses into two layers:
  a. Outer fibrous layer that forms sclera.
  b. Inner vascular layer that forms choroid.
- Choroid is anteriorly continuous with ciliary body and posteriorly with pia and arachnoid mater.
- Sclera is anteriorly continuous with substantia propria or stroma of the cornea and posteriorly with dura mater covering optic nerve.

Ciliary Body

- Ciliary body is a ring-shaped mass that divides eyeball separates aqueous humour from vitreous.
- It consists of *ciliary muscle* that controls shape of the lens.
- Ciliary body shows folding of epithelium called *ciliary processes* that secret the *aqueous humour*.
- Mesoderm surrounding the anterior part of optic cup forms *ciliary muscle* and connective tissues of ciliary body.

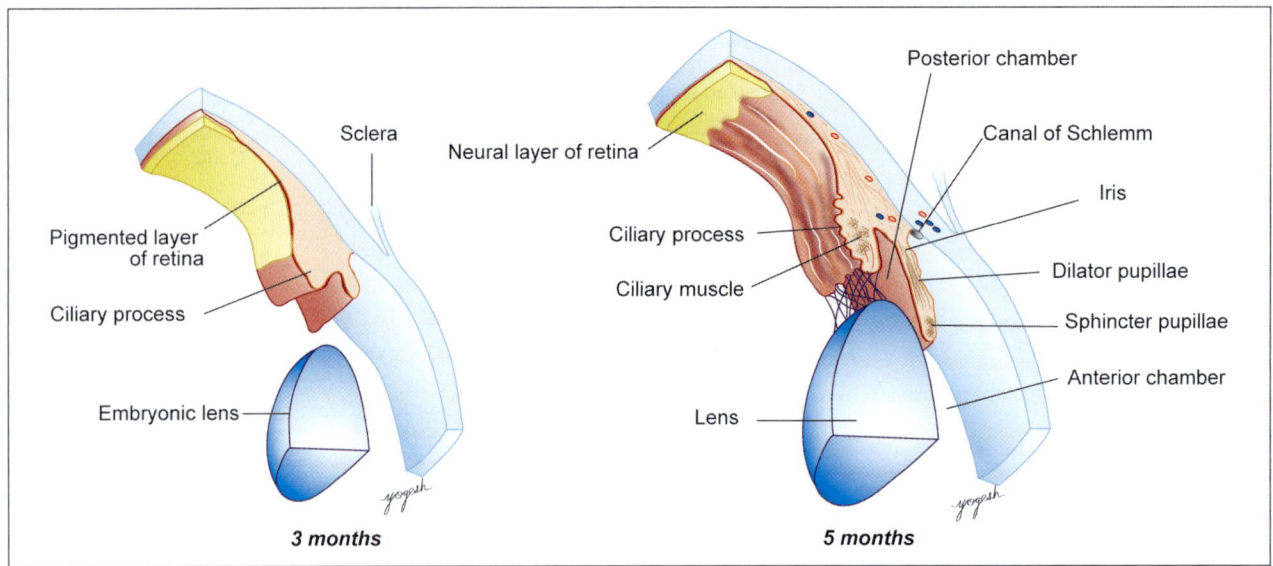

Fig. 23.7: Development of the iris and ciliary body

- Pigmented epithelial lining of inner aspect of ciliary body and ciliary processes is derived from outer layer of the optic cup; hence, continuous with pigmented layer of retina.
- The nonpigmented layer of epithelium covering deeper side of ciliary body is derived from inner layer of optic cup and continuous with neuronal layers of retina.

Iris

Q. Write short note on development of iris.

- Iris is a thin, circular structure in eyeball that controls size of the pupil.
- Iris shows anterior limiting layer, stroma, sphincter and dilator papillae muscles and posterior pigmented epithelium.
- Iris develops from anterior extension of optic cup.
- Epithelium (anterior and posterior) of iris is derived from double layered optic cup.
- Neuroectodermal cells of optic cup also give rise to muscles of the iris.
- Stoma of the iris is derived from neural crest cells.
- Colour of eye/pigmented layer of cornea depends on genetic constitution of an individual.

Anterior and Posterior Chambers of Eye

- Anterior and posterior chamber is similar to subarachnoid space of brain.[MCQ]
- Mesoderm located between lens and cornea split to form spaces. These spaces split into anterior and posterior chambers by developing *iris* and **pupillary membrane**.
- As pupillary membrane disappears, anterior chamber communicates with posterior chamber through pupil.

- Epithelium of ciliary process starts secreting *aqueous humour* that fills anterior and posterior chambers of eyeball.
- Sclera of sinus venosus forms a network of trabecular meshwork at sclerocorneal junction along the circumference of anterior chamber. These later form canal of Schlemm and drain aqueous humour. [Canal is named after Friedrich Schlemm (1795–1858), a German anatomist.]

Vitreous

- Vitreous occupies chamber of eyeball called *vitreous chamber*.
- Vitreous is a transparent, gelatinous mass that forms about 45th volume of the eyeball.
- Vitreous develops as follows:
  - *Primary vitreous humour* develops from neural crest cells of optic cup.
  - *Secondary vitreous humour* replaces the primary vitreous. Secondary vitreous humour is derived from inner layer of optic cup and lens vesicle.
- Vitreous humour is supplied by hyaloid artery that later gets obliterated.[Neet]

Accessory Structures of Eyeball

Extraocular Muscles

- Each eyeball has 6 extraocular muscles, namely superior rectus, inferior rectus, medial rectus, lateral rectus, superior oblique and inferior oblique muscles (levator palpebrae superioris muscle for eyelid).
- All extraocular muscles are derived from **preoccipital myotomes** and hence, supplied by 3rd, 4th and 6th cranial nerves.[Neet]

Development of Eye

Eyelids and conjunctival sac

- Eyelids are developed by folds of surface ectoderm that raise above and below the cornea.
- These ectodermal folds contain some mesoderm that gives raise to tarsal plate and other connective tissue of eyelids.
- Eyelashes and glands of eyelids develop from surface ectoderm.
- Surface ectoderm that lines inner surface of eyelids and covers eyeball form conjunctival sac.
- Eyelids remain fused till 28th week of IUL and later get separated.^MCQ

Lacrimal apparatus

- It consists of lacrimal gland, lacrimal sac and nasolacrimal ducts.
- Lacrimal gland is derived from 15 to 20 buds that grow at superolateral angle of conjunctival sac.
  – Nasolacrimal duct and lacrimal sac develop from naso-optic furrow (nasolacrimal furrow) (refer to Chapter 12, development of face).
  – Lacrimal canaliculi develop from canalisation of ectodermal buds that raise from medial margins of eyelids. Later these canaliculi develop communication with lacrimal sac.

CONGENITAL ANOMALIES OF EYE

1. *Anophthalmia* is an absence of eyeball due to failure of optic vesicle formation.
2. *Microphthalmia* is small eye due to under developed optic vesicle. It may be due to rubella virus, cytomegalovirus, toxoplasma or other intrauterine infections. PAX6 gene performs key-regulatory role in the development of eye. PAX6 gene mutation results in aniridia or microphthalmia.
3. *Cyclopia* is a presence of single median eye. It occurs due to fusion of two optic vesicles (synophthalmia). Single eye may be connected with face by a tubular stalk called *proboscis*. Inhibition of sonic hedgehog (SHH) gene may result in Cyclops.
4. *Coloboma of iris*: Due to failure of fusion of choroid fissure, iris shows a cleft on inferior side (keyhole appearance). This condition is called coloboma of iris (coloboma = missing part, Greek).
5. Persistent papillary membrane: Pupil may be covered partially or completely by persistent papillary membrane.
6. *Congenital aniridia* is complete absence of *iris* due to an arrest of development of optic cup.
7. *Congenital aphakia* is an absence of *lens* of eyeball due to failure of formation of lens vesicle.
8. *Coloboma of eyelid* is an absence of part of the eyelid.
9. Mutation of PAX2 gene results in optic nerve colobomas and renal aplasia.
10. Entropion is inward-turned eyelids, whereas ectropion is outward turned eyelids.
11. *Epicanthus* is a crescentic fold of skin that extends from upper eyelid to canthus. It is a feature of Mongolian races and Down syndrome (trisomy 21).
12. *Cryptophthalmos* is an absence of eyelids and palpebral fissures. The eyeball is covered by skin.
13. *Congenital ptosis* (drooping of eyelid) occurs due to failure of development of levator palpebrae superioris muscle.

Table 23.1 Development of eye

Part	Embryological source
1. Cornea	Epithelium: Surface ectoderm^Neet
	Other layers: Neural crest
2. Lens	Lens vesicle (surface ectoderm)
3. Retina	Optic cup (neuroectoderm)
4. Optic nerve	Optic stalk (neuroectoderm)
5. Sclera and choroid	Mesoderm surrounding optic cup
6. Ciliary body and muscle	Mesoderm
7. Iris	Mesoderm
8. Muscles of iris	Neuroectoderm optic cup
9. Extraocular muscles	Preoccipital myotomes
10. Eyelids, conjunctival sac	Surface ectoderm
11. Lacrimal glands	Surface ectoderm
12. Lacrimal sac and nasolacrimal duct	Ectoderm of naso-optic furrow

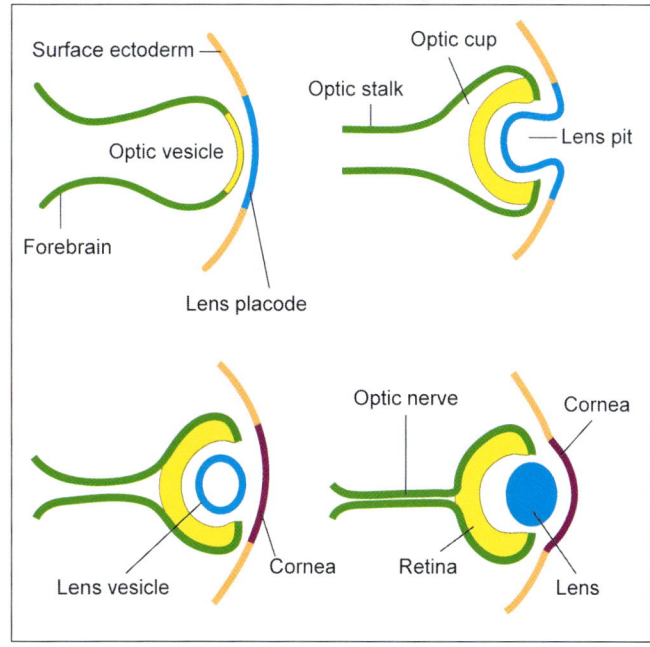

Practice Fig. 23.1: Development of eye

Some Interesting Facts

- The following parts of eye are also derived from neural crest cells: Trabecular meshwork, stroma of cornea, iris, ciliary body, choroid, melanocytes of conjunctiva, and muscle layer of orbital blood vessels, meningeal sheath of optic nerve, **sclera** and part of vitreous.[Neet]
- Epithelium of cornea and conjunctiva, crystalline lens, lacrimal and tarsal glands are derived from **surface ectoderm**.[Neet]
- Iris and ciliary body epitheliums, *epithelium and muscles of iris (constrictor and dilator pupillae)*, retina, vitreous optic nerve, *optic cup*, vesicle are derived from **neuroectoderm**.[Neet]
- Optic cup forms retina.[Neet]
- Melanocytes of iris develop from neural crest cells.[Neet]
- Ocular structures (sclera, iris, corneal stroma) develop from somatic layer of lateral plate mesoderm.[Neet]

CLINICAL EMBRYOLOGY

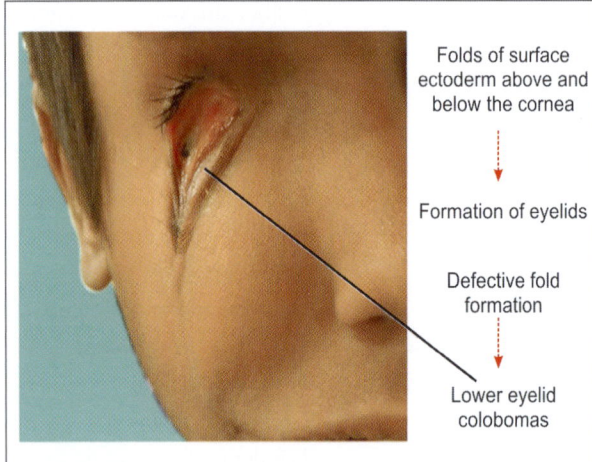

Clinical image 23.1: Lower eyelid colobomas is defect in the formation of eyelid. It is caused by failure of fusion of the mesodermal lid folds. As compared to upper lid colobomas lower lid defects are encountered less frequently but when they occur, they are seen in the lateral half of the lid in association with Treacher Collins syndrome (mandibulofacial dysostosis) which is autosomal dominant with variable penetrance and expressivity (Image courtesy: *Dr Rohit Rao*)

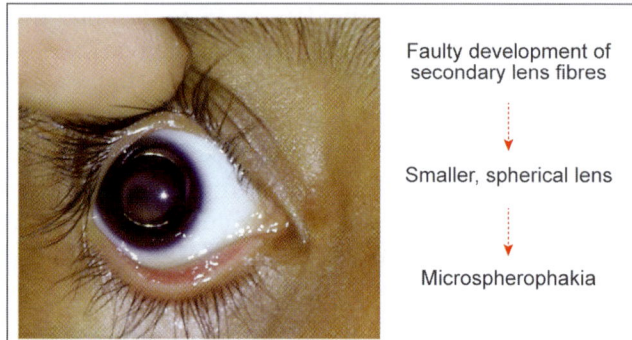

Clinical image 23.2: Microspherophakia. In microspherophakia, lens of the eye is smaller than normal and spherically shaped. With widely dilated pupil, entire lens equator can be visualised at the slit lamp examination. Faulty development of the secondary lens fibres during embryogenesis may produce microspherophakia. The spherical shape of the lens results in increased refractive power (highly myopic eye), causing secondary angle-closure glaucoma. Microspherophakia is most often seen as a part of Weill-Marchesani syndrome. This condition may also occur as an isolated hereditary abnormality or, occasionally, in association with Peters anomaly, Marfan syndrome, Alport syndrome, Lowe syndrome, or congenital rubella (Image courtesy: *Dr Rohit Rao*)

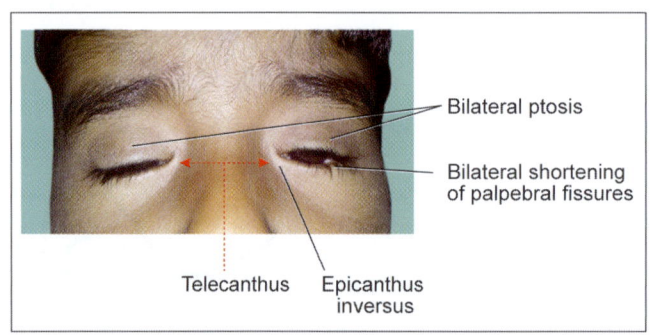

Clinical image 23.3: Blepharophimosis. It is an uncommon dysmorphic syndrome, which primarily affects the soft tissues of the mid-face It is a condition that shows bilateral shortening of palpebral fissures (eyelid opening) with bilateral ptosis and epicanthus inversus syndrome. In blepharophimosis, the eyes are also spaced more widely apart than usual (telecanthus). Autosomal dominant inheritance with up to 50% happened sporadically (Image courtesy: *Dr Rohit Rao*)

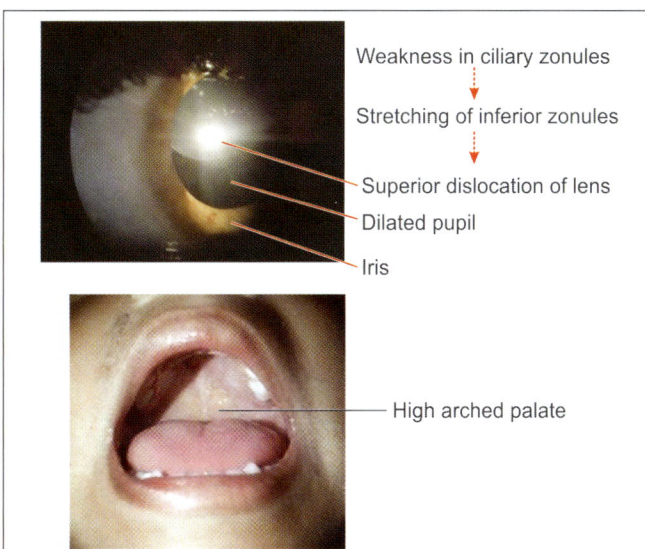

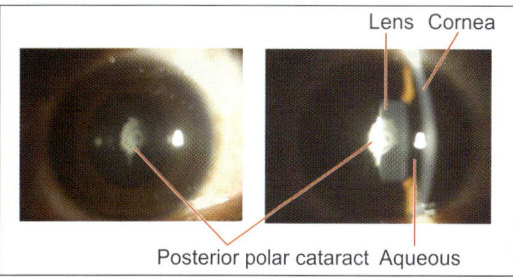

Clinical image 23.7: Congenital cataract. In the present case, congenital cataract is present in the form of posterior polar cataract. A dense plaque (disc-shaped opacity with onion-like ringed appearance like an onion) in the central posterior part of the lens is present (Image courtesy: *Dr Subashini K*)

Clinical image 23.4: Superior dislocation of lens may be due to Marfan syndrome. In Marfan syndrome, the lens dislocates superiorly because of weakness in the ciliary zonules (the connective tissue strands that suspend the lens within the eye), and stretching of inferior zonules. In the same case, high arched palate (that another typical feature of Marfan syndrome) is observed (Image courtesy: *Dr Rohit Rao*)

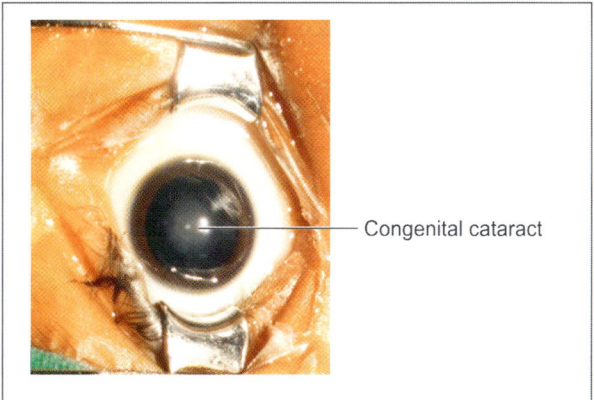

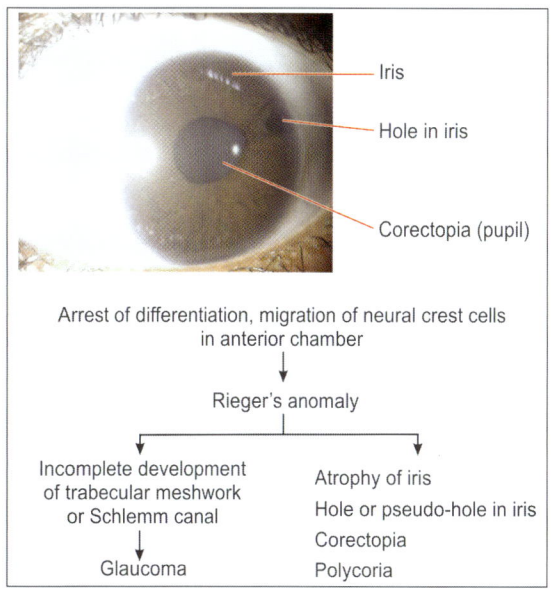

Clinical image 23.5: Congenital cataract. In the present case, congenital cataract is present in the form of lamellar or zonular form (the common morphological form in congenital cataract) (Image courtesy: *Dr Subashini K*)

Clinical image 23.8: Rieger's anomaly (anterior segment dysgenesis). Rieger's anomaly is a congenital anomaly of the eye caused by anterior segment dysgenesis. It shows atrophy of the iris stroma, with hole or pseudo-hole formation and corectopia (displacement of pupil from its normal central position) or polycoria (one pupillary opening in the iris). It is associated glaucoma (Image courtesy: *Dr Subashini K*)

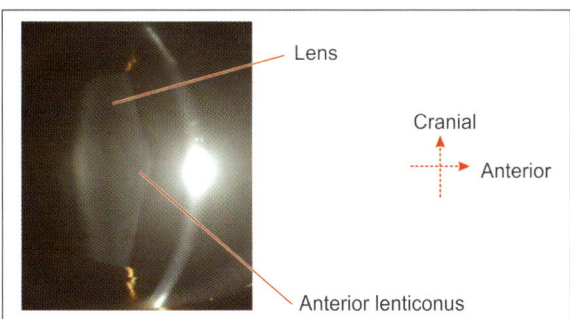

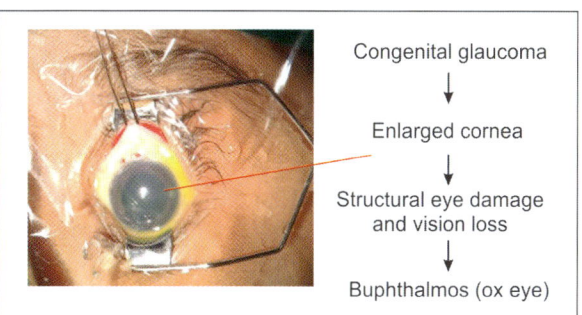

Clinical image 23.6: Anterior lenticonus. Lenticonus (a rare congenital anomaly) is characterised by a transparent, localised, conical protrusion on crystalline lens capsule, may be anterior or posterior. It causes a decrease in visual acuity and irregular refraction (Image courtesy: *Dr Subashini K*)

Clinical image 23.9: Buphthalmos (ox eye). Congenital glaucoma results in enlarged cornea and haze. Glaucoma is an elevated pressure within the eye that leads to structural eye damage and vision loss. Congenital glaucoma is also associated with horizontal breaks in the Descemet membrane called Haab's striae (Descemet's tears) (Image courtesy: *Dr Subashini K*)

24

Development of Ear

Chapter Outline

- Development of internal ear
  - Membranous labyrinth
  - Bony labyrinth
  - Histogenesis of internal ear
- Middle ear
- External ear
  - External acoustic meatus
  - Auricle
- Molecular regulation
- Developmental anomalies

INTRODUCTION

- Ear is the organ of special sense that helps in hearing as well as maintenance of equilibrium.
- Anatomically, ear has three parts: External ear, Middle ear and Internal ear.
- External ear includes auricle and external acoustic meatus. Tympanic membrane separates external ear from middle ear.
- Middle ear communicates anteriorly with nasopharynx through auditory tube and posteriorly with mastoid antrum through aditus.
- Internal ear consists of outer bony labyrinth and inner membranous labyrinth.
- Bony labyrinth lies in petrous part of temporal bone and it contains perilymph.
- Membranous labyrinth has cochlear duct, saccule, utricle and three semicircular ducts. Cochlear duct possesses organ of Corti that is responsible for hearing.
- Saccule and utricle possess maculae, whereas semicircular canals possess cristae ampullaris. Maculae and cristae ampullaris help to maintain equilibrium.
- Development of ear involves all three germ layers:
  - Surface ectoderm forms internal and external ear.
  - Endoderm forms middle ear.
  - Mesoderm forms connective tissue, cartilages bone (ossicles) and muscles of ear.

DEVELOPMENT OF INTERNAL EAR

- Inner ear develops from an ectodermal *otic vesicle* (Fig. 24.1, Scanning electron micrograph 24.1).
- Developmentally, internal ear consists of membranous labyrinth and bony labyrinth.

Membranous Labyrinth

Stages of Development (Flowchart 24.1)

- In the 4th week, surface ectoderm shows two thickenings called *otic placodes* (Fig. 24.1).
- Otic placode appears on each side of underlying rhombencephalon.
- Otic placode invaginates into underlying mesenchyme to form *otic pit*.
- Soon, otic pit forms *otic vesicle* or *otocyst* and lose the contact with surface ectoderm to move deep towards rhombencephalon.
- Oval-shaped otic vesicle gives rise to membranous labyrinth.
- Otocyst/otic vesicle is divided into (Fig. 24.2)
  1. Dorsal vestibular part
  2. Ventral cochlear part
- Cochlear part gives rise to saccule and cochlear duct (organ of Corti).
- Vestibular part gives rise to utricle, semicircular ducts, endolymphatic duct and sac.

Development of Ear

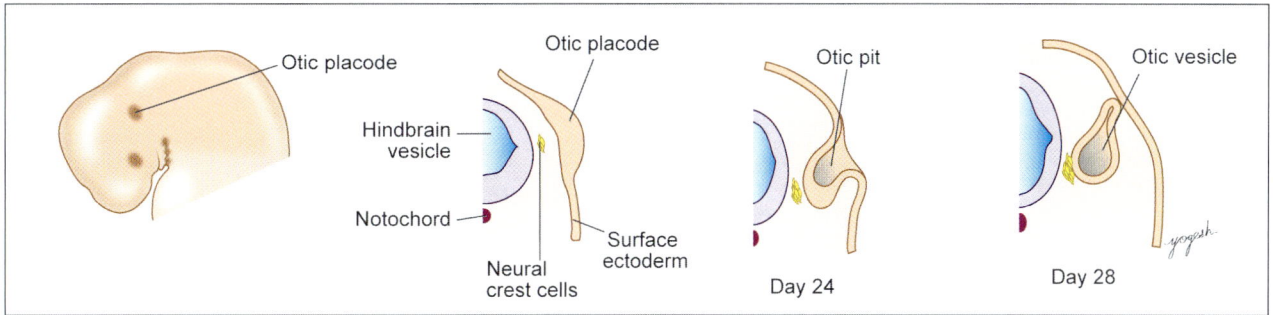

Fig. 24.1: Formation of otic vesicle

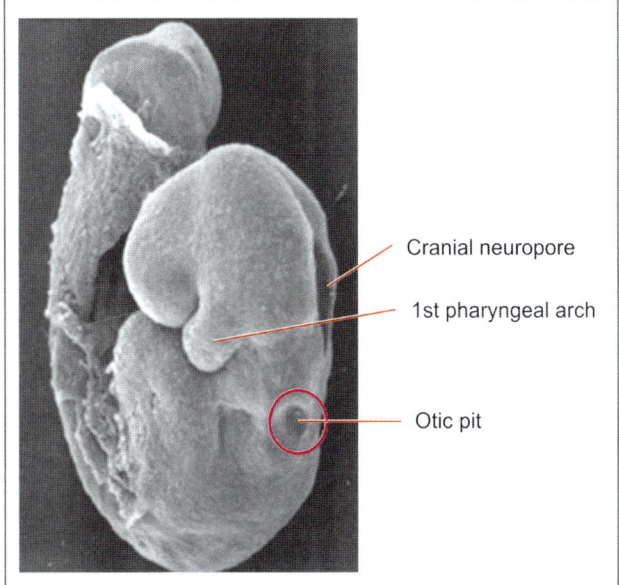

Scanning electron micrograph 24.1: The otic pit forms as this thickened (placodal) ectoderm invaginates. [Species: Mouse, approximate human age: 26 days, dorsolateral view]

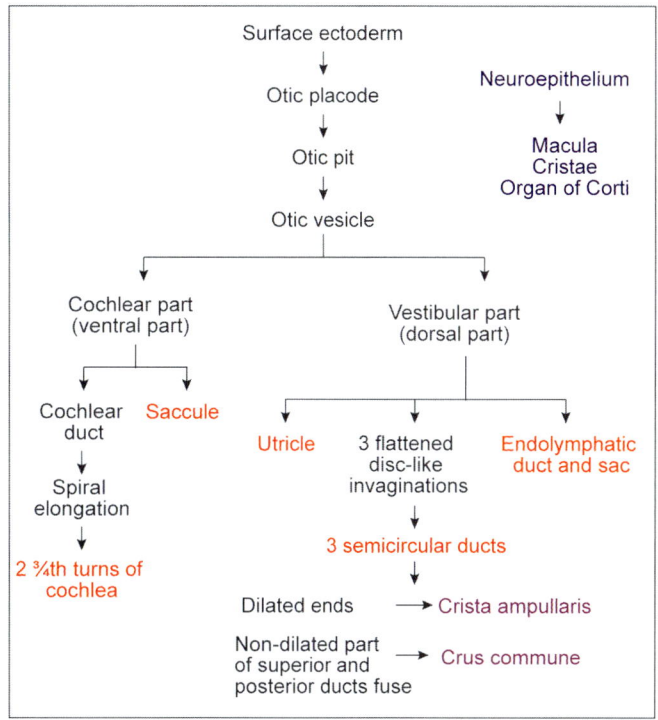

Flowchart 24.1: Development of membranous labyrinth. *Note:* Semicircular canals develop in the following sequence: First superior, then lateral (horizontal) followed by posterior

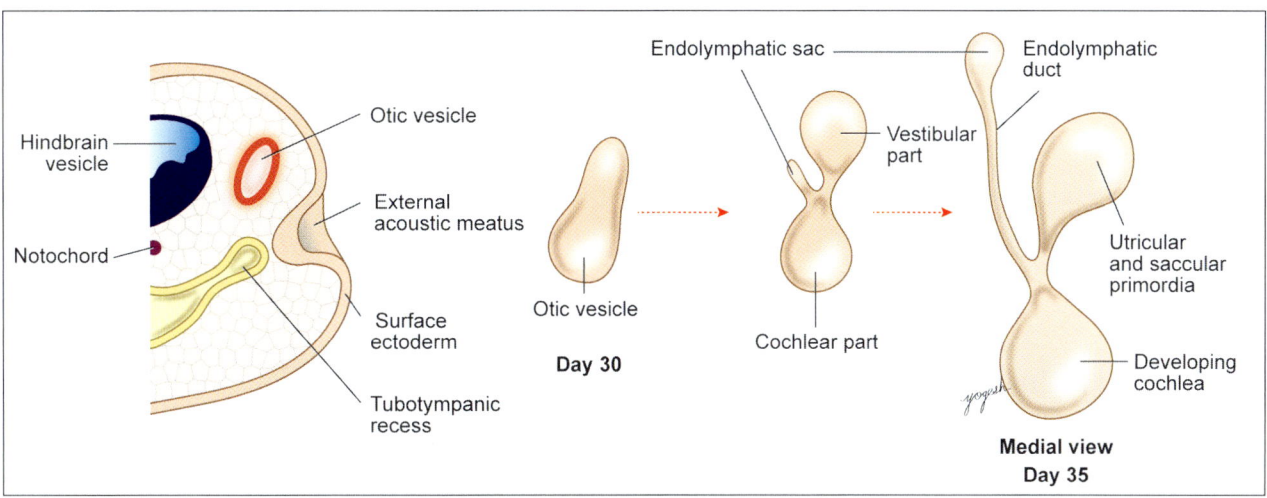

Fig. 24.2: Early development of otic vesicle

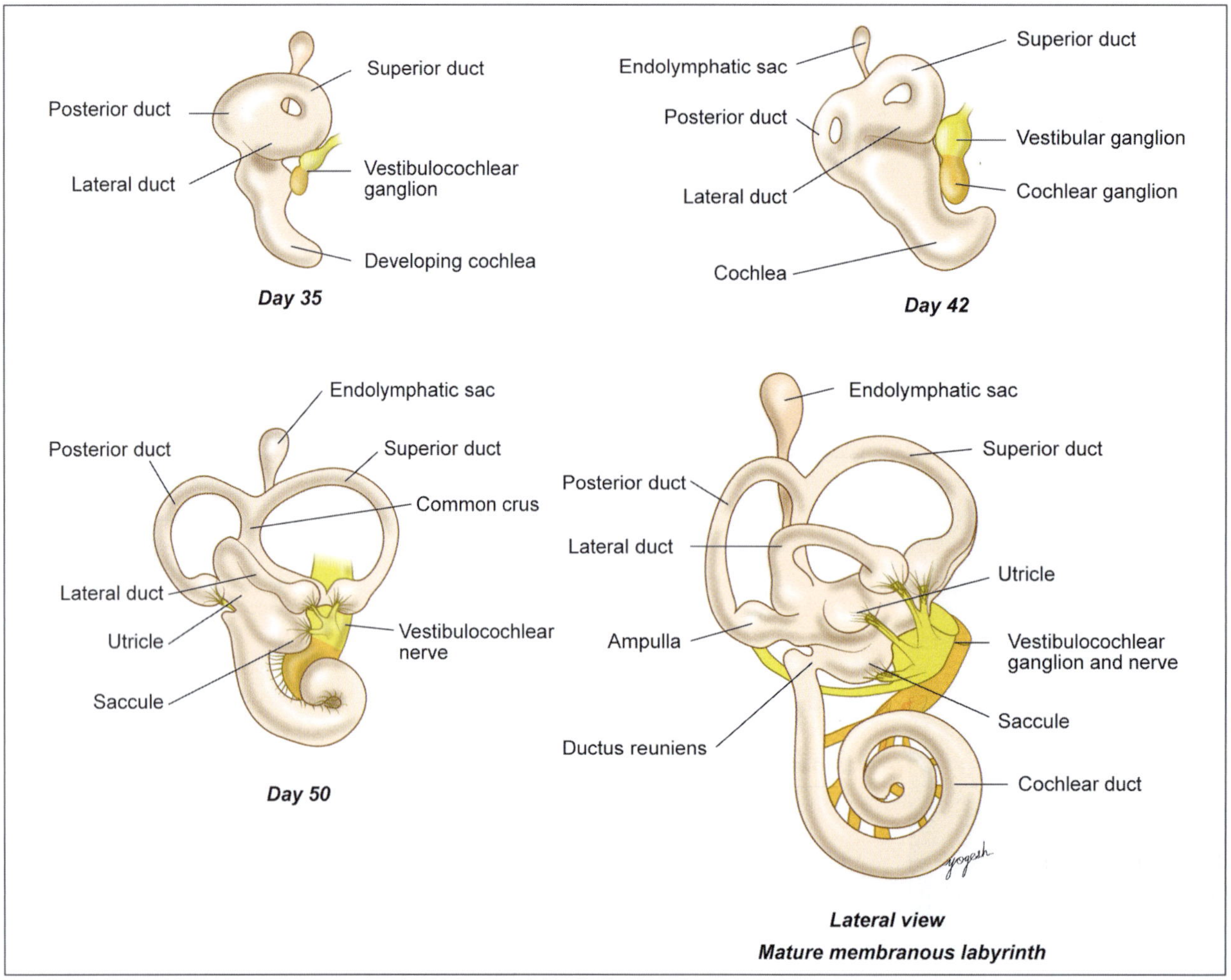

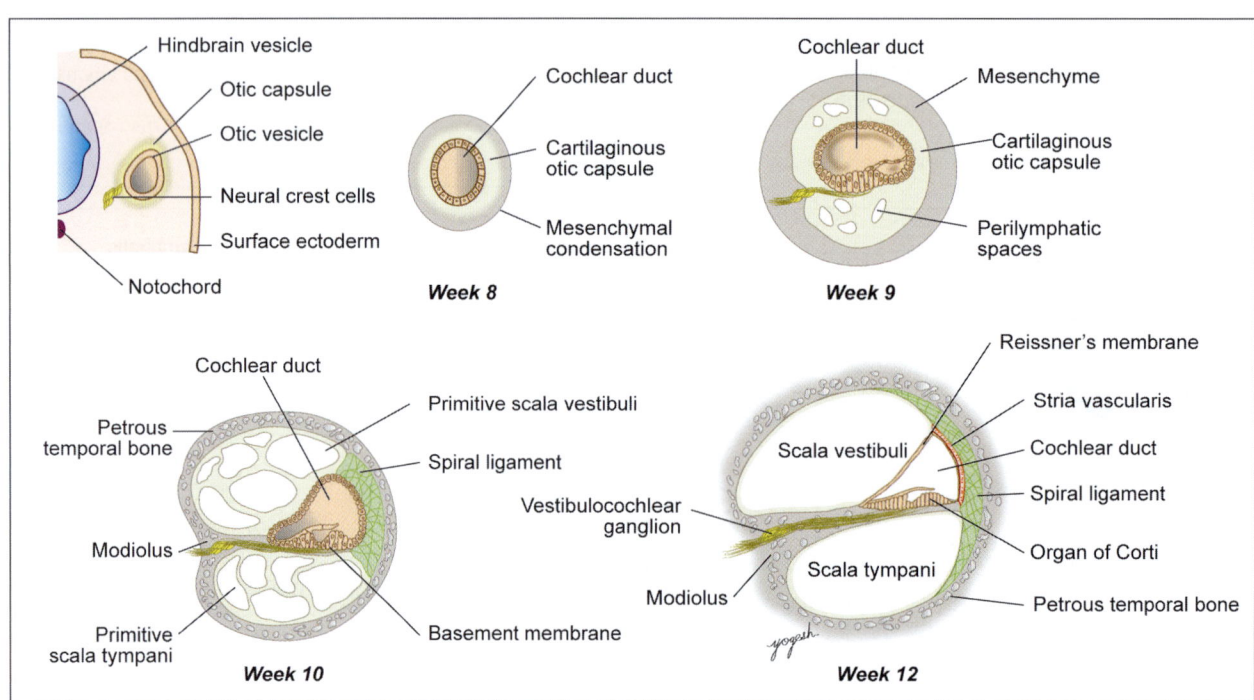

Fig. 24.3: Development of membranous labyrinth

Fig. 24.4: Development of cochlea

- Epithelium of membranous labyrinth modifies to form:
  1. Cristae of semicircular ducts for sense of equilibrium
  2. Macula of utricle for sense of equilibrium
  3. Organ of Corti of cochlea for hearing
  4. Macula of saccule for equilibrium
- Neural crest cells migrated towards otic vesicle give rise to bipolar neurons of vestibulo-cochlear ganglion.
- Peripheral process of bipolar neurons reaches the otic vesicle and get communicated with saccule, utricle, semicircular ducts and spiral organ of Corti (Fig. 24.3).
- Central processes of bipolar neurons grow towards vestibular and cochlear nuclei of hindbrain to form vestibulocochlear nerve.

Bony Labyrinth

- Mesenchymal tissue surrounding the otic vesicle (membranous labyrinth) condenses to form *otic capsule* (Fig. 24.4).
- Otic capsule soon gets converted into cartilage.
- Space between membranous labyrinth (otic vesicle) and otic capsule is filled with loose *periotic tissue*.
- Periotic tissue disappears leaving behind a space surrounding membranous labyrinth that soon get filled with *perilymph.*
- Membranous labyrinth becomes filled with *endolymph*.
- Periotic tissue, surrounding the otic vesicle and saccule degenerate to form a cavity called *vestibule*.
- Periotic tissue surrounding the semicircular ducts also disappear to form *semicircular canals*.
- Due to incomplete resorption of mesenchymal periotic tissue around cochlear duct, *scala tympani* and *scala vestibuli* (two spaces) are formed.
- Scala tympani is separated from cochlear duct by *basilar membrane*; whereas scala vestibuli is separated from cochlear duct by vestibular or *Reissner's membrane*.
- At the end of cochlea, scala vestibuli and scala tympani communicates with each other through an aperture called *helicotrema*.
- Cochlear duct is connected with the bony cochlear canal by spiral ligament.
- Vestibular membrane and basilar membrane meet at the *modiolous*.

Histogenesis of Internal Ear

Histogenesis of Semicircular Canals

- Auditory vesicle is lined by low columnar epithelium. Later, it becomes flattened except in ampullae.
- Cells in the ampulla produce *apical hair cells* and *cupula* (gelatinous mass). The hairs of hair cells and cupula form *crista* of the ampulla.
- In the utricle and saccule, hair cells with covering gelatinous mass form *maculae*.

Note: Cristae are more sensitive for rotational movements of head, whereas maculae are more sensitive for linear acceleration.

Histogenesis of Cochlea

- Cells of cochlear duct facing towards scala tympani get thickened in two areas and form outer and inner ridges separated by spiral sulcus.
  A. Outer ridge forms inner hair cells, 3–4 rows of outer hair cells, inner and outer rod cells.
  B. Inner ridge forms *membrana tectoria* (fibrillated gelatinous mass) that gives attachment to flagella of outer and inner hair cells.
- *Reissner's or vestibular membrane* is derived from dorsal surface of cochlear duct.
- External surface of cochlear duct forms a thick vascular zone, hence called *stria vascularis*.
- By 6th month of IUL, cochlear histogenesis completes.

MIDDLE EAR

- Middle ear cavity is endodermal in origin (Fig. 24.5).
- In 5th week, from the dorsal part of first pharyngeal pouch with a contribution from second pouch, a diverticulum called *tubotympanic recess* develops.
- Each tubotympanic recess grows laterally towards external ear.
- In 6th month of IUL, tubotympanic recess comes in contact with floor of first pharyngeal cleft (future external acoustic meatus). Still a thin rim of mesenchyme persists between endodermal pouch and ectodermal cleft. The combination of all 3 germ layers forms ear drum (tympanic membrane).
- Mesenchyme of the second arch is displaced laterally by mesenchyme of the third arch. Thus, third arch comes in contact with first arch.

- A narrow part of tubotympanic recess lies between the second and third arches and it forms the *auditory tube*.
- The lateral part of the tubotympanic recess widens to form *primary tympanic cavity*.
- Formation of definitive tympanic cavity
  - *Primary tympanic cavity* extends laterally to enclose ear ossicles, muscles, nerves and blood vessels to form *definitive ear cavity*.
  - Dorsal extension of tympanic cavity forms *tympanic antrum*.

Ear Ossicles

- By the end of 7th week, mesenchyme forms 3 condensations in the roof of tympanic cavity as follows:
  - Two from first arch (Meckel's cartilage) that later develops into malleus and incus.
  - One from second arch (Reichert's cartilage) that later develops into stapes.
- Ossicles remain embedded in the surrounding mesenchyme until 8 months.
- On degeneration of mesenchyme surrounding ossicles, mucous lining of primary tympanic cavity extends and envelopes the ossicles.

Muscles of Middle Ear

- Mesenchyme of the first arch forms *tensor tympani* muscle, and hence, supplied by trigeminal nerve (nerve of the 1st pharyngeal arch).
- Mesenchyme of the second arch forms *stapedius* muscle and hence, supplied by facial nerve (nerve of the 2nd pharyngeal arch).

Formation of Round and Oval Windows

- Parts of the bony labyrinth remain thin at two places:
  1. Opposite to stapes and this thin part of bony labyrinth forms *oval window* (fenestra vestibuli).
  2. Just below the stapes and this second thin part of bony labyrinth forms *round window* (fenestra cochleae).
- Fenestra vestibuli opens into the vestibule, whereas fenestra cochleae open into the scala tympani.
- Fenestra vestibuli gets closed by foot plate of stapes, whereas fenestra cochleae by a membrane called *secondary tympanic membrane*.

Formation of Tubal Tonsil

- Pharyngeal opening of tubotympanic recess is indicated by pharyngeal opening of the Eustachian (auditory) tube.
- The opening is surrounded by a considerable amount of lymphoid tissue, that forms a *tubal tonsil*.

EXTERNAL EAR

External Acoustic Meatus (Fig. 24.5)

- Dorsal part of the first pharyngeal cleft invaginates to form funnel-shaped portion called *primary meatus*.
- Primary meatus extends deep towards primary tympanic cavity.
- Medial cells of the primary meatus grow further to form as solid cord (medial plate).
- By 7th month, solid cord hollows out and touches primary tympanic cavity.
- On touching the primary tympanic cavity, the hollowed-out portion of solid cord forms *secondary meatus*.
- Cells of solid cord coming in touch with primary tympanic cavity form *outer (cuticular) layer of tympanic membrane*.
- The handle of malleus and chorda tympani nerve are trapped between ectoderm of meatal plug and endoderm of tympanic cavity and lies in the mesodermal components of tympanic membrane.
- Tympanic membrane lies horizontal at the birth and it faces downward forward and medially in later life.

Auricle (Fig. 24.6, Scanning electron micrograph 24.2)

- At about 6th week of IUL, 6 small tubercles or hillocks appear around the dorsal part of first pharyngeal cleft; 3 on cranial side called *mandibular tubercles* and 3 on caudal side called *hyoid tubercles*.
- These hillocks fuse and expand to form the definitive ear auricle (ear pinna) as follows:
  1. 1st hillock forms tragus
  2. 2nd hillock forms crus of helix
  3. 3rd hillock forms helix
  4. 4th hillock forms antihelix
  5. 5th hillock forms antitragus
  6. 6th hillock forms lower part of helix and ear lobule.
- The development of external ear is completed by 4th month.

Some Interesting Facts

- Middle ear, ear ossicles, mastoid antrum and internal ear assume adult size at birth.
- Internal ear appears earlier than middle and external ear (early in the 4th week).
- Failure of canalisation of meatal plate is the most common cause of congenital deafness.
- Mastoid air cells develop by the age of 2 years.

Development of Ear

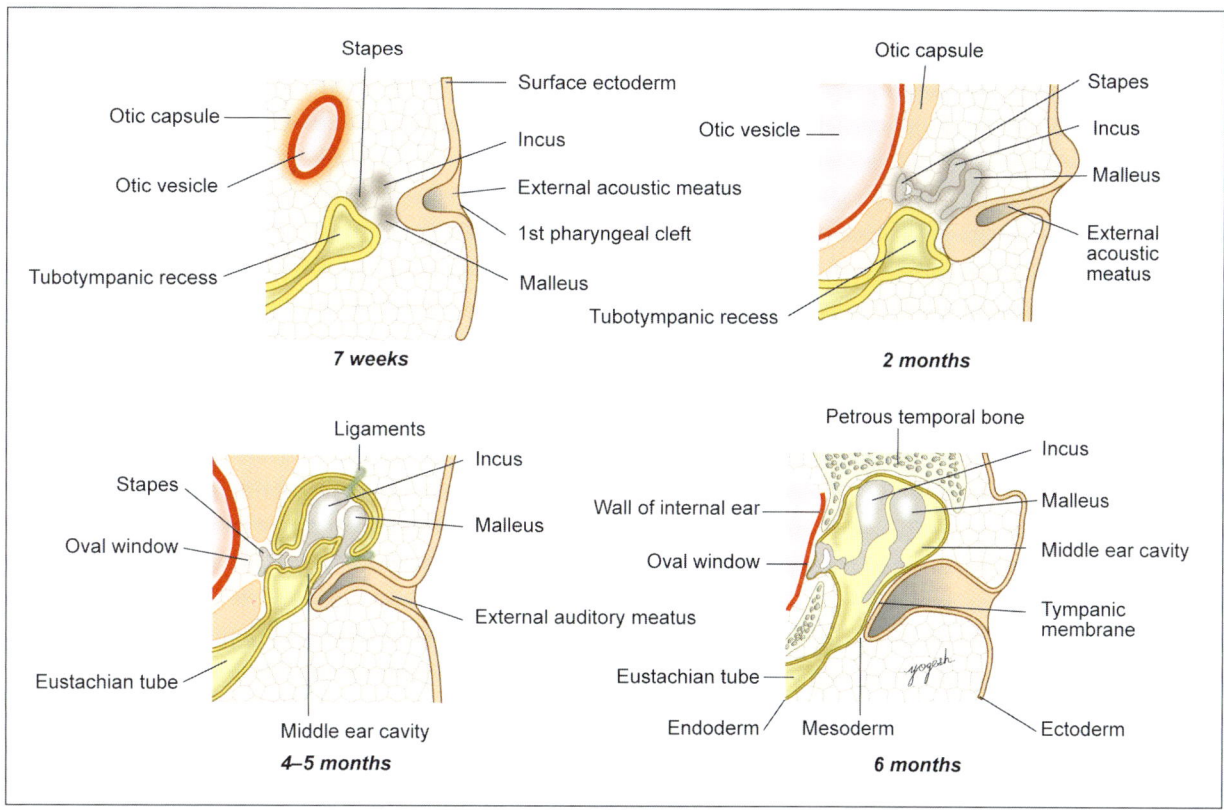

Fig. 24.5: Development of middle ear

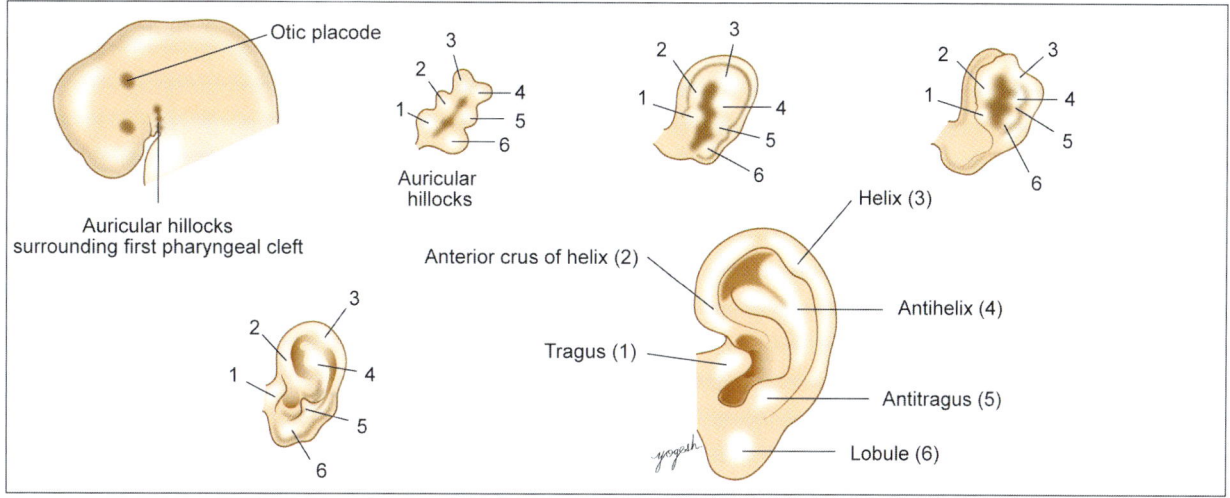

Fig. 24.6: Development of external ear

MOLECULAR REGULATION

Following proteins/genes or factors are important in the molecular regulation of ear development.
1. Wnt proteins and bone morphogenic proteins for development of otic placode.
2. Retinoic acid for anteroposterior differentiation of otic vesicle.
3. Wnt and SHH genes for membranous labyrinth.
4. Noggin and Pax2 genes for cochlea.

DEVELOPMENTAL ANOMALIES

External Ear

- Developmental anomalies may result from nonunion or absence of primordial hillocks. It may cause partial or total absence of auricle and isolated nodule.
- Abnormal position of ear
- Auricle migrates and changes its position due to developing mandible. Hence, mandibular malfor-

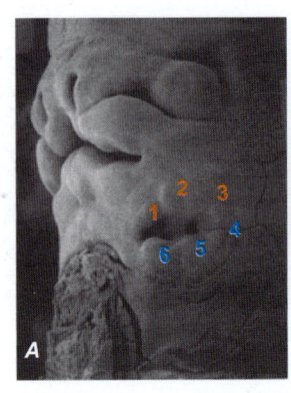 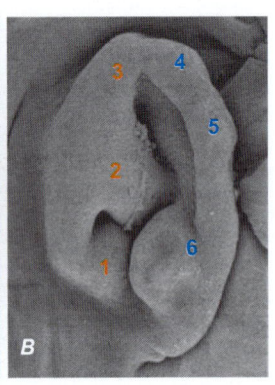

Scanning electron micrograph 24.2: Development of external ear at 6 weeks (A) and 9 weeks (B). The developing external ears are initially more caudal than the lower jaw. Growth of the lower jaw places the external ear in a relatively higher and more vertical orientation. Six hillocks fuse and expands to form the definitive ear auricle (ear pinna) as follows: 1st forms tragus, 2nd forms crus of helix, 3rd forms helix, 4th forms antihelix, 5th forms antitragus, 6th forms lower part of helix and ear lobule [Species: Human, lateral view]

mation (agnathia/micrognathia) results in abnormally low position of auricle. Hence, called *mandibulofacial dysostosis*.
- *Microtia* is suppressed development of auricle, whereas *anotia* is absence of auricle (Table 24.1).

External of Auditory Meatus

- Atresia of external auditory meatus may occur due to failure of meatal plate to canalise.
- Abnormal curvature of meatus: Tympanic membrane may not be fully visible due to congenitally accentuated curvature of meatus.

Middle ear

- Malformation of ossicles: Defective malleus and incus may be observed in 1st arch syndrome.
- *Congenital fixation of stapes*: Stapes may be congenitally fixed with the margins of the fenestra vestibuli. It results into severe conductive deafness.
- Abnormal course of facial nerve: Bulging facial canal in the middle ear may be present.

Internal Ear

- *Rubella virus infection*: Rubella infection in the second month of pregnancy affects mostly cochlear and vestibular development and to some extent organ of Corti. Hence, children born to a mother with rubella infection may perceive only deep frequency sounds.
- *Thalidomide* may cause malformations of semicircular canals.

Table 24.1 Development of ear

Adult structures	Embryonic source
External ear	
Auricle	6 Ectodermal hillocks *1st arch*: (1) Tragus, (2) crus of helix, (3) helix
	2nd arch: (4) Antihelix, (5) antitragus, (6) lobule
External acoustic meatus	1st pharyngeal cleft
Middle ear	
Middle ear cavity	Tubotympanic recess
Muscles	Tensor tympani—1st pharyngeal arch
	Stapedius—2nd pharyngeal arch
Ear ossicles	Malleus, incus—1st pharyngeal arch
	Stapes—2nd pharyngeal arch
Auditory tube, mastoid antrum	Tubotympanic recess
Tympanic membrane	Outer cuticular layer—ectoderm of 1st pharyngeal cleft
	Middle fibrous layer—mesoderm
	Inner mucous layer—endoderm of 1st pharyngeal pouch
Internal ear	
Membranous labyrinth	Otic vesicle
• Utricle, semicircular ducts, endolymphatic duct	Vestibular (dorsal) part of membranous labyrinth
• Saccule, ductus reuniens, cochlear duct	Cochlear (ventral) part of membranous labyrinth
Bony labyrinth	
• Vestibule, semicircular canals, scala tympani, scala vestibuli	Mesenchyme around otic vesicle (otic capsule)

25

Endocrine System

Chapter Outline

- Pituitary Gland
- Stages of development
- Clinical aspects
- Pineal gland
- Adrenal gland
  - Stages of development
  - Congenital anomalies
- Chromaffin cells

INTRODUCTION

- Endocrine glands are ductless gland. They secrete hormones directly into the blood.
- Hormones reach to the target organ through circulation and get attached to specific receptors for exerting a specific effect.
- The major endocrine glands are:
  1. Pituitary gland
  2. Pineal gland
  3. Thyroid gland
  4. Parathyroid gland
  5. Adrenal gland
  6. Islets of Langerhans in pancreas
  7. Testis and ovary
  8. Hypothalamus (in addition to many other functions, hypothalamus controls secretions of anterior pituitary gland)
- In this chapter, development of pituitary gland, pineal gland and adrenal gland is described. For development of thyroid gland and parathyroid gland, read Chapter 11, for pancreas read Chapter 15, for gonads read Chapter 21.

PITUITARY GLAND (HYPOPHYSIS CEREBRI)

- Pituitary gland is an unpaired endocrine gland located in a bony fossa called *sella turcica* of the sphenoid bone.
- It consists of two major parts: *adenohypophysis* (anterior pituitary) and *neurohypophysis* (posterior pituitary).

Summary (Examination Guide) (Figs 25.1 and 25.2, Flowchart 25.1, Practice Fig. 25.1)

- Anterior pituitary develops from Rathke's pouch that arises from ectoderm of stomodeum.
- Anterior lobe consists of pars distalis, pars intermedia and pars tuberalis.
- Cavity of the Rathke's pouch forms intraglandular cleft.
- Neurohypophysis develops from evagination of the floor of 3rd ventricle (diencephalon).

Stages of Development

1. Adenohypophysis develops form **Rathke's pouch**.
   - *Ectoderm* of stomodeum becomes thicker on day 21 of IUL. This thickened ectoderm invaginates and grows towards diencephalon in the form of *Rathke's pouch*.
   - By 2nd month of IUL, the Rathke's pouch loses its contact with stomodeum.
   - Cells of thick anterior wall of Rathke's pouch proliferate to form *pars distalis*, posterior thin wall forms *pars intermedia*.
   - The cavity of the pouch forms **intraglandular cleft** which is not recognisable in the adult human gland.

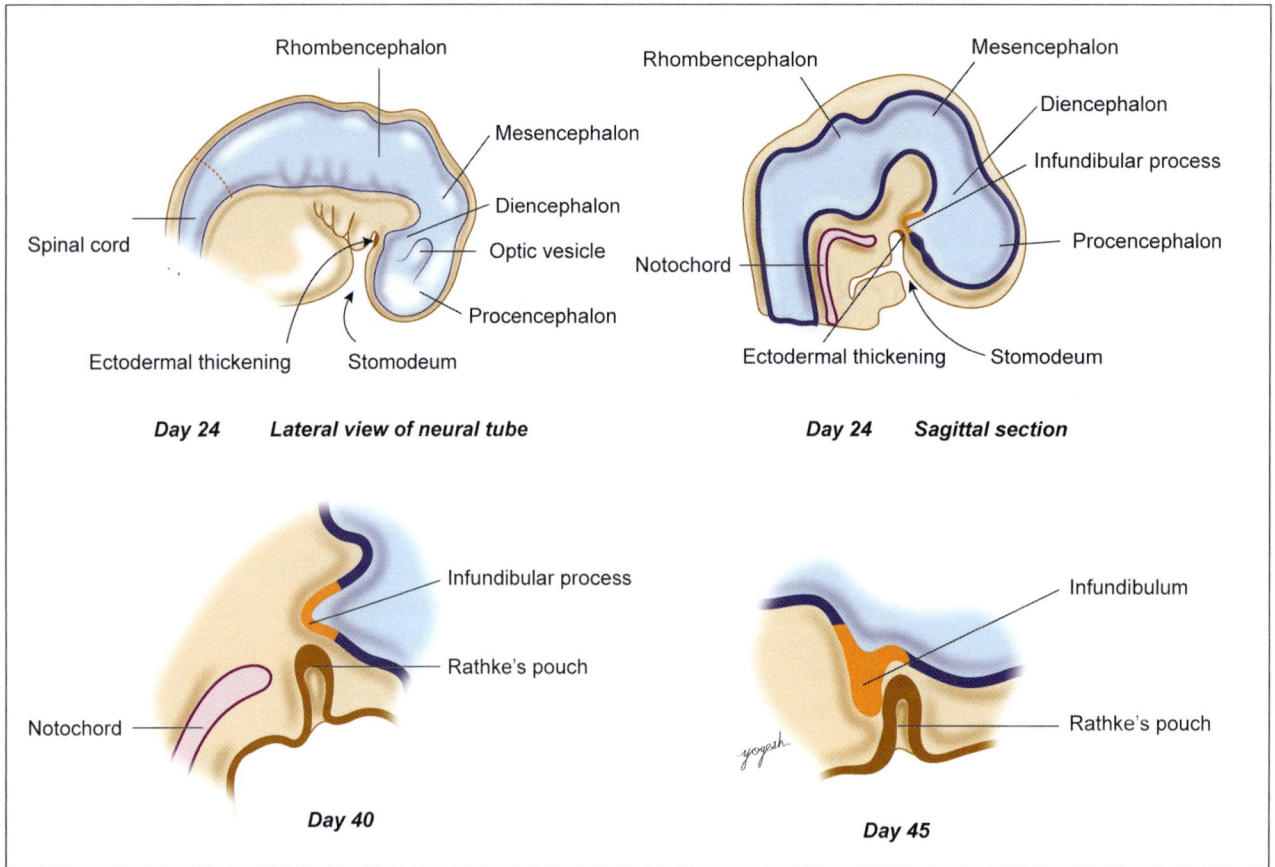

Fig. 25.1: Development of pituitary gland

- Upward proliferation of anterior wall forms *pars tuberalis*.
2. Neurohypophysis develops from **infundibular process of diencephalon**.
   - During 6th week of IUL, an infundibular process arises from the diencephalon in the floor of 3rd ventricle.
   - Infundibular process grows towards stomodeum (Rathke's pouch) and fuses with Rathke's pouch.
   - Infundibular process forms *pars nervosa* (posterior pituitary) neurohypophysis.
   - The connecting stalk between pars nervosa and diencephalon (later hypothalamus) forms *infundibulum*.
3. Histogenesis of pituitary gland
   - Histogenesis of pituitary gland begins in the 4th month of IUL.
   - Acidophils appear earlier followed by basophils and chromophobes.
   - Neuroglial cells start appearing in neurohypophysis by the 4th month. This is followed by axonal colonisation from supraoptic and paraventricular nuclei of hypothalamus.

Clinical Aspects

1. *Craniopharyngiomas*: Rathke's pouch passes through the craniopharyngeal canal from the stomodeum to the sella turcica and eventually loses contact with the stomodeum. *Remnants of Rathke's pouch* in craniopharyngeal canal may give rise to a tumour called *craniopharyngioma*. Craniopharyngioma is seen in relation to the sphenoid bone in the roof of nasopharynx. It may occur as childhood onset in 5–14 years of age or as adult onset in 50–70 years of age.
2. *Accessory pituitary gland*: It may be seen in relation to posterior wall of nasopharynx as pharyngeal hypophysis.
3. Pituitary agenesis or hypoplasia may be seen.

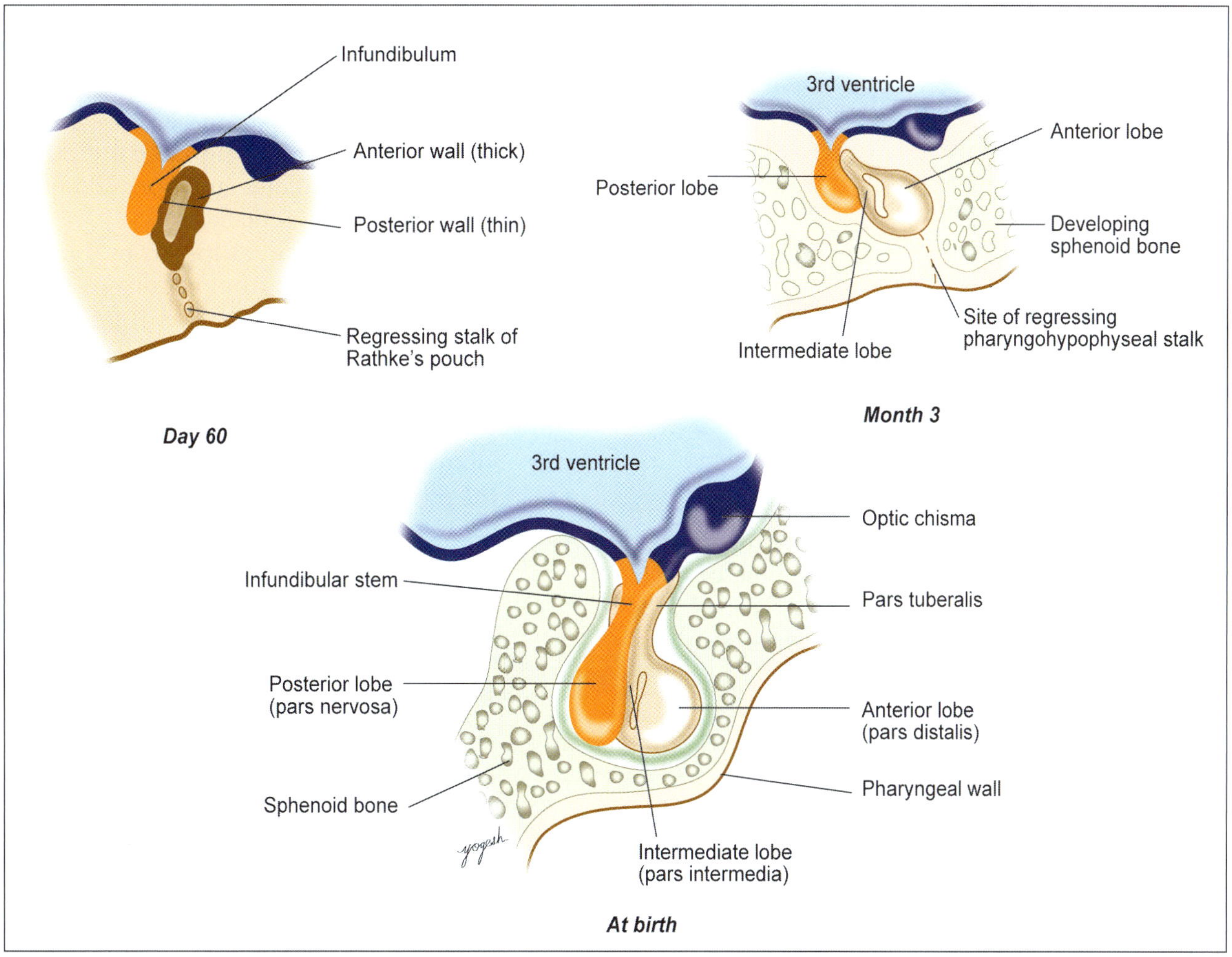

Fig. 25.2: Development of pituitary gland

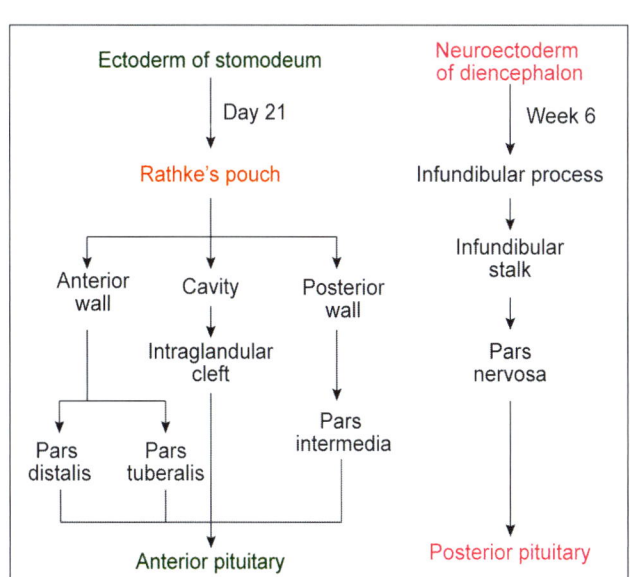

Flowchart 25.1: Development of pituitary gland

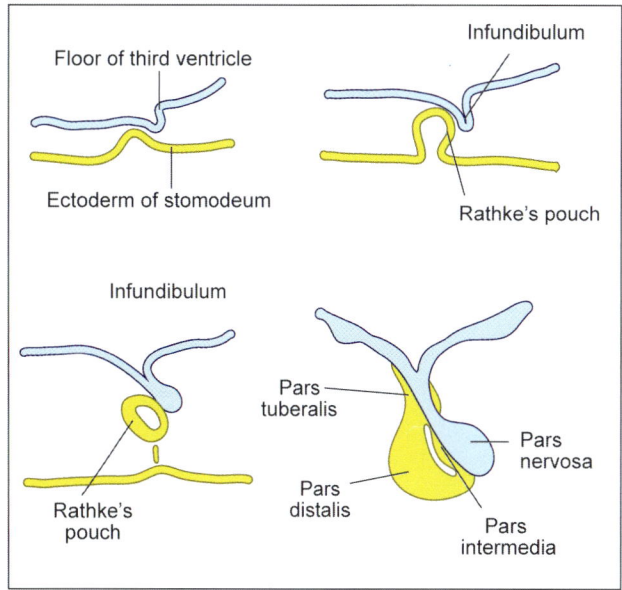

Practice Fig. 25.1: Development of pituitary gland

Human Embryology

> **Box 25.1:** Pineal gland (epiphysis cereberi)
> **Development of pineal gland**
> - Pineal gland is called third eye of human body or principal seat of soul.
> - Pineal gland develops as an evagination from diencephalon in the **roof** of 3rd ventricle.
> - Pineal gland is made up of pinealocytes (modified neuroglial cells).
> - Pinealocytes secrete melatonin hormone.
> - Melatonin inhibits the secretion of gonadotrophin releasing hormone (GnRH).

ADRENAL GLAND

- Adrenal glands (suprarenal glands) are the masses of glandular tissue located at upper pole of each kidney.
- Adrenal gland consists of superficial cortex and deep medulla.

Summary (Examination Guide) (Figs 25.3 to 25.5, Flowchart 25.2, Practice Fig. 25.2)

1. *Adrenal cortex*: It develops from coelomic epithelium (mesoderm) that forms suprarenal ridge. Initially formed foetal cortex gets replaced by definitive cortex which differentiates into zona glomerulosa, zona fasciculata, zona reticularis.
2. *Adrenal medulla*: It develops from sympatho-chromaffin cells derived from neural crest cells.

Stages of Development

Adrenal cortex is mesodermal in origin and medulla is neuroectodermal (neural crest) derivative.^{MCQ}

1. Development of adrenal cortex
   - In the 5th week of IUL, the *coelomic epithelium* in relation with developing gonad proliferates to form a *suprarenal ridge*.
   - In the 2nd month, the suprarenal ridge forms acidophilic cells that surround the primitive adrenal medulla. These acidophilic cells form *foetal cortex*.

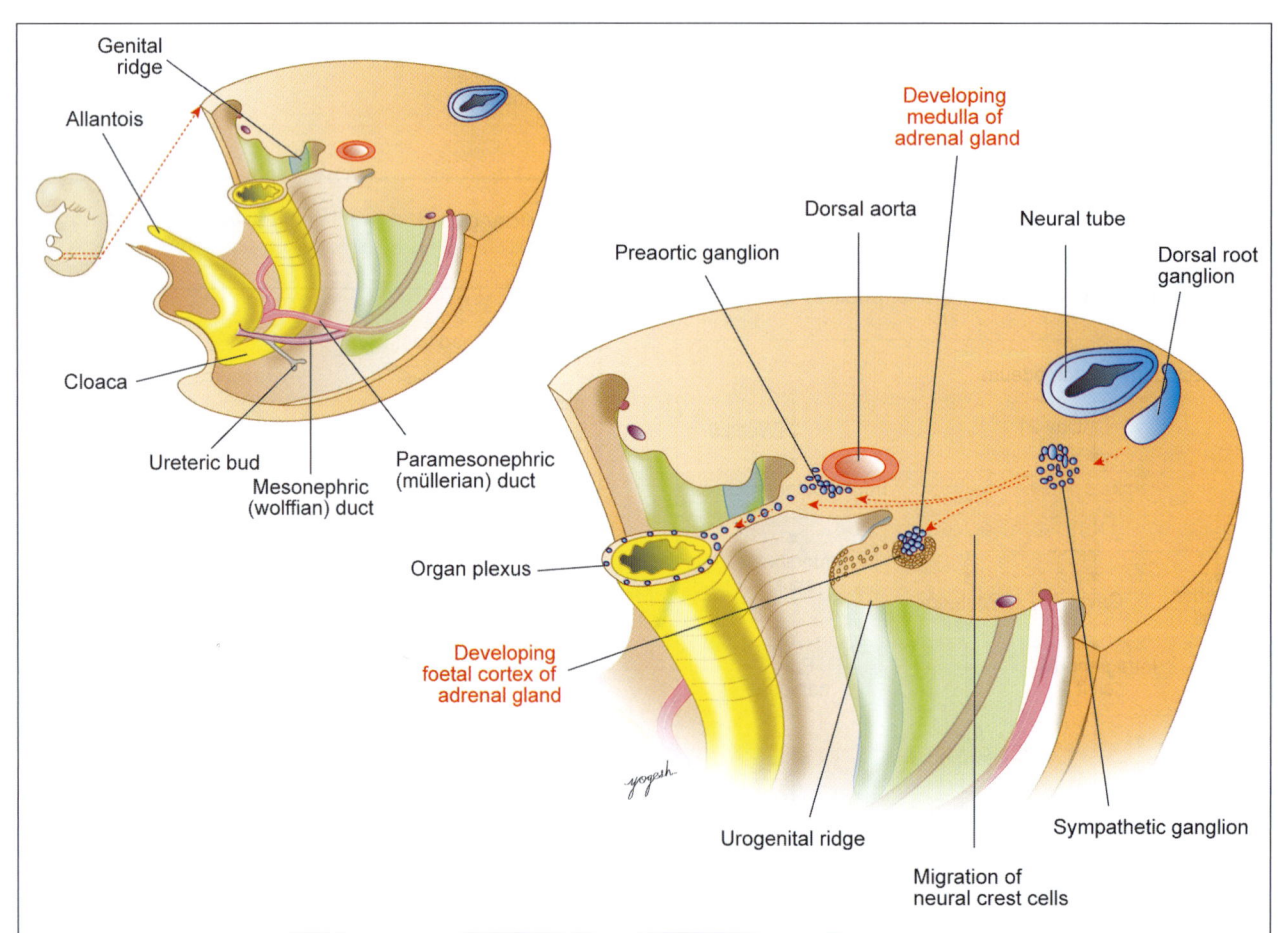

Fig. 25.3: Cross section of embryo showing developing adrenal gland

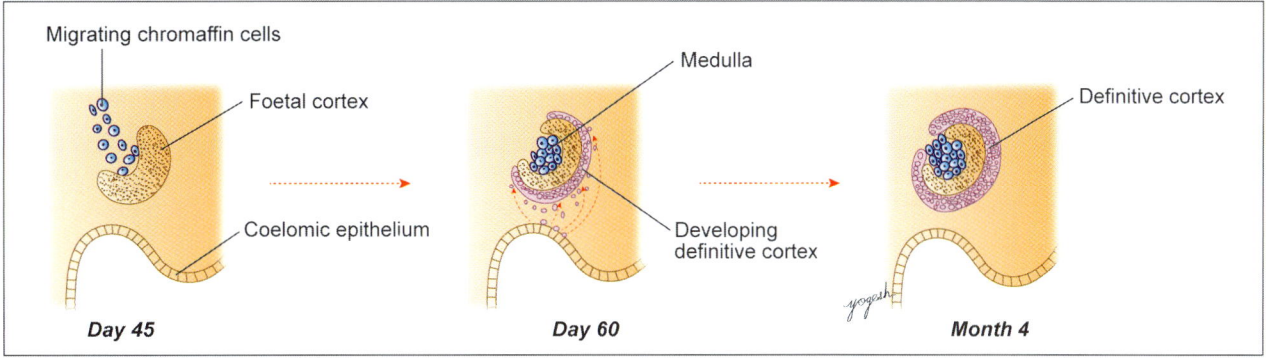

Fig. 25.4: Development of adrenal gland

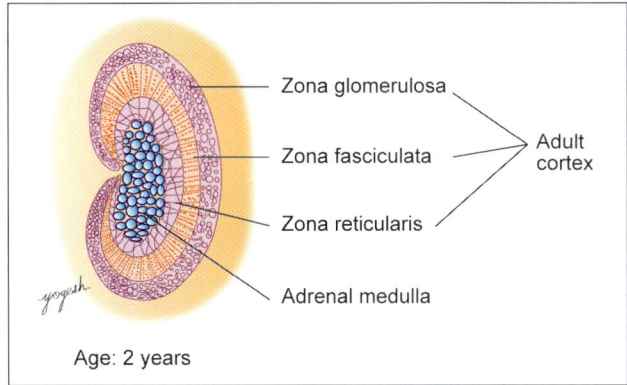

Fig. 25.5: Developed adrenal gland

Flowchart 25.2: Development of adrenal gland

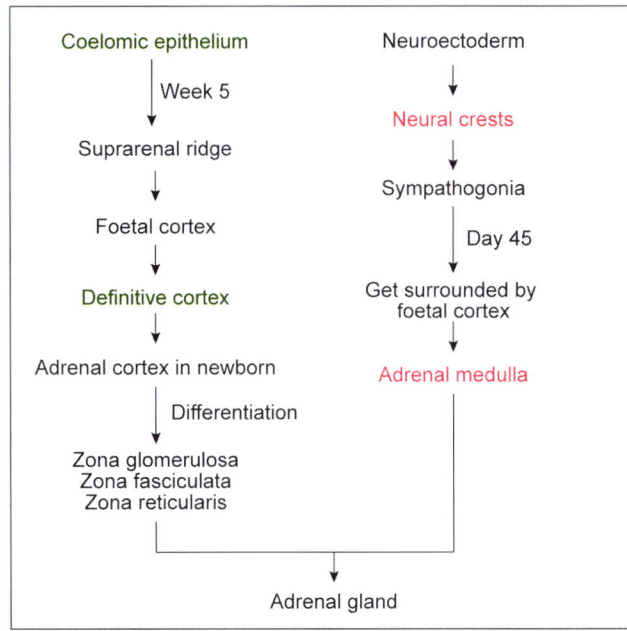

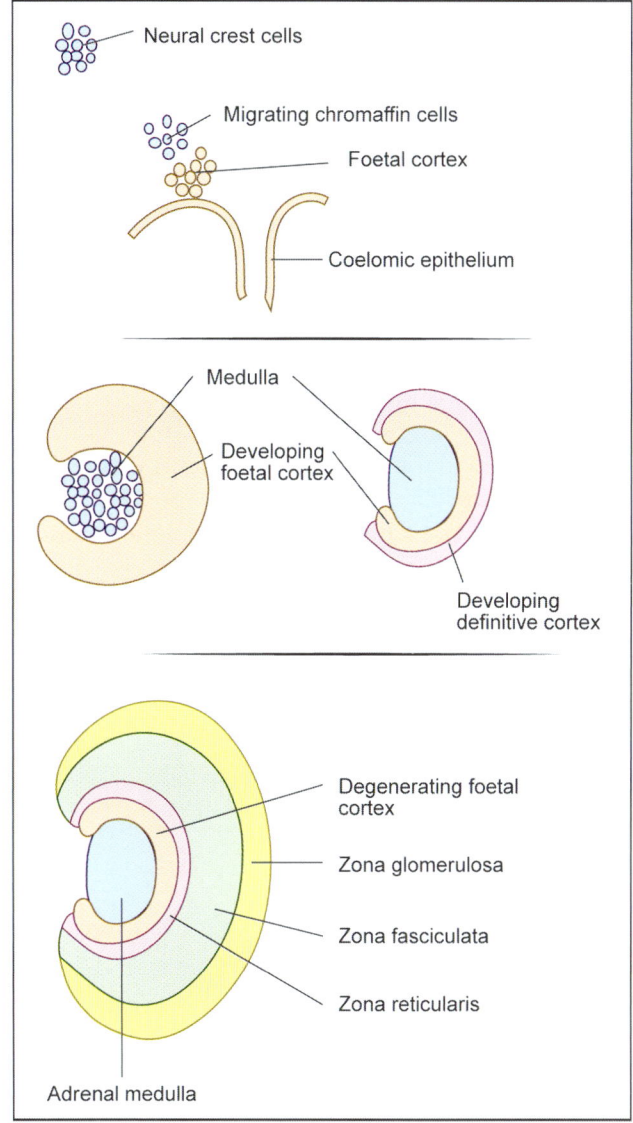

Practice Fig. 25.2: Development of adrenal gland

- In the 3rd month, a second wave of cells (small basophilic) arises from suprarenal ridge. These small basophilic cells surround foetal cortical cells and form *definitive cortex*.

2. Development of adrenal medulla
   - By the 45th day of gestation, sympathogonia accumulate near the foetal cortical cells. Sympathogonia arise from **neural crest cells** (neuroectoderm).
   - Sympathogonia invade foetal adrenal cortical cells and form clusters and cords of cells.
   - These sympathogonia differentiate to form *adrenal medulla*.
   - Differentiation of definitive cortex begins in foetal life.
   - At the birth, only zona glomerulosa and zona fasciculata are present.

3. Changes after birth
   - Foetal adrenal gland is 10–20 times larger than the adult adrenal gland.
   - At the birth, adrenal cortex forms only 15–20% of adrenal parenchyma.
   - The size of adrenal gland in foetus is almost of same size as that of the adult.
   - Foetal cortex regresses completely by the second year of life and thus, adrenal gland reduces in size.^MCQ
   - Zona reticularis appears at the end of the third year of life.^Neet
   - Preganglionic sympathetic neurons terminate in relation to cells of medulla.
   - *Note:* Cells of medulla correspond the postganglionic sympathetic neurons.

Congenital Anomalies

1. *Ectopic adrenal gland*: Ectopic adrenal tissue may be present deep to the renal capsule, or fused with the kidney or liver.
2. *Congenital adrenal hyperplasia*: It involves deficiency of 21 hydroxylase enzyme (essential for steroid hormone synthesis). It results in elevation of androgens and cause pseudointersexuality as follows:

   In male: It causes early development of secondary sexual characters and the condition is called adrenogenital syndrome.

   In female: It causes enlargement of clitoris and the condition is called pseudohermaphroditism.

Box 25.2: Chromaffin cells

- Chromaffin cells or pheochromocytes are neuroendocrine cells derived from neural crests.
- Staining property: These cells shows brown pigmentation on staining with chromium salts (affinity for chromium).
- *Note:* Enterochromaffin cells of Kulchitsky lie in gastroinstestinal tract. Though these cells have similar chemical property like adrenal medulla, but enterochromaffin cells are derived from endoderm.
- Location of chromaffin cells
   1. Para aortic bodies (organ of Zuckerkandl)
   2. Sympathetic ganglia
   3. Adrenal medulla
- *Pheochromocytoma* is a tumour of chromaffin cells. It produces a large quantities of adrenalin and noradrenalin. It causes hypertension.

26

Skeletal System and Limbs

Chapter Outline

- Formation of cartilage
- Formation of bone
  - Intramembranous ossification
  - Endochondral ossification
  - Development of typical long bone
  - Anomalies of bone formation
- Achondroplasia
- Development of axial skeleton
  - Development of vertebral column
  - Development of ribs
  - Development of sternum
  - Development of skull
- Costal element and transverse element
- Fontanelles
- Development of limbs
- Development of joints

INTRODUCTION

- Skeletal system consists of bones and cartilages that can be grouped into two parts:
  1. *Axial skeleton*: It includes skull, vertebrae, ribs and sternum.
  2. *Appendicular skeleton*: It includes pectoral and pelvic girdles and bones of upper and lower limbs.
- Skeletal system develops from intraembryonic mesoderm.
- The intraembryonic mesoderm is divided into paraxial, intermediate and lateral plate mesoderm.
- The *paraxial mesoderm* consists of
  - *Preotic part*: It lies cranial to otic capsules and forms unsegmented *somitomeres*.
  - *Postotic part*: It lies caudal to otic capsules and forms segmented *somites*.
- Each somite differentiates into dermatome for dermis of skin, myotome for skeletal muscles and sclerotome for vertebrae.
- For the details about somites, read Chapter 8.
- Dermatome forms dermis at the back of the head and trunk, whereas in other parts dermis is derived from the lateral plate mesoderm.^{Neet}

FORMATION OF CARTILAGE

- Cartilages are derived from mesenchymal tissue (Fig. 26.1).

Stages of Formation

1. *Mesenchymal cells* become closely packed (to form mesenchymal condensation) in the region of cartilage formation.
2. Mesenchymal cells differentiate to *chondroblasts*.
3. Chondroblasts deposit intercellular matrix and differentiate to form *chondrocytes*.
4. Depending on the type and amount of the fibres in the matrix, the following cartilages are formed:
   a. *Hyaline cartilage*: Fine collagen fibres in the matrix.
   b. *Elastic cartilage*: Elastic fibres in the matrix.
   c. *Fibrocartilage*: Dense collagen fibres in the matrix.
5. Mesenchymal cells surrounding the cartilage form *perichondrium*.

FORMATION OF BONE

- Bones are mesodermal derivatives (except in the facial skeleton—formed by neural crest contribution).
- The process of formation of bone is called *ossification*.

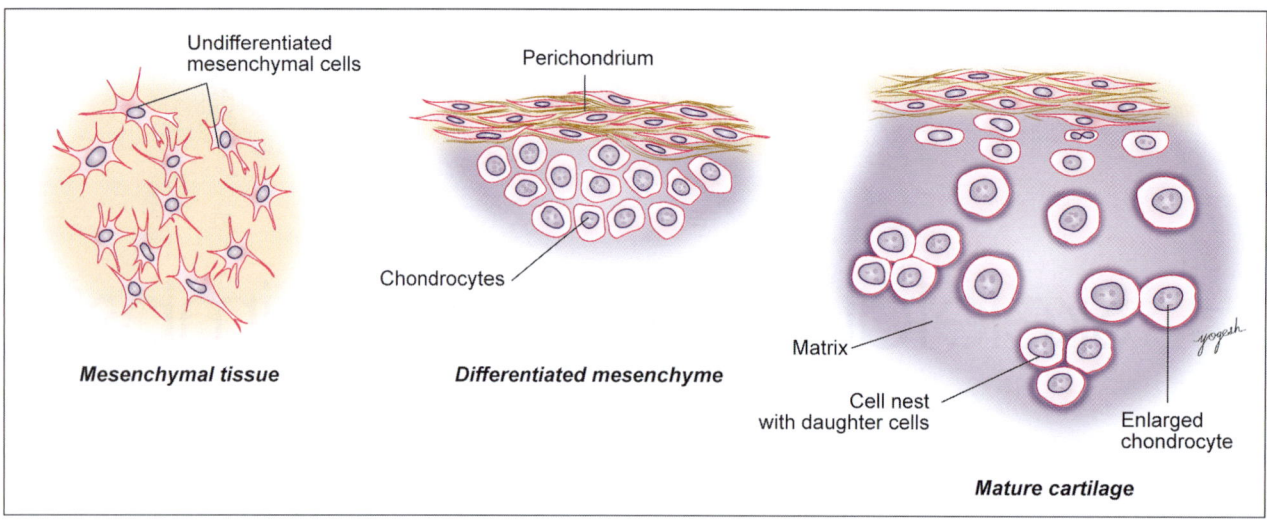

Fig. 26.1: Development of cartilage

- Ossification may be
  a. *Intramembranous ossification* that involves the direct conversion of mesenchymal tissue to bone.
  b. *Endochondral* (cartilaginous) ossification that involves the conversion of mesenchyme to a cartilage which is later replaced by bone.

Intramembranous Ossification

- In intramembranous ossification, the mesenchymal tissue forms bone (Fig. 26.2, Flowchart 26.1).

Steps of formation

1. Mesenchymal condensation: Star-shaped mesenchymal cells condense and differentiate to spindle-shaped fibroblasts that form a fibrous membrane.
2. Osteoid formation: Fibroblasts differentiate to osteoblasts that laydown the early bone matrix and forms uncalcified bone (osteoid).
3. Calcification of osteoid: Osteoblasts deposit calcium salts in intercellular matrix and thus converts osteoid into calcified bony spicules.
4. Formation of woven bone: Trapped osteoblasts in the matrix get differentiated to osteocytes. Spicules fuse with each other to form plates of compact bones. Arrangement of collagen bundles running in different directions produces woven bone appearance.
5. Formation of Haversian system: Waves of calcification and trapping of osteocyte processes in bony canaliculi forms Haversian system.
6. Stage of bone modelling and remodelling: Fusion of progressively growing bone give a primitive shape to a bone model. Continuous deposition and reabsorption of bone give the definitive shape to bone.

Flowchart 26.1: Intramembranous ossification

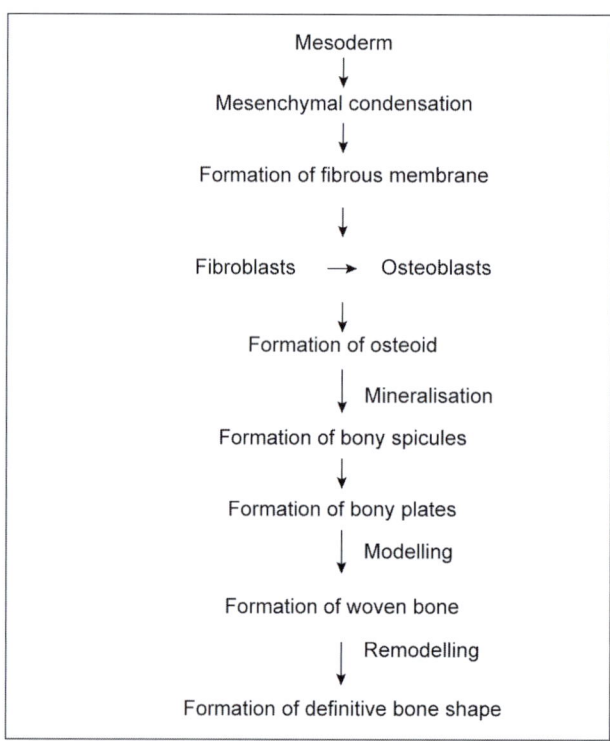

- Bones formed by membranous ossification are called *membranes bones*.
- Examples: Bones of skull vault, mandible, clavicle (partly).

Endochondral Ossification

- It involves conversion of mesenchymal tissue into cartilage that later replaced by bone (Fig. 26.3, Flowchart 26.2).

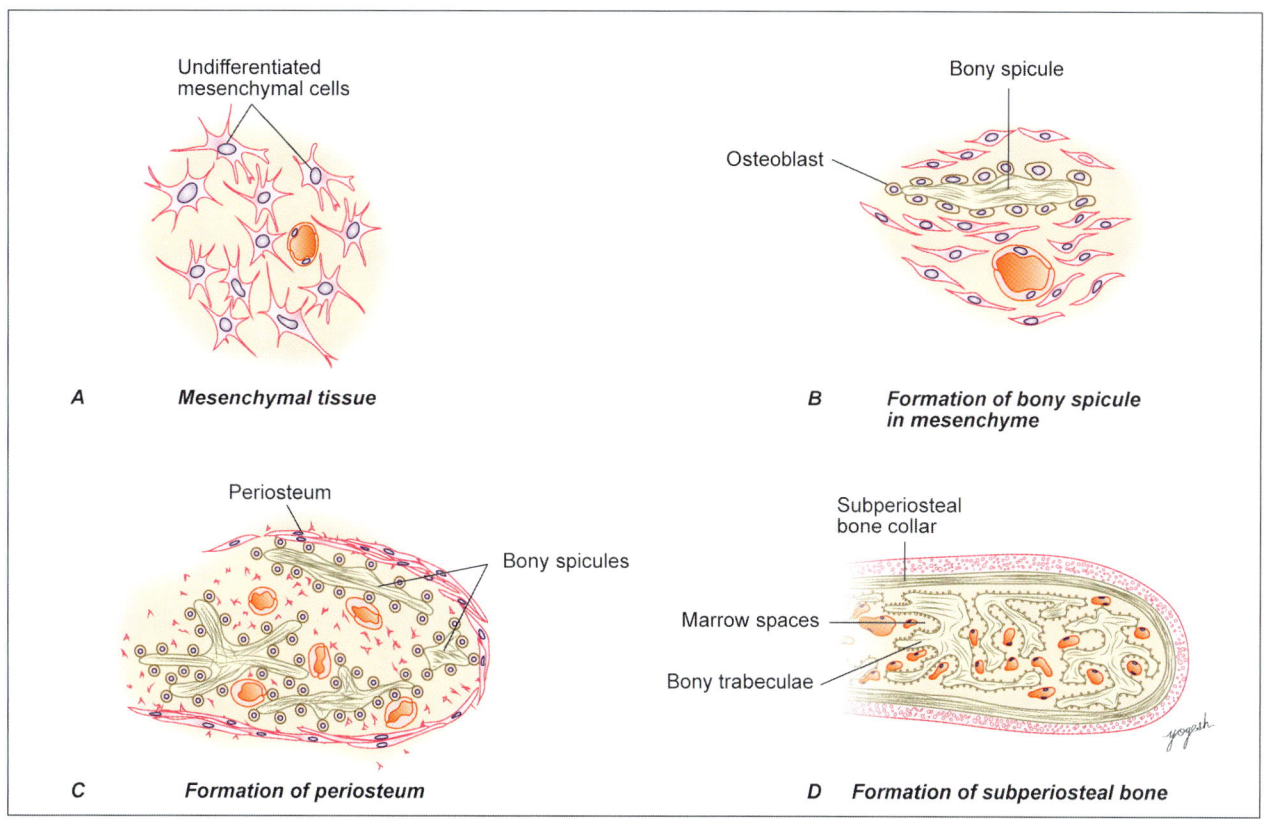

Fig. 26.2: Intramembranous ossification

- The bones developed by cartilaginous ossification are called *cartilaginous bones*.
- Examples: All long bones (except clavicle), base of the skull, vertebrae, ribs.

Stages of endochondral ossification

1. Mesenchymal condensation: Mesenchymal cells form condensed mesenchymal tissue at the site of bone formation.
2. Formation of cartilaginous model: At the site of mesenchymal condensation, chondroblasts appear and deposit hyaline cartilage. This cartilage is surrounded by a vascular mesenchyme that forms perichondrium.
3. Stage of cartilage hypertrophy: At the site of bone formation, the cells of cartilage increase in size (hypertrophy).
4. Stage of calcification: Hypertrophied cartilaginous cells start secretion of alkaline phosphatase and deposit calcium in intercellular matrix. Soon, chondrocytes lose nutritional source and die due to calcified matrix to leave behind *primary areolae*.
5. Formation of periosteal buds: Perichondral vessels and osteogenic cells invade calcified matrix to form periosteal bud.
6. Formation of secondary areolae: Periosteal bud removes calcified matrix from the wall of primary areolae and forms large cavities called secondary areolae.
7. Formation of osteoid: Osteogenic cells (osteoblasts) form a gelatinous matrix along the wall of secondary areolae. This newly formed mass is called *osteoid*.
8. Formation of bone lamella: Intercellular gelatinous matrix of osteoid gets calcified to develop a lamella of bone.
9. Formation of trabecular bone: Osteoblasts lay another layer of lamella over the first one and so on. Osteoblasts trapped in lamellae form osteocytes. The multilamellar portion is called trabecular bone.

Development of Typical Long Bone

Formation of long bone shows various stages as follows:

1. Stages of mesenchymal condensation
2. Formation of cartilaginous model
3. Stage of endochondral ossification
4. Stage of bone growth

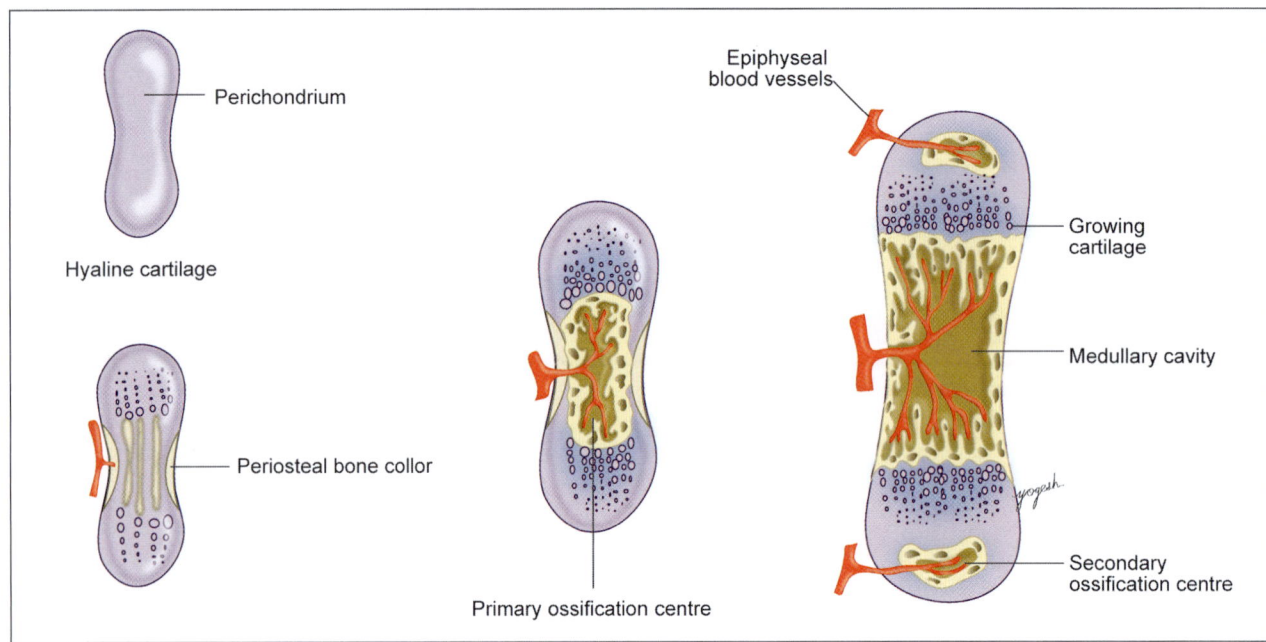

Fig. 26.3: Endochondral ossification (development of long bone)

5. Stage of remodelling
   - The calcification in the cartilaginous model of long bones starts in shaft at the *primary centre of ossification* (diaphysis).
   - On the appearance of the primary centre of ossification, the periosteum produces a calcified bone on the surface of cartilage by intramembranous ossification. This periosteal bone is called *periosteal collar*.
   - After the birth, cartilages at ends of the long bone starts ossification (secondary centres) to form *epiphysis*.
   - Diaphysis and epiphysis are separated by a plate of *epiphysis cartilage*.

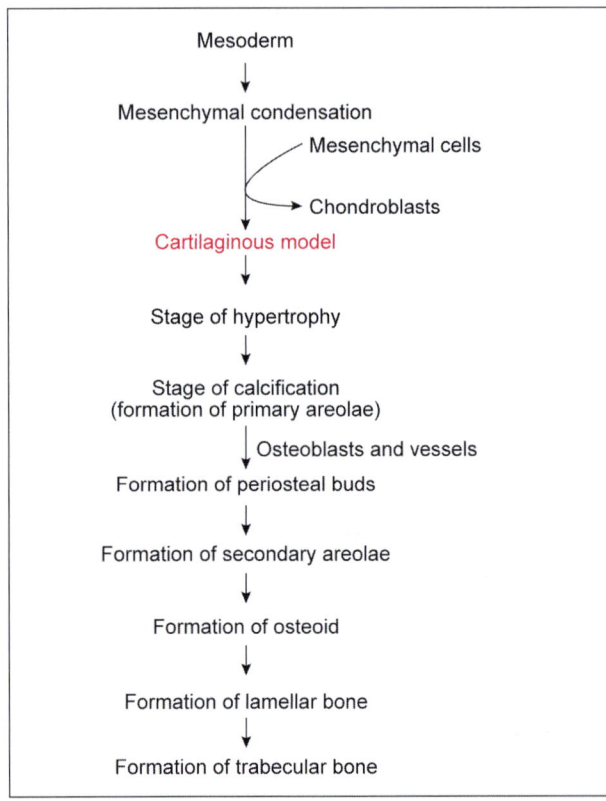

Flowchart 26.2: Endochondral ossification

Growth of long bone

1. **Increase in thickness and formation of bone marrow:** Periosteal collar increases in the thickness by deposition of more layers on outer surface of bone. Simultaneously, osteoblasts remove lamellae from the inner surface of bone, leaving behind a *bone marrow cavity*.
2. **Increase in length:** The length of bone increases by lengthening of epiphyseal cartilage and its simultaneous conversion into new bone.
   - In the developing bone, epiphysial cartilage shows the zone of resting cartilage, zone of proliferation, zone of calcification and zone of ossification (Fig. 26.4).
   - The terminal portion of diaphysis (active site of bone formation) is called *metaphysis*.
   - On completion of bone growth, epiphyseal cartilage stops proliferation and epiphysis fuses with diaphysis.
   - Cartilages show interstitial growth (deposition of intercellular substance), whereas bones show oppositional growth (growth on the surface and ends).

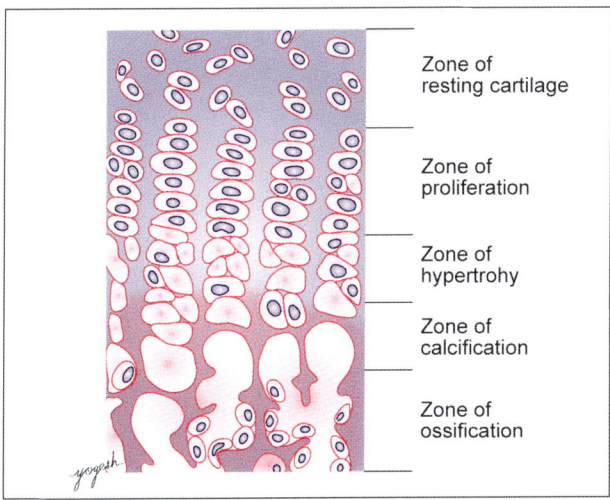

Fig. 26.4: Epiphyseal cartilage of developing bone

Box 26.1: Achondroplasia (dwarfism)

Q. Write short note on achondroplasia.
- It is a genetic disorder that causes dwarfism.

Cause
- It is inherited as autosomal dominant disease due to mutation of fibroblast growth factor receptor 3 (FGFR 3) gene

Signs and symptoms
The affected individual shows the following features:
- Disproportionate shortening (dwarf)
- Proportional large head
- Short-curved arms and legs
- Dorsal lordosis (convex curvature of vertebral column)
- Short fingers and toes

Some Interesting Facts

- Mandible, clavicle, occipital bone, temporal bone and sphenoid bone show membranocartilaginous ossification.
- Bones of cranial vault and facial bones are membranous bones.
- The clavicle is the first bone in the body to ossify.

Anomalies of Bone Formation

1. *Osteogenesis imperfecta* (brittle-bone disease): It involves lack of collagen type I fibres and defective calcification; hence, bones break easily. Other symphonies include short height, hearing loss, blue sclera and loose joints.[Neet]
2. Achondroplasia (Box 26.1).
3. *Cleidocranial dysostosis*: It is a congenital anomaly that involves partial or complete absence of clavicles. It also involves skull vault, causing large fontanelles and delayed closure of sutures. Due to the absence of clavicles, affected individual can bring both the shoulders close together.
4. Dyschondroplasias (enchondromatosis): It involves excessive proliferation of cartilages at growth plates in the long bones. These cartilages form abnormal cartilage masses with the metaphysis.

DEVELOPMENT OF AXIAL SKELETON

- Axial skeleton consists of skull, vertebrae, ribs and sternum.

Development of Vertebral Column

- Vertebral column develops from *sclerotomes* of somites (Figs 26.5 to 26.9).[MCQ]
- Development of vertebral column takes place in 3 essential stages: Precartilage stage, chondrification state, ossification state.

Precartilage stage
- Cells of sclerotome migrate in three directions as follows (Fig. 26.6):
  1. Ventromedial group
     It is divided into two portions:
     a. Densely arranged cells form intervertebral disc
     b. Loosely arranged cells fuse with the cells of underlying sclerotome to form centrum (body of vertebra), Thus, body of each vertebra develops from 2 adjacent sclerotomes.[MCQ]

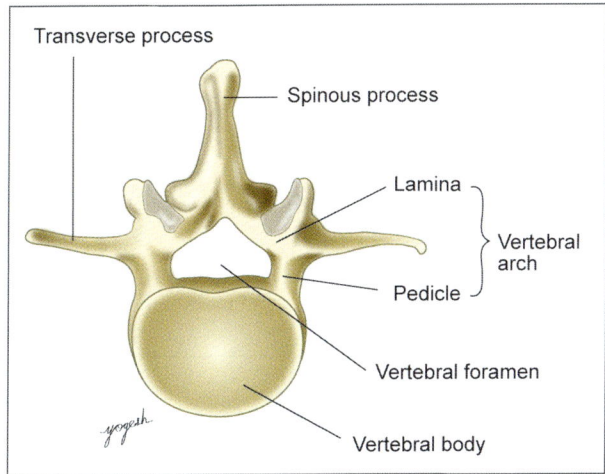

Fig. 26.5: Parts of typical vertebra

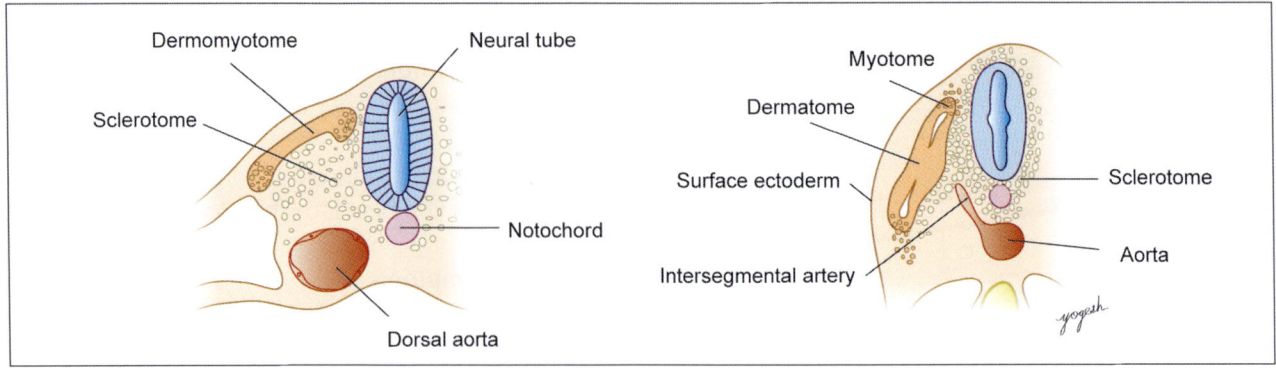

Fig. 26.6: Sclerotome

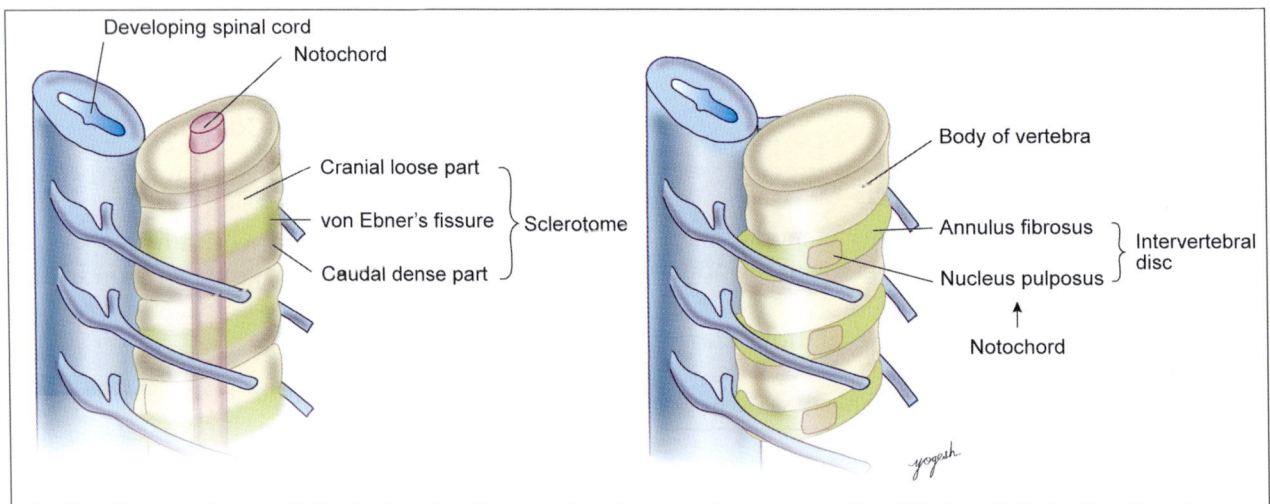

Fig. 26.7: Role of sclerotome in the formation of body of vertebrae

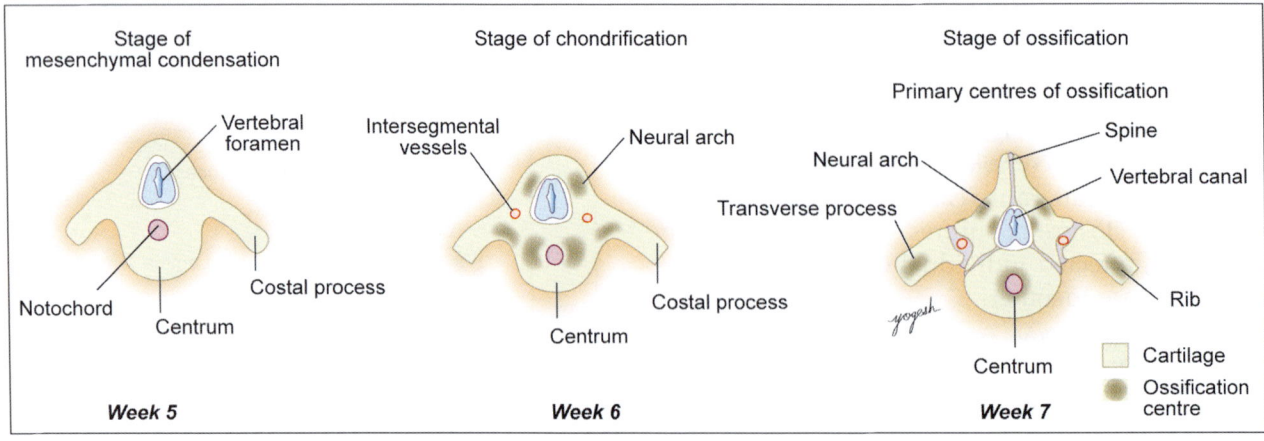

Fig. 26.8: Development of vertebra

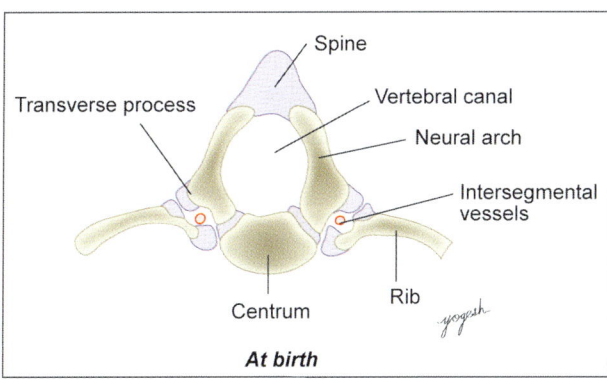

Fig. 26.9: Vertebra at birth

2. Dorsal group covers the neural tube and form vertebral arch and spine of vertebrae.
3. Venterolateral group forms costal elements.

- Notochord regresses slowly except at intervertebral disc, it forms nucleus pulposus.^{Neet}

Chondrification stage
- During the 6th week of IUL, chondrification of mesenchymal vertebrae begins.

Ossification stage
- Ossification of vertebrae begins in intrauterine life and continues up to 25 years of age.
- 3 primary centres: 1 for centrum, 1 for each half of the vertebral arch. At birth, each vertebra has 3 parts (body and two halves of vertebral arch) connected by cartilages (Fig. 26.8).
- 3–6 years: 2 halves vertebral arches fuse with each other as well as with centrum. Thus, vertebral arch (neural arch) of developing vertebra forms pedicel, laminae, spine and articular processes.
- Secondary centres: Total 5 centres: 1 for tip of each transverse process, 1 for tip of spinous process and 1 for upper and 1 for lower surface of body of vertebra (Fig. 26.10).

- 25 years: All secondary centres fuses with rest of the vertebra.
- Resegmentation of sclerotomes: Each sclerotome is divided into cranial and caudal portions by a transverse line called intrasegmental boundary or von Ebner's fissure. Later, the caudal segment of each sclerotome fuses with the cranial segment of the sclerotome caudal to it, with each of the two segments of the sclerotome contributing to a vertebra. This process is called resegmentation of the sclerotomes. Hence, the vertebrae are intersegmental in development.^{MCQ}
- At the intrasegmental boundary, the fibrous intervertebral discs develop. Notochordal cells form a gelatinous core called nucleus pulposus, whereas the surrounding annulus fibrosus develops from sclerotomal cells that are left in the region of the resegmentating sclerotome.
- The sclerotomes of the first four somites (occipital somites) fuse to form the occipital bone of skull. Eight cervical somites form only seven cervical sclerotomes. The sclerotome of the 1st cervical sclerotome fuses with the caudal half of the 4th occipital sclerotome and contributes to the base of the skull. The caudal half of the 1st cervical sclerotome fuses with the cranial half of the 2nd cervical sclerotome to form the 1st cervical vertebra (atlas).

> **Box 26.2:** Costal element and transverse element (Fig. 26.11)
>
> - Each vertebra shows transverse and costal elements that have different derivatives in different regions.
>
> Derivatives of costal element
> - In cervical region: Anterior root, anterior tubercle, costotransverse bar and posterior tubercle^{MCQ}
> - In thoracic region: Rib^{MCQ}
> - In lumbar region: Transverse process
> - In sacral region: Anterior 2/3rd of lateral mass
>
> Transverse element
> - In cervical region: Posterior root
> - In thoracic region: Transverse process^{MCQ}
> - In lumbar region: Mamillary process, accessory mamillary process^{MCQ}
> - In sacral region: Posterior 1/3rd of lateral mass

Congenital Anomalies of Vertebral Column

1. Spina bifida: Two halves of vertebral arch (neural arch) fail to fuse. For details, read Chapter 22. Spina bifida is the most serious vertebral defect. Rachischisis is the most serious form of spina bifida.^{MCQ}

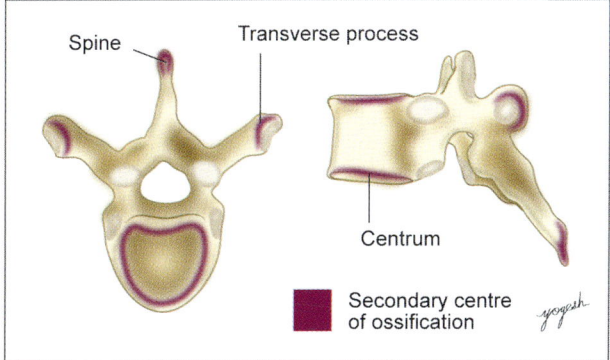

Fig. 26.10: Secondary centres of ossification for vertebra

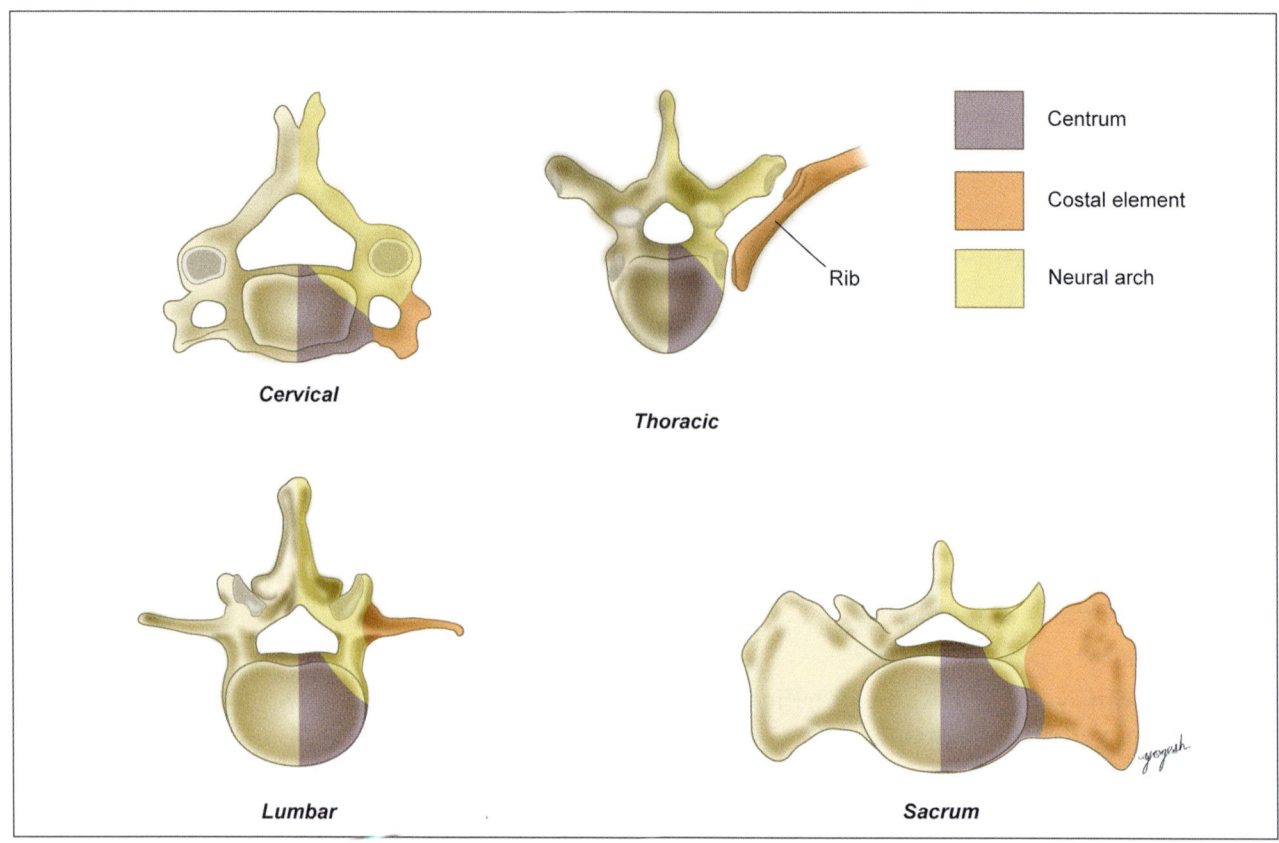

Fig. 26.11: Contribution of centrum, costal element and neural arch in the formation of vertebrae

2. **Hemivertebra:** Usually vertebral body ossifies from two primary centres. Failure of one of these primary centres may result in absence of half of the vertebral body (hemivertebra) and absence of corresponding rib. Hemivertebra is invariably associated with congenital scoliosis (lateral bending of vertebral column).
3. **Klippel-Feil syndrome:** It is congenital fusion of one or more cervical vertebra.^{Neet}
4. **Occipitalisation of atlas vertebra:** In this condition, atlas vertebra fuses with the occipital bone.
5. **Sacralisation of 5th lumbar vertebra:** It involves fusion of 5th lumbar vertebra with sacrum.
6. **Lumbarisation of 1st sacral vertebra:** It involves fusion of 1st sacral vertebra with 5th lumbar vertebra. Here, 1st sacral vertebra remains separated from rest of the sacrum.
7. **Spondylolisthesis:** It is a slippage (displacement) of vertebral body. Failure of formation of articular facet may cause spondylolisthesis. It commonly involves anterior displacement of 5th lumbar vertebra over the sacrum.

Development of Ribs

- Ribs are derived from ventral extensions of costal elements of the thoracic vertebrae.^{MCQ}
- Costal elements (arches) that later ossify to form the ribs.
- The mesenchyme near the junction of transverse process and costal arch undergo differentiation to form *costotransverse joint.*

Accessory ribs

- **Cervical rib:** It develops from costal element of the 7th cervical vertebra. It produces superior thoracic outlet syndrome due to compression of lower trunk of brachial plexus and subclavian artery.^{MCQ}
- **Lumbar rib:** It is occasionaly present but remains asymptomatic in most of the cases.

Development of Sternum

- Sternum develops from mesodermal condensation (lateral plate mesoderm) in the anterior body wall (Fig. 26.12).

Stages of development

1. **Formation of sternal bars:** In midline, the lateral plate mesoderm of anterior body wall forms two mesenchymal sternal bars that undergo chondrification and develop cartilaginous sternal bars.
2. **Formation of cartilaginous sternum model:** Two cartilaginous sternal bars fuse in the midline to form cartilaginous sternum model that has manubrium,

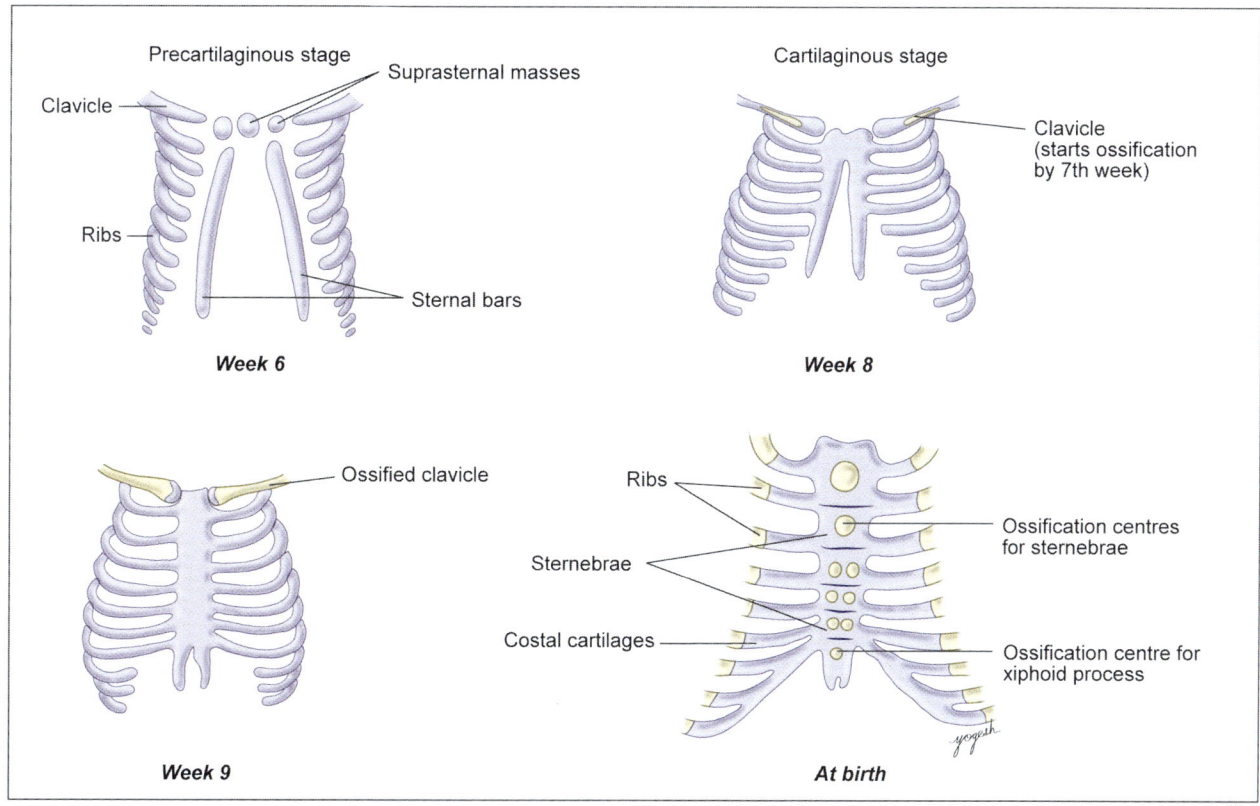

Fig. 26.12: Development of sternum

body and xiphoid process. Body consists of four fused segments called sternebrae.
3. Ossification of sternum
   - Ossification centres for sternum appear before birth except for the xiphoid (occurs in childhood).
   - For manubrium: A pair of ossification centres appears in 5th month of IUL
   - For body: 4 pairs of ossification centres appear in 6th, 7th, 8th, 9th month of IUL (from above downwards). Each pair of centres fuses to form sternebrae. Fusion of four sternebrae takes place from below upward and completes by 25 years of age.
   - For xiphoid process—centre appears in 3rd year of life and fuses with body by 40 years.

Abnormalities of sternum
1. Bifid sternum: Failure of fusion of two sternal bars may result in sternal foramen, sternal cleft, bifid sternum or bifid xiphoid process.
2. Funnel chest: Due to abnormally short central tendon of diaphragm, lower part of sternum and ribs are drawn inwards into the thorax. This condition is called *funnel chest*.[MCQ] Funnel chest is the most common congenital anomaly of the chest.
3. Pigeon chest (pectus carinatum): It involves forward projection of upper part of sternum and ribs.

Development of Skull (Cranium)
- Mesenchyme surrounding the developing brain condenses to form cranium (skull). Skull consists of
  1. Neurocranium: These bones enclose and protect the brain.
  2. Viscerocranium: These bones form facial skeleton.
- Neurocranium is divided into:
  – Chondrocranium: It forms bones of skull base.
  – Membranous neurocranium: It forms bones of skull vault.
- Viscerocranium is also divided into cartilaginous and membranous viscerocranium.

Chondrocranium (Fig. 26.13)
- At the 6th week of IUL, the cartilaginous neurocranium (chondrocranium) forms by fusion of several cartilages.
- Endochondral ossification starts forming the bones of skullbase.
- The cartilages are as follows:
  – Parachordal cartilage (basal plate) appears around the cranial end of notochord. It forms base of occipital bone and boundaries of foramen magnum.
  – Hypophyseal cartilage appears around the pituitary gland and forms body of sphenoid bone.

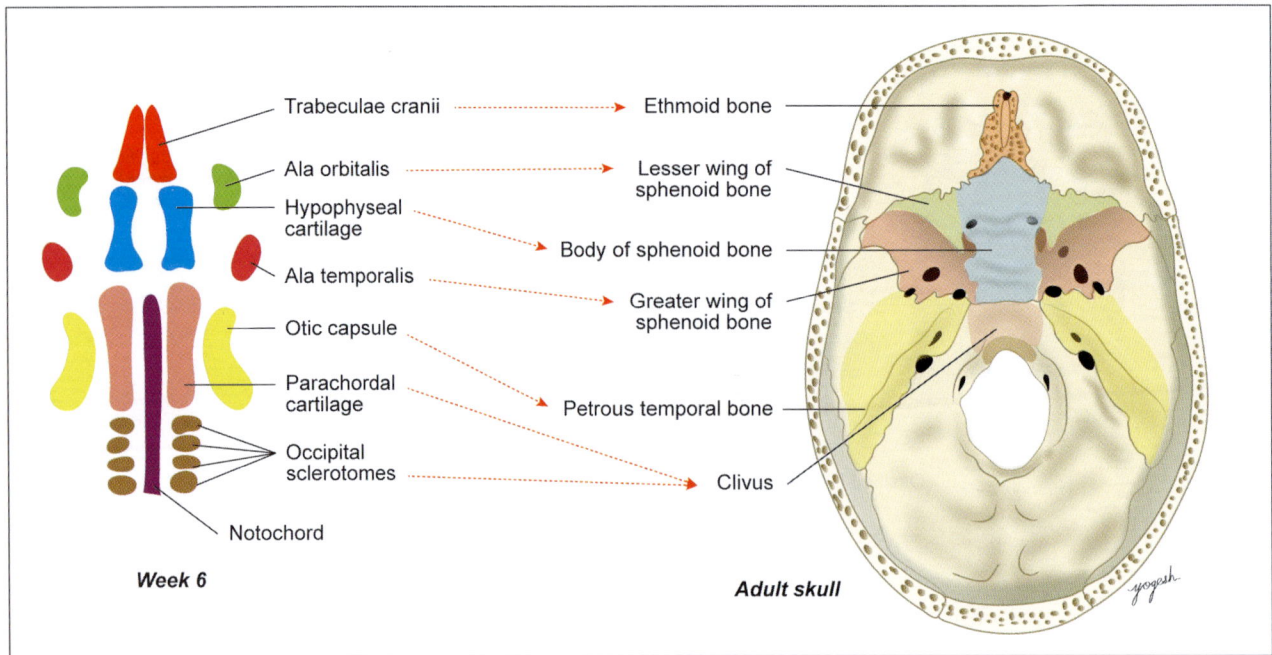

Fig. 26.13: Developmental components of chondrocranium and their derivatives

- Trabeculae crania form body of ethmoid bone.
- Ala orbitalis forms lesser wing of sphenoid bone.
- Otic capsule forms bony labyrinth, petrous and mastoid part of temporal bone.
- Nasal capsule contributes to ethmoid bone.
- Ala temporalis forms greater wing of sphenoid bone.

Membranous neurocranium
- Membranous ossification develops calvaria (cranial vault) on sides and top of the brain.
- The bones of skull vault are separated by sutures (fibrous joints).
- At 6 places, the sutures are wide and they form a gap called *fontanelles*. Modelling of foetal cranium during birth passage is possible due to the fontanelles.

Cartilaginous viscerocranium
- Cartilaginous viscerocranium is constituted by contribution from first and second pharyngeal arch cartilages as follows:
  a. First arch cartilage forms malleus and incus.^{MCQ}
  b. Second arch cartilage forms stapes and styloid process of temporal bone.^{MCQ}

Membranous viscerocranium
- Intramembranous ossification forms the following bones.
  Squamous part of temporal bone
  Maxillary and zygomatic bones
  Mandible (mandibular condyle and chin of mandible shows endochondral ossification)

Cranium in newborn
- In newborn, the cranium is large in proportion to that of the rest of body skeleton.
- In newborn, neurocranium is larger than viscerocranium because of:
  1. Underdeveloped jaw bone.
  2. Absence of paranasal air sinuses.
  3. Underdeveloped facial bones.

> **Box 26.3:** Fontanelles (Fig. 26.14)
> - Fontanelles are soft membrane gaps present in the skull vault of newborn.
> - These are 6 fontanelles at birth as follows:
>   - *Anterior fontanelle* between frontal and parietal bones. Anterior fontanelle is the largest fontanelle. ^{MCQ}
>   - *Posterior fontanelle* between occipital and parietal bones.
>   - *Anterolateral (sphenoid) fontanelle* between greater wing of sphenoid, squamous temporal, frontal and parietal bones.
>   - *Posterolateral (mastoid) fontanelle* between parietal, occipital, squamous temporal and occipital bones.
> - Closure of fontanelle
>   - All fontanelles close within 3–4 months after birth.
>   - Anterior fontanelle closes by 2–3 years of age.^{MCQ}

Contd.

Skeletal System and Limbs

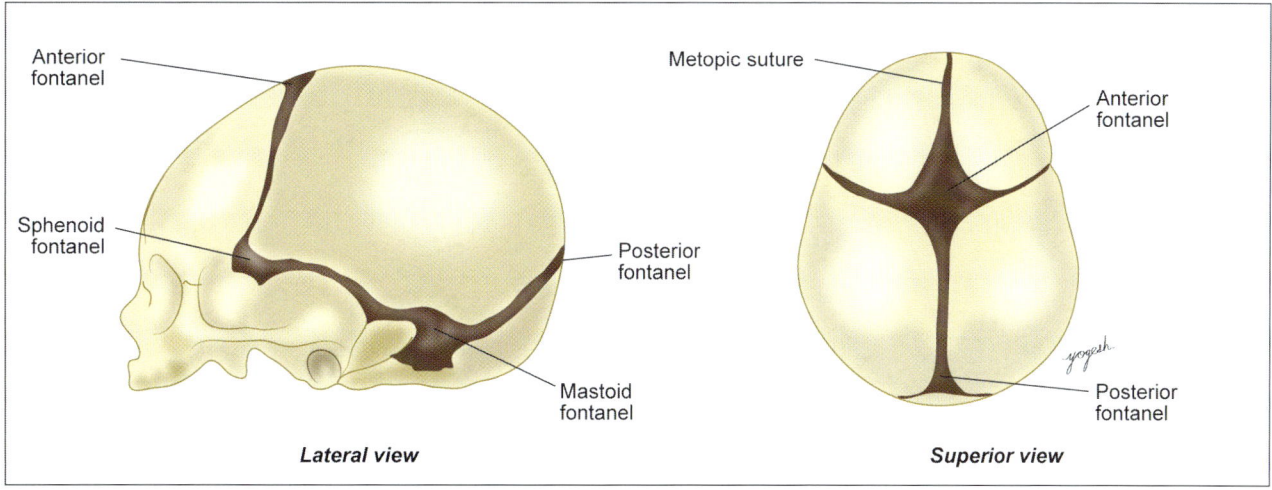

Fig. 26.14: Skull of the newborn showing fontanelles

Contd.

- Function of fontanelles
  - Allow moulding of skull during the birth passage of body.
  - Permit growth of skull bones to increase the cranial capacity.
  - Accommodate developing brain.
- Clinical aspects
  1. Closure of fontanelles gives an idea about the age of the newborn.
  2. Appearance of fontanelle gives an idea of intracranial pressure.
     - Bulging fontanelles indicate increased intracranial pressure.
     - Depressed fontanelles indicate dehydration cases.

Anomalies of Skull

1. Anencephaly: Major portion of brain, skull and scalp are absent in anencephaly. Anencephaly is most severe birth defect in stillborn babies.
2. Cleidocranial dysostosis: It involves absence of clavicle, nonclosure of metopic suture (between frontal bones), prominent forehead and abnormal teeth.
3. Scaphocephaly: Early closure of sagittal suture results in scaphocephaly. It shows boat-shaped skull (long narrow head).^{MCQ}
4. Brachycephaly: Early closure of coronal suture results in short skull (brachycephaly).
5. Plagiocephaly: Early closure of coronal and lambdoid sutures on one side results into grossly unequal curvatures of skull (plagiocephaly).
6. Trigonocephaly: Early closure of metopic suture results in triangular-shaped forehead (trigonocephaly).
7. Hydrocephalus: In this condition, the skull bones may be widely separated due to increased intracranial pressure.
8. Hand-Schüller-Christian disease: It is defect of reticuloendothelial system (Langerhans cell histiocytosis) associated with lytic bone lesions of the skull.^{Neet}

DEVELOPMENT OF LIMBS

Limbs develop from mesenchyme of limb buds as follows (Figs 26.15 and 26.16, SEM 26.1 and 26.2):

Formation of limb bud primordia

- At the end of 4th week, small elevations of limb bud primordia appear on the ventrolateral body wall.

Formation of limb bud

- In second month, limb primordia enlarge as paddle-shaped outgrowths on surface ectoderm to form *limb buds*.
- Forelimb bud grows faster than lower limb buds.

Formation of limbs

- In the 6th week, limb bud shows thickening at the tip called *apical ectodermal ridge*. Limb bud starts differentiation to form arm-forearm-hand and thigh-leg-foot in respective limb buds.
- Chondroblasts forms cartilaginous models for development of limb bones.
- Myoblasts form muscle masses.
- Hand differentiates to form palm and digits and foot differentiates to form sole and toes.

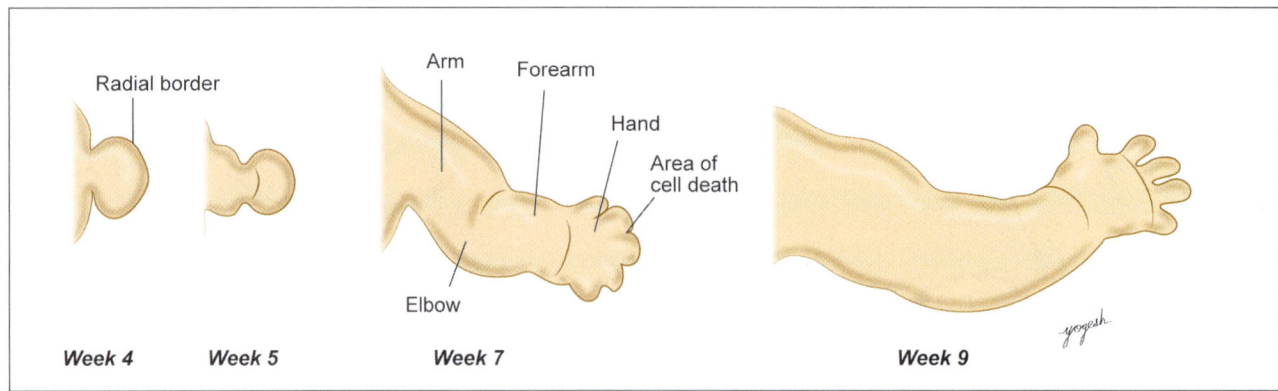

Fig. 26.15: Development of upper limb

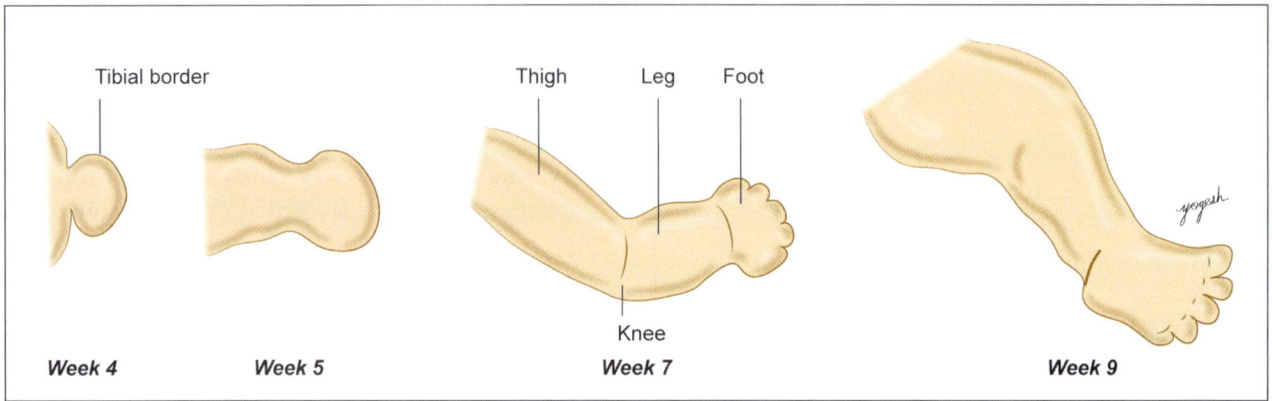

Fig. 26.16: Development of lower limb

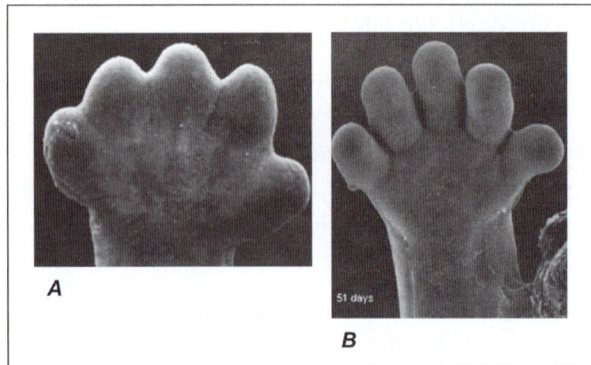

Scanning electron micrograph 26.1: Development of hand. During the seventh and eighth weeks of development the digits of hand become apparent: (A) 48 days; (B) 51 days. [Species: Human]

Rotation of limbs
- In the 7th week, upper limbs rotate laterally through 90° along their long axes and extensor surface comes to lie on dorsal aspects of the arm.
- Lower limbs rotate medially through 90° along their long axes and extensor surface comes to lie on ventral aspect of leg.

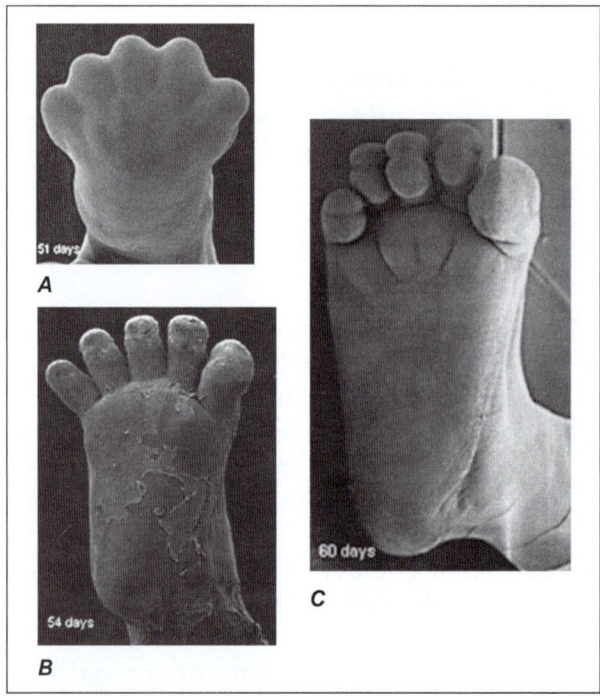

Scanning electron micrograph 26.2: Development of foot. Development of the foot is like that of the hand. It starts approximately 3–4 days later: (A) 51 days; (B) 54 days; (C) 60 days [Species: Human]

- Rotation makes preaxial border laterally in upper limb (thumb) and medially in lower limbs (greater toe).

Blood supply and nerve supply

- Limb buds are supplied by axis artery. For detailed development of axis artery of limbs, refer to Chapter 19.
- Dermatome is the area of skin supplied by a single spinal nerve.
- Upper limb receives supply from C4–8 and T1–2 spinal nerves.
- Lower limb receives supply from L2–5 and S1–2 spinal nerves.
- As the limb elongates, sensory nerves also migrate out.

Anomalies of Limbs

1. Amelia: It is complete absence of all four limbs.
2. Phocomelia: It involves rudimentary hands and feet that are directly attached to the trunk.^{MCQ}
3. Meromelia: It is shortening of all the segments of the limb.
4. Syndactyly (fused or webbed digits): It results due to failure of differentiation between two or more digits.^{MCQ}
5. Polydactyly (supernumerary digits): In this condition, there is an extra digit or phalanx on the hand or foot. Polydactyly is the most common anomaly of fingers and toes.
6. Brachydactyly: In this condition, there is an abnormal shortness of the fingers due to absence of phalynx.
7. Cleft hand or foot (Lobster-claw deformity): In this condition, one or more central digits are absent resulting in a wide cleft in hand or foot. Remaining digit may be separate or fused.
8. Club hand (congenital absence of radius): In this condition, radius is absent, ulna is bowed and hand deviates to lateral side.^{MCQ}
9. Club foot (talipes equinovarus): In this condition, the foot is turned inward and it remains inverted (adducted and plantar flexed).^{MCQ}
10. Congenital dislocation of hip: Due to lax joint capsule of hip joint and underdeveloped acetabulum at birth, dislocation of hip may occur. Its incidence is 1 in 1500 newborn and more common in females.
11. Sirenomelia (sympodia): In this condition, the lower limbs are fused. Foot may be separated or fused.^{MCQ}

DEVELOPMENT OF JOINTS

- The mesenchymal tissue between two bones differentiates to form joint.
- Type of joint depends on the differentiation of mesenchyme:
  - If mesenchyme differentiates into fibrous tissue—fibrous joint (syndesmosis).
  - If mesenchyme differentiates into cartilage—cartilaginous (primary or secondary cartilaginous joint).
  - If mesenchyme differentiates into three layers as outer two layers continuous with perichondrium of cartilages at ends of bones and middle layer degenerates to form joint cavity and synovial membrane—synovial joint.

CLINICAL EMBRYOLOGY

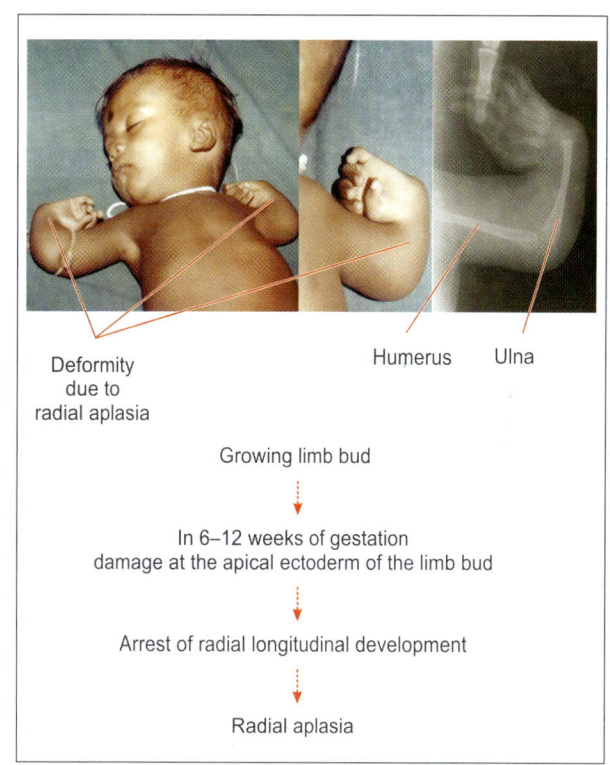

Clinical image 26.1: A case of bilateral radial aplasia (absence of radius). Incidence is 1 in 30,000 births and it occurs bilaterally in 50% of cases (Image courtesy: *Dr Kumaravel S*)

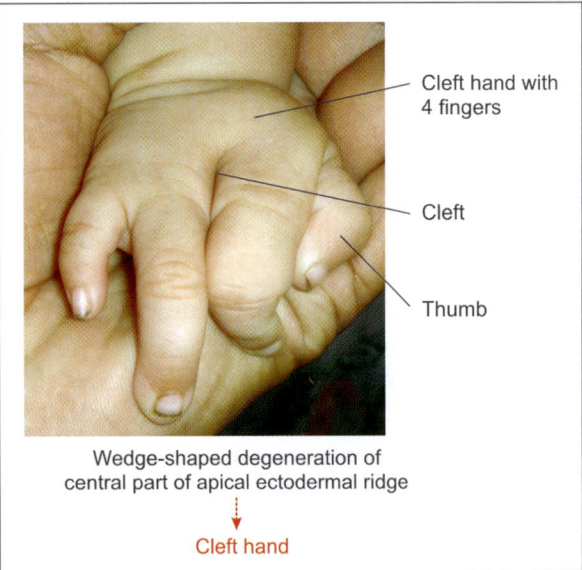

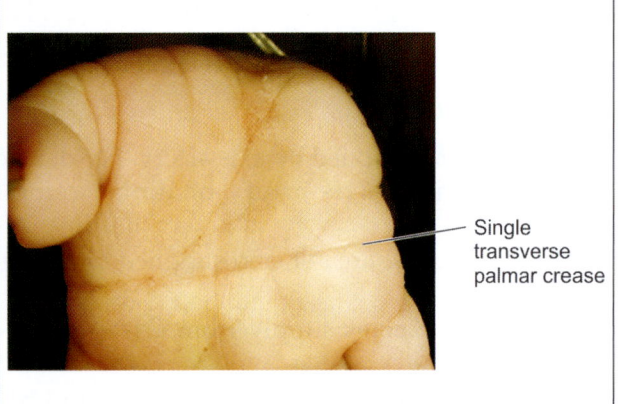

Clinical Image 26.2: Cleft hand of the right side with four fingers. Cleft hand (lobster-claw deformity) is characterised by the absence of 1 or more central digits of the hand and V-shaped cleft in the centre of the hand. Incidence is 1:10,000 to 1:90,000 and more common in males than in females (5:1). It is inherited as an autosomal dominant disorder in 70% cases (Image courtesy: *Dr Kumaravel S*)

Clinical image 26.3: Single transverse palmar crease. Usually, in humans, two transverse palmar creases are present (proximal and distal). In the present case, a single transverse palmar crease (Simian crease) formed by the fusion of the two palmar creases is present. Here, it is associated with Down Syndrome (facial features are not shown). It is present in 1.5% of the general population in at least one hand. The individual may be asymptomatic or may be associated with genetic chromosomal abnormalities such as Down syndrome, cri du chat syndrome, Klinefelter syndrome, Wolf-Hirschhorn syndrome, Noonan syndrome, Patau syndrome and Edward syndrome (Image courtesy: *Dr Kumaravel S*)

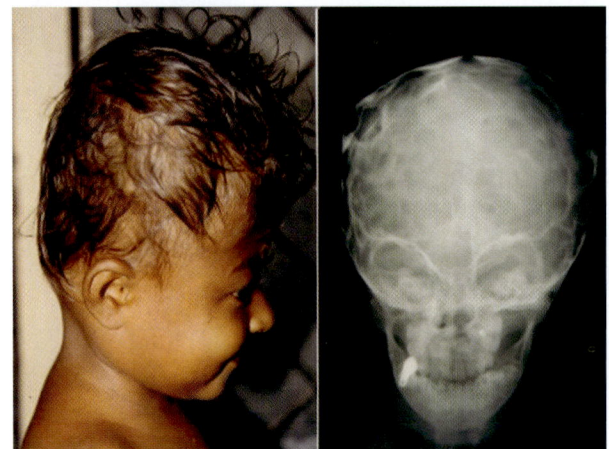

Clinical image 26.4: Scaphocephaly. Craniosynostosis involves premature ossification (fusion) of sutures. It causes alternation of the growth pattern of the skull and abnormal head shape. Scaphocephaly (premature fusion of sagittal sutures) is the most common craniosynostosis and is characterised by a long, narrow head that resembles an inverted boat (skaphe meaning 'light boat or skiff' and kephale meaning 'head' in Greek) (Image courtesy: *Dr Kumaravel S*)

27
Muscular System

Chapter Outline

- Development of skeletal muscles
  - Histogenesis of skeletal muscle
- Development of individual group muscle
  - Muscles of body wall
  - Extraocular muscles
  - Muscles of tongue
  - Muscles of pharyngeal arches
  - Muscles of limbs
  - Congenital anomalies of skeletal muscles
- Duchenne muscular dystrophy
- Development of smooth muscles
- Development of cardiac muscle

INTRODUCTION

- All the muscles of the body are derived from mesoderm except muscles of iris, arrector pili of skin and myoepithelial cells of glands. These are derived from ectoderm (neural crest).
- Muscles are classified as follows:
  A. Striated muscles: These show cytoplasmic striations of actin and myosin filaments. These are of two types:
    1. Skeletal muscles: These are responsible for the movement of bones and are derived from paraxial mesoderm (somites).
    2. Cardiac muscles: These are in myocardium and develop from splanchnopleuric mesoderm.
  B. Smooth muscles: These do not show cytoplasmic striations (hence, smooth) and develop from splanchnopleuric mesoderm.
- Skeletal muscles are voluntary, whereas cardiac and smooth muscles are involuntary.

DEVELOPMENT OF SKELETAL MUSCLES

- Skeletal muscles develop from somites.

Histogenesis of Skeletal Muscle

- Each *somite* has dorsolateral dermomyotome and venteromedial sclerotome
- Dermomyotome differentiates into superficial dermatome and deep myotome.
- Mesenchyme of myotome differentiates into *myoblasts* (primordial muscle cells).
- Myoblasts elongate and fuse at ends with each other to form multinucleated *myotube* (syncytium).
- Myotubes synthesize muscle proteins (actin, myosin, troponin and so on) and become muscle fibres. Muscle proteins push the nuclei to periphery (Fig. 27.1).
- Adjacent muscle fibres form bundles, fascicle and complete muscle.

Some Interesting Facts

1. Extraocular muscles develop from *preotic myotomes*.
2. Muscles of tongue (except palatoglossus) develop from *occipital myotomes*.
3. Skeletal muscle loses mitotic activity after birth, but they can undergo hypertrophy.

DEVELOPMENT OF INDIVIDUAL GROUP MUSCLE

The skeletal muscles can be grouped on the basis of development into the following groups:
1. Muscles of trunk (body wall)
2. Muscles of branchial arches

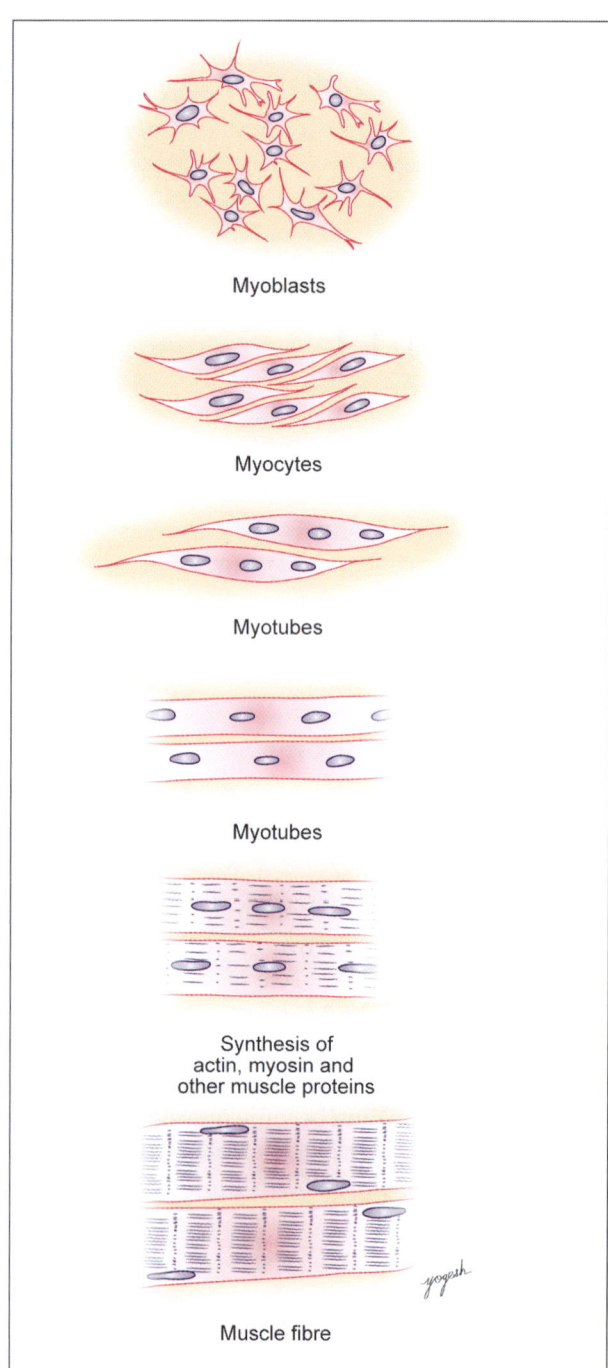

Fig. 27.1: Histogenesis of muscle fibre

3. Extraocular muscles
4. Muscles of tongue
5. Muscles of limbs

Muscles of Body Wall

- Muscles of body wall develop from myotomes of somites.
- Each myotome has two parts:
  A. Epaxial part (epimere): It is a smaller dorsal part. It forms extensor muscles of vertebral column; for example, erector spinae.
  B. Hypomere (hypaxial part): It is a larger ventral part. It forms the following muscles of the body wall:
    - Intercostal muscles
    - Muscles of anterior abdominal wall
    - Muscles of neck (longus coli, longus capitis and scalene muscles)
    - Muscles of ventral midline longitudinal column (rectus abdominis, rectus sternalis, infrahyoid muscles). These are also called strap muscles.
- Developmentally, scalene group of muscles corresponds to the intercostal muscles of thoracic cage.^{MCQ}
- Muscles of diaphragm correspond to transverse thoracic muscle (innermost muscle column).^{MCQ}
- Similarly, muscles of pelvic diaphragm develop from innermost muscle column.^{MCQ} Morphologically, medial fibres of levator ani represent the downward continuation of rectus abdominis muscle (longitudinal column).^{Neet}
- Nerve supply: Muscle of epimere are supplied by dorsal ramus of spinal nerve, whereas muscles of hypomere are supplied by ventral ramus of spinal nerve (Fig. 27.2).

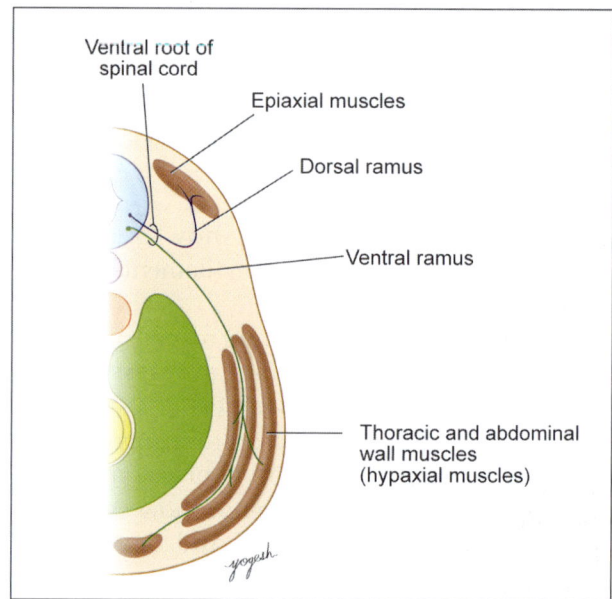

Fig. 27.2: Nerve supply of trunk muscles

Extraocular Muscles

- Extraocular muscles develop from 3 preotic myotomes (Fig. 27.3).^{MCQ}
- Nerve supply: $^{MCQ,\ Viva}$
  3rd cranial nerve: Inferior oblique, levator palpabrae superioris, medial rectus and inferior rectus.
  4th cranial nerve: Superior oblique.
  6th cranial nerve: Lateral rectus.

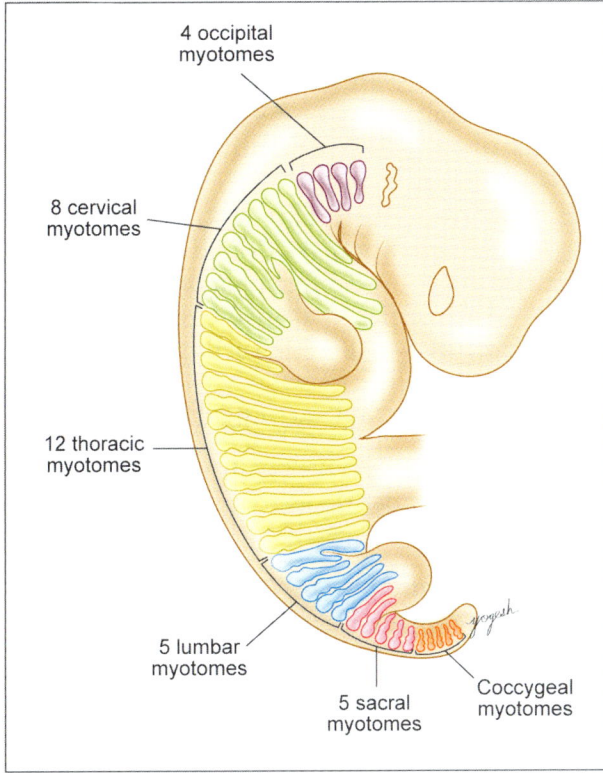

Fig. 27.3: Myotomes

Muscles of Tongue

- All the muscles of tongue (extrinsic and intrinsic) except palatoglossus are derived from 4 occipital myotomes.
- Hypoglossal nerve (precervical nerve) supplies the derivatives of occipital (precervical) myotomes.^{MCQ}
- Occipital myotomes migrate from cervical region to developing tongue along the epipericardial ridge. During migration, hypoglossal nerve transverses superficial to external and internal carotid arteries.^{Clinical fact}

Muscles of Pharyngeal Arches

- Muscles of pharyngeal arches develop from mesoderm of pharyngeal arches.
- The muscular derivatives of pharyngeal arches are as follows:^{High yielding facts, Neet}

  1st arch: Muscle of mastication (temporalis, masseter, lateral and medial pterygoid), tensor tympani, tensor veli palatini, anterior belly of digastric, mylohyoid
  2nd arch: Muscles of facial expression, posterior belly of digastric, stapedius, stylohyoid
  3rd arch: Stylopharyngeus
  4th arch: Cricothyroid, constrictors of pharynx, muscles of palate except tensor vili palatini
  6th arch: Intrinsic muscles of larynx except cricothyroid

Muscles of Limbs

- In the 5th week, myotomes of limb bud form anterior and posterior condensations.
- Anterior mesenchymal condensation forms flexor and pronator muscles in upper limb, whereas extensor and adductor muscles in lower limb.
- Posterior mesenchymal condensation forms extensor and supinator muscles in upper limb, whereas flexor and muscles in lower limb (Fig. 27.4).

Congenital Anomalies of Skeletal Muscles

1. Duchenne muscular dystrophy: Box 27.1.
2. A skeletal muscle may be partially or completely absent.
3. A muscle may show accessory head (origin).
4. Poland sequence is absence of pectoralis minor and partial absence of pectoralis major muscles. There may be absence or displaced nipple and areola, syndactyly (fused fingers) or brachydactyly (less number of fingers).
5. Congenital torticollis: Excessive stretching of sternocleidomastoid muscle during delivery causes shortening of this muscle (torticollis).^{MCQ}

Box 27.1: Duchenne muscular dystrophy (DMD)

Q. Write short note on Duchenne muscular dystrophy.

- DMD is a hereditary muscular dystrophy (progressive weakening of muscle)

Cause
- It is X-linked recessive disorder.
- Mutation of gene responsible for production of protein dystropin (essential for maintenance of cell membrane of muscle fibre).

Incidence
- 1 in 4000 males at birth.
- Most common type of muscular dystrophy.

Signs and symptoms
- Severe progressive muscle degeneration.
- Loss of ability to walk by 9–12 years of age.
- Death by the age of 20 years due to respiratory failure.

Treatment
- No cure treatment is available.
- Steroids can be given to slow down muscle dystrophy.
- Other supportive measure (breathing assistance, braces and so on) may be required.

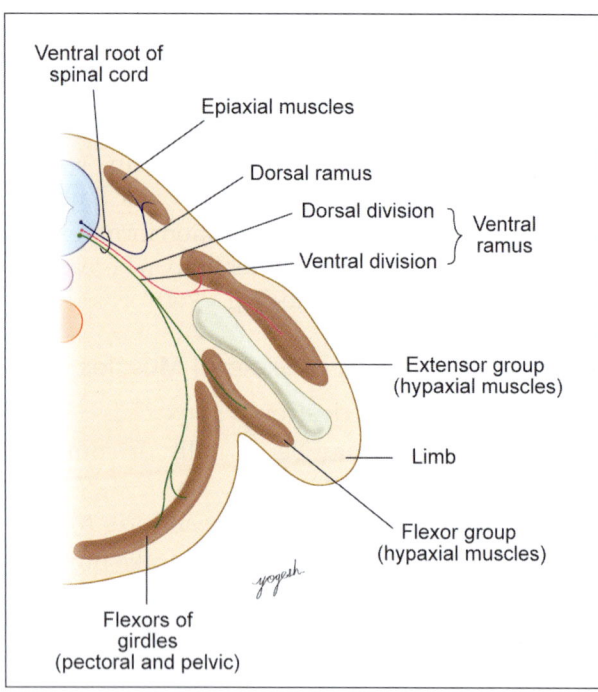

Fig. 27.4: Nerve supply of limb muscles

DEVELOPMENT OF SMOOTH MUSCLES

- Mesenchymal tissue differentiates into myoblast that later forms spindle-shaped smooth muscle cells.
- Smooth muscles are derived from the following sources:
  1. Splanchnopleuric mesoderm forms smooth muscles of gastrointestinal tract and respiratory tract.^{MCQ}
  2. Intermediate mesoderm forms smooth muscles in urogenital system.^{MCQ}
  3. Surrounding mesenchyme forms smooth muscles in developing vessels and lymph vessels.
  4. Neuroectoderm of optic cup forms muscles of iris (sphincter and dilator pupilae) and ciliaris muscle.^{MCQ}
  5. Arrector pili muscles of skin and myoepithelial cells of mammary gland are derived from ectoderm.^{MCQ}
  6. Serum response factor (SRF) (transcription protein) is responsible for differentiation of smooth muscle cell differentiation. Myocardin and myocardin-related transcription factors are cofactors that enhance the activity of SRF.

DEVELOPMENT OF CARDIAC MUSCLE

- The cardiac muscle develops from mesenchyme of myoepicardial mantle (part of splanchnic mesoderm).

Histogenesis of cardiac muscle

- In cardiac muscle development, each myoblast elongates and gives rise to numerous side branches.
- These side branches of adjacent cells come in contact with each other.
- At the point of contact, cell membrane modifies to form *intercalated disc*.
- Thus, cardiac muscle does not form true syncytium.

Some Interesting Facts
• First occipital myotome disappears soon after its formation.
• Rectus sternalis in thorax represents its abdominal counterpart rectus abdominis.^{Neet}
• Myoepithelial cells of secretory acini of glands, myoid cells of seminiferous tubules and myofibroblasts of healing wound are also contractile (non-muscular) cells.^{MCQ}

28

Foetal Period
Nine Weeks to Birth

Chapter Outline

- Growth of foetus
  - Changes in 3rd month
  - Changes in 4th month
  - Changes in 5th month
  - Changes in 6th month
  - Changes in 7th month
  - Changes in 8th month
  - Changes in 9th month
- Factor influencing growth

INTRODUCTION

- Embryologically prenatal period is divided into
  1. Germinal/ovular period: It consists of first three weeks of development after fertilisation.
  2. Embryonic period: It extends from 4th week to 8th week of development.^{Neet}
  3. Foetal period (organ growth): It extends from 9th week (3rd month) up to the termination of the pregnancy.

Gestation

- The period of development in the uterus, between conception and birth is called *gestation*.
- Length of gestational period: 280 days (40 weeks/ 9 months ± 7 days).
- Gestation means menstrual age in Latin.
- Gestational period (menstrual age) begins from 1st day of last menstrual phase prior to the conception.

Use of gestational period

- It can be used to calculate the expected date of delivery as follows:

  (Date of onset of last menstrual period) + 9 months 7 days = expected date of delivery (EDD)^{Viva}
- Thus, embryologically the age of foetus (fertilisation age) is 14 days less than the gestational age.
- *Note*: 14 days are considered as duration of the last menstrual cycle up to fertilisation.

GROWTH OF FOETUS

- In the foetal period, foetus grows rapidly to give shape of the newborn.
- All body parts undergo considerable growth and cellular and functional differentiation.
- Major events during foetal period are listed below.

Changes in 3rd Month (9–12 Weeks) (Fig. 28.1)

1. At beginning of the 3rd month, head is about half of the foetal size. Body grows in crown-to-rump (CR) length and doubles by the 12th week.
2. Face: Broad face, widely spaced eyes, low sets of ears, fused eyelids.
3. Limbs: By the 12th week, the upper limb develops to take their normal shape, but lower limbs lag.
4. External genitalia: It remains undifferentiated till 9th week.
5. Umbilical hernia: Intestinal loop returns the abdominal cavity by 10th week.^{MCQ}

Changes in 4th Month (13–16 Weeks) (Fig. 28.1)

1. Head: It becomes comparatively smaller due to growth of other body parts.
2. CR length: Length of foetus increases rapidly.
3. Limbs: Limbs increase in length. Lower limb obtains its normal shape. Movements of limbs can be seen on ultrasound examination.

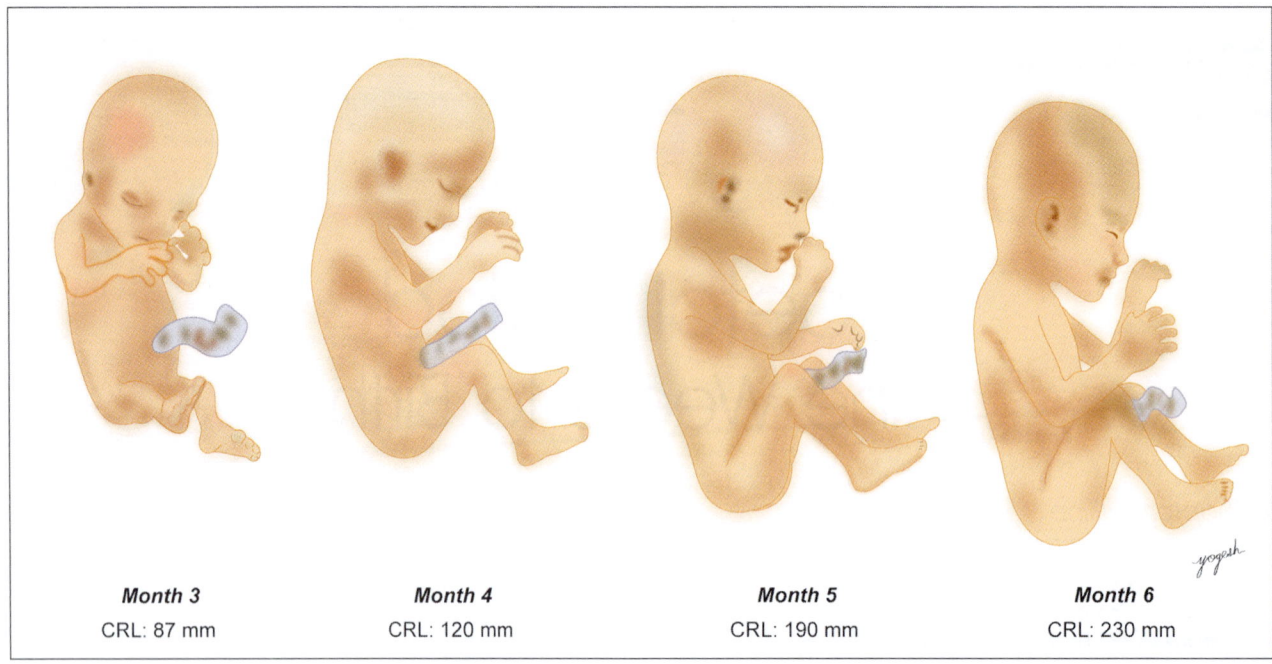

Fig. 28.1: Foetus of 3rd to 6th month of intrauterine life

Changes in 5th Month (17–20 Weeks) (Fig. 28.1)

1. CR length: Increases slowly up to 190 mm.
2. Quickening: Mother can feel foetal movements (quickening).
3. Vernix caseosa: Foetal skin is covered by greasy, chees-like material (*vernix caseosa*) secreted by sebaceous glands.^{MCQ}
4. Lanugo: By the end of 5th month, the foetus is fully covered by fine brown hairs (*lanugo*).^{MCQ}
5. Eyebrows and hairs on head become visible.

Changes in 6th Month (21–24 Weeks) (Fig. 28.1)

1. Skin: Due to the absence of subcutaneous tissue, skin is wrinkled, translucent and pink.
2. Lungs: Alveoli starts secreting surfactant.
3. Weight: Foetus starts getting weight.

Changes in 7th Month (25–29 Weeks) (Fig. 28.2)

1. Lungs: Foetus is *viable with supporting measures* as lung maturation is going on.
2. Blood formation: Bone marrow takes over the function of haematopoiesis from spleen.
3. CNS: Nervous system is matured to control respiration.

Changes in 8th Month (30–34 Weeks) (Fig. 28.2)

1. Skin: On the deposition of subcutaneous fat, skin becomes smooth.
2. Weight: Body weight increases rapidly.

Changes in 9th Month (35–38 Weeks) (Fig. 28.2)

1. Termination: Delivery takes place on 266 days (38 weeks) of fertilisation age or 280 days (40 weeks) of gestational age (after onset of last menstruation).^{Neet}
2. Testis: In male foetus, testes reach scrotum by the end of 9th month.^{Neet}
3. Fingernails: By 28th week, fingernails grow beyond fingertip.^{Neet}

FACTORS INFLUENCING GROWTH

Following factors play a major role in growth of the foetus:

1. Nutrition: Maternal nutrition has the highest impact on growth of the foetus. Maternal malnutrition causes foetal growth retardation.
2. Genetic factors: Growth depends on genetic constitution. Chromosomal/genetic abnormalities may lead to foetal growth retardation.
3. Placenta: Placental disorder affects the foetal growth due to insufficient uteroplacental blood flow.
4. Multiple pregnancies: Each foetus tends to be smaller than the normal single pregnancy due to distribution of available resources (nutrition and space).
5. Smoking, alcohol and drugs (thalidomide) may produce adverse foetal outcome.

Foetal Period: Nine Weeks to Birth

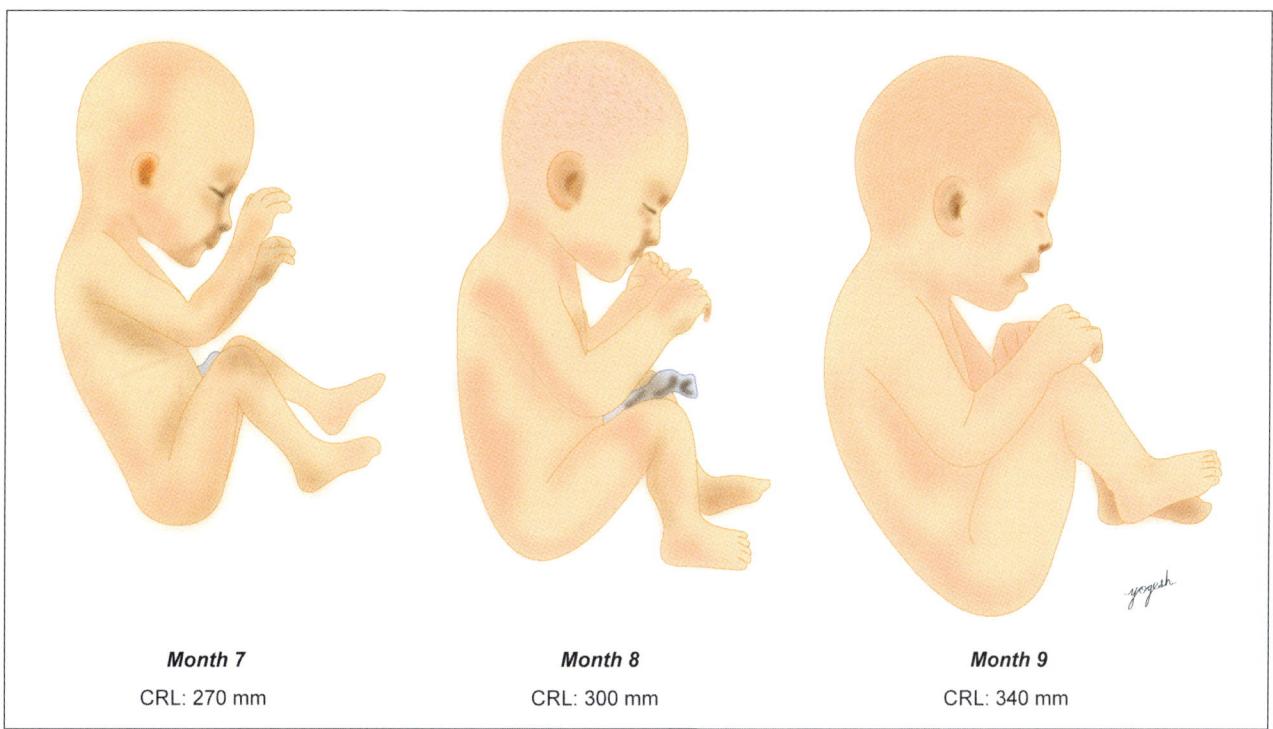

Month 7
CRL: 270 mm

Month 8
CRL: 300 mm

Month 9
CRL: 340 mm

Fig. 28.2: Foetus of 7th to 9th month of intrauterine life

CLINICAL EMBRYOLOGY

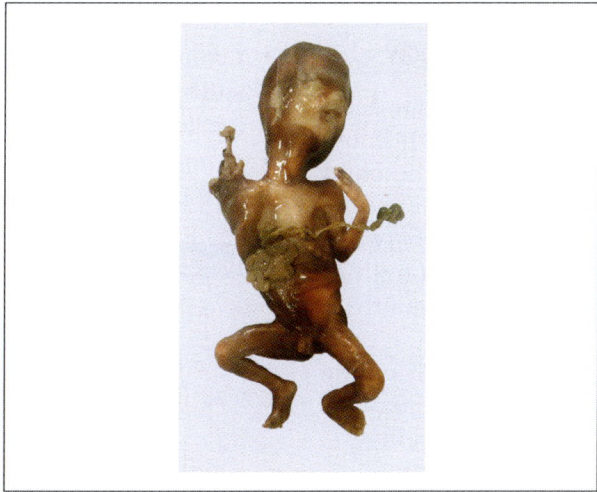

Clinical image 28.1: Foetus of second trimester (Image courtesy: *Dr Haritha Sagili*)

29
Clinical Applications and Ultrasonography in Embryology

Chapter Outline

Clinical applications in embryology
- Criteria for estimation of age in embryo
- Prenatal diagnosis
  - Amniocentesis
  - Chorionic villus sampling
  - Maternal blood screening
  - Percutaneous umbilical blood sampling
  - Fetoscopy

Ultrasonography in embryology
- Principle of ultrasonography
- Grey scale of ultrasound in obstetrics
- Ultrasound frequency
- Types
- Purpose of antenatal ultrasonography
- Classification of foetal sonographic examinations
- Indications for ultrasound examination
- Guidelines and parameters for ultrasonography

CLINICAL APPLICATIONS IN EMBRYOLOGY

- Obstetrics is the branch of the medicine that deals with the care of pregnant woman, unborn baby, labour and immediate period following the child birth.
- The period of development in the uterus, between conception and birth is called *gestation*. Length of gestational period: 280 days (40 weeks/9 months ± 7 days).
- During obstetrics practice, determination of the gestational age is important for the following reasons:
  1. For antenatal assessment of foetal well-being.
  2. For planning of termination of pregnancy.
  3. For taking decision about mode of delivery (normal vaginal or caesarean section).
  4. For taking decision about chorionic villus sampling or amniocentesis.
- Criteria for determination of age varies according to the age of the conceptus.

CRITERIA FOR ESTIMATION OF AGE IN EMBRYO

- The age of embryo (up to 8 weeks) can be determined by number of somites and crown to rump length.
- *Crown to rump length* (CR length): It is also called sitting length. It is measured from top of the skull (vertex) to the bottom of buttock (Table 29.1).
- *Crown to heel length* (CHL): It is measured from top of the skull (vertex) to the heel.

Table 29.1	Estimation of age in embryo	
Age (days)	Number of somites	CR length (mm)
20–21	1–7	1.5–3
22–23	7–13	2–3.5
24–25	13–19	2.5–4.5
26–27	19–24	3–5
28–30	24–35	4–6

Estimation of Age in Foetus (9–38 weeks)

- Foetal age can be determined by using the following parameters (Table 29.2):
  1. Crown to rump length (CR length)
  2. Foot length
  3. Weight of foetus

Clinical Applications and Ultrasonography in Embryology

Table 29.2 Foetal parameters for age estimation (approximate values)

Age (in weeks)	Crown to rump length (mm)	Weight (g)
9	50	8
10	61	14
12	87	45
16	120	200
20	190	460
24	230	820
28	270	1300
32	300	2100
36	340	2900
38	360	3400

PRENATAL DIAGNOSIS

- Pregnancy outcome depends on multiple factors such as genetic constitution, maternal factors and so on.
- Prenatal diagnosis is the application of available techniques to assess the status of foetus *in utero* and to detect the congenital malformations.
- The methods of prenatal diagnosis are classified as noninvasive methods, minimal invasive methods and invasive methods.
- Noninvasive methods include prenatal checkup and ultrasound examination. Minimal invasive techniques include maternal blood screening. Invasive methods include amniocentesis, chorionic villus sampling, fetoscopy, foetal blood sampling.

Amniocentesis

- Amniotic fluid (20 ml) is collected under ultrasound guidance during 14–20 weeks of IUL.
- Cells are assessed from amniotic fluid for chromosomal or genetic abnormalities.
- Amniotic fluid is also assessed for α-fetoprotein and other biochemical parameters.

Chorionic Villus Sampling (CVS)

- Chorionic villus tissue is collected under ultrasound guidance during 9–12 weeks of IUL.
- Cells are assessed for genetic and metabolic abnormalities.

Maternal Blood Screening

- Maternal blood screening (16 weeks onwards) includes assessment for circulating foetal cells, βhCG (human chorionic gonadotropin), α-fetoprotein, estriol and inhibin A.

Percutaneous Umbilical Blood Sampling

- It is performed under ultrasound guidance to collected foetal blood, usually in Rh incompatibility cases and for assessment of chromosomal aberrations.

Fetoscopy

- It is visualisation of the foetus using endoscope usually in second trimester to detect severe structural damage.
- For details about prenatal diagnosis, read *Principles of Clinical Genetics* by Dr Yogesh Sontakke.

ULTRASONOGRAPHY IN EMBRYOLOGY

- Ultrasonography is a non-invasive technique useful for prenatal assessment.
- *Ultrasound examination during pregnancy* was introduced in Sweden in 1973.

PRINCIPLE OF ULTRASONOGRAPHY

- In ultrasound examination, transducer generates ultrasound waves and record echoes generated by medium (here, tissue).
- Transducer has piezoelectric material that can generate ultrasound of typical wavelength (2–18 MHz) on electric stimulus.
- The material on the surface of transducer enables the sound to be transmitted efficiently into the body.
- To enhance the transmission, water-based gel is placed between the skin and the transducer probe.
- Returning sound waves (echoes) vibrate the transducer that in turn generates electric pulses.
- These electric pulses are carried to the scanner that generates the image depending on the time required for the sound wave to come back from the object (for example, uterus), strength of the echo and focal length of phased array.
- Depending on the strength of the echoes, scanner generates different shades of grey to produce an image.
- 2D image (slice of body) can be generated by sweeping or rotating transducer mechanically. 3D images can be generated by acquiring a series of adjacent 2D images.
- *Doppler ultrasonography* is useful to study blood flow and muscle motion of foetus.[Neet] In Doppler ultrasonography, the different detected speeds are represented in colour for easy interpretation.
- Doppler shifts cells fall in audible sounds. It is represented by audibly distinctive pulsing sound (*pulsed Doppler*) to measure the velocity.

- In Doppler ultrasonography, use of specific colour has not set with any standard. Some use red for artery, whereas some use red to indicate flow towards transducer.
- World Health Organization (1988) declared that diagnostic ultrasound is safe (harmless) and capable of providing clinically relevant information about most parts of the body and even ultrasound is safe for foetus.

GREY SCALE OF ULTRASOUND IN OBSTETRICS

- On ultrasonography, substance may be
  - Hyperechoic: It gives white colour on screen. For example, fat containing tissue.
  - Hypoechoic: It gives grey scale. For example, soft tissue.
  - Anechoic: It gives black colour. For example, clear fluid (amniotic fluid), blood vessels.
  - Acoustic shadow: Gas does not echo sound waves; hence, it produces black colour.
- Bones appear as black (anechoic) with bright hyperechoic rim as ultrasound does not penetrate the bone.[MCQ]
- Cartilage appears white (hyperechoic) as ultrasound penetrates cartilage.[MCQ]
- Usually Doppler shows red for flow towards probe and blue for flow away from probe. (BART: Blue away, red toward). [MCQ]
- Muscles are hypoechoic, whereas other connective tissues are hyperechoic.

ULTRASOUND FREQUENCY

- High frequency probes (10–15 MHz) are suitable for superficial structures (2–4 cm depth).
- Mid frequency probes (5–10 MHz) are suitable deeper structures (5–6 cm).
- Low frequency probes (2–5 MHz) are suitable for more deeper structures (~10 cm depth).
- With decreasing frequency of probe; quality of image also decreases.

TYPES

According to the method of ultrasonography technique, it is classified as:
A. *Transabdominal sonography*: It is performed across the abdominal wall.
B. *Transvaginal sonography*: It is performed through vagina. It is also called endovaginal sonography.

PURPOSE OF ANTENATAL ULTRASONOGRAPHY

- The ultrasonography during pregnancy is targeted for the following purposes:
  1. Confirmation of pregnancy (presence of gestational sac).
  2. Estimation of gestational age of foetus.
  3. Detection of multiple pregnancies.
  4. Detection of foetal anomalies.
  5. Monitoring of foetal growth and development.
  6. Detection of ectopic pregnancy.
  7. To guide surgical procedures (amniocentesis, chorionic villus sampling).

CLASSIFICATION OF FOETAL SONOGRAPHIC EXAMINATIONS

A. First trimester Examination

- It includes evaluation of presence, size, location and number of gestational sac(s).
- The gestation sac is examined for presence of a yolk sac and embryo/foetus.

B. Second and Third Trimester Examination

- It includes an evaluation of foetal well-being, foetal presentation/position, volume of amniotic fluid, cardiac activity, placental position and foetal morphometric parameters (biometry).

C. Limited Examination

- It includes a specific targeted examination. For example, foetal heart activity in bleeding patient.

D. Specialised Examinations

- It includes detailed anatomic examination for suspected anomaly on the basis of history.

INDICATIONS FOR ULTRASOUND EXAMINATION

First Trimester Ultrasound Examination

Indications for the first trimester ultrasound examination include:
1. Confirmation of the pregnancy.
2. Detection of the ectopic pregnancy.
3. Detection for cause of vaginal bleeding.
4. Determination of gestational age.
5. Detection of multiple gestation.
6. Confirmation of cardiac activity.

- Gestational sac is seen in 3rd–5th week after menstruation.^MCQ
- Embryonic cardiac activity is identifiable by 6–6.5 weeks (embryonic length 2 mm or more).^Neet
- In addition to above indications, adnexal masses, uterus and cervix are also screened for presence of any abnormalities.

Second and Third Trimester Examination

Indications for second and third trimester ultrasound examination include:
1. Evaluation of foetal anatomy, growth and anomalies.
2. Determination of gestational age.
3. Evaluation of abdominal pain, vaginal bleeding, ectopic pregnancy.
4. Evaluation of foetal presentation, position of placenta, amniotic fluid abnormalities, premature rupture of membranes.
5. Evaluation of hydatidiform mole, uterine abnormalities
6. To guide amniocentesis and chorionic villus sampling.

GUIDELINES AND PARAMETERS FOR ULTRASONOGRAPHY

Some important parameters and guidelines for the ultrasound examination in obstetrics are as follows (Table 29.3):
1. To visualise cervix and internal os, transvaginal ultrasound may be helpful.
2. Gestational sac
   - It can be detected during 3–5th week after menstruation.
   - Mean diameter of gestational sac is useful for the determination of gestational age.
   - Growth rate of gestational sac is 1 mm per day.
   - It is suitable only up to gestational sac diameter 14 mm for gestational age determination, after that embryo can be identified.^MCQ
3. Yolk sac
   - It becomes visible by 5th–6th week and useful only for confirmation of pregnancy.^MCQ
   - It becomes 6 mm by 10th week (maximum size), then gradually decreases in size and becomes nondetectable by the end of third week.
4. **Crown to rump length (CRL)** (Clinical image 29.1)
   - It is the distance between highest point of skull and lowest point of buttocks.
   - It is most accurate for gestational age determination in **first** trimester.
   - It is suitable up to 84 mm size, after that biparietal diameter is useful.^MCQ
5. In second and third trimester, gestational age determination depends on biparietal diameter, head circumference, abdominal circumference and femur length. Use of multiple parameters is recommended.
6. **Biparietal diameter:** It is the diameter of axial plane through skull of the foetus (embryo) (Clinical image 29.2).
7. **Head circumference**: It is obtained in the same plane of biparietal diameter. The tracings for head circumference should follow the outer perimeter of skull (Clinical image 29.2).
8. **Abdominal circumference**: It should be measured at the level of bifurcation of portal vein or at the level of stomach (Clinical image 29.3).
9. **Femur length:** For measurement of the femur length, both femoral condyle should be visualised simultaneously. The ultrasound transducer should be perpendicular to the long axis of the femur. It is measured from tip of the greater trochanter to the lateral epicondyle (Clinical image 29.4).

Further Reading
- Babuta S, Chauhan S, Garg R, Bagarhatta M. Assessment of fetal gestational age in different trimester from ultrasonographic measurements of various foetal biometric parameters. *J ASI* 2013;60: 40–46.
- Butt K, Lin K. Determination of gestational age by ultrasound. *J Obstet Gynaecol Can* 2014;36(2):171–181.
- Handlock FP, Deter RL, Harrist RB, et al. Estimating foetal age: Computer-assisted analysis of multiple fetal growth parameters. *Radiology* 1984;152:497–501.
- Handlock FP, Deter RL, Harrist RB, et al. Foetal head circumference: Accuracy of real time ultrasound measurement of term. *Perinatol Nenatal* 1982;6: 97–100.
- Handlock FP, Deter RL, Harrist RB, et al. Foetal head circumference: Relation to menstrual age. *AJR* 1982; 139: 367–370.
- Ihnatsenka B, Boezaarrt AP. Ultrasound: Basic understanding and learning the language. *Int J Shoulder Surg* 2010; 4(3):55–62.
- Obstetrics ultrasound examinations by the America Institute of Ultrasound in Medicine. 2013.

Table 29.3	Foetal parameters in second and third trimester (Handlock)			
Gestational age (weeks)	BPD (mm)	Head circumference (mm)	Abdominal circumference (mm)	Femur length (mm)
13	21	82	60	11
16	32	124	99	20
20	46	177	150	33
24	59	224	197	44
28	71	266	240	54
32	81	301	281	62
36	89	328	318	70
38	92	338	336	74

BPD: Biparietal diameter.

CLINICAL EMBRYOLOGY

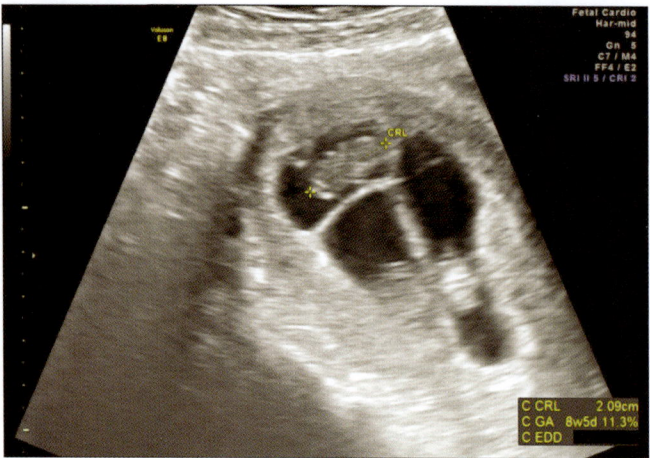

Clinical image 29.1: Ultrasonographical measurement of crown to rump length (CRL). It is the distance between highest point of skull and lowest point of buttocks. It is most accurate for gestational age determination in first trimester (Image courtesy: *Dr Mamatha Gowda*)

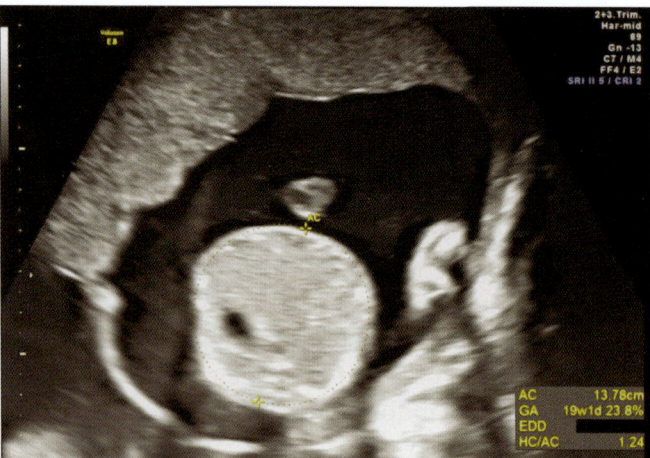

Clinical image 29.3: Ultrasonographical measurement of abdominal circumference (AC) (Image courtesy: *Dr Mamatha Gowda*)

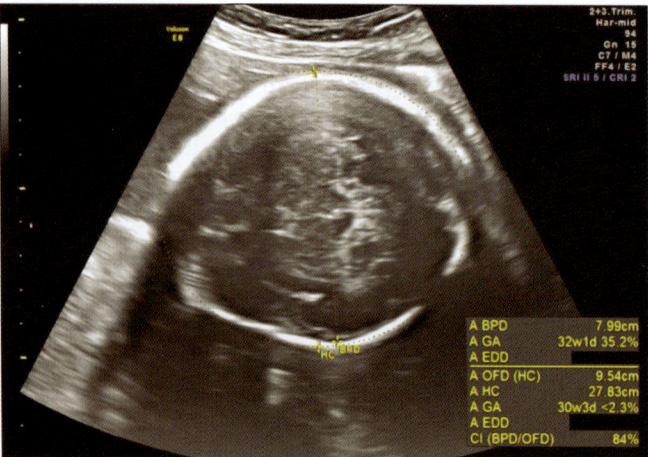

Clinical image 29.2: Ultrasonographical measurement of biparietal diameter (BPD) and head circumference (HC). BPD is the diameter of axial plane through skull of the foetus (embryo). Head circumference is obtained in the same plane of biparietal diameter. The tracings for head circumference should follow the outer perimeter of skull (Image courtesy: *Dr Mamatha Gowda*)

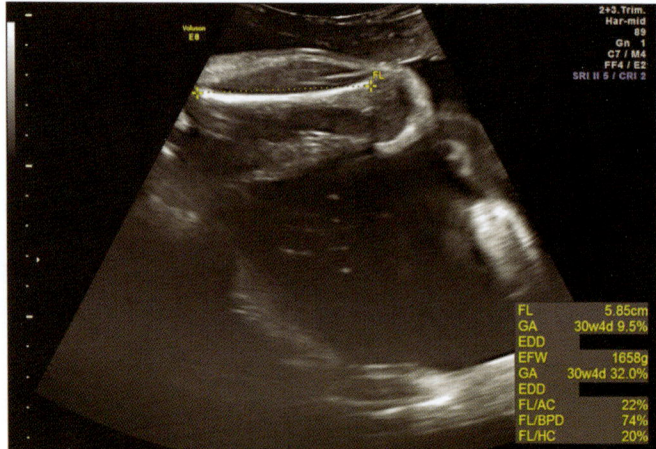

Clinical image 29.4: Ultrasonographical measurement of femur length: For measurement of the femur length, both femoral condyle should be visualised simultaneously. The ultrasound transducer should be perpendicular to the long axis of the femur. It is measured from tip of the greater trochanter to the lateral epicondyle (Image courtesy: *Dr Mamatha Gowda*)

30

Multiple Pregnancy (Twinning)

Chapter Outline

- Classification of twins
  - Dizygotic twins
  - Monozygotic twins
- Classification of twins according to degree of separation
  - Dichorionic diamniotic twins
  - Monochorionic diamniotic twins
  - Monochorionic monoamniotic twins
  - Conjoined twins

INTRODUCTION

- As in human, only one ovum is released in one menstrual cycle, usually, *singleton pregnancy* is seen.
- When the mother gives birth to **two or more** offspring in a single pregnancy, it is called *multiple pregnancy*. Multiple pregnancy, in dogs, cats and so many other mammals is common.
- When the mother gives birth to two offspring in a single pregnancy, it is called *twinning*.
- *In vitro* fertilisation enhances chances of multiple pregnancy (incidence of twins in IVF: 21 twins /1000 births).*Clinical fact*

CLASSIFICATION OF TWINS

- Multiple pregnancy is classified as per the number of offspring born as follows:
  1. Twins: 2 offspring
  2. Triplet: 3 offspring
  3. Quadruplets: 4 offspring
  4. Quintuplets: 5 offspring
- Multiple pregnancy can be classified according to the genetic relationship of the offspring as follows:
  1. *Monozygotic twins*: These twins are produced by fertilisation of *single ovum* by one sperm (one zygote).
  2. *Dizygotic twins*: These twins are produced by fertilisation of *two different oocytes* by *two different sperms* (two zygotes).
  3. *Trizygotic twins*: These are produced by fertilisation of multiple ova by different sperms (3 zygotes).
- Differences between monozygotic and dizygotic twins are listed in Table 30.1.

Some Interesting Facts

- **Superfecundation**: In polyovulatory animal, multiple ova are discharged and may get fertilised by sperms from *different male partners*. In such case, resultant foetuses are of *same* gestational age.
- **Superfoetation:** In some animals, ova released during pregnancy, may get fertilised and produce another offspring of *different* gestational age.

Dizygotic (Fraternal) Twins

Q. Write short note on dizygotic twins.

- *Definition*: Dizygotic twins are produced by the fertilisation of two different ova by two different sperms (two zygotes) (Fig. 30.1).
- Fraternal means unlike.
- Incidence: 7–10 per 1000 births, incidence increases with age.

Features

- The dizygotic twins are phenotypically dissimilar, even may have different gender (one male and other female offspring).
- The dizygotic twins are genetically dissimilar.

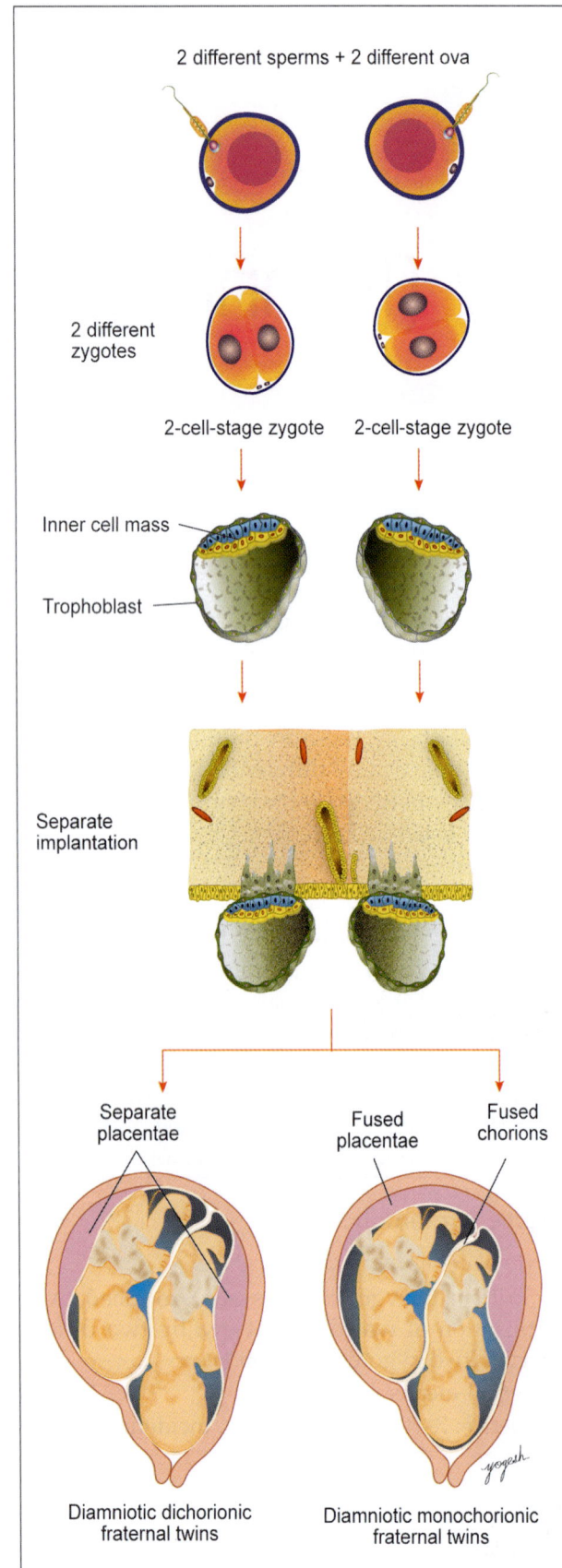

Fig. 30.1: Fraternal twins

- Dizygotic twins do not share placenta (except occasionally), chorion and amnion.
- They have two different gestational sacs.
- As placentae may be close to each other, occasionally fused placentae may be observed.
- About 2/3rd of human twins are dizygotic.

Monozygotic (Identical) Twins

Q. Write short note on monozygotic twins.

- *Definition*: Monozygotic twins are produced by fertilisation of one oocyte by one sperm (single zygote). The resultant zygote forms blastocyst with inner cell mass. This inner cell mass (embryoblast) divides into two parts and produce monozygotic twins (Fig. 30.2).
- Incidence: 3 in 1000 births.

Features
1. Monozygotic twins are phenotypically similar (they have same gender).
2. They are genetically similar.
3. They may share placenta, amniotic cavity and chorionic sac.
4. About 1/3rd of human twins are monozygotic twins.

CLASSIFICATION OF TWINS ACCORDING TO DEGREE OF SEPARATION

- Monozygotic twins can be classified based on degree of separation as follows:

1. Dichorionic Diamniotic Twins

- These are also called bichorial, diamniotic twins.
- In monozygotic twins, after first few divisions, cells of zygote get separated and form two embryos with separate chorionic and amniotic sac.
- *Note*: Dizygotic twins are also dichorionic, diamniotic.
- **Up to 3rd day** of fertilisation, separation of cells results in dichorionic and diamniotic twins.
- These twins have separate placenta.
- Incidence is 25% of twin pregnancies.

2. Monochorionic Diamniotic Twins

- They are also called monochorial, diamniotic twins.
- Mechanism: If separation of inner cells mass of blastocyst takes place on **4th–7th day**, monochorionic diamniotic twins are produced.
- These twins have a common chorionic sac and single placenta but two amniotic sacs.
- Incidence is 70–75% of twin pregnancies.

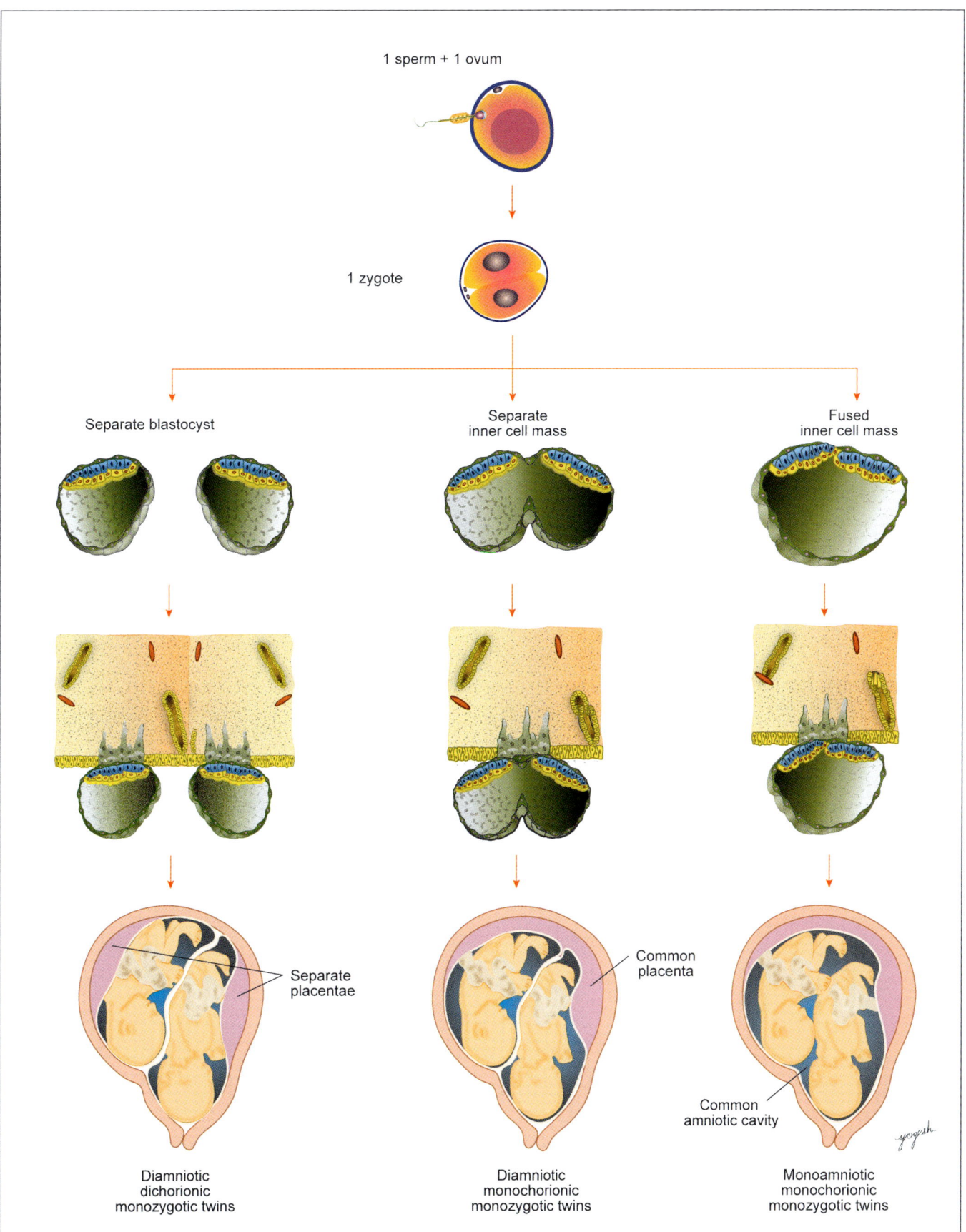

Fig. 30.2: Monozygotic twins

3. Monochorionic Monoamniotic Twins

- They are also called monochorial, monoamniotic twins.
- Mechanism: If the separation of inner cell mass takes place on **9th day** of fertilisation, in monochorionic monoamniotic twins are produced.
- They have common placenta, chorionic cavity and amniotic cavity.
- Incidence is 1–2% of monozygotic twin pregnancies.

4. Conjoined (Siamese) Twins (Fig. 30.3)

- If the separation occurs **after 12th day** of fertilisation, monozygotic twins form conjoined twins.
- Conjoined twins have joined bodies.

Classification of conjoined twins

Based on the site and extent of fusion, conjoined twins are classified as follows:
1. Craniopagus: Fusion of heads (skulls).
2. Thoracopagus: Fusion of anterior thoracic walls and abdominal walls up to umbilicus.
3. Omphalopagus: Fusion of lower abdominal walls.
4. Cephalothoracopagus: Fusion of head and thoracic walls.
5. Pyopagus: Fusion of sacral regions.
6. Ischiopagus: Fusion at the pelvis. These twins are classically joined with the vertebral axis at 180° (Clinical image 30.1).
7. Parasitic twin: Conjoined twin that have one large and another smaller (parasitic) twin.

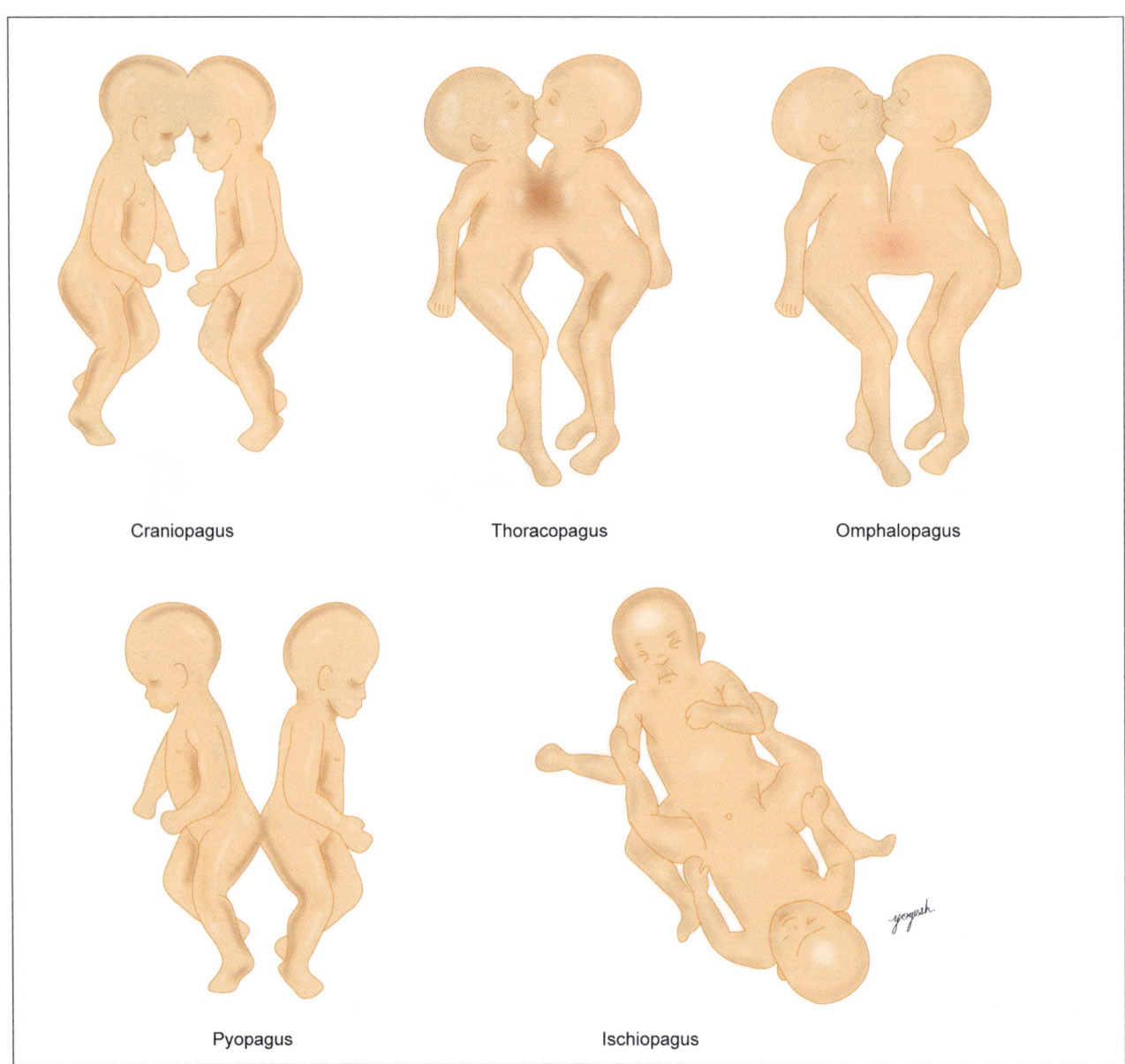

Fig. 30.3: Conjoined twins

Multiple Pregnancy (Twinning)

Q. List the differences between monozygotic and dizygotic twins.

Table 30.1	Differences between monozygotic and dizygotic twins	
Origin	Monozygotic twins	Dizygotic twins
Cause	1 sperm + 1 ovum = 1 zygote	2 different sperms + 2 different ova = 2 different zygotes
Incidence	More common	Less common
Phenotype	Similar	Dissimilar
Genotype	Similar	Dissimilar
Sex	Similar	May or may not be similar
Placenta	Single, shared by twins	Different placentae
Chorionic sac	May be single	Always different
Amniotic sac		

CLINICAL EMBRYOLOGY

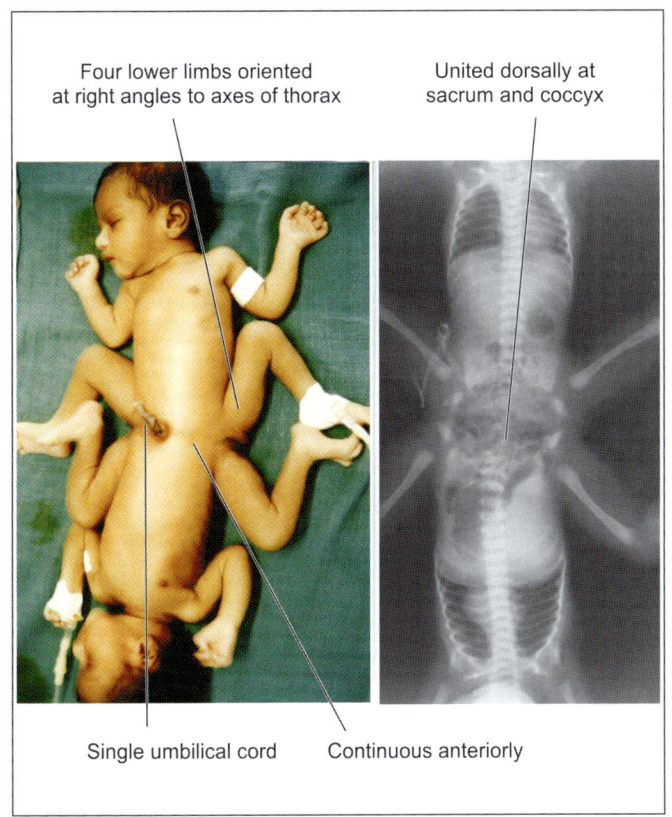

Clinical image 30.1: Ischiopagus tetrapus twins (phenotype on the left and radiological features on the right). Ischiopagus twins are united dorsally at the sacrum and coccyx. The twins are classically joined with the vertebral axis at 180°. Ischiopagus tetrapus (quadripus) shows four lower limbs and they are continuous anteriorly with each other. Limbs are oriented at right angles to the axes of the thorax. Ischiopagus dipus shows two shared lower limbs, ischiopagus tripus twins have three shared lower limbs. *Note:* In pygopagus, twins are joined ventrally at the buttocks and facing away from each other. Parapagus twins are joined side-by-side (Image courtesy: *Dr Kumaravel S*)

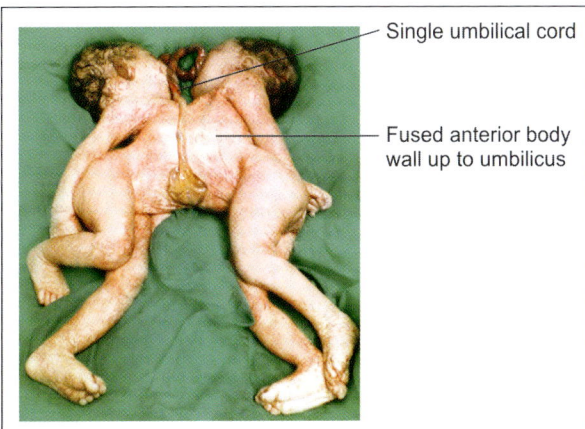

Clinical image 30.2: Conjoined twins: Thoracopagus. Thoracopagus is the most common form of conjoined twins. It involves fusion of anterior thoracic wall up to the umbilicus. A common pericardial sac is present in 90% of thoracopagus twins and conjoined hearts in 75% cases (Image courtesy: *Dr Haritha Sagili*)

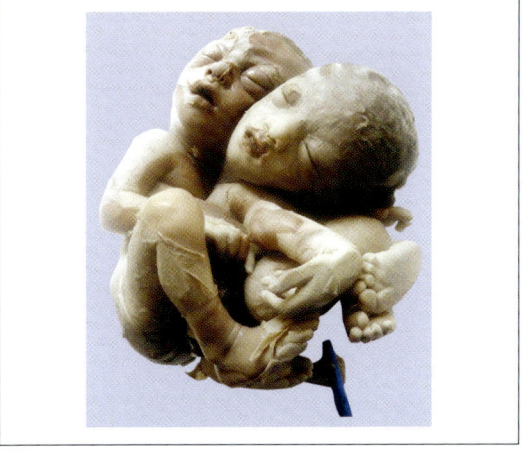

Clinical image 30.3: Conjoined twins: Thoracopagus. It involves fusion of anterior thoracic wall up to the umbilicus (Image courtesy: *Dr Mamatha Gowda*)

Annexures

ANNEXURE I

EMBRYONIC REMNANTS *Neet, High yielding fact*

Remnant after birth	Embryonic source
Ligamentum arteriosum	Ductus arteriosus
Ligamentum teres hepatis	Left umbilical vein
Fossa ovalis	Septum primum
Annulus fossa ovalis	Septum secundum
Ligamentum venosum	Ductus venosus
Meckel's diverticulum	Vitellointestinal duct
Median umbilical ligament	Urachus
Medial umbilical ligament	Distal part of umbilical arteries
Superior vesicle artery	Proximal part of umbilical arteries
Superior aberrant ductules Inferior aberrant ductules Tubules of paradidymis Efferent ductules of testis	Mesonephric tubules in male
Tubules of epoöphoron Tubules of paroöphoron	Mesonephric tubules in female
Duct of epoöphoron (Gartner's duct)	Mesonephric duct in female
Organ of Rosenmuller (epoöphoron)	Mesonephric tubules
Appendix of testis, prostatic utricle	Paramesonephric ducts in male

ANNEXURE II

PLACENTA PREVIA

Q. Write short note on placenta previa.

Definition: If the placenta is implanted partially or completely over the lower uterine segment, it is called placenta previa. Previa means *in front of* (Latin). Here, it indicates the position of placenta in relation to the internal os cervix uteri.

Incidence
0.5–1% hospital deliveries.
Incidence increases with increasing maternal age beyond 35.

Types
There are four types of the placenta previa depending on encroachment over lower uterine segment as follows:

Type I (low-lying): Only a lower margin of placenta encroaches on to the lower uterine segment.

Type II (marginal): Placenta encroaches the margin of internal os but does not cover it.

Type III (incomplete or partial central): Placenta covers the internal os partially.

Type IV (central or total): Placenta completely covers the internal os.

Diagnosis: Ultrasonographical examination is useful for detection of placenta previa.

Complications: Placenta previa is one of the commonest causes of antepartum haemorrhage (bleeding from the genital tract after 28 weeks of the pregnancy but before birth of the baby).

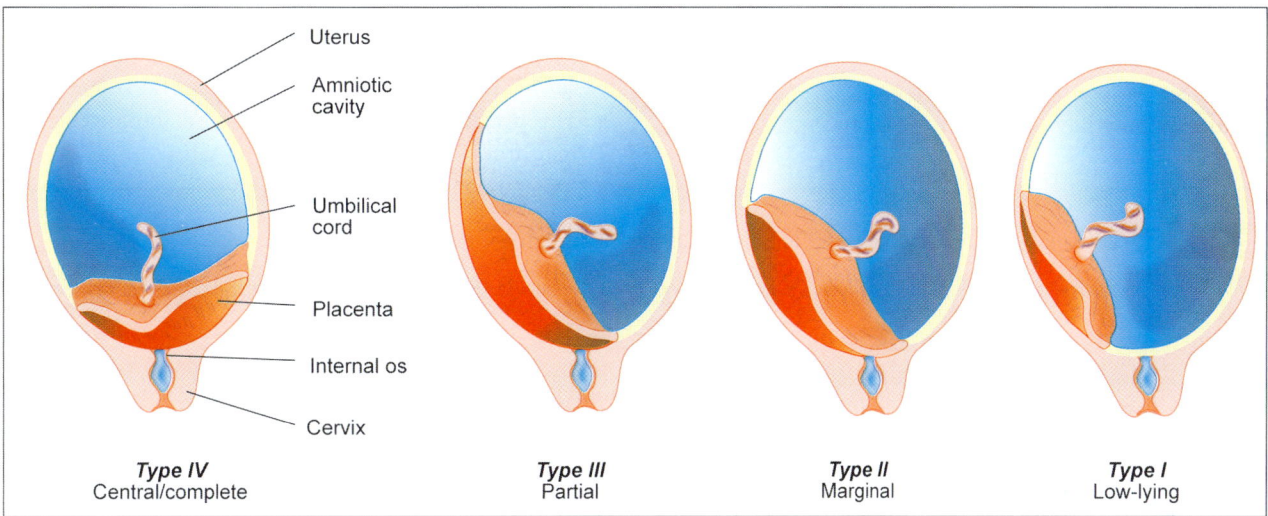

Fig. AII.1: Placenta previa

ANNEXURE III

HERMAPHRODITE

Q. Write short note on hermaphroditism.

Hermaphrodite

- A *hermaphrodite* is a person who phenotypically (physical characteristics) does not entirely resemble male or female and shows the characteristics of both the sexes. Hence, also called *intersex*.
- Hermaphrodites include ambiguous external genitalia and mosaic karyotypes (46,XX/46,XY, 46,XX/47,XXY or 45,X/XY mosaic).

True Hermaphrodites

- The *true hermaphroditism* is a rare condition. This individual has both testes and ovaries (usually combined as ovotestes) and external ambiguous genitalia (neither completely male nor completely female).
- Both testes and ovaries are usually nonfunctional.
- Genotype: Mostly 46,XX in 80% cases or 46,XX/46,XY mosaics or may have SRY translocations.
- The uterus is present and breasts are frequently developed. Most of these individuals are brought up as females. Most of these individuals menstruate except in XY mosaic cases.

Pseudohermaphrodite

- It is defective sexual development due to mutations or chromosomal anomalies affecting autosomes or sex chromosomes.
- Pseudohermaphrodites have gonads of one sex and external genitalia and genital tract of another sex.
- For example:
  1. Male pseudohermaphrodites: These are genetically male (46,XY) individuals with testes and external genitalia that resembles female.
  2. Female pseudohermaphrodite: These are genetically female (46,XX) individuals with ovaries and external genitalia that resembles male.
- Pseudohermaphrodites usually have abnormal levels of sex hormones or anomalies in the sex hormone receptors.
- The differences between male and female pseudohermaphrodites are listed in Table AIII.1.

Table AIII.1	Differences between male and female pseudohermaphrodites	
Feature	Male pseudohermaphrodite	Female pseudohermaphrodite
Gonads	Testes	Ovaries
Genotype	46,XY	46,XX
Phenotype	Male	Female
External genitalia	Resemble that of female	Resemble that of male
Phallus	Phallus remains rudimentary and looks like clitoris.	Excessive enlargement of clitoris resembling penis.
Labioscrotal swellings	Scrotal swellings fail to fuse, giving an appearance of labia majora.	Partial fusion of labia majora, giving an appearance of a scrotum.
Cause	Lack of androgen receptors (hence androgens produced by foetal testes are ineffective in inducing differentiation of male genitalia).	Congenital adrenal hyperplasia with excessive production of androgens. Excessive production of androgens masculinises external genitals.

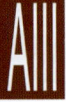

ANNEXURE IV

DERIVATIVES OF NEURAL CREST CELLS *Neet, High yielding facts*

Dorsal Mass

A. Neuroblast cells
- Dorsal root ganglia
- Sensory ganglia of V, VII, IX and X cranial nerves
- Skeletal elements of pharyngeal arches
- Odontoblast of teeth
- Parafollicular cells of thyroid gland

B. Spongioblast cells
- Satellite cells in ganglion
- Schwann cells

C. Pluripotent cells
- Melanocytes

Ventral mass

A. Sympatho-chromaffin organ
B. Sympathoblasts
- Sympathetic ganglionic neurons
- Parasympathetic ganglionic neurons (ciliary, pterygopalatine, submandibular and otic)

C. Chromaffin cells
- Chromaffin cells of medulla of adrenal gland
- Para-aortic body
- Argentaffin cells in respiratory system
- Enterochromaffin cells in gut

Other derivatives

- Facial bones and vault of skull
- Dermis of face and neck
- Muscles of ciliary body
- Sclera and choroids of eyeball
- Substantia propria and posterior epithelium of cornea
- Pharyngeal arch cartilages
- Semilunar valves in heart
- Spiral and bulbar septum in heart

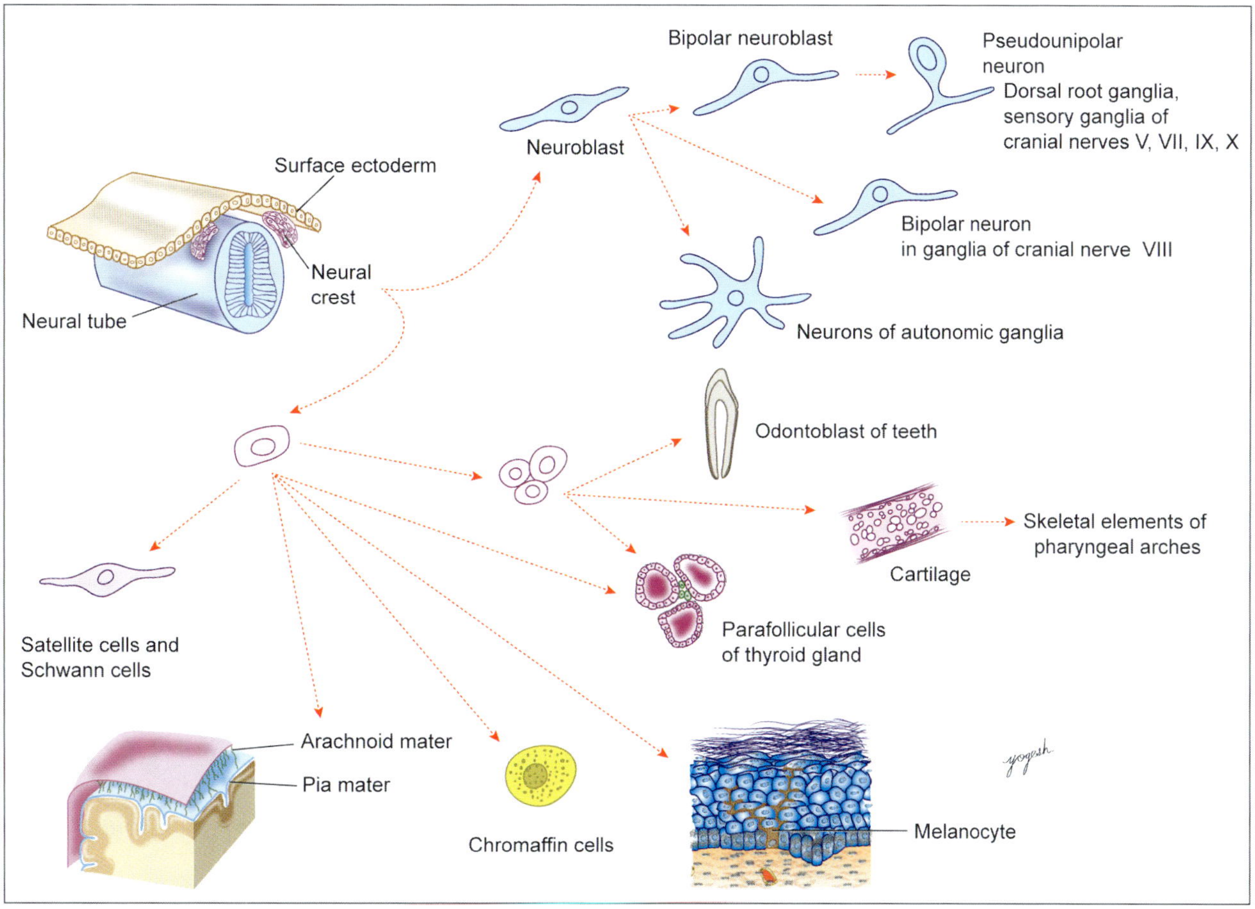

Fig. AIV.1: Derivatives of neural crest cells

Index

Abdominal circumference 303
Abembryonic pole 30
Accessory pancreatic tissue 148
Achalasia cardia 128
Achondroplasia 283
Acrosomal cap 10
Adenohypophysis 273
Adrenal cortex 276
Adrenal gland 276
   ectopic 276
Adrenal medulla 276
Adrenogenital syndrome 276
Agenesis 72
Aglossia 123
Agnathia 115, 272
Albinism 88
Allantois 55, 211
Allocortex 251, 252
Allograft 47
Alpha keratin 91
Amastia 94
Amelia 291
Ameloblasts 118
Amelogenesis imperfecta 120
Amenorrhoea 22
   primary 22
   secondary 22
Amnioblasts 40
Amniocentesis 83, 301
Amnio-ectodermal junction 40, 68
Amnion 82
Amnion nodosum 83
Amniotic cavity 40
Amniotic fluid 82, 83
Amniotic fluid index 83
Anal
   canal 135
   folds 226
   membrane 226
   pit 136
Anaphase 3
Androgen insensitivity 230
Anencephaly 241, 253, 255, 289
Angiogenesis 66, 184
Angora 89
Ankyloglossia 123
Ankyloglossia superior 123
Annulus ovalis 174
Anodontia 120
Anonychia 92
Anophthalmia 263
Anorchism 220
Anotia 107, 272
Anovulation 14, 22
Anterior lenticonus 265
Anterior nares 112
Anterior pituitary 273
Anti-müllerian substance 216
Anus
   ectopic 137
   imperforate 137, 139
Aorta
   arch of 186
   dorsal 185, 186
   ventral 186

Aortic body 101
Aortic sac 186
Apical ectodermal ridge 290
Aplasia 72
Aplasia of skin 88
Appendix 135
Apple-peel atresia 135
Aqueous humour 261
Archicerebellum 249
Archipallium 251, 252
Areola 94
Arnold-Chiari malformation 253
Artery/ies
   accessory renal 209
   axis artery of upper limb 191
   basilar 191
   coeliac 131, 188
   common carotid 102, 186
   external carotid 186, 187
   first aortic arch 186
   gonadal 188
   hyoid 102, 186
   inferior mesenteric 188, 208
   intercostal 188
   internal carotid 186, 187
   internal iliac 82
   lateral sacral 188
   left pulmonary 102
   lumbar 188
   maxillary 102, 186
   median sacral 188
   of arches 102
   phrenic 188
   pulmonary 186, 186
   renal 188, 205
   right pulmonary 102
   right 7th intersegmental 188
   right subclavian 102
   somatic intersegmental 188
   stapedial 102, 186
   subclavian 186
   superior mesenteric 131, 132, 188
   suprarenal 188
   umbilical 81, 185, 189
   vertebral 190
   vitelline 185
Artificial insemination 38
Aspermia 11
Asplenia 148
Asthenozoospermia 11
Astrocytes 237, 238
Astrocytoblast 238
Athelia 94
Atresia 72
Atrial septal defects 176
Atrioventricular canal 173
Atrophy 72
Auditory tube 270
Auricle 270
Autosomes 312
AV cushions 173
AV node 179

Axial skeleton 283
Axon 237
Azoospermia 11
Azygous lobe 155

Barr body 48, 216
Bile canaliculi 142
Billings method 13
Biparietal diameter 303
Bird-beak deformity 128
Blastocoel 29
Blastocyst 31
Blastomeres 28
Blastopore 51
Blepharophimosis 264
Blood island 66
Bone
   bone marrow cavity 282
   cartilaginous 281
   formation of 279
   long 281
   morphogenic proteins 143, 176, 236
Bowman's capsule 205
Brachycephaly 289
Brachydactyly 291
Brainstem functional
      columns of 242
Branchial arch 96
Brittle-bone disease 283
Bronchial tree 149
Bronchopulmonary segments 152
Bulbo-pontine extension 244
Bulboventricular chamber 177
Bulboventricular loop 171
Bulbus cordis 170, 177
Bundle of His 179
Buphthalmos 265
Butterfly children 94

Caecal bud 135
Caecum 135
Camerous fluid 82
Canal
   inguinal 219
   nasopalatine 115
   neurenteric 55
   notochordal 55
   of Nuck 222
   of Schlemm 262
   pericardio-peritoneal 149, 159
   pleuroperitoneal 152
   uterovaginal 205, 223
   vesicourethral 203
Capacitation 9, 25
Cardiac muscle 296
Cardiogenic area 168
Cardiospasm 128
Caroli's disease 143
Carotid body 101
Cartilage
   arytenoid 100, 151
   corniculate 100, 151
   cricoid 100, 151
   cuneiform 100, 151
   elastic 279
   epiglottic 100, 151

   fibrocartilage 279
   formation of 279
   hyaline 279
   Meckel's 99, 270
   Reichert's 100, 270
   second arch 100
   third arch 100
   thyroid 100, 151
Caudal
   dysgenesis 57
   intestinal portal 126
   pharyngeal complex 105
Cavity
   chorionic 42
   exocoelomic 41
   oral 117
   pleural 149, 158
C-cells 105
Cells
   alpha 147
   apical hair 269
   basket 249
   beta 147
   chromaffin 276
   delta 147
   endothelial precursor 66
   enterochromaffin cells of Kulchitsky 276
   ependymal 238
   gamma 147
   glial 238
   glomus 236
   Golgi 249
   granule 249
   Hofbauer 81
   Kupffer's 141
   Langerhans 86, 88
   Leydig 217, 219
   Merkel 86, 87
   microglial 238
   myoepithelial 90, 92
   neural crest 235
   neuroblast 237
   osteogenic 281
   parafollicular 105
   pluripotent 1
   primitive haematopoietic stem 66
   primordial germ 215
   Purkinje 249
   Schwann 240
   Sertoli 204, 216, 218
   stellate 249
   sympathochromaffin 276
   totipotent 1
Cementoblasts 119
Cementum 119
Central artery of retina 257
Central vein of retina 257
Cephalothoracopagus 308
Cerebellar
   cortex 247, 249
   hemispheres 247
   nuclei 247
   peduncle inferior 249

peduncle middle   245, 249
peduncles superior   249
plate   247
primordium   249
Cerebellum   247, 249
Cerebral aqueduct of Sylvius   235, 246
Cerebral hemisphere   250
Cerebral peduncles   246
Cerebrum   250
Cetrorelix   35
Cheeks   110, 111
Chemotaxis   25
Chondroblasts   279
Chondrocytes   279
Chorda-mesoderm   52
Chordomas   55
Chorion   42, 74
Chorion frondosum   77
Chorion laeve   77
Chorionic villi   77
   anchoring   77
   definitive   56
   development of   56
   primary   56
   secondary   56
   tertiary   56
Chorionic villus sampling   301
Choroid   261
Choroid plexus   245
Choroid plexus of 3rd ventricle   250
Choroidal fissure   257
Christmas tree intestinal atresia   135
Chromosomes   2
   sex   312
   structure   2
Ciliary body   261
Ciliary processes   261
Circulation
   fetoplacental   56
   foetal   198
   uteroplacental   41, 75
Circumvallate papillae   122
Cleavage   28
Cleft
   foot   291
   hand   291, 292
   intra-tonsillar   105
   lip   114, 255
   palate   115, 255
   pharyngeal first   269
Cleidocranial dysostosis   283, 289
Clitoris   226, 227
Cloaca   126, 135, 203, 211
Cloacal exstrophy   138
Club hand   291
Clubfoot   291, 292
Coarctation of aorta   188
Coelom extraembryonic   42, 64
Coelom intraembryonic   64, 158
Coelomic cavity   64
Coelomic ducts   158
Coeur en sabot   181
Collecting tubules   205
Collodion babies   87
Coloboma of eyelid   263
Commissure
   anterior   253
   habenular   253
   hippocampal   253
   posterior   253
Conceptus   2
Conducting system of heart   179
Congenital adrenal hyperplasia   276
Congenital alopecia   90

Congenital aniridia   263
Congenital aphakia   263
Congenital cataract   259, 265
Congenital hepatic fibrosis   143
Congenital hydrocephalus   255
Congenital hypertrophic pyloric
   stenosis   131
Congenital lymphedema   201
Congenital megacolon   136
Congenital ptosis   263
Congenital retinal detachment   261
Congenital umbilical hernia   134
Conjunctival sac   263
Connecting stalk   42, 68
Conus cordis   177
Convergence   54
Copper-T   46
Copula of His   122
Cornea   257
Corona radiata   15
Corpus albicans   20
Corpus callosum   253
Corpus haemorrhagicus   19
Corpus luteum   12
Corpus striatum   250
Cortrioculare biventricularae   176
Costal element   285
Cotton wool babies   94
Cotyledons   73
CR length   300
Cranial intestinal portal   126
Craniopagus   308
Craniopharyngiomas   274
Craniosynostosis   292
Crown to heel length   300
Crown to rump length   300, 303
Crus cerebri   246
Cryptamagna   105
Cryptophthalmos   263
Cryptorchidism   220, 214, 220, 229
Cumulus ovaricus   12
Cupula   269
Cuticle   91
Cycle menstrual   16
Cycle ovarian   16
Cycle uterine   16
Cyclopia   263
Cyst
   branchial   102
   branchial cleft   108
   Gartner's   204
   paratubal   204
   thyroglossal   107
   urachal   56, 213
Cystic hygromas   201
Cystic lymphangioma   201
Cytokinesis   4
Cytotrophoblast   32
Cytotrophoblast shell   56, 74, 76

Dandy-Walker malformation   253
Decidua   48, 74
   basalis   48, 74, 77
   capsularis   74
   decidua vera   74
   reflexa   74
Decidual reaction   74
Dental cuticle of Nasmyth   119
Dental
   epithelium inner   119
   epithelium outer   119
   lamina   118
   papilla   118
Dentate gyrus   252
Dentigerous cyst   121
Dentine   119
Dentinogenesis imperfecta   121

Dermal papilla   88
Dermatoglyphics   88
Dermatome   65, 88, 279, 293
Dermis   86, 88
Dermomyotome   65, 293
Deutoplasm   14, 168
Development   1
Dextrocardia   175
Diaphragm
   development of   161
   eventration of   163
Diastematomyelia   254
Diencephalon   233, 249, 250
Diplotene   4
Distal convoluted tubules   205
Diverticulum
   allantoenteric   55
   duodenal   131
   ilei   134
   Meckel's   134
Doppler foetoscope   199
Doppler pulsed   301
Dorsal mesocardium   171
Dorsal root ganglia   238
Double aortic arches   188
Down regulation   35
Duchenne muscular dystrophy   295
Duct/s
   accessory pancreatic   145
   archinephric   204
   carotid   187
   ejaculatory   204, 219
   Gartner's   204, 223
   genital   222
   hepatic   142
   lactiferous   93
   Leydig's   204
   main pancreatic   145
   mesonephric   204, 222
   müllerian   205, 223
   nasolacrimal   110, 263
   nephric   204
   of Cuvier   172, 192, 194
   of Luschka   121
   omphaloenteric   68
   paramesonephric   205, 223
   semicircular   266
   thyroglossal   107, 122
   vitellointestinal   68, 84, 132
   wolffian   204
Ductus
   aorticus   187
   arteriosus   102, 186, 188, 198
   caroticus   187
   venosus   194, 198
Duodenal atresia   131
Duodenal stenosis   131
Duodenum   130
Dwarfism   283
Dyschondroplasias   283
Dyskeratosis congenita   92
Dysmenorrhoea   22

Ear drum   270
Ear
   external   270
   internal   266
   middle   269
   ossicles   99, 270
E-Cadherin   54, 55
Ectoderm definitive   51
Ectoderm
   differentiation of   61
   surface   62
Ectopia cordis   175, 182
Ectopia vesicae   213, 214
Ectopic testis   220
Ectopic thyroid tissue   107
EDD   297

Eisenmenger's complex   181
Elephant trunk sign   138
Emboly   54
Embryoblast   29
Embryotroph   42
Enamel   119
Enamel knot   121
Enamel organ   118
Encephalocele   241, 253–256
Enchondromatosis   283
Endocardial cushion defect   176
Endoderm definitive   51
Endoderm   9
Endolymph   269
Endometrium   18
Enterocystoma   134
Epiblast   40
Epiboly   54
Epi-branchial placodes   102
Epicanthus   263
Epidermal ridges   87
Epidermis   86
Epidermolysis bullosa   94
Epididymis   204, 219
   appendix of   204
Epiglottis   122
Epiphysis   281
Epiphysis cereberi   276
Epispadias   228
Epithalamus   250
Epithelial cell rests of Malassez   121
Epithelium coelomic   205
Epithelium of lens   259
Epitrichium   87
Eponychium   91
Epoöphoron   204, 223
Erythropoiesis   185
Eustachian tube   270
Exomphalos   134
Expected date of delivery   297
External acoustic meatus   102, 270
External capsule   251
Eyelid colobomas   264
Eyelids   263

Face
   development of   109
   developmental anomalies of   115
Facial colliculus   246
Factor/s
   fibroblast growth   2, 8, 55,
      142, 236
   hepatocyte growth   220, 227
   hepatocyte nuclear
      transcription   143
   oocyte maturation inhibitor   11
   testis-determining   216, 217
   transforming growth factor β   236
   zinc-finger transcription   54
Fallot tetralogy   180, 227
Femur length   303
Fertilisation   24
Fetoscopy   301
Foetus as graft   47
Fifth pouch   105
Filum terminale   239
Fimbria   223, 252
First arch   99
First pouch   105
Fistula
   branchial   102
   cervical   102, 103
   congenital rectovesical   213
   congenital vesicovaginal   213
   rectal   137
   recto-urethral   137
   recto-vaginal   137, 225
   recto-vesical   137
   thyroglossal   107

Index

tracheoesophageal 128, 152
umbilical faecal 134
urachal 56, 213
vesicovaginal 225
vitelline 134
flocculonodular lobe 247
foetal cotyledons 78
foetal heartbeat 198
fold/s
  head 67
  lateral 67
  of Rathke 135
  tail 67
  vestibular 151
  vocal 151
Folding cephalocaudal 66
Folding of embryo 66
Folic acid 241
Follicle
  Graafian 12
  primary 12
  secondary 12
  tertiary 12
Fontanelles 288
Foramen
  caecum 107, 122
  Magendie 235
  of Luschka 121, 235, 245
  of Morgagni 164
  ovale 174, 198
  primum 174
  secundum 174
Fornix 253
Fossa incisive 115
Fossa ovalis 174
Fourth arch 101
Fourth pouch 105
Fourth ventricle 235, 244
Frontal air sinus 113
Frontal lobe 251
Funnel chest 287
Furcula of His 121

Galea capitis 10
Gallbladder
  agenesis of 144
  development of 144
  double 144
  floating 144
  intrahepatic 144
  septate 144
  sessile 144
Gamete intrafallopian transfer 38
Gametogenesis 6
Ganirelix 35
Gastroschisis 135, 139
Gastrulation 49
  cellular basis of 54
  definition 49
Gene
  ABCA12 95
  PAX6 263
  Snail 54
  SOXG 104
  SRY 216
  TBX5 181
  WT1 209
Genital ridge 203, 216
Genital swellings 226
Genital tubercle 226
Genomic imprinting 48
Germ disc
  bilaminar 40
  midline structures of 66
  trilaminar 49
Gland/s
  apocrine 90, 91
  bulbourethral 215
  holocrine 91

mammary 92
Meibomian 91
merocrine 90
parathyroid 106
parotid 124
pineal 276
pituitary 273
preputial 91
salivary 124
sebaceous 91
Skene's 204
sublingual 124
submandibular 124
sweat apocrine 90, 91
sweat eccrine 90
tarsal 19
Tyson's 91
Glans penis 226
Glomeruli (kidney) 205
Glossoptosis 104
Gonad 216
Gonadal ridge 216
Grey horn 238
Grey matter 238
Growth 1
  accretionary 1
  auxetic 1
  multiplicative 1
Gubernaculum ovarii 221
Gubernaculum testis 219
Gynecomastia 94

Haab's striae 265
Habenular commissure 250
Habenular nuclei 250
Haemangioblasts 66
Hair 88
Hand-Schüller-Christian disease 289
Harelip 114
Harlequin foetuses 88
Harlequin ichthyosis 95
Hartmann's pouch 144
Hassall's corpuscles 105
Hatching 37
Haversian system 280
Head circumference 303
Heart field 168
Heart tubes 169
Helicotrema 269
Hemifacial microsomia 107
Hemiglossia 123
Hemivertebra 286
Hensen's node 49
Hepatic bud 142
Hepatic sinusoids 142
Hepatic trabeculae 142
Hepatocardiac channel 195
Hermaphrodite 312
Hernia
  congenital diaphragmatic 164
  congenital hiatal 162
  congenital inguinal 220
  parasternal 162
  physiological umbilical 82, 132
  proboscoid umbilical 167
  retrosternal 162
Hertwig epithelial root sheath 121
Hippocampal cortex 252
Hippocampus 252
Hirschsprung's disease 136
Holoprosencephaly 56, 256
Holt-oram syndrome 181
Hormone/s
  anti-müllerian 204, 216, 224
  follicle stimulating 35
  gonadotropin-releasing 35
  human chorionic gonadotropin 81
  luteinising 21, 35
  melatonin 276

oestrogen 21
progesterone 21
Hyaline membrane disease 156
Hyaloid vessels 257
Hydatid of Morgagni 204
Hydatidiform mole 30
Hydrocephalus 241, 289
Hydrocoele congenital 220
Hydrometrocolpos 229
Hydroureter 210
Hymen
  imperforate 225, 229
  orifice of 223
Hyoid bone 100
Hyperspermia 11
Hypertelorism 115
Hypertrichosis 89
Hypoblast 40
Hypobranchial eminence 100, 122
Hypomenorrhoea 22
Hyponychium 91
Hypophysis cerebri 273
Hypospadias 228
Hypothalamus 250
Hyrtl's anastomosis 82

Ichthyosis 88
Implantation 31
Implantation abnormal 31
In vitro fertilisation 34
Incus 99, 270
Indomethacin 188
Induction 5
Induism griseum 252
Infantile haemangioma 95
Inferior colliculus 246
Inferior vena cava 196
Infracardiac bursa 165
Inguinal bursa 219
Iniencephaly 241
Insula 252
Intermaxillary segment 113
Internal capsule 251
Intersex 312
Interventricular foramina of Monro 235
Intervillous space 76, 77
Intestinal atresia 131
Intestinal portal
  anterior 67
  posterior 67
Intracytoplasmic sperm injection 37
Intra-hepatic biliary atresia 143
Intra-tonsillar cleft 105
Intrauterine devices 46
Involution 106
Iris 262
  coloboma of 263
Ischiopagus 308
Islets of Langerhans 145
IVC double 196
IVC preureteric 196

Keratin 87
Kidney
  ascent of 207
  blood supply of 207
  development of 205
  horseshoe 208
  lobulated 209
  mesonephric 206
  metanephric 206
  pancake 209
  polycystic 209
  pronephric 206
  rotation of 207
  secretory part of 205
Koller's sickle 52

Labia majora 227
Labia minora 227
Labyrinth
  bony 269
  membranous 266
Lacrimal apparatus 263
Lacrimal sac 110
Lacunar spaces 43
Lamina
  alar 237
  basal 237
  terminalis 250
Langerhans cell histiocytosis 289
Lanugo 89
Larygoptosis 151
Laryngeal web
Laryngocele 151
Laryngotracheal groove 121, 127, 149
Larynx 149, 150
Lateral thyroid element 105
Layer ependymal cell 237
Layer
  Langhans 78
  mantle 236
  marginal 237
Left atrium 172
Left venous valve 172
Lens 258
  dislocation 265
Leptomeninges 253
Leptotene 4
Lesser omentum 141
Lesser sac 130, 164
Leuprorelin 35
LH surge 21
Ligament
  anterior ligament of malleus 99
  broad ligament of uterus 223
  coronary 130, 141
  falciform 130, 141
  gastrosplenic 130, 148
  lienorenal 130, 148
  median umbilical 56, 211
  of ovary 221
  of Treitz 135
  round ligament of uterus 221
  sphenomandibular 99
  stylohyoid 100
  triangular 130, 141
Ligamentous arteriosus 102, 186, 188
Ligamentum teres hepatis 82
Limbic lobe 252
Limbs 290
Lingual swellings 122
Liquor amnii 82
Liquor folliculi 12
Liver 141
  histogenesis of 143
Lobe of Wrisberg 155
Lobster-claw deformity 291, 292
Loop of Henle 205
Lower lip 110
Lung
  buds 149
  congenital polycystic 156
  ectopic 156
  sequestration of 156
Lunula 91
Luschka 121
Luteinisation 20
Lymphatic system 199

Macroglossia 123
Macrostomia 115
Macula of saccule 267
Major histocompatibility complex 47
Male external genitalia 226
Malleus 99, 270
Malrotation 135

Mamillary body 250
Mammary ridge 92
Mandible 99
Mandibulofacial dysostosis 104, 272
Mater
   arachnoid 239
   dura 239
   pia 239
Maternal blood screening 301
Maternal inheritance 28
Maxilla 99, 110
Maxillary air sinus 113
Mechanism of menstrual bleeding 20
Meconium 137
Meconium ileus 137
Meconium stained liquor 137
Medulla oblongata 242
Medullary plate 57, 231
Medullary velum 249
Meiosis 4
Melanoblasts 87
Melanocytes 86, 87, 89
Membranatectoria 269
Membrane
   anal 62, 126, 135, 136, 211
   basilar 269
   bucconasal 112
   buccopharyngeal 51, 62, 109, 117, 126
   exocoelomic 41
   Heuser 41, 84
   hymenal 223
   membrane cloacal 52, 62, 126, 135
   Nitabuch's 78
   oral 51
   oropharyngeal 62
   pharyngeal 98
   pleuropericardial 158, 159
   pleuroperitoneal 158
   Riessner's 269
   tympanic 98, 102
   urogenital 62, 126, 135, 211
   vestibular 269
   vitelline 14
Meningocele 241, 255
Menometrorrhagia 22
Menopause 16
Menorrhagia 22
Menstrual cycle 16, 17
Meromelia 291
Mesencephalon 233, 246
Mesenteries 164
Mesoderm
   axial 52
   extraembryonic 41, 42
   intermediate 58, 64, 203
   intraembryonic 51
   lateral plate 58, 64, 88, 203
   paraxial 58, 63, 203, 279
   somatopleuric 42, 64
   splanchnopleuric 42, 64
Mesodermal differentiation 63
Mesoduodenum 131
Mesogastrium dorsal 128
Mesogastrium ventral 128, 142
Mesonephric tubules 222
Mesonephros 206
Mesovarium 221
Metameres 64
Metanephric blastema 205, 206
Metanephric vesicle 207
Metanephros 206
Metaphase 3
Metaphysis 282
Metencephalon 234
Metrorrhagia 22
Microcephaly 253
Microglossia 123

Micrognathia 272
Microphthalmia 263
Microspherophakia 264
Microstomia 115
Microtia 107, 271
Midbrain 246
Milk lines 92
Mitosis 3
Mittelschmerz 14
Modiolous 269
Monorchism 220
Montgomery's areolar tubercles 91
Morula 29
Mouth cavity 117
Müllerian tubercle 223
Multiple pregnancy 305
Muscle/s
   anterior belly of digastric 100, 295
   arrector pili 88
   ciliary 261
   constrictor of pharynx 101, 295
   cricothyroid 101, 295
   extraocular 294
   intrinsic muscles of larynx 101
   lateral pterygoid 100, 295
   lateral rectus 246
   masseter 100, 295
   medial pterygoid 100, 295
   mylohyoid 100, 295
   of body wall 294
   of facial expression 101
   of limbs 295
   of mastication 100
   of palate 101, 295
   of pharyngeal arches 295
   of tongue 295
   posterior belly of digastric 101, 295
   skeletal 293
   smooth 296
   stapedius 101, 270, 295
   stylohyoid 101, 295
   stylopharyngeus 101, 295
   temporalis 100, 295
   tensor tympani 100, 270, 295
   tensor veli palatine 100, 295
Myelencephalon 234
Myelination 240
Myelinogenesis 240
Myelomeningocele 241, 254
Myeloschisis 241
Myoblasts 293
Myocele 65
Myoepicardial mantle 168
Myotome 65, 293
   occipital 122, 293
   preoccipital 262
   preotic 293
Myotube 293

Nafarelin acetate 35
Nails 91
Nasal pit 109
Nasal placodes 109
Nasal septum 112
Nasolacrimal groove 110
Naso-optic furrow 110
Neocerebellum 249
Neonatal milk 94
Neopallium 251
Nephrogenic cord 203
Nerve
   chorda tympani 101, 122
   facial 101
   glossopharyngeal 101, 122
   hypoglossal 122, 295
   mandibular 100, 101, 110, 122
   maxillary 110
   olfactory 112
   ophthalmic 110
   optic 261
   post-trematic 101
   pre-trematic 101
   recurrent laryngeal 101, 151
   superior laryngeal 101, 151
   vagus 101, 123
Neural crest 57, 231
   derivatives of 236
   process of formation 57
Neural folds 57, 231
Neural groove 57, 231
Neural plate 57, 61, 231
Neural tube 231
   defects 240
   differentiation of 233
   flexure of 234
   formation of 57
Neuroblast 237
Neurocranium 287
Neuroectoderm 61, 231
Neurohypophysis 250, 274
Neuron pseudounipolar 237
Neuropore 57
   caudal (posterior) 57, 233
   cranial (anterior) 57, 233
Neurulation 57, 231
Nipple 94
Nodal gene 52
Non-disjunction 4
Nose 111, 112
Nostrils 112
Notochord 52, 55, 231
Notochordal plate 55
Notochordal process 52
Nucleus
   amibuguus 244
   cochlear 245
   cuneatus 245
   dentate 249
   dorsal nucleus of vagus 244
   Edinger-Westphal 246
   emboliform 249
   fastigial 249
   globose 249
   gracilis 245
   hypoglossal 244
   inferior salivatory 244
   lacrimatory 246
   mesencephalic nucleus of V nerve 246
   motor nucleus of V nerve 246
   motor nucleus of VI nerve 246
   oculomotor 246
   of spinal tract of V nerve 246
   olivary 244
   pontine 246
   pulposus 55
   red 246
   spinal nucleus of trigeminal 244
   superior salivatory 246
   tractus solitarius 244–246
   trochlear 246
   vestibular 245

Oblique facial cleft 115
Oblique vein of left atrium 172, 195
Oblique vein of Marshall 195
Occipital lobe 251
Occipital myotomes 295
Odontoblasts 118
Oesophageal atresia 128
Oesophageal stenosis 128
Oesophagus 127
Olfactory bulb 252
Olfactory epithelium 112
Olfactory tract 252
Oligodendroblast 238, 240
Oligohydramnios 83
Oligomenorrhoea 22
Oligoovulation 14, 22
Oligozoospermia 11
Omental bursa 164
Omentum greater 130
Omentum lesser 130
Omphalocele 134, 138
Omphalopagus 308
Ontogeny 1
Oocyte
   cryopreservation 38
   primary 6, 11
   retrieval 35
   secondary 6, 12
Oogonia 6, 11
Optic cup 257
Optic stalk 257
Optic vesicle 257
Oral fissure 110
Organ of Corti 266
Organ of Rosenmüller 223
Organ of Zuckerkandl 276
Organiser 5, 121
Organiser embryonic 55
Organiser Primary 5
Organiser Secondary 5
Organiser Spemann 55
Organiser Tertiary 5
Orthopantomogram 125
Ossification 279
   cartilaginous 280
   endochondral 280
   intramembranous 280
   membrano-cartilaginous 283
   primary centre of 282
Osteoblasts 281
Osteogenesis imperfecta 283
Osteoid 280
Ostium secundum defects 176
Otic pit 266
Otic placodes 266
Otocyst 266
Ovary 221
Overriding of aorta 180
Ovulation 13
Ovum 14
Ox eye 265

Pachytene 4
Palate 112
Palatine tonsil 105
Paleocerebellum 249
Paleopallium 251, 252
Pancreas
   annular 147
   development of 145
   divided 147
Pancreatic buds 145
Pancreatic divisum 147
Paraaortic bodies 276
Paranasal air sinuses 113
Paraoöphoron 204, 223
Parietal lobe 251
Pars cystica 142
Pars distalis 274
Pars hepatica 142
Pars intermedia 274
Pars tuberalis 274
Parthenogenesis 28
Patent ductus arteriosus 188
Patent vitellointestinal duct 140
Pectinate line 136
Pectus carinatum 287
Penile raphe 227
Penis primitive 226
Pericardial bar 52, 64
Pericardial cavity 158
Pericardial sac 64, 158
Pericardium 179
Perichondrium 279
Periderm 86, 87

Index

Perilymph 269
Perineal body 211
Period
    embryonic 2, 61, 297
    fertile 16
    foetal 2
    germinal 2, 297
    of egg 2
    organogenic 61
    ovular 297
Perionychium 91
Periosteal collar 281
Periotic tissue 269
Peritoneal cavity 159
Phallus 227
Pharyngeal
    apparatus 97
    arch 96, 97, 98
        nerves of 101
    bursa 121
    clefts 96, 97, 102
    pouches 96, 97, 104
    tonsil 121
Pharynx 121
Phase
    follicular 17, 18
    luteal 18
    menstrual 17, 18
    oestrogenic 19
    post-ovulatory 18, 19
    progestational 19
    proliferative 17, 18, 19
    secretory 17
Pheochromocytoma 276
Philtrum 111
Phocomelia 182, 291
Phrygian cap 144
Phylogeny 1
Piebaldism 88
Pigeon chest 287
Pineal body 250
Pinealocytes 276
Pituitary gland accessory 274
Pituitary suppression 35
Placenta 73
    accrete 79
    basal plate 74
    battledore 78
    bidiscoid 78
    chorionic plate 74
    circumvallate 78
    development of 74
    discoid 78
    foetal surface 73
    functions of 80
    increta 79
    lobed 78
    maternal surface 73
    membranacea 78
    percreta 79
    phylogeny of 79
    previa 31, 311
    succenturiate 78
    velamentous 78
Placental barrier 77
Placental septae 73
Plagiocephaly 289
Pleura 152
Pleural cavity 159
Plexus Auerbach's 128
Plexus Meissner's 128
Poland sequence 295
Polar body 12
Polycystic liver disease 143
Polydactyly 291
Polyhydramnios 83, 128
Polymastia 94
Polymenorrhoea 22
Polyspermy 27

Polysplenia 148
Polythelia 94
Pons 245
Pontine flexure 235, 245
Postaxial polydactyly 292
Posterior nares 112
Posterior pituitary 274
Pouch of Luschka 121
Prechordal plate 43, 46
    ectopic pregnancy 31
Pre-maxilla 99
Prenatal diagnosis 301
Prepuce 227
Primary areolae 281
Primary lens fibres 258
Primary tympanic cavity 270
Primitive anorectal canal 126
Primitive anterior nares 109
Primitive atrium 170
Primitive gonads 215
Primitive groove 51
Primitive knot 49
Primitive node 49
Primitive pit 51
Primitive rectum 126, 135, 203, 211
Primitive streak 49
Primitive urogenital sinus 126, 135
Primitive ventricle 170
Primordial follicle 221
Primordial germ cells 6
Probe patency 177
Proboscis 115, 263
Process
    frontonasal 109, 111
    lateral nasal 112, 119
    lateral palatine 114
    mandibular 99, 109
    maxillary 99, 109
    medial nasal 109, 111
    median palatine 114
    odontoblastic 119
    styloid 100
Processes Tomes 119
Processus vaginalis 219
Proctodeum 135, 136
Prometaphase 3
Pronephros 206
Prophase 3
Prosencephalon 233, 250
Prostaglandin inhibitor 188
Prostaglandins 188
Prostate 225
Prostatic utricle 205, 224
Proximal convoluted tubules 205
Pseudoclitoris 230
Pseudohermaphrodite female 312
Pseudohermaphrodite male 230, 312
Pseudohermaphroditism 276
Pseudointersexuality 276
Puberty 16
Pulmonary stenosis 180
Pulp canal 119
Pupillary membrane 262
Purkinje fibres 179
Pyopagus 308

Rachischisis 241, 254
Radial aplasia 291
Rami chorii 77
Ramuli chorii 77
Raspberry tumour 134
Ratio lecithin:sphingomyelin 83
Rathke's pouch 274
Rauber's sickle 52
Reaction
    acrosome 27
    decidual 20, 33, 48
Renal agenesis 207
Renal collar 196
Renal corpuscles 207

Renal pelvis 205
Rete testis 217
Retina 260
Retrognathia 104, 115
Rhombencephalic isthmus 244
Rhombencephalon 233
Rhombic lip 245
Rib/s 286
Riedel's lobe 143
Rieger's anomaly 265
Right
    aortic arch 188
    atrium 172
    venous value 172
    ventricular hypertrophy 180
Rohr's fibrinoid stria 78
Rotation of gut 132

SA node 179
Sacrococcygeal teratoma 55
Scala tympani 269
Scala vestibuli 269
Scaphocephaly 289, 292
Sclera 261
Sclerotome 65, 283, 293
Scoliosis 286
Scrotum 219
Sebum 91
Second arch 101
Second pouch 105
Secondary lens fibres 259
Secondary tympanic membrane 270
Sella turcica 273
Semen liquefaction of 25
Semicircular canals 269
Seminal vesicles 204, 219
Seminiferous tubules 217
Septum
    aortico-pulmonary 177, 178
    interatrial 173
    intermedium 173
    interventricular 177
    pellucidum 253
    primum 173
    primum defect 176
    secundum 174
    sinus 172
    spiral 177
    spurium 172
    transversum 64, 142, 159, 161
    urorectal 126, 203
Serotina 74
Sex cords 221
Sign double-bubble 131
Simian crease 292
Sinovaginal bulbs 223
Sinus
    cervical 102
    definitive urogenital 203, 211
    primitive urogenital 203
    transverse 171
    urachal 56, 213
    urogenital 211
    venarum 175
    venosus 170, 172, 192
Sirenomelia 57, 291
Situs inversus 54
Sixth arch 101
Skeleton appendicular 279
Skeleton axial 279
Skin 86
Skull 287
Somite 64, 65, 279
Somites preotic 64
Somitomeres 64, 279
Sonography
    transabdominal 302
    transvaginal 302
Sperm washing 36

Spermatids 8
Spermatocyte primary 7
Spermatocyte secondary 8
Spermatocytosis 7
Spermatogenesis 7
Spermatogonia 6, 7
    type A dark 7
    type B 7
Spermatozoa 6
    abnormal 11
    structure of 10
Spermiation 9
Spermiogenesis 8, 9
Spina bifida 241, 285
Spina bifida occulta 241, 254
Spina bifida anterior 241
Spinal cord 236
    functional columns of 239
    lateral horn of 238
    positional changes 238
Spinal ganglia 238
Spinal nerve
    motor roots of 238
    sensory roots of 238
Spinnbarkeit 13
Spleen
    accessory 148
    development of 148
    hypoplastic 148
    lobulated 148
Splenculi 148
Split cord malformation 254
Spondylolisthesis 286
Spongioblast 237, 238
Stapes 100
Stellate reticulum 119
Stem villus 77
Stenosis tracheal 152
Sternal bars 286
Sternebrae 287
Sternum 286
    bifid 287
Stomach 128
Stomodeum 96, 109, 117
Stratum
    basale 18, 87
    compactum 18
    corneum 87
    functionale 18
    germinativum 87
    granulosum 12, 87
    spinosum 87
    spongiosum 18
Strawberry mark 95
Stria vascularis 269
Substantia nigra 246
Sulcus
    bulboventricular 171
    labio-gingival 117
    limitans 237
    linguo-gingival 117
    terminalis (tongue) 122
Superfecundation 305
Superfoetation 305
Superior colliculus 246
Superior vena cava 195
    double 195
    left 195
Suprarenal ridge 276
Surfactant 156
Surgical sperm extraction 37
Suspensory ligament of
    duodenum 135
Syncytiotrophoblast 32
Syndactyly 291
Syndrome
    22q11.2 deletion 103
    branchio-otorenal 207
    coloboma 207

DiGeorge's 103
Eagle-Barrel 214
first arch 103
Goldenhar 107
Gorlin 88
Holt-Oram 181
infant respiratory distress 156
Klippel-Fail 286
meconium aspiration 137
Menkes 90
mermaid 57
nevoid basal cell carcinoma 88
oculo-auriculo-vertebral 107
ovarian hyperstimulation 35
Pierre Robin 104
Potter 83
premenstrual 22
Prune belly 214
Shprintzen 103
Taussig-Bing 181
Townes-Brock 207
Treacher Collins 103
velocardiofacial 103
Zinsser-Cole-Engman 92
Syringomyelia 241

Talipes equinovarus 291
Teeth
   anomalies of 120
   deciduous 120
   development of 118
   milk 118
   natal 120
   permanent 120
   successional 118
   super-added 118
   time of eruption 120
Telachoroidea 245
Telencephalic flexure 235
Telencephalon 233
Telophase 3
Temporal bone 99
Temporal lobe 251
Teratogenic agents 55
Teratoma 6
   ovarian 222
Teratozoospermia 11
Test tube baby 34
Testis
   descent of 219
   development of 217
Testosterone 217
Thalamus 250
Theca externa 12
Theca interna 12
Third arch 101
Third pouch 105
Thoracopagus 308, 309
Thymic element 105
Thymic involution 106
Thymocytes 106
Thymus 105
Thyroglossal cyst carcinoma 107
Thyroid gland
   anomalies of 107
   development of 106
   infrahyoid 107
   intralingual 107
   lingual 107, 123
   suprahyoid 107
Tongue 121
   bifid 123
   development of 121
   tie 123
Tonsil capsule of 105
Tonsillar crypts 105
Tooth impacted 120
Tooth milk 120
Torticollis 295
Tourneux fold 135
Trabeculae 75
Trachea 149, 151
   agenesis of 152
   lobe 152
Tracheal bronchus 152
Tracheoesophageal septum 149
Transverse element 285
Trichorrhexis nodosa 90
Trigonocephaly 289
Trophoblast 29
   lacunar stage of 41
   mural 30
Trophectoderm 29
Truncus arteriosus 170, 177
Truncus chorii 77
Tubal tonsil 270
Tube auditory 105
Tube/s
   eustachian 105
   fallopian 223
   uterine 205, 223
Tuberculum impar 107, 122
Tubotympanic recess 105, 269
Tunica albuginea 219
Tunica vaginalis 219
Turner's syndrome 230
Twin reversed-arterial perfusion 182
Twinning 305
Twins
   acardiac 182
   conjoined 308
   dichorionic diamniotic 306
   dizygotic 305
   fraternal 305
   ischiopagus tetrapus 309
   monochorionic diamniotic 306
   monochorionic monoamniotic 308
   monozygotic 305, 306
   parasitic 308
   Siamese 308
   trizygotic 305
Tympanic antrum 270
Tympanic membrane 270

Ultimobranchial body 105
Ultrasonography 301
Umbilical cord 42, 81
Umbilical ring 81
Upper lip 110
Urachus 56, 211
Ureter 209
   blind 210
   development of 209
   ectopic 210
Ureteric bud 205, 206
Urethra 204, 213
Urethra penile 226
Urethral folds 226
Urethral plate 227
Urinary bladder 210
   development of 210
   exstrophy 214
   hourglass 213
   trigone 204, 210
Urogenital membrane 226
Urorectal septum 135
Uterus 205, 223
   anomalies of 224
   bicornuate 224
   development of 224
   didelphys 224
   double 224
   septate 224
   unicornuate 224
Utricle 266
Uvula 115

Vacteral association 157
Vagina 205, 223, 224
   agenesis of 225
   atresia of 225
   musculina 205
Valve
   aortic 179
   atrioventricular 178
   bicuspid 179
   mitral 179
   of heart 178
   pulmonary 179
   tricuspid 179
Vas deferens 204, 219
Vasculogenesis 66, 184
Vein
   accessory hemizygous 197
   anterior cardinal 185, 192, 194
   azygous 172, 192, 197
   brachiocephalic 195
   caval 192
   cervicothoracic 195
   common cardinal 172, 185, 192, 194
   hemizygous 197
   hepatic 193
   iliac 195
   internal jugular 195
   left umbilical 82
   omphalomesenteric 192
   portal 93, 192
   posterior cardinal 185, 192, 194, 195
   primary head 194
   pulmonary 175
   right umbilical 81
   somatic 192, 194
   subcardinal 195
   supracardinal 195
   thoracolumbar 195
   umbilical 141, 172, 185, 192, 193
   vitelline 141, 172, 185, 192
Ventricle 177
   lateral 235
   of larynx 151
   third 235
Ventricular septal defects 180
Ventriculoradial syndrome 182
Vermiform appendix 135
Vermis 247
Vernix caseosa 87
Vertebral column 283
Vesicle
   forebrain 109
   otic 266
   umbilical 68, 84
Vesiculaprostatica 205
Vestibular fold 151
Vestibule of vagina 227
Vagina septate 225
Villi 43
   anchoring 56
   floating 77
   free 56, 77
   primary 75
   primary stem 43
   secondary 75
   tertiary 75
   zones of 77
Vimentin 54
Viscerocranium 287
Vitelline block 27
Vitelline cyst 134
Vitiligo 88
Vitreous 87
Vitreous chamber 262
Vocal fold 151

Webbed neck 230
Wharton's jelly 81
White matter 238
Wilms tumour 209
Window oval 270
Window round 270
Witch's milk 94
Wnt proteins 271
Woven bone 280

X chromosome
   inactivation 48
   methylation of 48
Xiphoid process 287

Yolk sac 41, 43, 47, 84
Yolk stalk 132

Zona fasciculata 276
Zona glomerulosa 276
Zona pellucida 12, 15, 31
Zona reticularis 276
Zygomatic bone 99
Zygosis 131
Zygote 24, 28
Zygote intrafallopian transfer 38
Zygotene 4